Seventh Edition

Medical Terminology

A LIVING LANGUAGE

Seventh Edition

Medical Terminology

A LIVING LANGUAGE

Bonnie F. Fremgen, PhD
Former Associate Dean
Allied Health Program
Robert Morris College
Chicago, IL

Suzanne S. Frucht, PhD
Associate Professor Emeritus
Northwest Missouri State University
Maryville, MO

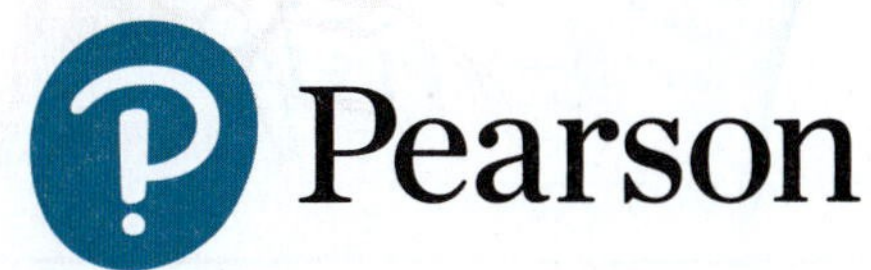

330 Hudson Street, New York, NY 10013

Vice President, Portfolio Management: Julie Levin Alexander
Director of Portfolio Management: Marlene McHugh Pratt
Portfolio Manager: John Goucher
Content Producer: Melissa Bashe
Portfolio Management Assistant: Lisa Narine
Development Editor: Danielle Doller
Vice President, Content Production and Digital Studio: Paul DeLuca
Vice President, Product Marketing: David Gesell
Senior Field Marketing Manager: Brittany Hammond
Product Marketing Manager: Rachele Strober
Operations Specialist: MaryAnn Gloriande
Cover Design: Studio Montage
Interior Designer: Pam Verros
Creative Digital Lead: Mary Siener
Cover Art: Sebastian Kaulitzki/Shutterstock
Director, Digital Studio, Health Science: Amy Peltier
Digital Studio Producer, e-text 2.0: Ellen Viganola and Allison Longley
Full-Service Project Management: Joanna Stein, SPi Global
Composition: SPi Global
Editorial Project Manager: Meghan DeMaio, SPi Global
Digital Content Team Lead: Brian Prybella
Digital Content Project Lead: William Johnson
Printer/Binder: LSC Communications, Inc.
Cover Printer: LSC Communications
Text Font: Meridien Com 11/13

DEDICATION

To my husband for his love and encouragement.

Bonnie Fremgen

To my granddaughter, Adrienne, who every day brings a smile to my face.

To Danielle Doller, whose incredible editing skills (and friendship) have made each edition of this text better.

I would like to extend a special thank you to Garnet Tomich who added to her normal workload by taking on the immense task of double-checking the pronunciations of every term in this edition and updating them as needed to ensure consistency.

Suzanne Frucht

Credits and acknowledgments for content borrowed from other sources and reproduced, with permission, in this textbook appear on appropriate page within text.

Library of Congress Cataloging-in-Publication Data

Names: Fremgen, Bonnie F., author. | Frucht, Suzanne S., author.
Title: Medical terminology : a living language / Bonnie F. Fremgen, Suzanne S. Frucht.
Description: Seventh edition. | Hoboken, New Jersey : Pearson Education, 2017. | Includes bibliographical references and index.
Identifiers: LCCN 2017041703 | ISBN 9780134701202 | ISBN 0134701208
Subjects: | MESH: Medicine | Terminology
Classification: LCC R123 | NLM W 15 | DDC 610.1/4--dc23
LC record available at https://lccn.loc.gov/2017041703

7 2022

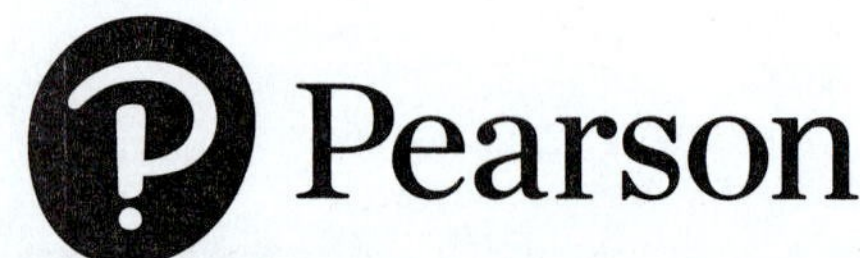

www.pearsonhighered.com

ISBN-10: 0-13-470120-8
ISBN-13: 978-013-470120-2

Welcome!

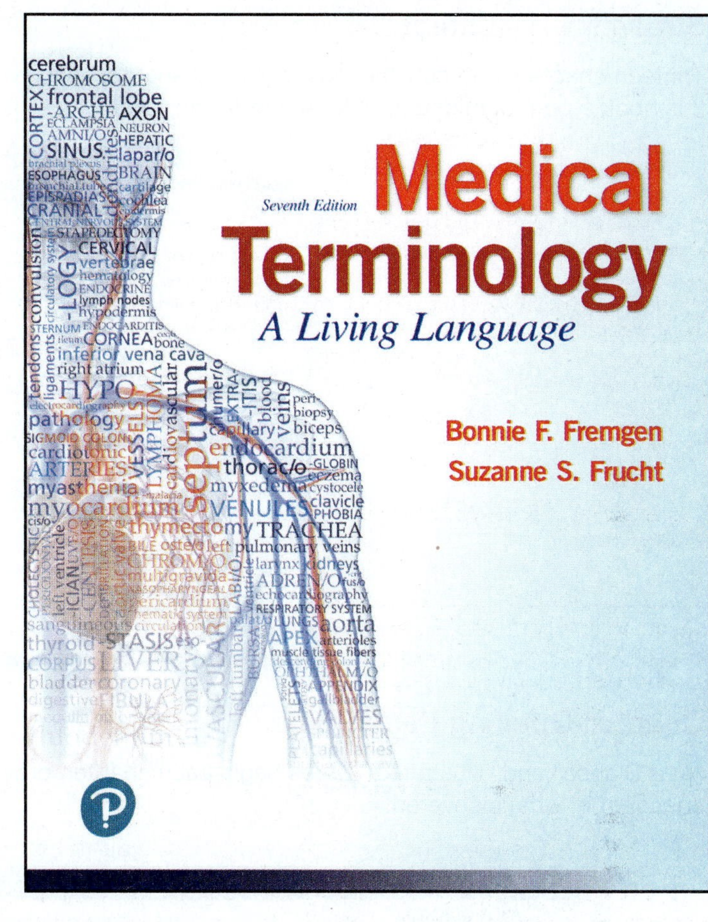

Welcome to the fascinating study of Medical Terminology: A Living Language—a vital part of your preparation for a career as a health professional. We are glad that you have joined us. Throughout your career, in a variety of settings, you will use medical terminology to communicate with coworkers and patients. Employing a carefully constructed learning system, ***Medical Terminology: A Living Language*** has helped thousands of readers gain a successful grasp of Medical Terminology: A Living Language within a real-world context.

In developing this book we had seven goals in mind:

1. To provide you with a clear introduction to the basic rules of using word parts to form medical terms.
2. To use phonetic pronunciations that will help you easily pronounce terms by spelling out the word part according to the way it sounds.
3. To help you understand medical terminology within the context of the human body systems. Realizing that this book is designed for a terminology course and not an anatomy and physiology course, we have aimed to stick to only the basics.
4. To help you develop a full range of Latin and Greek word parts used to build medical terms so that you will be able to interpret unfamiliar terms you encounter in the future.
5. To help you visualize Medical Terminology: A Living Language with an abundance of real-life photographs and accurate illustrations.
6. To provide you with a wealth of practice applications throughout and at the end of each chapter to help you review and master the content as you go along.
7. To create rich multimedia practice opportunities for you by way of MyLab Medical Terminology.

Please turn the page to get a visual glimpse of what makes this book an ideal guide to your exploration of medical terminology.

A Guide to What Makes This Book Special

Streamlined Content

Thirteen chapters and only the most essential anatomy and physiology coverage make this book a perfect midsized fit for a one-term course.

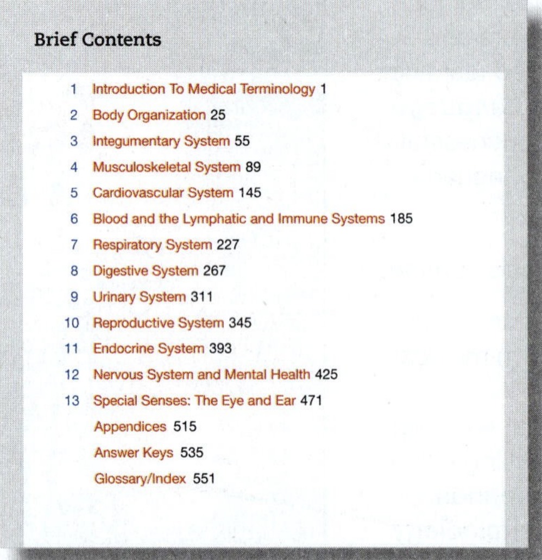

Brief Contents

Chapter-Opening Page Spreads

"At a Glance" and "Illustrated" pages begin each chapter, providing a quick, visual snapshot of what's covered.

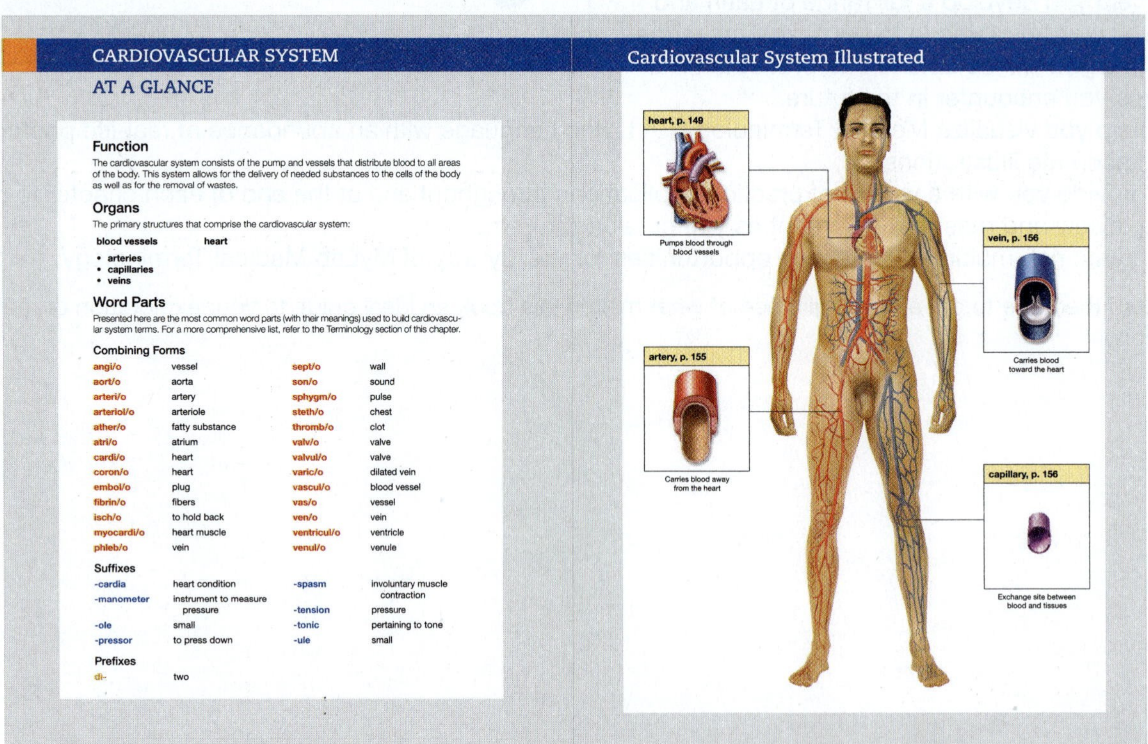

CARDIOVASCULAR SYSTEM

AT A GLANCE

Function

The cardiovascular system consists of the pump and vessels that distribute blood to all areas of the body. This system allows for the delivery of needed substances to the cells of the body as well as for the removal of wastes.

Organs

The primary structures that comprise the cardiovascular system:

blood vessels **heart**

- **arteries**
- **capillaries**
- **veins**

Word Parts

Presented here are the most common word parts (with their meanings) used to build cardiovascular system terms. For a more comprehensive list, refer to the Terminology section of this chapter.

Combining Forms

angi/o	vessel	sept/o	wall
aort/o	aorta	son/o	sound
arteri/o	artery	sphygm/o	pulse
arteriol/o	arteriole	steth/o	chest
ather/o	fatty substance	thromb/o	clot
atri/o	atrium	valv/o	valve
cardi/o	heart	valvul/o	valve
coron/o	heart	varic/o	dilated vein
embol/o	plug	vascul/o	blood vessel
fibrin/o	fibers	vas/o	vessel
isch/o	to hold back	ven/o	vein
myocardi/o	heart muscle	ventricul/o	ventricle
phleb/o	vein	venul/o	venule

Suffixes

-cardia	heart condition	-spasm	involuntary muscle contraction
-manometer	instrument to measure pressure	-tension	pressure
-ole	small	-tonic	pertaining to tone
-pressor	to press down	-ule	small

Prefixes

di-	two

Cardiovascular System Illustrated

heart, p. 149
Pumps blood through blood vessels
vein, p. 156
Carries blood toward the heart
artery, p. 155
Carries blood away from the heart
capillary, p. 156
Exchange site between blood and tissues

Anatomy & Physiology

Prior to being introduced to terms associated with an organ system, the anatomy and physiology of that body system is described in concise and easy to understand language. Information coverage begins with the overall function and the organs that comprise the system. Then each organ is addressed with its structure and how it contributes to the function of that system. Having a grasp of this basic level of information before being introduced to terms associated with each system makes it easier for students to understand the pathologic, diagnostic, and therapeutic terms.

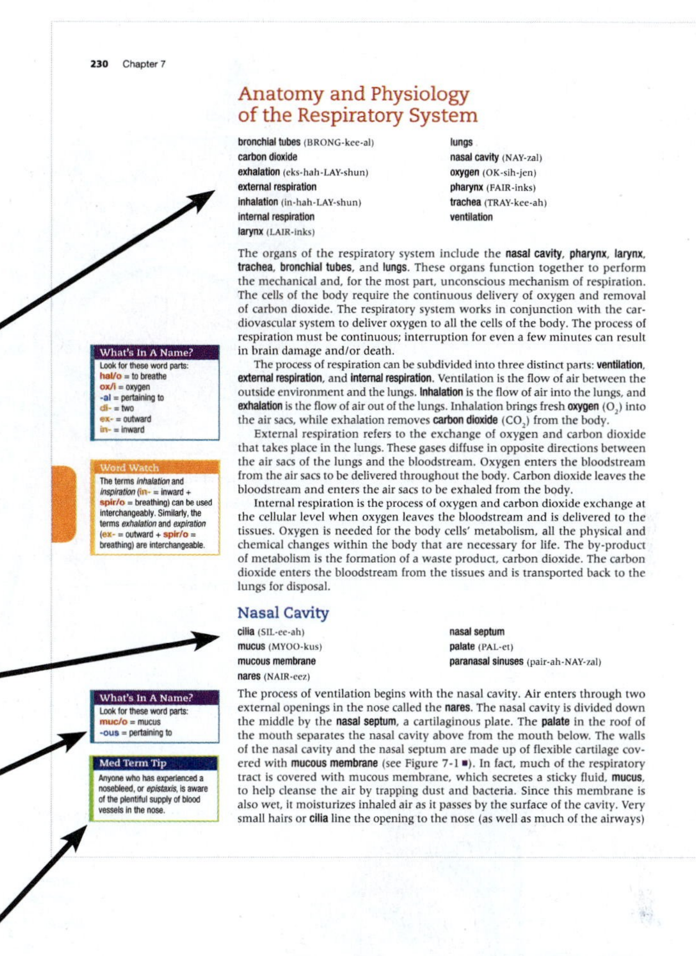

230 Chapter 7

Anatomy and Physiology of the Respiratory System

bronchial tubes (BRONG-kee-al)
carbon dioxide
exhalation (eks-hah-LAY-shun)
external respiration
inhalation (in-hah-LAY-shun)
internal respiration
larynx (LAIR-inks)
lungs
nasal cavity (NAY-zal)
oxygen (OK-sih-jen)
pharynx (FAIR-inks)
trachea (TRAY-kee-ah)
ventilation

The organs of the respiratory system include the **nasal cavity**, **pharynx**, **larynx**, **trachea**, **bronchial tubes**, and **lungs**. These organs function together to perform the mechanical and, for the most part, unconscious mechanism of respiration. The cells of the body require the continuous delivery of oxygen and removal of carbon dioxide. The respiratory system works in conjunction with the cardiovascular system to deliver oxygen to all the cells of the body. The process of respiration must be continuous; interruption for even a few minutes can result in brain damage and/or death.

The process of respiration can be subdivided into three distinct parts: **ventilation**, **external respiration**, and **internal respiration**. Ventilation is the flow of air between the outside environment and the lungs. **Inhalation** is the flow of air into the lungs, and **exhalation** is the flow of air out of the lungs. Inhalation brings fresh **oxygen** (O_2) into the air sacs, while exhalation removes **carbon dioxide** (CO_2) from the body.

External respiration refers to the exchange of oxygen and carbon dioxide that takes place in the lungs. These gases diffuse in opposite directions between the air sacs of the lungs and the bloodstream. Oxygen enters the bloodstream from the air sacs to be delivered throughout the body. Carbon dioxide leaves the bloodstream and enters the air sacs to be exhaled from the body.

Internal respiration is the process of oxygen and carbon dioxide exchange at the cellular level when oxygen leaves the bloodstream and is delivered to the tissues. Oxygen is needed for the body cells' metabolism, all the physical and chemical changes within the body that are necessary for life. The by-product of metabolism is the formation of a waste product, carbon dioxide. The carbon dioxide enters the bloodstream from the tissues and is transported back to the lungs for disposal.

What's In A Name?
Look for these word parts:
hal/o = to breathe
ox/i = oxygen
-al = pertaining to
di- = two
ex- = outward
in- = inward

Word Watch
The terms *inhalation* and *inspiration* (in- = inward + spir/o = breathing) can be used interchangeably. Similarly, the terms *exhalation* and *expiration* (ex- = outward + spir/o = breathing) are interchangeable.

Nasal Cavity

cilia (SIL-ee-ah)
mucus (MYOO-kus)
mucous membrane
nares (NAIR-eez)
nasal septum
palate (PAL-et)
paranasal sinuses (pair-ah-NAY-zal)

The process of ventilation begins with the nasal cavity. Air enters through two external openings in the nose called the **nares**. The nasal cavity is divided down the middle by the **nasal septum**, a cartilaginous plate. The **palate** in the roof of the mouth separates the nasal cavity above from the mouth below. The walls of the nasal cavity and the nasal septum are made up of flexible cartilage covered with **mucous membrane** (see Figure 7-1 ■). In fact, much of the respiratory tract is covered with mucous membrane, which secretes a sticky fluid, **mucus**, to help cleanse the air by trapping dust and bacteria. Since this membrane is also wet, it moisturizes inhaled air as it passes by the surface of the cavity. Very small hairs or **cilia** line the opening to the nose (as well as much of the airways)

What's In A Name?
Look for these word parts:
muc/o = mucus
-ous = pertaining to

Med Term Tip
Anyone who has experienced a nosebleed, or *epistaxis*, is aware of the plentiful supply of blood vessels in the nose.

Key Terms

Every subsection starts with a list of key terms that will be covered in that section. This sets the stage for comprehension and mastery.

EXPANDED! Pronunciations

Every chapter includes sound-it-out pronunciations to help students say medical terms accurately.

Color-Coded Word Parts

Red combining forms, blue suffixes, and gold prefixes allow for quick recognition throughout the book.

Informative and Interesting Sidebars

- The popular **Med Term Tip** feature offers tidbits of noteworthy information about medical terms that engage learners.
- **Word Watch** points out words that have a similar sound or similar spelling, and also alerts students about abbreviations that have more than one meaning.
- **What's In A Name?** reinforces the breakdown of terms into word parts.

Medically Accurate Illustrations

Concepts come to life with vibrant, clear, and scientifically precise images.

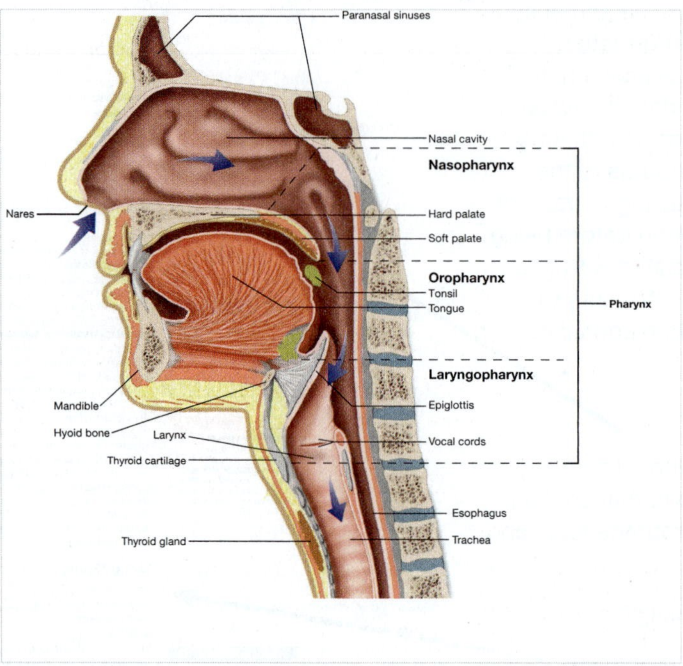

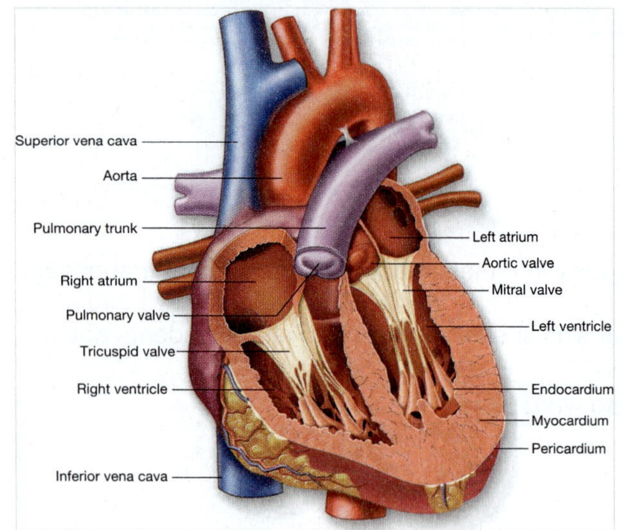

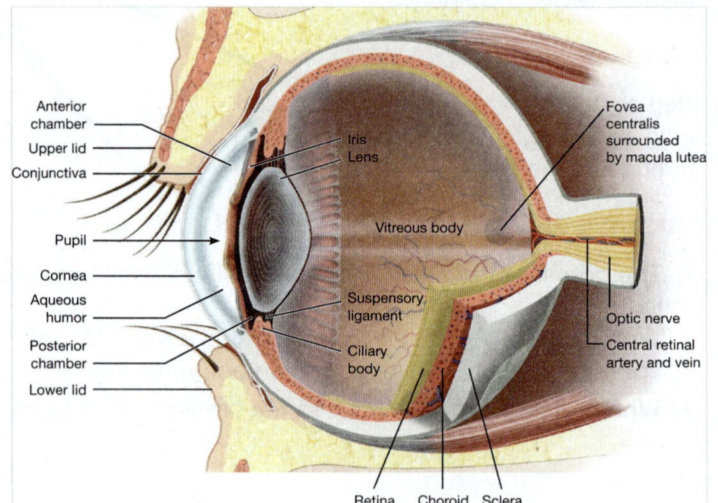

Terminology Tables

Terms are categorized and presented in a clear, logical, color-coded format that eases the learning process. The major categories include Pathology, Adjective Forms, Diagnostic Procedures, Therapeutic Procedures, Pharmacology, and Abbreviations. Each major category table is further subdivided into smaller subsections of related terms, thereby making learning easier. Also, the three-column format of the tables allows for the term (with pronunciation and/or abbreviation), word parts (if appropriate), and definitions to be displayed. The Pharmacology table also includes drug name examples in a fourth column.

Terminology

Word Parts Used to Build Eye Terms

The following lists contain the combining forms, suffixes, and prefixes used to build terms in the remaining sections of this chapter.

Combining Forms

aden/o	gland	emmetr/o	correct, proper	opt/o	eye, vision
ambly/o	dull, dim	esthesi/o	sensation, feeling	optic/o	eye, vision
angi/o	vessel	glauc/o	gray	papill/o	optic disk
bi/o	life	ir/o	iris	phac/o	lens
blast/o	immature	irid/o	iris	phot/o	light
blephar/o	eyelid	kerat/o	cornea	pneum/o	air
chromat/o	color	lacrim/o	tears	presby/o	old age
conjunctiv/o	conjunctiva	macul/o	macula lutea	pupill/o	pupil
corne/o	cornea	mi/o	lessening	retin/o	retina
cry/o	cold	myc/o	fungus	scler/o	sclera
cycl/o	ciliary body	mydr/i	widening	stigmat/o	point
cyst/o	sac	nyctal/o	night	ton/o	tone
dacry/o	tears	ocul/o	eye	uve/o	choroid
dipl/o	double	ophthalm/o	eye	xer/o	dry

Suffixes

-al	pertaining to	-logy	study of	-pexy	surgical fixation
-algia	pain	-malacia	abnormal softening	-phobia	fear
-ar	pertaining to	-meter	instrument to measure	-plasty	surgical repair
-ary	pertaining to	-metrist	specialist in measuring	-plegia	paralysis
-atic	pertaining to	-metry	process of measuring	-ptosis	drooping
-ectomy	surgical removal	-oma	tumor; mass	-rrhagia	abnormal flow condition
-edema	swelling	-opia	vision condition	-scope	instrument for viewing
-graphy	process of recording	-opsia	vision condition	-scopy	process of visually examining
-ia	condition	-osis	abnormal condition	-tic	pertaining to
-ic	pertaining to	-otomy	cutting into	-tropia	turned condition
-ician	specialist	-pathy	disease		
-ism	state of				
-itis	inflammation				

Prefixes

a-	without	exo-	outward	intra-	within
an-	without	extra-	outside of	micro-	small
anti-	against	hemi-	half	mono-	one
de-	without	hyper-	excessive	myo-	to shut
eso-	inward				

Abbreviations

#	number	ii	two
BCC	basal cell carcinoma	iii	three
bid	two times a day	MM	malignant melanoma
BX, bx	biopsy	oint	ointment
C&S	culture and sensitivity	qid	four times a day
decub	decubitus ulcer	SCC	squamous cell carcinoma
Derm, derm	dermatology	SG	skin graft
FS	frozen section	SLE	systemic lupus erythematosus
I&D	incision and drainage	STSG	split-thickness skin graft
i	one	Subc, Subq	subcutaneous
ID	intradermal	tid	three times a day
		UV	ultraviolet
		x	times

Word Watch

Be careful when using the abbreviation *ID* meaning *intradermal* and *I&D* meaning *incision and drainage*.

Pharmacology

Vocabulary

Term	Word Parts	Definition
cumulative action		Action that occurs in body when drug is allowed to accumulate or stay in body
prophylaxis (proh-fih-LAK-sis)	pro- = before -phylaxis = protection	Prevention of disease; for example, antibiotic can be used to prevent occurrence of bacterial infection

Drugs

Classification	Word Parts	Action	Examples
antibiotic (an-tih-bye-AW-tik)	anti- = against bi/o = life -tic = pertaining to	Kills bacteria causing respiratory infections	ampicillin; amoxicillin, Amoxil; ciprofloxacin, Cipro
antihistamine (an-tih-HIST-ah-meen)	anti- = against	Blocks effects of histamine released by body during allergy attack	fexofenadine, Allegra; loratadine, Claritin; diphenhydramine, Benadryl
antitussive (an-tih-TUSS-iv)	anti- = without tuss/o = cough	Relieves urge to cough	hydrocodon, Hycodan; dextromethorphan, Vicks Formula 44
bronchodilator (BRONG-koh-dye-lay-ter)	bronch/o = bronchus	Relaxes muscle spasms in bronchial tubes; used to treat asthma	albuterol, Proventil, Ventolin; salmeterol, Serevent
corticosteroids (kor-tih-koh-STAIR-oydz)	cortic/o = outer layer, cortex	Reduces inflammation and swelling in respiratory tract	fluticasone, Flonase; mometasone, Nasonex; triamcinolone, Azmacort
decongestant (dee-kon-JES-tant)	de- = without	Reduces stuffiness and congestion throughout respiratory system	oxymetazoline, Afrin, Dristan, Sinex; pseudoephedrine, Drixoral, Sudafed

Med Term Tip

There are three accepted pronunciations for the prefix anti-, "an-tih," "an-tee," and "an-tye."

Pathology (continued)

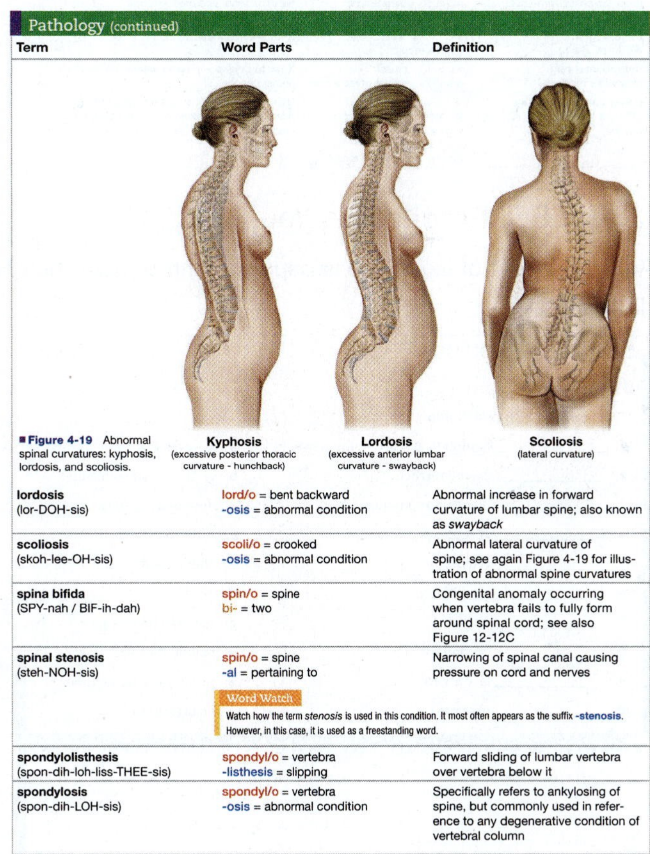

■ **Figure 4-19** Abnormal spinal curvatures: kyphosis, lordosis, and scoliosis.

Term	Word Parts	Definition
lordosis (lor-DOH-sis)	lord/o = bent backward -osis = abnormal condition	Abnormal increase in forward curvature of lumbar spine; also known as *swayback*
scoliosis (skoh-lee-OH-sis)	scoli/o = crooked -osis = abnormal condition	Abnormal lateral curvature of spine; see again Figure 4-19 for illustration of abnormal spine curvatures
spina bifida (SPY-nah / BIF-ih-dah)	spin/o = spine bi- = two	Congenital anomaly occurring when vertebra fails to fully form around spinal cord; see also Figure 12-12C
spinal stenosis (steh-NOH-sis)	spin/o = spine -al = pertaining to	Narrowing of spinal canal causing pressure on cord and nerves
spondylolisthesis (spon-dih-loh-liss-THEE-sis)	spondyl/o = vertebra -listhesis = slipping	Forward sliding of lumbar vertebra over vertebra below it
spondylosis (spon-dih-LOH-sis)	spondyl/o = vertebra -osis = abnormal condition	Specifically refers to ankylosing of spine, but commonly used in reference to any degenerative condition of vertebral column

Word Watch

Watch how the term *stenosis* is used in this condition. It most often appears as the suffix **-stenosis**. However, in this case, it is used as a freestanding word.

Therapeutic Procedures

Term	Word Parts	Definition
Medical Procedures		
autologous transfusion (aw-TALL-oh-gus / trans-FYOO-zhun)	auto- = self	Procedure for collecting and storing patient's own blood several weeks prior to actual need; can then be used to replace blood lost during surgical procedure
blood transfusion (trans-FYOO-zhun)	trans- = across fus/o = pouring -ion = action	Artificial transfer of blood into bloodstream **Med Term Tip** Before a patient receives a blood transfusion, the laboratory performs a **type and cross-match**. This test first double-checks the blood type of both the donor's and recipient's blood. Then a cross-match is performed. This process mixes together small samples of both bloods and observes the mixture for adverse reactions.
bone marrow transplant (BMT)		Patient receives red bone marrow from donor after patient's own bone marrow has been destroyed by radiation or chemotherapy
homologous transfusion (hoh-MALL-oh-gus / trans-FYOO-zhun)	homo- = same	Replacement of blood by transfusion of blood received from another person
packed red cells		Transfusion in which most of plasma, leukocytes, and platelets have been removed, leaving only erythrocytes
plasmapheresis (plaz-mah-fah-REE-sis)	-apheresis = removal, carry away	Method of removing plasma from body without depleting formed elements; whole blood is removed and cells and plasma are separated; cells are returned to patient along with donor plasma transfusion
whole blood		Transfusion of a mixture of both plasma and formed elements

Diagnostic Procedures (continued)

Term	Word Parts	Definition
Pap (Papanicolaou) **smear** (pap-ah-NIK-oh-lao)		Test for early detection of cancer of the cervix named after developer of test, George Papanicolaou, a Greek physician; a scraping of cells is removed from the cervix for examination under microscope
pregnancy test (PREG-nan-see)		Chemical test that can determine pregnancy during first few weeks; can be performed in physician's office or with home-testing kit
vaginal smear wet mount (VAJ-in-al)	vagin/o = vagina -al = pertaining to	Microscopic examination of cells obtained by swabbing vaginal wall; used to diagnose candidiasis
Diagnostic Imaging		
hysterosalpingography (HSG) (hiss-ter-oh-sal-pin-GOG-rah-fee)	hyster/o = uterus salping/o = uterine tube -graphy = process of recording	Taking of X-ray after injecting radiopaque material into uterus and uterine tubes
mammogram (MAM-oh-gram)	mamm/o = breast -gram = record	X-ray record of the breast
mammography (mam-OG-rah-fee)	mamm/o = breast -graphy = process of recording	X-ray to diagnose breast disease, especially breast cancer
pelvic ultrasonography (PEL-vik / ul-trah-son-OG-rah-fee)	pelv/o = pelvis -ic = pertaining to ultra- = beyond son/o = sound -graphy = process of recording	Use of high-frequency sound waves to produce image or photograph of an organ, such as uterus, ovaries, or fetus

Adjective Forms of Anatomical Terms

Term	Word Parts	Definition
conjunctival (kon-junk-TYE-val)	conjunctiv/o = conjunctiva -al = pertaining to	Pertaining to conjunctiva
corneal (KOR-nee-al)	corne/o = cornea -al = pertaining to **Word Watch** Be careful using the combining forms core/o meaning *pupil* and corne/o meaning *cornea*.	Pertaining to cornea
extraocular (eks-trah-OK-yoo-lar)	extra- = outside of ocul/o = eye -ar = pertaining to	Pertaining to being outside the eyeball; for example, the extraocular eye muscles
intraocular (in-trah-OK-yoo-lar)	intra- = within ocul/o = eye -ar = pertaining to	Pertaining to within eye
iridal (IR-id-al)	irid/o = iris -al = pertaining to	Pertaining to iris
lacrimal (LAK-rim-al)	lacrim/o = tears -al = pertaining to	Pertaining to tears
macular (MAK-yoo-lar)	macul/o = macula lutea -ar = pertaining to	Pertaining to macula lutea
ocular (OK-yoo-lar)	ocul/o = eye -ar = pertaining to	Pertaining to eye
ophthalmic (off-THAL-mik)	ophthalm/o = eye -ic = pertaining to	Pertaining to eye
optic (OP-tik)	opt/o = eye, vision -ic = pertaining to	Pertaining to eye or vision
optical (OP-tih-kal)	optic/o = eye, vision -al = pertaining to	Pertaining to eye or vision
pupillary (PYOO-pih-lair-ee)	pupill/o = pupil -ary = pertaining to	Pertaining to pupil
retinal (RET-ih-nal)	retin/o = retina -al = pertaining to	Pertaining to retina
scleral (SKLAIR-al)	scler/o = sclera -al = pertaining to	Pertaining to sclera
uveal (YOO-vee-al)	uve/o = choroid -al = pertaining to	Pertaining to choroid layer of eye

UPDATED! Practice As You Go

An assortment of exercises is peppered throughout the chapters to assess students' understanding of the material discussed.

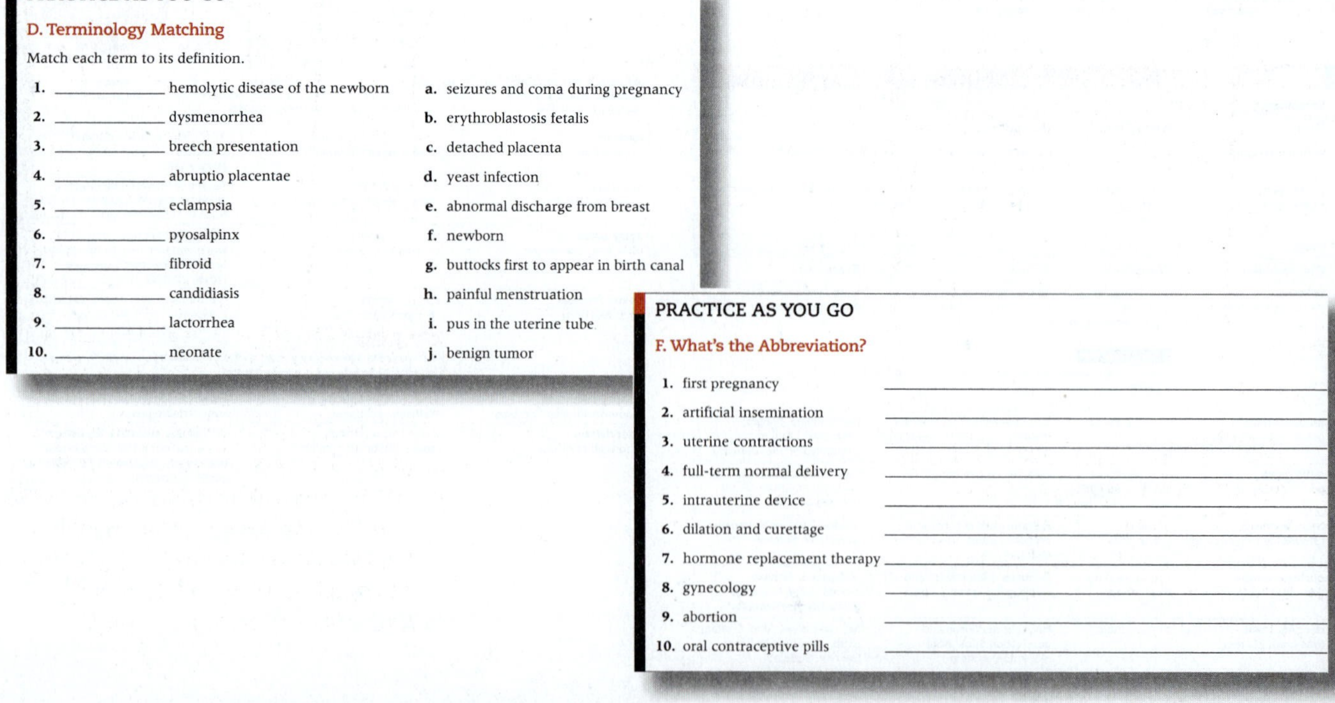

PRACTICE AS YOU GO

D. Terminology Matching

Match each term to its definition.

1. ____________ hemolytic disease of the newborn
2. ____________ dysmenorrhea
3. ____________ breech presentation
4. ____________ abruptio placentae
5. ____________ eclampsia
6. ____________ pyosalpinx
7. ____________ fibroid
8. ____________ candidiasis
9. ____________ lactorrhea
10. ____________ neonate

a. seizures and coma during pregnancy
b. erythroblastosis fetalis
c. detached placenta
d. yeast infection
e. abnormal discharge from breast
f. newborn
g. buttocks first to appear in birth canal
h. painful menstruation
i. pus in the uterine tube
j. benign tumor

PRACTICE AS YOU GO

F. What's the Abbreviation?

1. first pregnancy ____________
2. artificial insemination ____________
3. uterine contractions ____________
4. full-term normal delivery ____________
5. intrauterine device ____________
6. dilation and curettage ____________
7. hormone replacement therapy ____________
8. gynecology ____________
9. abortion ____________
10. oral contraceptive pills ____________

Chapter Review

Real-World Applications—Three critical thinking activities allow students to apply their medical knowledge to true-to-life scenarios:

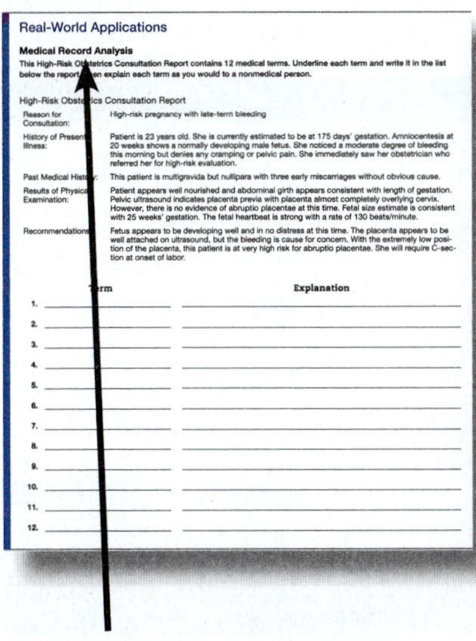

Real-World Applications

Medical Record Analysis

This High-Risk Obstetrics Consultation Report contains 12 medical terms. Underline each term and write it in the list below the report. Then explain each term as you would to a nonmedical person.

High-Risk Obstetrics Consultation Report

Reason for Consultation:	High-risk pregnancy with late-term bleeding
History of Present Illness:	Patient is 23 years old. She is currently estimated to be at 175 days' gestation. Amniocentesis at 20 weeks shows a normally developing male fetus. She noticed a moderate degree of bleeding this morning but denies any cramping or pelvic pain. She immediately saw her obstetrician who referred her for high-risk evaluation.
Past Medical History:	This patient is multigravida but nullipara with three early miscarriages without obvious cause.
Results of Physical Examination:	Patient appears well nourished and abdominal girth appears consistent with length of gestation. Pelvic ultrasound indicates placenta previa with placenta almost completely overlying cervix. However, there is no evidence of abruptio placentae at this time. Fetal size estimate is consistent with 25 weeks' gestation. The fetal heartbeat is strong with a rate of 130 beats/minute.
Recommendations:	Fetus appears to be developing well and in no distress at this time. The placenta appears to be well attached on ultrasound, but the bleeding is cause for concern. With the extremely low position of the placenta, this patient is at very high risk for abruptio placentae. She will require C-section at onset of labor.

	Term	Explanation
1.		
2.		
3.		
4.		
5.		
6.		
7.		
8.		
9.		
10.		
11.		
12.		

1) Medical Record Analysis

Exercises that challenge students to read examples of real medical records and then to apply their medical terminology knowledge in answering related questions.

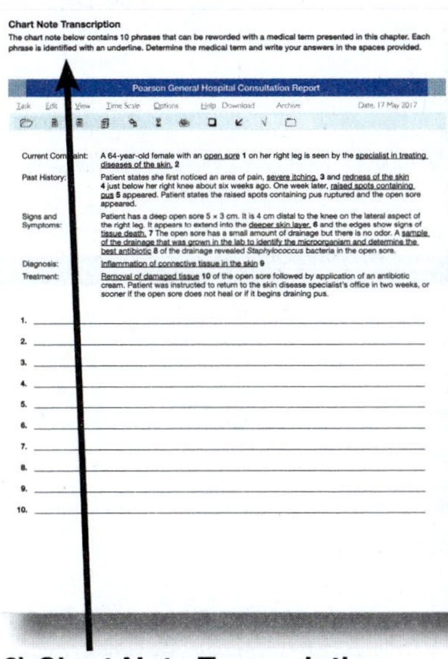

Chart Note Transcription

The chart note below contains 10 phrases that can be reworded with a medical term presented in this chapter. Each phrase is identified with an underline. Determine the medical term and write your answers in the spaces provided.

Pearson General Hospital Consultation Report

Task Edit View Time Scale Options Help Download Archive Date: 17 May 2017

Current Complaint:	A 64-year-old female with an open sore 1 on her right leg is seen by the specialist in treating diseases of the skin. 2
Past History:	Patient states she first noticed an area of pain, severe itching, 3 and redness of the skin 4 just below her right knee about six weeks ago. One week later, raised spots containing pus 5 appeared. Patient states the raised spots containing pus ruptured and the open sore appeared.
Signs and Symptoms:	Patient has a deep open sore 5 × 3 cm. It is 4 cm distal to the knee on the lateral aspect of the right leg. It appears to extend into the deeper skin layer, 6 and the edges show signs of tissue death. 7 The open sore has a small amount of drainage but there is no odor. A sample of the drainage that was grown in the lab to identify the microorganism and determine the best antibiotic 8 of the drainage revealed *Staphylococcus* bacteria in the open sore.
Diagnosis:	Inflammation of connective tissue in the skin 9
Treatment:	Removal of damaged tissue 10 of the open sore followed by application of an antibiotic cream. Patient was instructed to return to the skin disease specialist's office in two weeks, or sooner if the open sore does not heal or if it begins draining pus.

1. ______
2. ______
3. ______
4. ______
5. ______
6. ______
7. ______
8. ______
9. ______
10. ______

2) Chart Note Transcription

Slice-of-real-life exercise that asks students to replace lay terms in a medical chart with the proper medical term.

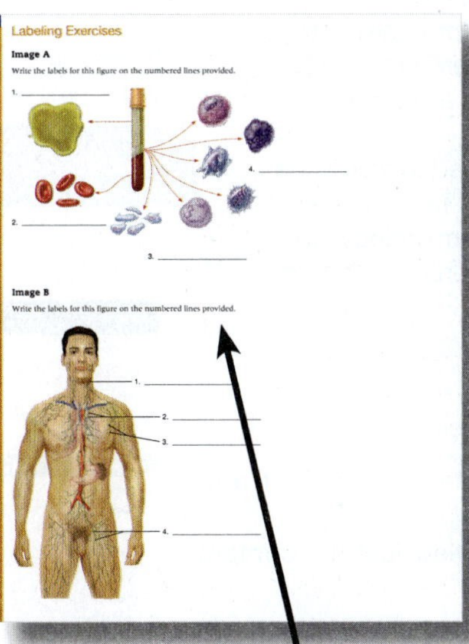

Labeling Exercises

Image A

Write the labels for this figure on the numbered lines provided.

1. ______ 2. ______ 3. ______ 4. ______

Image B

Write the labels for this figure on the numbered lines provided.

1. ______ 2. ______ 3. ______ 4. ______

Additionally, **Labeling Exercises** provide a visual challenge to reinforce students' grasp of anatomy and physiology concepts.

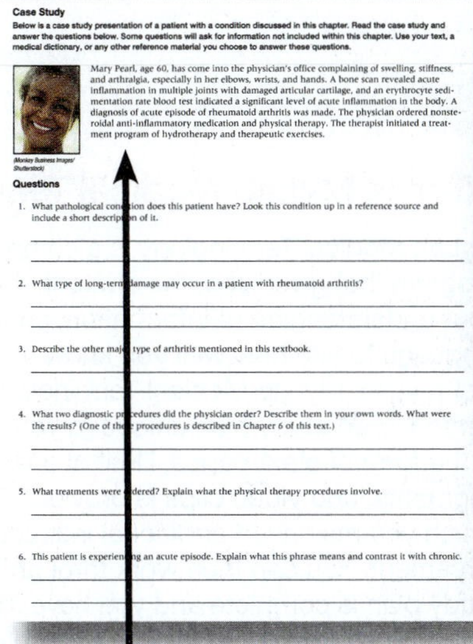

Case Study

Below is a case study presentation of a patient with a condition discussed in this chapter. Read the case study and answer the questions below. Some questions will ask for information not included within this chapter. Use your text, a medical dictionary, or any other reference material you choose to answer these questions.

Mary Pearl, age 60, has come into the physician's office complaining of swelling, stiffness, and arthralgia, especially in her elbows, wrists, and hands. A bone scan revealed acute inflammation in multiple joints with damaged articular cartilage, and an erythrocyte sedimentation rate blood test indicated a significant level of acute inflammation in the body. A diagnosis of acute episode of rheumatoid arthritis was made. The physician ordered nonsteroidal anti-inflammatory medication and physical therapy. The therapist initiated a treatment program of hydrotherapy and therapeutic exercises.

(Monkey Business Images/Shutterstock)

Questions

1. What pathological condition does this patient have? Look this condition up in a reference source and include a short description of it.
2. What type of long-term damage may occur in a patient with rheumatoid arthritis?
3. Describe the other major type of arthritis mentioned in this textbook.
4. What two diagnostic procedures did the physician order? Describe them in your own words. What were the results? (One of these procedures is described in Chapter 6 of this text.)
5. What treatments were ordered? Explain what the physical therapy procedures involve.
6. This patient is experiencing an acute episode. Explain what this phrase means and contrast it with chronic.

3) Case Study

Scenarios that use critical thinking questions to help students develop a firmer understanding of the terminology in context.

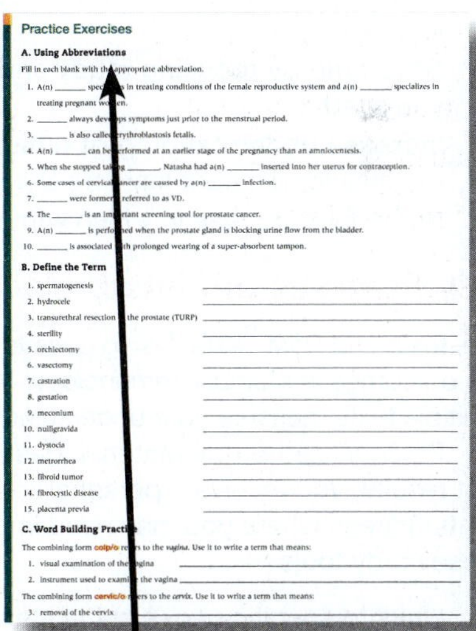

Practice Exercises

A. Using Abbreviations

Fill in each blank with the appropriate abbreviation.

1. A(n) ______ specializes in treating conditions of the female reproductive system and a(n) ______ specializes in treating pregnant women.
2. ______ always develops symptoms just prior to the menstrual period.
3. ______ is also called erythroblastosis fetalis.
4. A(n) ______ can be performed at an earlier stage of the pregnancy than an amniocentesis.
5. When she stopped taking ______, Natasha had a(n) ______ inserted into her uterus for contraception.
6. Some cases of cervical cancer are caused by a(n) ______ infection.
7. ______ were formerly referred to as VD.
8. The ______ is an important screening tool for prostate cancer.
9. A(n) ______ is performed when the prostate gland is blocking urine flow from the bladder.
10. ______ is associated with prolonged wearing of a super-absorbent tampon.

B. Define the Term

1. spermatogenesis ______
2. hydrocele ______
3. transurethral resection of the prostate (TURP) ______
4. sterility ______
5. orchiectomy ______
6. vasectomy ______
7. castration ______
8. gestation ______
9. meconium ______
10. nulligravida ______
11. dystocia ______
12. metrorrhea ______
13. fibroid tumor ______
14. fibrocystic disease ______
15. placenta previa ______

C. Word Building Practice

The combining form **colp/o** refers to the *vagina*. Use it to write a term that means:

1. visual examination of the vagina ______
2. instrument used to examine the vagina ______

The combining form **cervic/o** refers to the *cervix*. Use it to write a term that means:

3. removal of the cervix ______

Practice Exercises—A wide array of updated workbook exercises at the end of each chapter serve as a fun and challenging study review. A larger variety of question types leads to a more engaging assessment of student understanding of concepts like spelling, adjective formation, and anatomy and physiology.

MyLab Medical Terminology™

What is MyLab Medical Terminology?

MyLab Medical Terminology is a comprehensive online program that gives you, the student, the opportunity to test your understanding of information, concepts and medical language to see how well you know the material. From the test results, MyLab Medical Terminology builds a self-paced, personalized study plan unique to your needs. Remediation in the form of etext pages, illustrations, exercises, audio segments, and video clips is provided for those areas in which you may need additional instruction, review, or reinforcement. You can then work through the program until your study plan is complete and you have mastered the content. MyLab Medical Terminology is available as a standalone program or with an embedded etext.

MyLab Medical Terminology is organized to follow the chapters and learning outcomes in *Medical Terminology: A Living Language*. With MyLab Medical Terminology, you can track your own progress through your entire med term course.

How do Students Benefit?

Here's how MyLab Medical Terminology helps you.

- Keep up with information presented in the text and lectures.
- Save time by focusing study and review just the content you need.
- Increase understanding of difficult concepts with study material for different learning styles.
- Remediate in areas in which you need additional review.

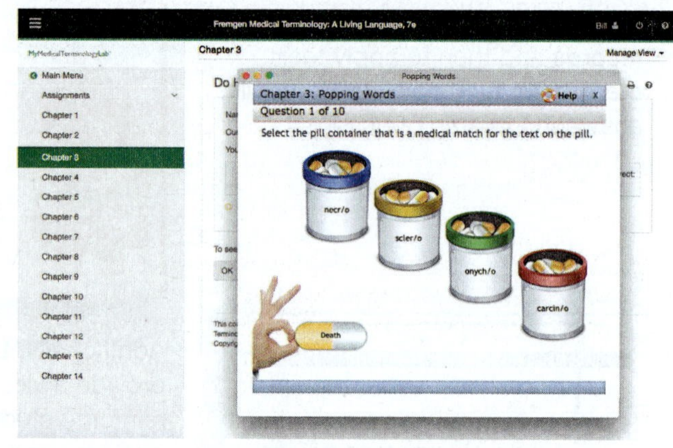

Key Features of MyLab Medical Terminology

Pre-Tests and Post-Tests. Using questions aligned to the learning outcomes in *Medical Terminology: A Living Language*, multiple tests measure your understanding of topics.

Personalized Study Material. Based on the topic pre-test results, you receive a personalized study plan, highlighting areas where you may need improvement. It includes these study tools

- Links to specific pages in the etext
- Images for review
- Interactive exercises
- Animations and video clips
- Audio glossary
- Access to full Personalized Study Material

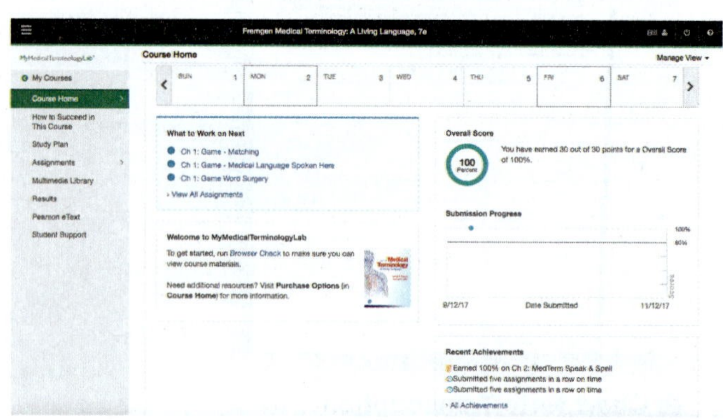

How do Instructors Benefit?

- Save time by providing students with a comprehensive, media-rich study program.
- Track student understanding of course content in the program gradebook.
- Monitor student activity with viewable student assignments.

Preface

Since the first edition of ***Medical Terminology: A Living Language*** was published it has been noted for its "clean" and logical format that promotes learning. In this revised edition, we have built upon this strength by enhancing many features to make this text an ideal choice for semester- or quarter-length courses.

Features of this Edition

This new seventh edition contains features that facilitate student mastery, while maintaining the best aspects of previous editions. Each chapter is arranged in a similar format and the content is organized with an emphasis on maintaining consistency and accuracy.

We have revised ***Medical Terminology: A Living Language*** so that it provides for an even more valuable teaching and learning experience. Here are the enhancements we have made:

- Based on market feedback, we have taken the content that appeared in the special topics chapter in previous editions, and have now broken it up and interspersed this material throughout the book to better correspond with the body systems organization of the text. We hope this change will make incorporating this information easier into your course.
- All of the phonetic pronunciations have been reviewed and revised as needed to ensure consistency and to provide the most commonly used pronunciation.
- The beginning of the Terminology section in each chapter includes an even more comprehensive list of all combining forms, suffixes, and prefixes used to build terms in the remaining sections of the chapter.
- For this seventh edition, every term presented in the book has been evaluated for its currency and additional terms have been added throughout to reflect the newest technologies and procedures.
- **Practice As You Go**, our popular "speed bump" feature scattered throughout the chapters, has been expanded to appear more frequently throughout each chapter to allow the reader to get a quick check on their grasp of the content presented by using a combination of short-answer exercises. Answers are provided at the back of the book.
- End-of-Chapter Practice Exercises have been revamped to better emphasize terminology usage rather than simple recall of word parts. In addition to the rewriting of many standard question types, new exercises have been added to the end of each chapter to provide students an engaging opportunity to assess their skills in:
  - spelling
  - building medical terms
  - using abbreviations
  - defining medical terms
  - understanding true-to-life scenarios
  - labeling drawings of human anatomy

Organization of the Book

Introductory Chapters

Chapter 1 contains information necessary for an understanding of how medical terms are formed. This includes learning about word roots, combining forms, prefixes, and suffixes, and general rules for building medical terms. Readers will learn about terminology for medical records, the different healthcare settings, and about Pharmacology and the elements of a prescription. Chapter 2 presents terminology relating to the body organization, including organs and body systems. Here readers will first encounter word-building tables, a feature found in each remaining chapter that lists medical terms and their respective word parts. Chapter 2 also includes a discussion about the routes used to introduce drugs into the body.

Body Systems Chapters

Chapters 3–13 are organized by body system. Each chapter begins with the System At a Glance feature, which lists combining forms, prefixes, and/or suffixes with their meanings and is followed by a System Illustrated overview of the organs in the system. The anatomy and physiology section is divided into the various components of the system, and each subsection begins with a list of key medical terms accompanied by a phonetic pronunciation guide. Key terms are boldfaced the first time they appear in the narrative for easy recognition. The Terminology section of each chapter begins with a list of all word parts used within the chapter. For ease of learning, the medical terms are divided into five separate sections: adjective forms of anatomical terms, pathology, diagnostic procedures, therapeutic procedures, and pharmacology. The word parts used to build terms are highlighted within each table. An abbreviations section then follows to complete each chapter.

Appendices

The appendices contain helpful reference lists of word parts and definitions provided in the text. This information is intended for quick access and includes three appendices: Word Parts Arranged Alphabetically and Defined, Word Parts Arranged Alphabetically by Definition, and Abbreviations.

Answer Keys

A comprehensive listing of answers is provided in the back of the book for all of the Practice As You Go exercises, as well as the Chapter Review section's Real-World Applications activities, Practice Exercises, and Labeling Exercises. Students should use these answer keys to check their answers as they complete each chapter to better assess any areas that may need additional study.

Glossary/Index

Lastly, all of the key terms in the book appear again in the combination glossary/index at the end of the text. In addition to providing a page reference for each entry, complete definitions of key terms are also presented for quick access.

About the Authors

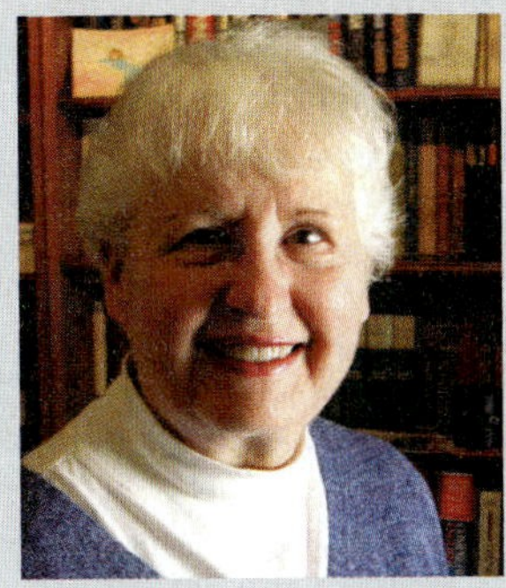

Bonnie F. Fremgen

Bonnie F. Fremgen, PhD, is a former Associate Dean of the Allied Health Program at Robert Morris College and was vice president of a hospital in suburban Chicago. She was also director of continuing education at three Chicago area hospitals. She has taught medical law and ethics courses as well as clinical and administrative topics. In addition, Dr. Fremgen has served as an advisor for students' career planning. She has broad interests and experiences in the healthcare field, including hospitals, nursing homes, and physicians' offices as well as responsibility for departments of social services, home health care, discharge planning, quality assurance, and hospital-wide education. She currently has two patents on a unique circulation-assisting wheelchair.

Dr. Fremgen holds a nursing degree as well as a master's in healthcare administration. She received her PhD from the College of Education at the University of Illinois. Dr. Fremgen has performed postdoctoral studies in Medical Law at Loyola University Law School in Chicago. She has authored five textbooks with Pearson. Dr. Fremgen has also taught ethics at the University of Notre Dame, South Bend, Indiana; University of Detroit, Detroit, Michigan; and Saint Xavier University, Chicago, Illinois.

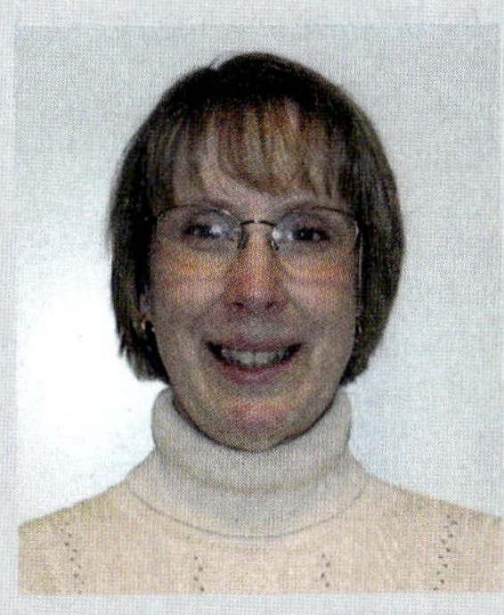

Suzanne S. Frucht

Suzanne S. Frucht is an Associate Professor Emeritus of Anatomy and Physiology at Northwest Missouri State University (NWMSU). She holds baccalaureate degrees in biological sciences and physical therapy from Indiana University, an MS in biological sciences at NWMSU, and a PhD in molecular biology and biochemistry from the University of Missouri–Kansas City.

For 14 years Dr. Frucht worked full time as a physical therapist in various healthcare settings, including acute care hospitals, extended care facilities, and home health. Based on her educational and clinical experience she was invited to teach medical terminology part time in 1988 and became a full-time faculty member three years later as she discovered her love for the challenge of teaching. Dr. Frucht has taught a variety of courses including medical terminology, human anatomy, human physiology, and animal anatomy and physiology. She received the Governor's Award for Excellence in Teaching in 2003. After retiring from teaching in 2008, she continues to be active in student learning through teaching medical terminology as an online course and writing medical terminology texts and anatomy and physiology laboratory manuals.

About the Illustrators

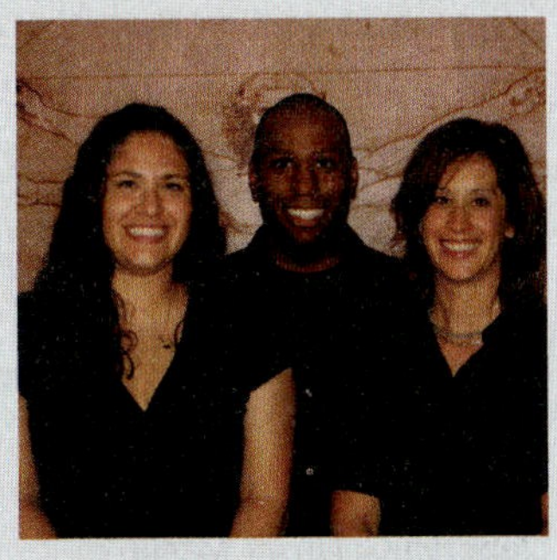

Marcelo Oliver is president and founder of Body Scientific International LLC. He holds an MFA degree in Medical and Biological Illustration from the University of Michigan. For the past 15 years, his passion has been to condense complex anatomical information into visual education tools for students, patients, and medical professionals. For seven years Oliver worked as a medical illustrator and creative director developing anatomical charts used for student and patient education. In the years that followed, he created educational and marketing tools for medical device companies prior to founding Body Scientific International, LLC.

Body Scientific's lead artists in this publication were medical illustrators Liana Bauman and Katie Burgess. Both hold a Master of Science degree in Biomedical Visualization from the University of Illinois at Chicago. Their contribution to the publication was key in the creation and editing of artwork throughout.

Our Development Team

We would like to express deep gratitude to the over 120 colleagues from schools across the country who have provided us with many hours of their time over the years to help us tailor this book to suit the dynamic needs of instructors and students. These individuals have reviewed manuscript chapters and illustrations for content, accuracy, level, and utility. We sincerely thank them and feel that ***Medical Terminology: A Living Language*** has benefited immeasurably from their efforts, insights, encouragement, and selfless willingness to share their expertise as educators.

Reviewers of the Seventh Edition

Pamela A. Dobbins, MS
Shelton State Community College
Natural Sciences-Biology
Tuscaloosa, Alabama

Pamela J. Edwards, MA, CCMA, CBCS, NRCMA
Lone Star College System
Business and Social Sciences Division
Conroe, Texas

Gerry Gordon, BA, CPC, CPB
Daytona College
Medical Billing and Coding, Adjunct Faculty
Ormond Beach, Florida

Marleshia D. Hall, PhD
Shelton State Community College
Department of Natural Sciences
Tuscaloosa, Alabama

Timothy J. Jones, BA, MA
Oklahoma City Community College
Health Professions
Oklahoma City, Oklahoma

Tammie Petersen RNC-OB, BSN
Austin Community College
Health Sciences
Austin, Texas

Amy Bolinger Snow, MS
Greenville Technical College
Biological Sciences Department
Greenville, South Carolina

Reviewers of Earlier Editions

Yvonne Alles, MBA, RMT
Davenport University
Grand Rapids, Michigan

Rachael C. Alstatter, Program Director
Southern Ohio College
Fairfield, Ohio

Steve Arinder, BS, MPH
Meridian Community College
Meridian, Mississippi

K. William Avery, BSMT, JD, PhD
City College
Gainesville, Florida

Beverly A. Baker, DA, CST
Western Iowa Technical Community College
Sioux City, Iowa

Michael Battaglia, MS
Greenville Technical College
Taylors, South Carolina

Nancy Ridinger Bean, Health Assistant Instructor
Wythe County Vocational School
Wytheville, Virginia

Deborah J. Bedford, CMA, AAS
North Seattle Community College
Seattle, Washington

Barbara J Behrens, PTA, MS
Mercer County Community College
Trenton, New Jersey

Pam Besser, PhD
Jefferson Community and Technical College
Louisville, Kentucky

Norma J. Bird, MEd, BS, CMA
Idaho State University College of Technology
Pocatello, Idaho

Trina Blaschko, RHIT
Chippewa Valley Technical College
Eau Claire, Wisconsin

Richard T. Boan, PhD
Midlands Technical College
Columbia, South Carolina

Susan W. Boggs, RN, BSN, CNOR
Piedmont Technical College
Greenwood, South Carolina

Bradley S. Bowden, PhD
Alfred University
Alfred, New York

Jeannie Bower, BS, NRCAMA
Central Penn College
Summerdale, Pennsylvania

Joan Walker Brittingham
Sussex Tech Adult Division
Georgetown, Delaware

Phyills J. Broughton, Curriculum Coordinator
Pitt Community College
Greenville, North Carolina

Barbara Bussard, Instructor
Southwestern Michigan College
Dowagiac, Michigan

Toni Cade, MBA, RHIA, CCS
University of Louisiana at Lafayette
Lafayette, Louisiana

Nicole Claussen, MS, CST, FAST
Rolla Technical Institute
Rolla, Missouri

Gloria H. Coats, RN, MSN
Modesto Junior College
Modesto, California

Linda A. Costarella, ND
Lake Washington Institute of Technology
Kirkland, Washington

Lyndal M. Curry, MA, RP
University of South Alabama
Mobile, Alabama

Nancy Dancs, PT
Waukesha County Technical College
Pewaukee, Wisconsin

Theresa H. deBeche, RN, MN, CNS
Louisiana State University at Eunice
Eunice, Louisiana

Bonnie Deister, MS, BSN, CMA-C
Broome Community College
Binghamton, New York

Antoinette Deshaies, RN, BSPA
Glendale Community College
Glendale, Arizona

Pamela Dobbins, MS, BS, AAS
Shelton State Community College
Tuscaloosa, Alabama

Carole DuBose, LPN, CST
Choffin School of Surgical Technology
Youngstown, Ohio

Carol Eckert, RN, MSN
Southwestern Illinois College
Belleville, Illinois

Pamela Edwards, MA, NRCMA
Lone Star College System
The Woodlands, Texas

Jamie Erskine, PhD, RD
University of Northern Colorado
Greeley, Colorado

Robert Fanger, MS
Del Mar College
Corpus Christi, Texas

Mildred K. Fuller, PhD, MT (ASCP), CLS(NCA)
Norfolk State University
Norfolk, Virginia

Deborah Galanski-Maciak
Davenport University
Grand Rapids, Michigan

Debra Getting, Practical Nursing Instructor
Northwest Iowa Community College
Sheldon, Iowa

Ann Queen Giles, MHS, CMA
Western Piedmont Community College
Morganton, North Carolina

Brenda L. Gleason, MSN
Iowa Central Community College
Fort Dodge, Iowa

Steven B. Goldschmidt, DC, CCFC
North Hennepin Community College
Brooklyn Park, Minnesota

Linda S. Gott, RN, MS
Pensacola High School
Pensacola, Florida

Martha Grove, Staff Educator
Mercy Regional Health System
Cincinnati, Ohio

Kathryn Gruber
Globe College
Oakdale, Minnesota

Karen R. Hardney, MSEd
Chicago State University
Chicago, Illinois

Mary Hartman, MS, OTR/L
Genesee Community College
Batavia, New York

Joyce B. Harvey, PhD, RHIA
Norfolk State University
Norfolk, Virginia

Beulah A. Hofmann, RN, BSN, MSN, CMA
Ivy Tech Community College of Indiana
Greencastle, Indiana

Kimberley Hontz, RN
Antonelli Medical and Professional Institute
Pottstown, Pennsylvania

Dolly Horton, CMA (AAMA), EdD
Asheville Buncombe Technical Community College
Asheville, North Carolina

Pamela S. Huber, MS, MT (ASCP)
Erie Community College
Williamsville, New York

Eva I. Irwin
Ivy Tech State College
Indianapolis, Indiana

Susan Jackson, EdS
Valdosta Technical College
Valdosta, Georgia

Mark Jaffe, DPM, MHSA
Nova Southeastern University
Ft. Lauderdale, Florida

Carol Lee Jarrell, MLT, AHI
Brown Mackie College
Merrillville, Indiana

Holly Jodon, MPAS, PA-C
Gannon University
Erie, Pennsylvania

Virginia J. Johnson, CMA
Lakeland Academy
Minneapolis, Minnesota

Marcie C. Jones, BS, CMA
Gwinnett Technical Institute
Lawrenceville, Georgia

Robin Jones, RHIA
Meridian Community College
Meridian, Mississippi

Rebecca Keith, PT, MSHS
Arkansas State University
Jonesboro, Arkansas

Gertrude A. Kenny, BSN, RN, CMA
Baker College of Muskegon
Muskegon, Michigan

Dianne K. Kuiti, RN
Duluth Business University
Duluth, Minnesota

Andrew La Marca, EMT-P
Mobile Life Support Services
Middletown, New York

Francesca L. Langlow, BS
Delgado Community College
New Orleans, Louisiana

Julie A. Leu, CPC
Creighton University
Omaha, Nebraska

Norma Longoria, BS, COI
South Texas Community College
McAllen, Texas

Jeanne W. Lovelock, RN, MSN
Piedmont Virginia Community College
Charlottesville, Virginia

Jan Martin, RT(R)
Ogeechee Tech College
Statesboro, Georgia

Leslie M. Mazzola, MA
Cuyahoga Community College
Parma, Ohio

Michelle C. McCranie, CPhT
Ogeechee Technical College
Statesboro, Georgia

Lola McGourty, MSN, RN
Bossier Parish Community College
Bossier City, Louisiana

Patricia Moody, RN
Athens Technical College
Athens, Georgia

Bridgit R. Moore, EdD, MT (ASCP), CPC
McLennan Community College
Waco, Texas

Christine J. Moore, MEd
Armstrong Atlantic State University
Savannah, Georgia

Catherine Moran, PhD
Breyer State University
Birmingham, Alabama

Connie Morgan
Ivy Tech State College
Kokomo, Indiana

Katrina B. Myricks
Holmes Community College
Ridgeland, Mississippi

Pam Ncu, CMA
International Business College
Fort Wayne, Indiana

Judy Ortiz MHS, MS, PA-C
Pacific University
Hillsboro, Oregon

Tina M. Peer, BSN, RN
College of Southern Idaho
Twin Falls, ID

Dave Peruski, RN, MSA, MSN
Delta College
University Center, Michigan

Lisa J. Pierce, MSA, RRT
Augusta Technical College
Augusta, Georgia

Sister Marguerite Polcyn, OSF, PhD
Lourdes College
Sylvania, Ohio

Vicki Prater, CMA, RMA, RAHA
Concorde Career Institute
San Bernardino, California

Carolyn Ragsdale CST, BS
Parkland College
Champaign, Illinois

LuAnn Reicks, RNC, BS, MSN
Iowa Central Community College
Fort Dodge, Iowa

Linda Reigel
Glenville State College
Glenville, West Virginia

Shiela Rojas, MBA
Santa Barbara Business College
Santa Barbara, California

Ellen Rosen, RN, MN
Glendale Community College
Glendale, California

Georgette Rosenfeld, PhD, RRT, RN
Indian River State College
Fort Pierce, Florida

Brian L. Rutledge, MHSA
Hinds Community College
Jackson, Mississippi

Sue Shibley, MEd, CMT, CCS-P, CPC
North Idaho College
Coeur d'Alene, Idaho

Misty Shuler, RHIA
Asheville Buncombe Technical Community College
Asheville, North Carolina

Patricia A. Slachta, PhD, RN, ACNS-BC, CWOCN
Technical College of the Lowcountry
Beaufort, South Carolina

Donna J. Slovensky, PhD, RHIA, FAHIMA
University of Alabama at Birmingham
Birmingham, Alabama

Connie Smith, RPh
University of Louisiana at Monroe School of Pharmacy
Monroe, Louisiana

Karen Snipe, CPhT, ASBA, MAEd
Trident Technical College
Charleston, South Carolina

Janet Stehling, RHIA
McLennan College
Lorena, Texas

Karen Stenback, MFA, CHHC
Antelope Valley College
Lancaster, California

Donna Stern
University of California San Diego
La Jolla, California

Jodi Taylor, AAS, LPN, RMA
Terra State Community College
Fremont, Ohio

Annmary Thomas, MEd, NREMT-P
Community College of Philadelphia
Philadelphia, Pennsylvania

Lenette Thompson, CST, AS
Piedmont Technical College
Greenwood, South Carolina

Scott Throneberry, BS, NREMTP
Calhoun Community College
Decatur, Alabama

Maureen Tubbiola, MS, PhD
St. Cloud State University
St. Cloud, Minnesota

Marilyn Turner, RN, CMA
Ogeechee Technical College
Statesboro, Georgia

Marianne Van Deursen, MS, Ed, CMA (AAMA), MLT
Warren County Community College
Washington, New Jersey

Joan Ann Verderame, RN, MA
Bergen Community College
Paramus, New Jersey

Twila Wallace, MEd
Central Community College
Columbus, Nebraska

Kathy Wallington
Phillips Junior College
Campbell, California

Linda Walter, RN, MSN
Northwestern Michigan College
Traverse City, Michigan

Jean Watson, PhD
Clark College
Vancouver, Washington

Twila Weiszbrod, MPA
College of the Sequoias
Visalia, California

Sara J. Wellman, RHIT
Indiana University Northwest
Gary, Indiana

Leesa Whicker, BA, CMA
Central Piedmont Community College
Charlotte, NC

Lynn C. Wimett, RN, ANP, EdD
Regis University
Denver, Colorado

Kathy Zaiken, PharmD
Massachusetts College of Pharmacy and Health Sciences
Boston, Massachusetts

Judith Zappala, MT, ASCP, MBA
Middlesex Community College
Lowell, Massachusetts

Carole A. Zeglin, MSEd, BS, MT, RMA (AMT)
Westmoreland County Community College
Youngwood, Pennsylvania

A Commitment to Accuracy

As a student embarking on a career in healthcare you probably already know how critically important it is to be precise in your work. Patients and coworkers will be counting on you to avoid errors on a daily basis. Likewise, we owe it to you—the reader—to ensure accuracy in this book. We have gone to great lengths to verify that the information provided in ***Medical Terminology: A Living Language*** is complete and correct. To this end, here are the steps we have taken:

1. **Editorial Review—**We have assembled a large team of developmental consultants (listed on the preceding pages) to critique every word and every image in this book. Multiple content experts have read each chapter for accuracy.
2. **Medical Illustrations—**A team of medically trained illustrators was hired to prepare many of the pieces of art that grace the pages of this book. These illustrators have a higher level of scientific education than the artists for most textbooks, and they worked directly with the authors and members of our development team to make sure that their work was clear, correct, and consistent with what is described in the text.
3. **Accurate Ancillaries—**Realizing that the teaching and learning ancillaries are often as vital to instruction as the book itself, we took extra steps to ensure accuracy and consistency within these components. We assigned some members of our development team to specifically focus on critiquing every bit of content that comprises the instructional ancillary resources to confirm accuracy.

While our intent and actions have been directed at creating an error-free text, we have established a process for correcting any mistakes that may have slipped past our editors. Pearson takes this issue seriously and therefore welcomes any and all feedback that you can provide along the lines of helping us enhance the accuracy of this text. If you identify any errors that need to be corrected in a subsequent printing, please notify us. Thank you for helping Pearson to reach its goal of providing the most accurate medical terminology textbooks available. Any corrections can be sent to us through your institution's Pearson representative or please mail them to:

Pearson Health Science Editorial
Medical Terminology Corrections
211 River Street
4th Floor
Hoboken, NJ 07030

Contents

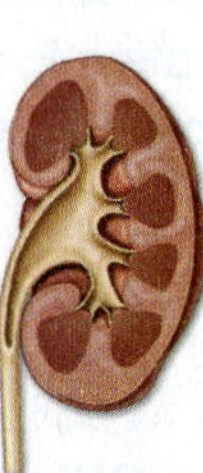

12 Nervous System and Mental Health 425

13 Special Senses: The Eye and Ear 471

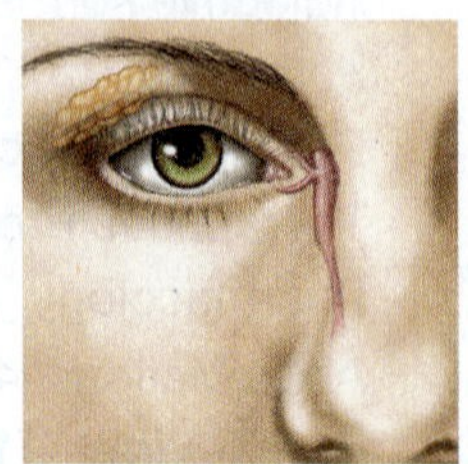

Appendices 515

Chapter 1

Introduction to Medical Terminology

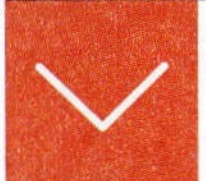

Learning Objectives

Upon completion of this chapter, you will be able to

1. Discuss the four parts of medical terms.
2. Recognize word roots and combining forms.
3. Identify the most common prefixes and suffixes.
4. Define word building and describe a strategy for translating medical terms.
5. State the importance of correct spelling of medical terms.
6. State the rules for determining singular and plural endings.
7. Discuss the importance of using caution with abbreviations.
8. Recognize the documents found in a medical record.
9. Recognize the different healthcare settings.
10. Understand the importance of confidentiality.
11. Describe how drugs are named and classified.
12. Read and understand all abbreviations and notations in a written prescription.

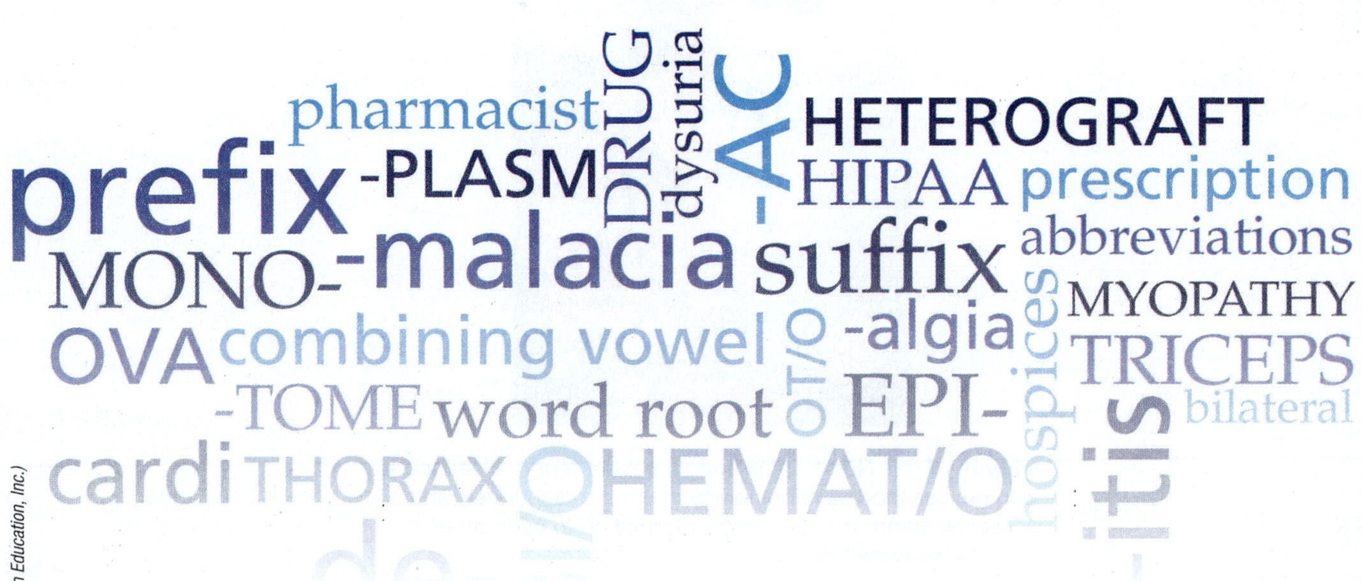

(Pearson Education, Inc.)

MEDICAL TERMINOLOGY

AT A GLANCE

Learning medical terminology can initially seem like studying a strange new language. However, once you understand some of the basic rules about how medical terms are formed using word building, it will become much like piecing together a puzzle. This chapter discusses the general guidelines for forming words; an understanding of word roots, combining forms, prefixes, and suffixes; pronunciation; and spelling. Chapter 2 introduces you to terms that are used to describe the body as a whole. Chapters 3–13 each focus on a specific body system and present new combining forms, prefixes, and suffixes, as well as exercises to help you gain experience building new medical terms. Additionally, sprinkled throughout all chapters are "Med Term Tips" to assist in clarifying some of the material, "Word Watch" boxes to point out terms that may be particularly confusing, and "What's In A Name?" boxes to highlight the word parts found in the text. Key terms (with their pronunciations) are listed at the beginning of the section in which they are discussed, and each chapter contains numerous pathological, diagnostic, treatment, and surgical terms. Use these lists as an additional study tool for previewing and reviewing terms.

Understanding medical terms requires being able to put words together or build words from their parts. It is impossible to memorize thousands of medical terms; however, once you understand the basics, you can distinguish the meaning of medical terms by analyzing their prefixes, suffixes, and word roots. Remember that there will always be some exceptions to every rule, and medical terminology is no different. We attempt to point out these exceptions where they exist. Most medical terms, however, do follow the general rule that there is a **word root** (indicated by a red color) or fundamental meaning for the word, a **prefix** (indicated by a gold color) and a **suffix** (indicated by a blue color) that modify the meaning of the word root, and sometimes a **combining vowel** to connect other word parts. You will be amazed at the seemingly difficult words you will be able to build and understand when you follow the simple steps in word building (see Figure 1-1 ■).

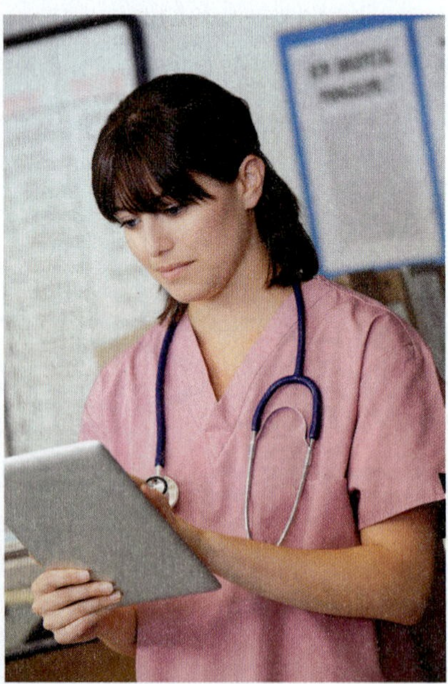

■ **Figure 1-1** Nurse completing a patient report. Healthcare workers use medical terminology in order to accurately and efficiently communicate patient information to each other.
(Monkey Business Images/Shutterstock)

Building Medical Terms From Word Parts

Four different word parts or elements can be used to construct medical terms:

1. The **word root** is the foundation of the word. — **cardi** ogram = *record of the heart*
2. A **prefix** is at the beginning of the word. — **peri** cardium = *around the heart*
3. A **suffix** is at the end of the word. — card **itis** = *inflammation of the heart*
4. The **combining vowel** is a vowel (usually *o*) that links the word root to another word root or a suffix. — cardi **o** my **o** pathy = *disease of the heart muscle*

Med Term Tip

Medical terms are built from word parts:

Word Part	Example (Meaning)
Word root	**cardi** *(heart)*
Prefix	**peri-** *(around)*
Suffix	**-itis** *(inflammation)*

When these components are put together, the word *pericarditis* is formed, meaning *inflammation around the heart.*

The following sections on word roots, combining vowels and forms, prefixes, and suffixes consider each of these word parts in more detail and present examples of some of those most commonly used.

PRACTICE AS YOU GO

A. Complete the Statement

1. The four components of a medical term are ____________________, ____________________, ____________________, and ____________________.
2. The combination of a word root and the combining vowel is called a(n) ____________________.
3. The vowel that connects two word roots or a suffix with a word root is usually a(n) ____________________.
4. A word part used at the end of a word root to change the meaning of the word is called a(n) ____________________.
5. A(n) ____________________ is used at the beginning of a word to indicate number, location, or time.

Word Roots

The word root is the foundation of a medical term and provides the general meaning of the word. The word root often indicates the body system or part of the body being discussed, such as **cardi** for *heart.* At other times, the word root may be an action. For example, the word root **cis** means *to cut* (as in incision).

A term may have more than one word root. For example, **osteoarthritis** (oss-tee-oh-ar-THRY-tis) combines the word root **oste** meaning *bone* and **arthr** meaning *joint.* When the suffix **-itis**, meaning *inflammation,* is added, we have the entire word, meaning an *inflammation involving bone at a joint.*

Combining Vowel/Form

A combining vowel makes it possible to pronounce long medical terms with ease and to combine several word parts. This is most often the vowel *o.* Combining vowels are utilized in two places: between a word root and a suffix or between two word roots.

To decide whether or not to use a combining vowel between a word root and a suffix, first look at the suffix. If it begins with a vowel, do not use the combining vowel. If, however, the suffix begins with a consonant, then use a combining vowel. For example: To combine **arthr** with **-scope** will require a combining vowel: **arthroscope** (AR-throh-skohp). But to combine **arthr** with **-itis** does not require a combining vowel: **arthritis** (ar-THRY-tis).

The combining vowel is typically kept between two word roots, even if the second word root begins with a vowel. For example, in forming the term **gastroenteritis** (gas-troh-en-ter-EYE-tis), the combining vowel is kept between the two word roots **gastr** and **enter** (gastrenteritis is incorrect). As you can tell from pronouncing these two terms, the combining vowel makes the pronunciation easier.

When writing a word root by itself, its **combining form** is typically used. This consists of the word root and its combining vowel written in a word root/vowel form, for example, **cardi/o.** Since it is often simpler to pronounce word roots when they appear in their combining form, this format is used throughout this book.

Med Term Tip

Remember to break down every word into its components (prefix, word root/combining form, and suffix) when learning medical terminology. Do not try to memorize every medical term. Instead, figure out how the word is formed from its components. In a short time you will be able to do this automatically when seeing a new term.

Common Combining Forms

What follows are some commonly used word roots in their combining form, their meaning, and examples of their use. Review the examples to observe when a combining vowel was kept and when it was dropped according to the rules presented above.

COMBINING FORM	MEANING	EXAMPLE (DEFINITION)
bi/o	life	biology (study of life)
carcin/o	cancer	carcinoma (cancerous tumor)
cardi/o	heart	cardiac (pertaining to the heart)
chem/o	chemical	chemotherapy (treatment with chemicals)
cis/o	to cut	incision (process of cutting into)
dermat/o	skin	dermatology (study of the skin)
enter/o	small intestine	enteric (pertaining to the small intestine)
gastr/o	stomach	gastric (pertaining to the stomach)
gynec/o	female	gynecology (study of females)
hemat/o	blood	hematic (pertaining to the blood)
immun/o	protection	immunology (study of protection)
laryng/o	larynx	laryngeal (pertaining to the voice box)
nephr/o	kidney	nephromegaly (enlarged kidney)
neur/o	nerve	neural (pertaining to a nerve)
ophthalm/o	eye	ophthalmic (pertaining to the eye)
ot/o	ear	otic (pertaining to the ear)
path/o	disease	pathology (study of disease)
pulmon/o	lung	pulmonary (pertaining to the lungs)
rhin/o	nose	rhinoplasty (surgical repair of the nose)

PRACTICE AS YOU GO

B. Name That Term

Use the suffix **-logy** to write a term for each medical specialty.

1. heart ______________________
2. stomach ______________________
3. skin ______________________
4. eye ______________________
5. immunity ______________________
6. kidney ______________________
7. blood ______________________
8. female ______________________
9. nerve ______________________
10. disease ______________________

Prefixes

Adding a prefix to the front of a term forms a new medical word. Prefixes frequently provide information about the location of an organ, the number of parts, or time (frequency). For example, the prefix **bi-** stands for two of something, such as **bilateral** (bye-LAT-er-al), meaning *to have two sides*. However, not every term will have a prefix.

Common Prefixes

What follows are some of the more common prefixes, their meanings, and examples of their use. When written by themselves, prefixes are followed by a hyphen.

PREFIX	MEANING	EXAMPLE (DEFINITION)
a-	without	aphasia (without speech)
an-	without	anoxia (without oxygen)
anti-	against	antibiotic (against life)
auto-	self	autograft (a graft from one's own body)
brady-	slow	bradycardia (slow heartbeat)
de-	without	depigmentation (without pigment)
dys-	painful; difficult; abnormal	dysuria (painful urination); dyspnea (difficulty breathing); dystrophy (abnormal development)

PREFIX	MEANING	EXAMPLE (DEFINITION)
endo-	within; inner	endoscope (instrument to view within); endocardium (inner lining of heart)
epi-	above	epigastric (above the stomach)
eu-	normal	eupnea (normal breathing)
ex-	outward	exostosis (condition of outward, or projecting, bone)
extra-	outside of	extracorporeal (outside of the body)
hetero-	different	heterograft (graft [like a skin graft] from another species)
homo-	same	homograft (graft [like a skin graft] from the same species)
hyper-	excessive	hypertrophy (excessive development)
hypo-	below; insufficient	hypodermic (below the skin); hypoglycemia (insufficient blood sugar)
in-	not; inward	infertility (not fertile); inhalation (to breathe in)
inter-	between	intervertebral (between the vertebrae)
intra-	within	intravenous (within a vein)
macro-	large	macrotia (having large ears)
micro-	small	microtia (having small ears)
neo-	new	neonatology (study of the newborn)
para-	beside; abnormal; two like parts of a pair	paranasal (beside the nose); paresthesia (abnormal sensation); paraplegia (paralysis of two like parts of a pair [the legs])
per-	through	percutaneous (through the skin)
peri-	around	pericardial (around the heart)
post-	after	postpartum (after birth)
pre-	before	preoperative (before a surgical operation)
pro-	before	prolactin (before milk)
pseudo-	false	pseudocyesis (false pregnancy)
re-	again	reinfection (to infect again)
retro-	backward; behind	retrograde (to move backward); retroperitoneal (behind the peritoneum)
sub-	under	subcutaneous (under the skin)
tachy-	fast	tachycardia (fast heartbeat)
trans-	across	transurethral (across the urethra)
ultra-	beyond	ultrasound (beyond sound [high-frequency sound waves])
un-	not	unconscious (not conscious)

Word Watch

Be extremely careful with prefixes; many have similar spellings but very different meanings. For example:

inter- means *between;* **intra-** means *inside*

per- means *through;* **peri-** means *around*

re- means *again;* **retro-** means *behind*

Number Prefixes

What follows are some common prefixes pertaining to the number of items or measurement, their meanings, and examples of their use.

PREFIX	MEANING	EXAMPLE (DEFINITION)
bi-	two	bilateral (two sides)
hemi-	half	hemiplegia (paralysis of one side/half of the body)
mono-	one	monoplegia (paralysis of one extremity)
multi-	many	multigravida (woman with many [two or more] pregnancies)
nulli-	none	nulligravida (woman with no pregnancies)
pan-	all	pansinusitis (inflammation of all the sinuses)
poly-	many	polymyositis (inflammation of many muscles)
quadri-	four	quadriplegia (paralysis of all four limbs)
semi-	partial	semiconscious (partially conscious)
tetra-	four	tetraplegia (paralysis of all four limbs)
tri-	three	triceps (muscle with three heads)

PRACTICE AS YOU GO

C. Prefix Practice

Circle the prefixes in the following terms and then define them in the spaces provided.

1. tachycardia ______________________________
2. pseudocyesis ______________________________
3. hypoglycemia ______________________________
4. intercostal ______________________________
5. eupnea ______________________________
6. postoperative ______________________________
7. monoplegia ______________________________
8. subcutaneous ______________________________

Suffixes

A suffix is attached to the end of a word to add meaning, such as a condition, disease, or procedure. For example, the suffix **-itis**, meaning *inflammation,* when added to **cardi** forms the new word **carditis** (kar-DYE-tis), meaning *inflammation of the heart.* Every medical term *must* have a suffix. Most often the

Med Term Tip

Remember, if a suffix begins with a vowel, the combining vowel is dropped; for example, *mastitis* rather than *mastoitis*.

suffix is added to a word root, as in carditis above; however, terms can also be built from a suffix added directly to a prefix, without a word root. For example, the term **dystrophy** (DIS-troh-fee), meaning *abnormal development*, is built from the prefix **dys-** (meaning *abnormal*) and the suffix **-trophy** (meaning *development*).

Common Suffixes

What follows are some common suffixes, their meanings, and examples of their use. When written by themselves, suffixes are preceded by a hyphen.

SUFFIX	MEANING	EXAMPLE (DEFINITION)
-algia	pain	gastralgia (stomach pain)
-cele	protrusion	cystocele (protrusion of the bladder)
-cyte	cell	erythrocyte (red cell)
-dynia	pain	cardiodynia (heart pain)
-ectasis	dilation	bronchiectasis (dilated bronchi)
-gen	that which produces	pathogen (that which produces disease)
-genic	producing	carcinogenic (cancer producing)
-ia	condition	bradycardia (condition of slow heart)
-iasis	abnormal condition	lithiasis (abnormal condition of stones)
-ism	state of	hypothyroidism (state of low thyroid)
-itis	inflammation	dermatitis (inflammation of skin)
-logist	one who studies	cardiologist (one who studies the heart)
-logy	study of	cardiology (study of the heart)
-lytic	destruction	thrombolytic (clot destruction)
-malacia	abnormal softening	chondromalacia (abnormal cartilage softening)
-megaly	enlarged	cardiomegaly (enlarged heart)
-oma	tumor, mass	carcinoma (cancerous tumor)
		hematoma (mass of blood)
-opsy	view of	biopsy (view of life)
-osis	abnormal condition	cyanosis (abnormal condition of being blue)
-pathy	disease	myopathy (muscle disease)
-plasm	formation	neoplasm (new formation)
-plegia	paralysis	laryngoplegia (paralysis of larynx)
-ptosis	drooping	blepharoptosis (drooping eyelid)
-rrhage	abnormal flow	hemorrhage (abnormal flow of blood)
-rrhagia	abnormal flow condition	cystorrhagia (abnormal flow from the bladder)
-rrhea	discharge	rhinorrhea (discharge from the nose)
-rrhexis	rupture	hysterorrhexis (ruptured uterus)

SUFFIX	MEANING	EXAMPLE (DEFINITION)
-sclerosis	hardening	arteriosclerosis (hardening of an artery)
-stenosis	narrowing	angiostenosis (narrowing of a vessel)
-therapy	treatment	chemotherapy (treatment with chemicals)
-trophy	development	hypertrophy (excessive development)

Adjective Suffixes

The following suffixes are used to convert a word root into an adjective. Each of these suffixes is usually translated as *pertaining to*.

SUFFIX	MEANING	EXAMPLE (DEFINITION)
-ac	pertaining to	cardiac (pertaining to the heart)
-al	pertaining to	duodenal (pertaining to the duodenum)
-an	pertaining to	ovarian (pertaining to the ovary)
-ar	pertaining to	ventricular (pertaining to a ventricle)
-ary	pertaining to	pulmonary (pertaining to the lungs)
-atic	pertaining to	lymphatic (pertaining to lymph)
-eal	pertaining to	esophageal (pertaining to the esophagus)
-iac	pertaining to	chondriac (pertaining to cartilage)
-ic	pertaining to	gastric (pertaining to the stomach)
-ical	pertaining to	chemical (pertaining to a chemical)
-ile	pertaining to	penile (pertaining to the penis)
-ine	pertaining to	uterine (pertaining to the uterus)
-ior	pertaining to	superior (pertaining to above)
-nic	pertaining to	embryonic (pertaining to an embryo)
-ory	pertaining to	auditory (pertaining to hearing)
-ose	pertaining to	adipose (pertaining to fat)
-ous	pertaining to	intravenous (pertaining to within a vein)
-tic	pertaining to	acoustic (pertaining to hearing)

Surgical Suffixes

The following suffixes indicate surgical procedures.

SUFFIX	MEANING	EXAMPLE (DEFINITION)
-centesis	puncture to withdraw fluid	arthrocentesis (puncture to withdraw fluid from a joint)
-ectomy	surgical removal	gastrectomy (surgical removal of the stomach)
-ostomy	surgically create an opening	colostomy (surgically create an opening for the colon [through the abdominal wall])
-otomy	cutting into	thoracotomy (cutting into the chest)

Med Term Tip

Surgical suffixes have very specific meanings:
-otomy means *to cut into*
-ostomy means *to surgically create an opening*
-ectomy means *to cut out* or *remove*

SUFFIX	MEANING	EXAMPLE (DEFINITION)
-pexy	surgical fixation	nephropexy (surgical fixation of a kidney)
-plasty	surgical repair	dermatoplasty (surgical repair of the skin)
-rrhaphy	to suture	myorrhaphy (suture together muscle)
-tome	instrument to cut	dermatome (instrument to cut skin)

Procedural Suffixes

The following suffixes indicate procedural processes or instruments.

SUFFIX	MEANING	EXAMPLE (DEFINITION)
-gram	record	electrocardiogram (record of heart's electricity)
-graphy	process of recording	electrocardiography (process of recording the heart's electrical activity)
-meter	instrument for measuring	audiometer (instrument for measuring hearing)
-metry	process of measuring	audiometry (process of measuring hearing)
-scope	instrument for viewing	gastroscope (instrument for viewing stomach)
-scopic	pertaining to visually examining	endoscopic (pertaining to visually examining within)
-scopy	process of visually examining	gastroscopy (process of visually examining the stomach)

PRACTICE AS YOU GO

D. Combining Form and Suffix Practice

Join a combining form and a suffix to build words with the following meanings.

1. study of lungs ____________________
2. nose discharge ____________________
3. abnormal softening of a kidney ____________________
4. enlarged heart ____________________
5. cutting into the stomach ____________________
6. inflammation of the skin ____________________
7. surgical removal of the voice box ____________________
8. surgical repair of a joint ____________________

Word Building

Word building consists of putting together two or more word elements to form a variety of terms. Prefixes and suffixes may be added to a combining form to create a new descriptive term. For example, adding the prefix **hypo-** (meaning *below*) and the suffix **-ic** (meaning *pertaining to*) to the combining form **derm/o** (meaning *skin*) forms **hypodermic** (high-poh-DER-mik), which means *pertaining to below the skin*.

Interpreting Medical Terms

The following strategy is a reliable method for puzzling out the meaning of an unfamiliar medical term.

STEP	EXAMPLE
1. Divide the term into its word parts.	gastr/o/enter/o/logy
2. Define each word part.	**gastr** = stomach
	o = combining vowel, no meaning
	enter = small intestine
	o = combining vowel, no meaning
	-logy = study of
3. Combine the meaning of the word parts.	stomach, small intestine, study of

Med Term Tip

To gain a quick understanding of a term, it may be helpful to you to read from the end of the word (or the suffix) back to the beginning (the prefix), and then pick up the word root. For example, *pericarditis* reads inflammation (**-itis**) around (**peri-**) the heart (**cardi/o**).

Pronunciation

You may hear different pronunciations for the same terms depending on where a person was born or educated. As long as it is clear which term people are discussing, differing pronunciations are acceptable. Some people are difficult to understand over the telephone or on a transcription tape. If you have any doubt about a term being discussed, ask for the term to be spelled. For example, it is often difficult to hear the difference between the terms **abduction** and **adduction**. However, since the terms refer to opposite directions of movement, it is very important to double-check if there is any question about which term is being used.

Each new term in this book is introduced in boldface type, with the phonetic or "sounds like" pronunciation in parentheses immediately following. The part of the word that should receive the greatest emphasis during pronunciation appears in capital letters, for example, **pericarditis** (pair-ih-kar-DYE-tis). Each term presented in this book is also pronounced on the accompanying MyLab Medical Terminology website (*www.mymedicalterminologylab.com*). Listen to each word, then pronounce it silently to yourself or out loud.

Spelling

Although you may hear differing pronunciations of the same term, there is only one correct spelling. If you have any doubt about the spelling of a term or of its meaning, always look it up in a medical dictionary. If only one letter of the word is changed, it can make a critical difference for the patient. For example, imagine the problem that could arise if you note for insurance purposes that a portion of a patient's **ileum**, or small intestine, was removed when in reality he had surgery for removal of a piece of his **ilium**, or hipbone.

Med Term Tip

If you have any doubt about the meaning or spelling of a word, look it up in a medical dictionary. Even experienced medical personnel still need to look up a few words. It is never acceptable to "make up" your own spelling for a term.

Some words have the same beginning sounds but are spelled differently. Examples include:

Sounds like *si*

psy	**psychiatry** (sigh-KIGH-ah-tree)
cy	**cytology** (sigh-TALL-oh-jee)

Sounds like *dis*

dys	**dyspepsia** (dis-PEP-see-ah)
dis	**dislocation** (dis-loh-KAY-shun)

Singular and Plural Endings

Many medical terms originate from Greek and Latin words. The rules for forming the singular and plural forms of some words follow the rules of these languages rather than English. For example, the heart has a left atrium and a right atrium for a total of two *atria*, not two *atriums*. Other words, such as *virus* and *viruses*, are changed from singular to plural by following English rules. Each medical term needs to be considered individually when changing from the singular to the plural form. The following examples illustrate how terms that follow Greek and Latin rules are pluralized. Throughout the book, unusual or unexpected plural forms will be included with the term definition.

WORDS ENDING IN	SINGULAR	PLURAL
-a	vertebra	vertebrae
-ax	thorax	thoraces
-ex or -ix	appendix	appendices
-is	metastasis	metastases
	epididymis	epididymides
-ma	sarcoma	sarcomata
-nx	phalanx	phalanges
-on	ganglion	ganglia
-um	ovum	ova
-us	nucleus	nuclei
-y	biopsy	biopsies

PRACTICE AS YOU GO

E. Make It Plural

Change the following singular terms to plural terms.

1. metastasis ____________
2. ovum ____________
3. nucleus ____________
4. phalanx ____________
5. appendix ____________
6. vertebra ____________

Abbreviations

Abbreviations are commonly used in the medical profession as a way of saving time. However, some abbreviations can be confusing, such as *SM* for simple mastectomy and *sm* for small. Using incorrect abbreviations can result in problems for a patient, as well as with insurance records and processing. If you have any concern that you will confuse someone by using an abbreviation, spell out the word instead. It is never acceptable to use made-up abbreviations. All types of healthcare facilities will have a list of approved abbreviations, and it is extremely important that you become familiar with this list and follow it closely. Throughout this book abbreviations are included, when possible, immediately following terms. Additionally, a list of common abbreviations for each body system is provided in each chapter. Finally, Appendix III offers a complete alphabetical listing of all the abbreviations used in this text.

The Medical Record

The **medical record** or chart documents the details of a patient's hospital stay. Each healthcare professional that has contact with the patient in any capacity completes the appropriate report of that contact and adds it to the medical chart. This results in a permanent physical record of the patient's day-to-day condition, when and what services he or she received, and the response to treatment. Each institution adopts a specific format for each document and its location within the chart. This is necessary because each healthcare professional must be able to locate quickly and efficiently the information he or she needs in order to provide proper care for the patient. The medical record is also a legal document. Therefore, it is essential that all chart components be completely filled out and signed. Each page must contain the proper patient identification information: the patient's name, age, gender, physician, admission date, and identification number.

While the patient is still in the hospital, a unit clerk is usually responsible for placing documents in the proper place. After discharge, the medical records department ensures that all documents are present, complete, signed, and in the correct order. If a person is readmitted, especially for the same diagnosis, parts of this previous chart can be pulled and added to the current chart for reference (see Figure 1-2 ■). Physicians' offices and other outpatient care providers such as clinics and therapists also maintain a medical record detailing each patient's visit to their facility.

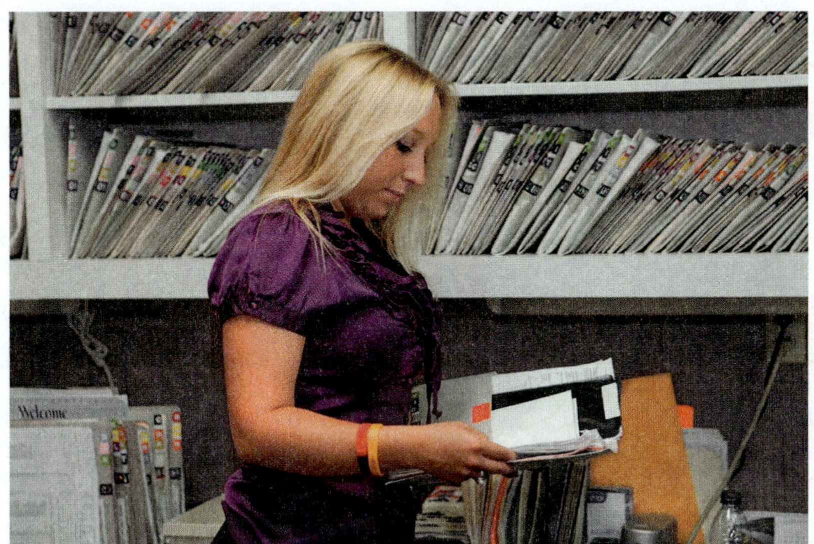

■ **Figure 1-2** Health information professionals maintain accurate, orderly, and permanent patient records. Medical records are stored securely and available for future reference. *(B. Franklin/ Shutterstock)*

The digital revolution has also impacted healthcare with the increasing use of the **Electronic Medical Record** (EMR). A software program allows for entering of patient information via a computer or tablet, which then organizes and stores the data. Information is entered either at a centralized workstation or by using mobile devices at the point of care. Once digitally stored, the information may be analyzed and monitored to detect and prevent potential errors. Since the records are digitally stored, they can be accessed and shared between healthcare providers easily, which reduces unnecessary repetition of tests and inadvertent medication errors. Table 1-1 ■ includes the most common elements of a paper chart with a brief description.

■ **TABLE 1-1 Elements of the Medical Record**

Component	Description
History and Physical	Written or dictated by admitting physician; details patient's history, results of physician's examination, initial diagnoses, and physician's plan of treatment
Physician's Orders	Complete list of care, medications, tests, and treatments physician orders for patient
Nurse's Notes	Record of patient's care throughout the day; includes vital signs, treatment specifics, patient's response to treatment, and patient's condition
Physician's Progress Notes	Physician's daily record of patient's condition, results of physician's examinations, summary of test results, updated assessment and diagnoses, and further plans for patient's care
Consultation Reports	Reports given by specialists whom physician has asked to evaluate patient
Ancillary Reports	Reports from various treatments and therapies patient has received, such as rehabilitation, social services, or respiratory therapy
Diagnostic Reports	Results of diagnostic tests performed on patient, principally from clinical lab (e.g., blood tests) and medical imaging (e.g., X-rays and ultrasound)
Informed Consent	Document voluntarily signed by patient or a responsible party that clearly describes purpose, methods, procedures, benefits, and risks of a diagnostic or treatment procedure
Operative Report	Report from surgeon detailing an operation; includes pre- and postoperative diagnosis, specific details of surgical procedure itself, and how patient tolerated procedure
Anesthesiologist's Report	Relates details regarding substances (such as medications and fluids) given to patient, patient's response to anesthesia, and vital signs during surgery
Pathologist's Report	Report given by pathologist who studies tissue removed from patient (e.g., bone marrow, blood, or tissue biopsy)
Discharge Summary	Comprehensive outline of patient's entire hospital stay; includes condition at time of admission, admitting diagnosis, test results, treatments and patient's response, final diagnosis, and follow-up plans

PRACTICE AS YOU GO

F. Medical Records Matching

Match each definition to its medical record element.

_____ **1.** physician's orders	**a.** written after patient care is completed
_____ **2.** discharge summary	**b.** includes vital signs
_____ **3.** ancillary reports	**c.** lists medications to be given to patient
_____ **4.** consultation reports	**d.** written by specialists
_____ **5.** nurse's notes	**e.** location of rehabilitation reports

Healthcare Settings

The use of medical terminology is widespread. It provides healthcare professionals with a precise and efficient method of communicating very specific patient information to one another, regardless of whether they are in the same type of facility (see Figure 1-3 ■). See Table 1-2 ■ for descriptions of the different types of settings where medical terminology is used.

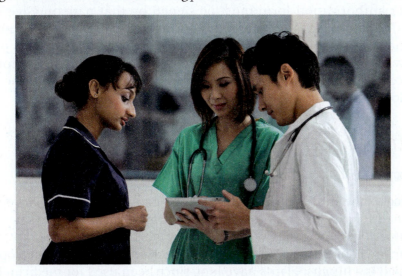

■ **Figure 1-3** Medical team reviewing patient's medical record on a tablet. *(Stuart Jenner/ Shutterstock)*

■ **TABLE 1-2** Healthcare Settings

Healthcare Setting	Description
Acute Care or General Hospitals	Provide services to diagnose (laboratory, diagnostic imaging) and treat (surgery, medications, therapy) diseases for a short period of time; in addition, they usually provide emergency and obstetrical care
Specialty Care Hospitals	Provide care for very specific types of diseases (e.g., psychiatric hospital)
Nursing Homes or Long-Term Care Facilities	Provide long-term care for patients needing extra time to recover from illness or injury before returning home or for persons who can no longer care for themselves
Ambulatory Care Centers, Surgical Centers, or Outpatient Clinics	Provide services not requiring overnight hospitalization; services range from simple surgeries to diagnostic testing or therapy
Physicians' Offices	Provide diagnostic and treatment services in a private office setting
Health Maintenance Organization (HMO)	Provides wide range of services by a group of primary-care physicians, specialists, and other healthcare professionals in a prepaid system
Home Health Care	Provides nursing, therapy, personal care, or housekeeping services in patient's own home
Rehabilitation Centers	Provide intensive physical and occupational therapy; includes inpatient and outpatient treatment
Hospices	Provide supportive treatment to terminally ill patients and their families

PRACTICE AS YOU GO

G. Healthcare Settings

Match each setting listed on the left with a setting listed on the right that provides similar services.

_____ **1.** long-term care facility — **a.** ambulatory care center

_____ **2.** outpatient clinic — **b.** general hospital

_____ **3.** acute care hospital — **c.** nursing home

Confidentiality

Anyone working with medical terminology and involved in the medical profession must have a firm understanding of confidentiality. Any information or record relating to a patient must be considered privileged. This means that there is a moral and legal responsibility to keep all information about the patient confidential. If there is a request to supply documentation relating to a patient, the proper authorization form must be signed by that patient. Give only the specific information that the patient has authorized. The Health Insurance Portability and Accountability Act of 1996 (HIPAA) set federal standards providing patients with more protection of their medical records and health information, better access to their own records, and greater control over how their health information is used and to whom it is disclosed.

Pharmacology

pharmacology (far-mah-KALL-oh-jee)

Pharmacology is the study of the origin, characteristics, and effects of drugs. Drugs are obtained from many different sources. Some drugs, such as vitamins, are found naturally in the foods we eat. Others, such as hormones, are obtained from animals. Penicillin and some of the other antibiotics are developed from mold, which is a fungus. Plants have long since been used for medicinal healing purposes and continue to be a source of many of today's modern medicines. Many drugs, such as those used in chemotherapy, are synthetic, meaning they are developed by artificial means in a laboratory.

Med Term Tip

The terms *drug* and *medication* have the same meaning. However, the general public often uses the term *drug* to refer to a narcotic type of medication. The term can also mean illegal chemical substances. For purposes of medical terminology, use of the word *drug* means *medication.*

Drug Names

brand name
chemical name
generic name
nonproprietary name (non-proh-PRYE-ah-tair-ee)
pharmaceutical (far-mah-SOO-tih-kal)
pharmacist (FAR-mah-sist)
proprietary name (proh-PRYE-ah-tair-ee)
trademark

All drugs are chemicals. The **chemical name** describes the chemical formula or molecular structure of a particular drug. For example, the chemical name for ibuprofen, an over-the-counter pain medication, is 2-*p*-isobutylphenyl propionic acid. Just as in this case, chemical names are usually very long, so a shorter name is given to the drug. This name is the **generic** or **nonproprietary name**, and it is recognized and accepted as the official name for a drug.

Each drug has only one generic name, such as ibuprofen, and this name is not subject to copyright protection, so any **pharmaceutical** manufacturer may use it. However, the pharmaceutical company that originally developed the drug has exclusive rights to produce it for 20 years. After that time, any manufacturer may produce and sell the drug. When a company manufactures a drug for sale, it must choose a **brand name**, or **proprietary name**, for its product. This is the company's **trademark** for the drug. For example, ibuprofen is known by several brand names, including Motrin™, Advil™, and Nuprin™. All three contain the same ibuprofen; they are just marketed by different pharmaceutical companies. (See Table 1-3 ■ for examples of different drug names.)

What's In A Name?

Look for these word parts:
chem/o = drug
pharmac/o = drug
-ary = pertaining to
-ical = pertaining to
-ist = specialist
-logy = study of
non- = not

Generic drugs are usually priced lower than brand name drugs. A physician can indicate on a prescription if the **pharmacist** may substitute a generic drug for

TABLE 1-3 Examples of Different Drug Names

Chemical Name	Generic Name	Brand Names
2-*p*-isobutylphenyl propionic acid	Ibuprofen	Motrin™
		Advil™
		Nuprin™
Acetylsalicylic acid	Aspirin	Anacin™
		Bufferin™
		Excedrin™
S-2-[1-(methylamino) ethyl] benzenemethanol hydrochloride	Pseudoephedrine hydrochloride	Sudafed™
		Actifed™
		Nucofed™

a brand name. The physician may prefer that a particular brand name drug be used if he or she believes it to be more effective than the generic drug.

Legal Classification of Drugs

controlled substances
Drug Enforcement Administration
over-the-counter drug
prescription (prih-SKRIP-shun)
prescription drug (prih-SKRIP-shun)

A **prescription drug** can only be ordered by licensed healthcare practitioners such as physicians, dentists, or physician assistants. These drugs must include the words "Caution: Federal law prohibits dispensing without prescription" on their labels. Antibiotics, such as penicillin, and heart medications, such as digoxin, are available only by prescription. A **prescription** is the written explanation to the pharmacist regarding the name of the medication, the dosage, and the times of administration. A licensed practitioner can also submit a prescription order electronically (if it is not a controlled substance) or orally to a pharmacist.

A drug that does not require a prescription is referred to as an **over-the-counter** (OTC) **drug**. Many medications or drugs can be purchased without a prescription, for example, aspirin, antacids, and antidiarrheal medications. However, taking aspirin along with an anticoagulant, such as coumadin, can cause internal bleeding in some people, and OTC antacids interfere with the absorption of the prescription drug tetracycline into the body. It is better for the physician or pharmacist to advise the patient on the proper OTC drugs to use with prescription drugs.

Med Term Tip

It is critical that patients receive the correct drug, but it is not possible to list or remember all the drug names. You must acquire the habit of looking up any drug name you do not recognize in the *Physician's Desk Reference (PDR)*. Every medical office or medical facility should have either an electronic or hard copy of this book.

Certain drugs are classified as **controlled substances** if they have a potential for being addictive (habit forming) or can be abused. The **Drug Enforcement Administration** (DEA) enforces the control of these drugs. Some of the more commonly prescribed controlled substances are:

- butabarbital
- chloral hydrate
- codeine
- diazepam
- oxycontin
- morphine
- phenobarbital
- secobarbital

Controlled drugs are classified as Schedule I through Schedule V, indicating their potential for abuse with I being most addictive and V being the least addictive drugs. The differences between each schedule are listed in Table 1-4 ■.

■ **TABLE 1-4** Schedule for Controlled Substances

Classification	Meaning
Schedule I	Drugs with the highest potential for addiction and abuse; they are not accepted for medical use; examples are heroin and LSD
Schedule II	Drugs with a high potential for addiction and abuse accepted for medical use in the United States; examples are codeine, cocaine, morphine, opium, and secobarbital
Schedule III	Drugs with a moderate to low potential for addiction and abuse; examples are butabarbital, anabolic steroids, and acetaminophen with codeine
Schedule IV	Drugs with a lower potential for addiction and abuse than Schedule III drugs; examples are chloral hydrate, phenobarbital, and diazepam
Schedule V	Drugs with a low potential for addiction and abuse; an example is low-strength codeine combined with other drugs to suppress coughing

PRACTICE AS YOU GO

H. True or False

_____ **1.** The nonproprietary name is also called the generic name.

_____ **2.** A drug's chemical name is the company's trademark for its product.

_____ **3.** Controlled substances have a potential for being addictive.

_____ **4.** A drug may have many generic names, but only one brand name.

_____ **5.** OTC drugs do not require a prescription.

How to Read a Prescription

Med Term Tip

Many abbreviations have multiple meanings, such as od, which can mean overdose (od) or right eye (OD), depending on whether the letters are lowercase or uppercase. Care must be taken when reading abbreviations since some may be written too quickly, making them difficult to decipher. Never create your own abbreviations. When in doubt, confirm with the prescriber.

A prescription is not difficult to read once you understand the symbols that are used. Symbols and abbreviations based on Latin and Greek words are used to save time for the physician. For example, the abbreviation po, meaning *to be taken by mouth,* comes from the Latin term *per os,* which means *by mouth.*

See Figure 1-4 ■ for an example of a prescription. In this sample, the prescribed drug (Rx) is Tagamet (a medication to reduce stomach acid) in the 800 milligram (mg) size. The instructions on the label are to say (Sig) to take 1 (ṫ) by mouth (po) three times a day (tid). The pharmacist is to dispense (disp) 30 tablets (#30). The prescription concludes by informing the pharmacist to refill the prescription two times, and he or she may substitute with another medication. Each prescription must contain the date, physician's name, address, and Drug Enforcement Administration number as well as the patient's name and date of birth. The physician must also sign his or her name at the bottom of the prescription. A blank prescription cannot be handed to a patient.

The physician's instruction to the patient will be placed on the label. The pharmacist will also include instructions about the medication and alert the patient to side effects that may need to be reported to the physician. Additionally, any special instructions regarding the medication (i.e., take with meals, do not take along with dairy products, etc.) are supplied by the pharmacist.

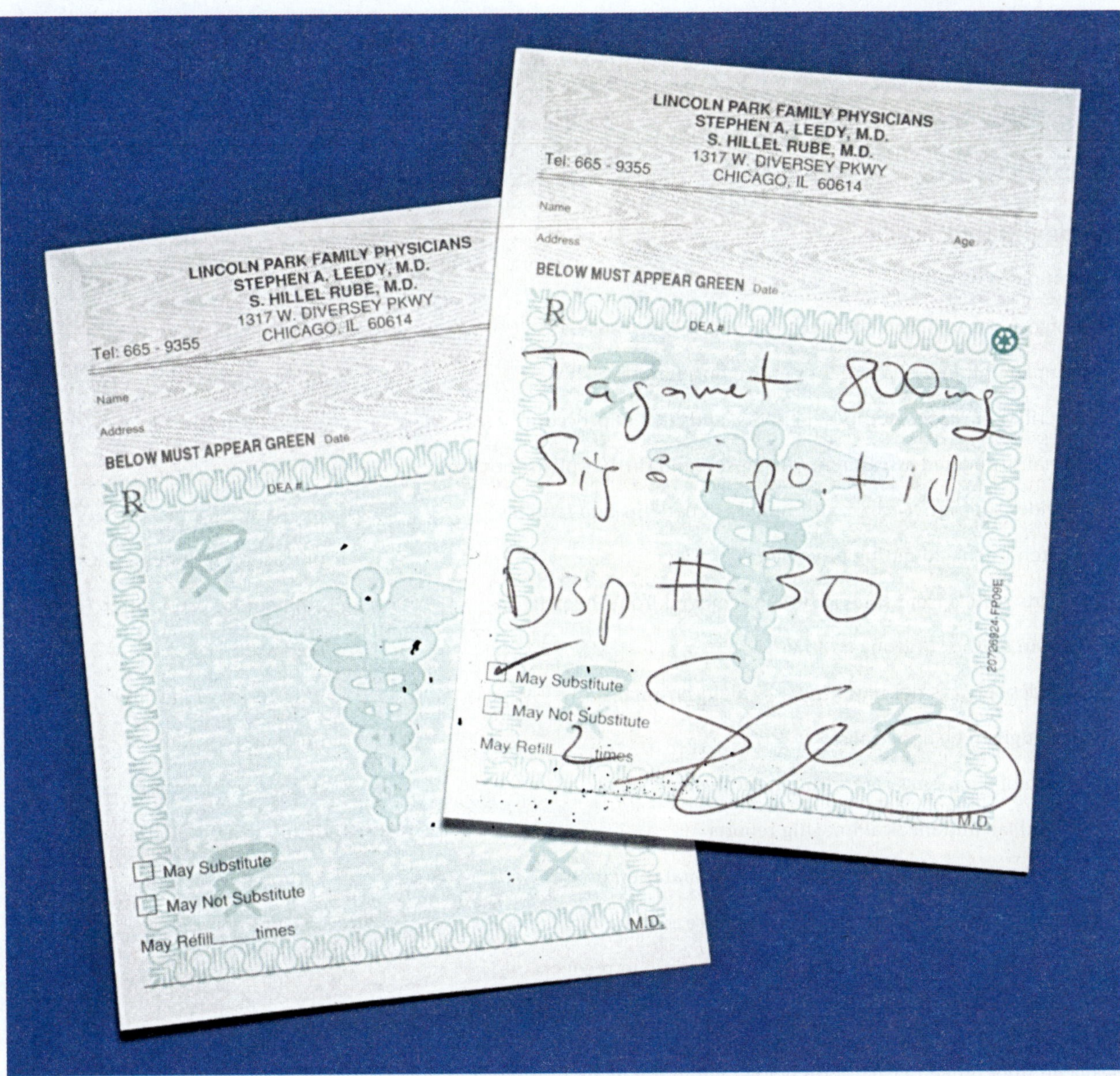

Figure 1-4 A sample prescription written by a physician. *(Michal Heron/Pearson Education, Inc.)*

PRACTICE AS YOU GO

I. Prescription Abbreviation Matching

_____ **1.** milligram — **a.** disp

_____ **2.** by mouth — **b.** i̇̄

_____ **3.** three times a day — **c.** Sig

_____ **4.** dispense — **d.** po

_____ **5.** label instructions — **e.** mg

_____ **6.** one — **f.** tid

Chapter Review

Practice Exercises

A. Terminology Matching

Match each definition to its term.

1. ________ Provides services for a short period of time
2. ________ Complete outline of a patient's entire hospital stay
3. ________ Describes purpose, methods, benefits, and risks of procedure
4. ________ Contains updated assessment, diagnoses, and further plans for care
5. ________ Provides supportive care to terminally ill patients and families
6. ________ Written by the admitting physician
7. ________ Reports results from study of tissue removed from the patient
8. ________ Written by the surgeon
9. ________ Provides services not requiring overnight hospital stay
10. ________ Report given by a specialist
11. ________ Record of a patient's care throughout the day
12. ________ Clinical lab and medical imaging reports
13. ________ Provides intensive physical and occupational therapy
14. ________ Report of treatment/therapy the patient received
15. ________ Provides care for patients who need more time to recover

a. rehabilitation center
b. nurse's notes
c. ancillary report
d. hospice
e. discharge summary
f. physician's progress notes
g. ambulatory care center
h. diagnostic report
i. long-term care facility
j. informed consent
k. history and physical
l. acute care hospital
m. pathologist's report
n. consultation report
o. operative report

B. Prefix Practice

The prefix has been underlined in each term below. Fill in the blank in the term's definition with the meaning of that prefix.

Term	Definition
1. aphasia	____________ speech
2. bradycardia	____________ heartbeat
3. anoxia	____________ oxygen
4. eupnea	____________ breathing
5. hypertrophy	____________ development
6. intervertebral	pertaining to ____________ the vertebrae
7. preoperative	____________ an operation
8. subcutaneous	pertaining to ____________ the skin

Term	Definition
9. unconscious	________ conscious
10. polymyositis	inflammation of ________ muscles
11. intravenous	pertaining to ________ a vein
12. extracorporeal	pertaining to ________ of the body
13. bilateral	pertaining to ________ sides
14. pansinusitis	inflammation of ________ the sinuses
15. epigastric	pertaining to ________ the stomach
16. antibiotic	pertaining to ________ life
17. tachycardia	________ heartbeat
18. hypoglycemia	________ blood sugar
19. percutaneous	pertaining to ________ the skin
20. pericardial	pertaining to ________ the heart

C. Suffix Practice

The suffix has been underlined in each term below. Fill in the blank in the term's definition with the meaning of that suffix.

Term	Definition
1. cardiology	________ the heart
2. laryngoplegia	________ of the larynx
3. rhinorrhea	________ from the nose
4. angiostenosis	________ of a vessel
5. chemotherapy	________ with chemicals
6. duodenal	________ the duodenum
7. pathogen	________ disease
8. thrombolytic	clot ________
9. biopsy	________ life
10. gastrectomy	________ of the stomach
11. arteriosclerosis	________ of an artery
12. uterine	________ the uterus
13. gastralgia	stomach ________
14. nephropexy	________ of a kidney
15. audiometry	________ hearing
16. acoustic	________ hearing
17. dermatoplasty	________ of the skin
18. thoracotomy	________ the chest
19. gastroscope	________ the stomach
20. cardiac	________ the heart

D. Building Medical Terms

Build a medical term by combining the word parts requested in each question.

For example, use the combining form for *spleen* with the suffix meaning *enlargement* to form a word meaning *enlargement of the spleen* (answer: *splenomegaly*).

1. combining form for *heart* ______
   suffix meaning *abnormal softening* ______
   ______ term meaning *abnormal softening of the heart*

2. word root form for *stomach* ______
   suffix meaning *to surgically create an opening* ______
   ______ term meaning *surgically creating an opening into the stomach*

3. combining form for *nose* ______
   suffix meaning *surgical repair* ______
   ______ term meaning *surgical repair of the nose*

4. prefix meaning *excessive* ______
   suffix meaning *development* ______
   ______ term meaning *excessive development*

5. combining form meaning *disease* ______
   suffix meaning *the study of* ______
   ______ term meaning *the study of disease*

6. word root meaning *nerve* ______
   suffix for *tumor/mass* ______
   ______ term meaning *nerve tumor*

7. combining form meaning *stomach* ______
   combining form meaning *small intestine* ______
   suffix meaning *study of* ______
   ______ term meaning *study of stomach and small intestine*

8. word root meaning *ear* ______
   suffix meaning *inflammation* ______
   ______ term meaning *ear inflammation*

9. prefix meaning *chemical* ______
   suffix meaning *treatment* ______
   ______ term meaning *chemical treatment*

10. combining form meaning *cancer* ______
    suffix meaning *that which produces* ______
    ______ term meaning *that which produces cancer*

E. Define the Combining Form

1. **bi/o** ______
2. **carcin/o** ______

3. **cardi/o** ______________________________

4. **chem/o** ______________________________

5. **cis/o** ______________________________

6. **dermat/o** ______________________________

7. **enter/o** ______________________________

8. **gastr/o** ______________________________

9. **gynec/o** ______________________________

10. **hemat/o** ______________________________

11. **immun/o** ______________________________

12. **laryng/o** ______________________________

13. **nephr/o** ______________________________

14. **neur/o** ______________________________

15. **ophthalm/o** ______________________________

16. **ot/o** ______________________________

17. **path/o** ______________________________

18. **pulmon/o** ______________________________

19. **rhin/o** ______________________________

F. Making Plurals

For each singular term below, write the plural form.

1. diagnosis ______________________________

2. diverticulum ______________________________

3. bursa ______________________________

4. bronchus ______________________________

5. artery ______________________________

G. Complete the Statement

1. The reference book containing important information regarding medications is the ______________________________.

2. A person specializing in the dispensing of medications is a ______________________________.

3. The accepted official name for a drug is the ______________________________ name.

4. The trade name for a drug is the ______________________________ name.

5. The chemical name represents ______________________________.

6. The federal agency that enforces controls over the use of drugs causing dependency is the ______________________________.

H. Prescription Practice

Write out the following prescription instructions in the space provided. Some of the abbreviations were introduced in this chapter. Refer to Appendix III for unfamiliar abbreviations.

1. Pravachol, 20 mg, Sig. ī q noc, #30, refill 3x, no sub.

   ____

2. Lanoxin, 0.125 mg, Sig. īīī stat, then īī q am, #100, refills prn.

   ____

3. Synthroid, 0.075 mg, Sig. ī daily, #100, refill x4.

   ____

4. Norvasc, 5 mg, Sig. ī q am, #60, 0 refills.

   ____

MyLab Medical Terminology™

MyLab Medical Terminology is a premium online homework management system that includes a host of features to help you study. Registered users will find:

- A multitude of activities and assignments built within the MyLab platform
- Powerful tools that track and analyze your results—allowing you to create a personalized learning experience
- Videos and audio pronunciations to help enrich your progress
- Streaming lesson presentations (Guided Lectures) and self-paced learning modules
- A space where you and your instructors can check your progress and manage your assignments

Chapter 2

Body Organization

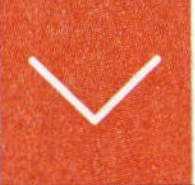

Learning Objectives

Upon completion of this chapter, you will be able to

1. Recognize the combining forms introduced in this chapter.
2. Correctly spell and pronounce medical terms and anatomical structures relating to body structure.
3. Discuss the organization of the body in terms of cells, tissues, organs, and systems.
4. Describe the common features of cells.
5. Define the four types of tissues.
6. List the major organs found in the 12 organ systems and their related medical specialties.
7. Describe the anatomical position.
8. Define the body planes.
9. Identify regions of the body.
10. List the body cavities and their contents.
11. Locate and describe the nine anatomical and four clinical divisions of the abdomen.
12. Define directional terms.
13. Build body organization medical terms from word parts.
14. Describe routes used to introduce drugs into the body.
15. Interpret abbreviations associated with body organization.

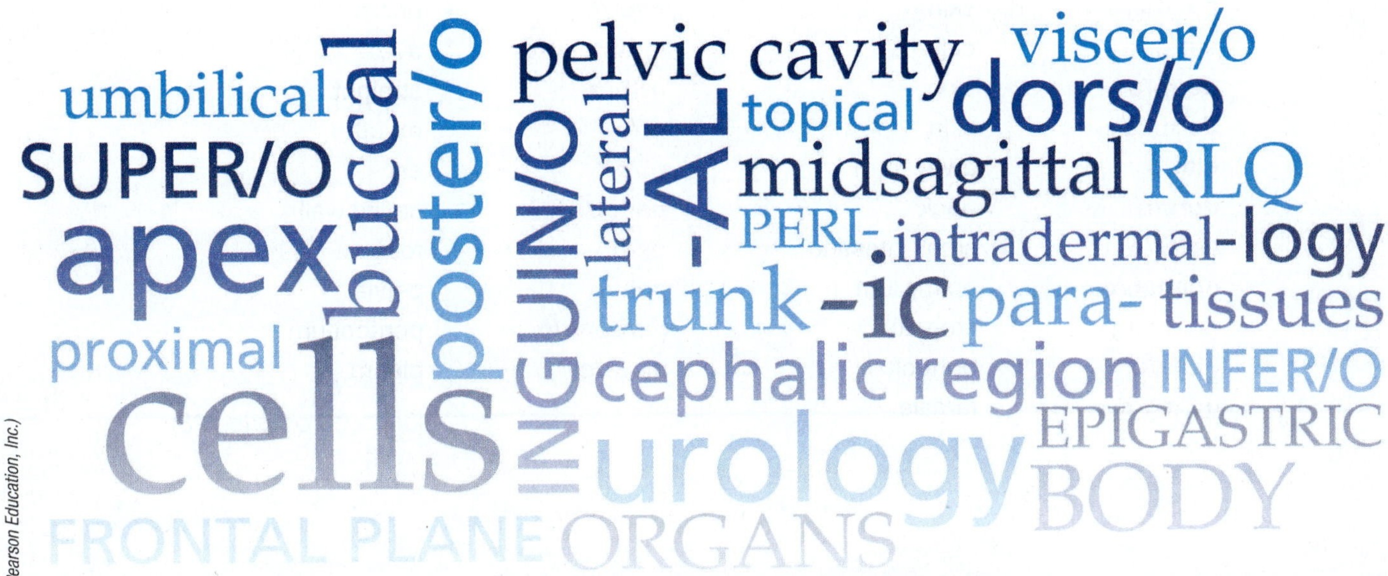

(Pearson Education, Inc.)

BODY ORGANIZATION

AT A GLANCE

Arrangement

The body is organized into levels; each is built from the one below it. In other words, the body as a whole is composed of systems, a system is composed of organs, an organ is composed of tissues, and tissues are composed of cells.

Levels

The major body structural levels from smallest to largest are:

cells **tissues** **organs** **systems** **body**

Word Parts

Presented here are some of the more common combining forms used to build body organizational terms.

Combining Forms

abdomin/o	abdomen	**hal/o**	to breathe
adip/o	fat	**hemat/o**	blood
aer/o	air	**hist/o**	tissue
anter/o	front	**immun/o**	protection
brachi/o	arm	**infer/o**	below
bucc/o	cheek	**inguin/o**	groin
cardi/o	heart	**laryng/o**	larynx
caud/o	tail	**later/o**	side
cephal/o	head	**lingu/o**	tongue
cervic/o	neck	**lumb/o**	loin (low back)
chondr/o	cartilage	**lymph/o**	lymph
crani/o	skull	**medi/o**	middle
crin/o	to secrete	**muscul/o**	muscle
crur/o	leg	**nephr/o**	kidney
cutane/o	skin	**neur/o**	nerve
cyt/o	cell	**ophthalm/o**	eye
derm/o	skin	**orth/o**	straight
dermat/o	skin	**or/o**	mouth
dist/o	away from	**ot/o**	ear
dors/o	back	**pariet/o**	cavity wall
enter/o	small intestine	**ped/o**	foot
epitheli/o	epithelium	**pelv/o**	pelvis
gastr/o	stomach	**peritone/o**	peritoneum
glute/o	buttock	**pleur/o**	pleura
gynec/o	female		

(*continued on page 28*)

Body Organization Illustrated

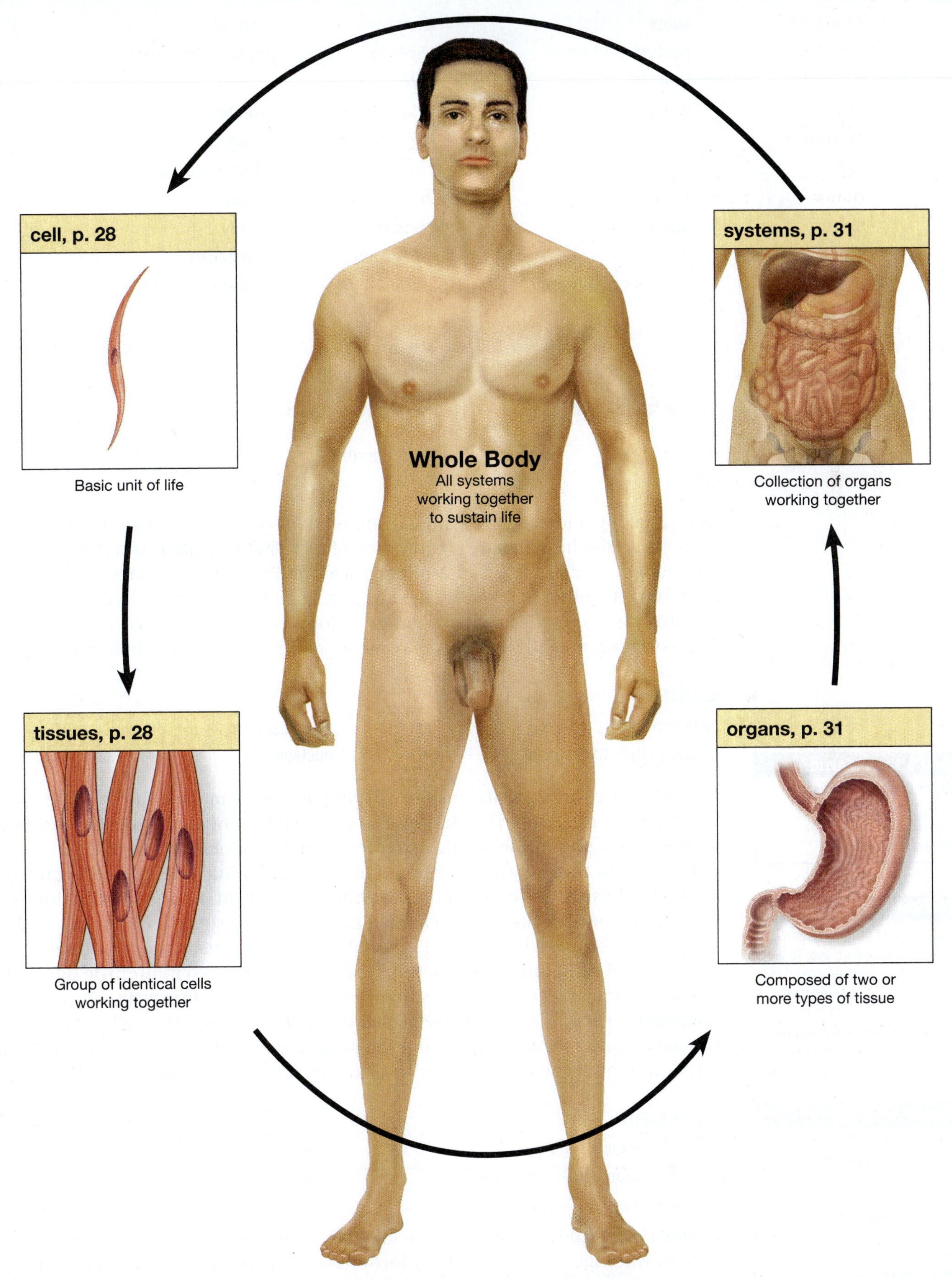
cell, p. 28
Basic unit of life
tissues, p. 28
Group of identical cells working together
organs, p. 31
Composed of two or more types of tissue
systems, p. 31
Collection of organs working together
Whole Body
All systems working together to sustain life

(continued from page 26)

poster/o	back	**thorac/o**	chest
proct/o	rectum and anus	**topic/o**	a specific area
proxim/o	near to	**ur/o**	urine
pub/o	genital region	**urin/o**	urine
pulmon/o	lung	**vagin/o**	vagina
rect/o	rectum	**vascul/o**	blood vessel
rhin/o	nose	**ven/o**	vein
spin/o	spine	**ventr/o**	belly
super/o	above	**vertebr/o**	vertebra
thec/o	sheath (meninges)	**viscer/o**	internal organ

Levels of Body Organization

body
cells
organs
systems
tissues

Before taking a look at the whole human body, we need to examine its component parts. The human **body** is composed of **cells, tissues, organs**, and **systems**. These components are arranged in a hierarchical manner. That is, parts from a lower level come together to form the next higher level. In that way, cells come together to form tissues, tissues come together to form organs, organs come together to form systems, and all the systems come together to form the whole body.

Cells

cell membrane
cytology (sigh-TALL-oh-jee)
cytoplasm (SIGH-toh-plazm)
nucleus

What's In A Name?
Look for these word parts:
cyt/o = cell
-logy = study of
-plasm = formation

The cell is the fundamental unit of all living things. That is to say, it is the smallest structure of a body that has all the properties of being alive: responding to stimuli, engaging in metabolic activities, and reproducing itself. All the tissues and organs in the body are composed of cells. Individual cells perform functions for the body such as reproduction, hormone secretion, energy production, and excretion. Special cells are also able to carry out very specific functions, such as contraction by muscle cells and electrical impulse transmission by nerve cells. The study of cells and their functions is called **cytology**. No matter the difference in their shape and function, at some point during their life cycle, all cells have **cytoplasm**, a **nucleus**, and a **cell membrane** (see Figure 2-1 ■). The cell membrane is the outermost boundary of a cell. It encloses the cytoplasm, the watery internal environment of the cell, and the nucleus, which contains the cell's DNA.

Med Term Tip
Cells were first seen by Robert Hooke over 300 years ago. To him, the rectangular shapes looked like prison cells, so he named them cells. It was a common practice for early anatomists to name an organ solely on its appearance.

Tissues

connective tissue
epithelial tissue (ep-ih-THEE-lee-al)
histology (hiss-TALL-oh-jee)
muscular tissue
nervous tissue

What's In A Name?
Look for these word parts:
epitheli/o = epithelium
hist/o = tissue
muscul/o = muscle
-al = pertaining to
-ar = pertaining to
-logy = study of
-ous = pertaining to

Histology is the study of tissue. When like cells group together and function together to perform a specific activity, they form tissue. The body has four types of tissue: **muscular tissue, epithelial tissue, connective tissue**, and **nervous tissue** (see Figure 2-2 ■).

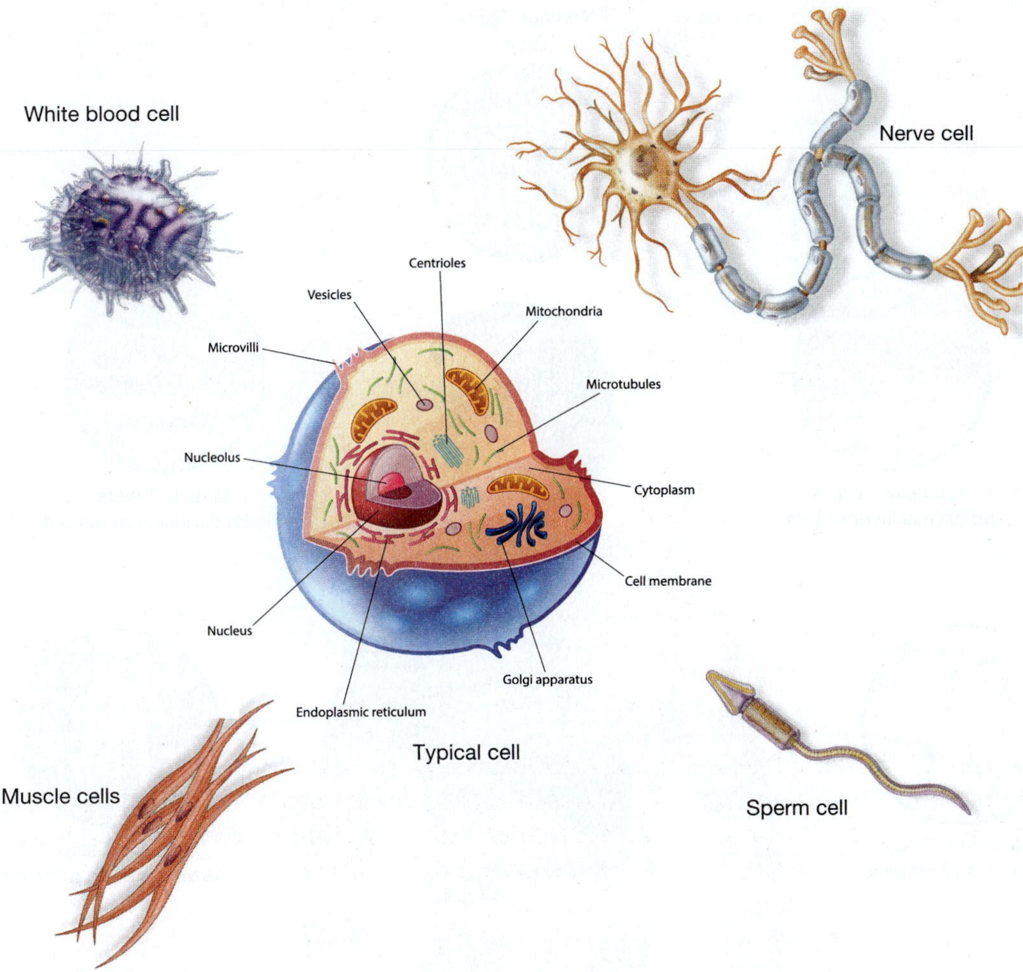

Figure 2-1 Typical cell (in center) illustrates three main cellular structures: cell membrane, nucleus, and cytoplasm. Examples of four cells with very different shapes are located around the typical cell. Although each cell has a cell membrane, nucleus, and cytoplasm, each has a unique shape depending on its location and function.
(La Gorda/Shutterstock)

Muscular Tissue

cardiac muscle
smooth muscle
muscle fibers
skeletal muscle

Muscular tissue produces movement in the body through contraction, or shortening in length, and is composed of individual muscle cells called **muscle fibers**. Muscle tissue forms one of three basic types of muscles: **skeletal muscle**, **smooth muscle**, or **cardiac muscle**. Skeletal muscle attaches to bone. Internal organs, such as the intestine, uterus, and blood vessels, contain smooth muscle. Only the heart contains cardiac muscle.

What's In A Name?
Look for these word parts:
cardi/o = heart
-ac = pertaining to
-al = pertaining to

Epithelial Tissue

epithelium (ep-ih-THEE-lee-um)

Epithelial tissue, or **epithelium**, is found throughout the body and is composed of close-packed cells that form the covering for and lining of body structures. For example, both the top layer of skin and the lining of the stomach are epithelial tissue (see Figure 2-2). In addition to forming a protective barrier, specialized epithelial tissues absorb substances (such as nutrients from the intestine), secrete substances (such as sweat glands), or excrete wastes (such as the kidney tubules).

Med Term Tip
The term *epithelium* comes from the prefix **epi-** meaning *on top of* and the combining form **theli/o** meaning *nipple* (referring to any projection from the surface).

■ Figure 2-2 The appearance of different types of tissues—muscle, epithelial, nervous, connective—and their location within the body.

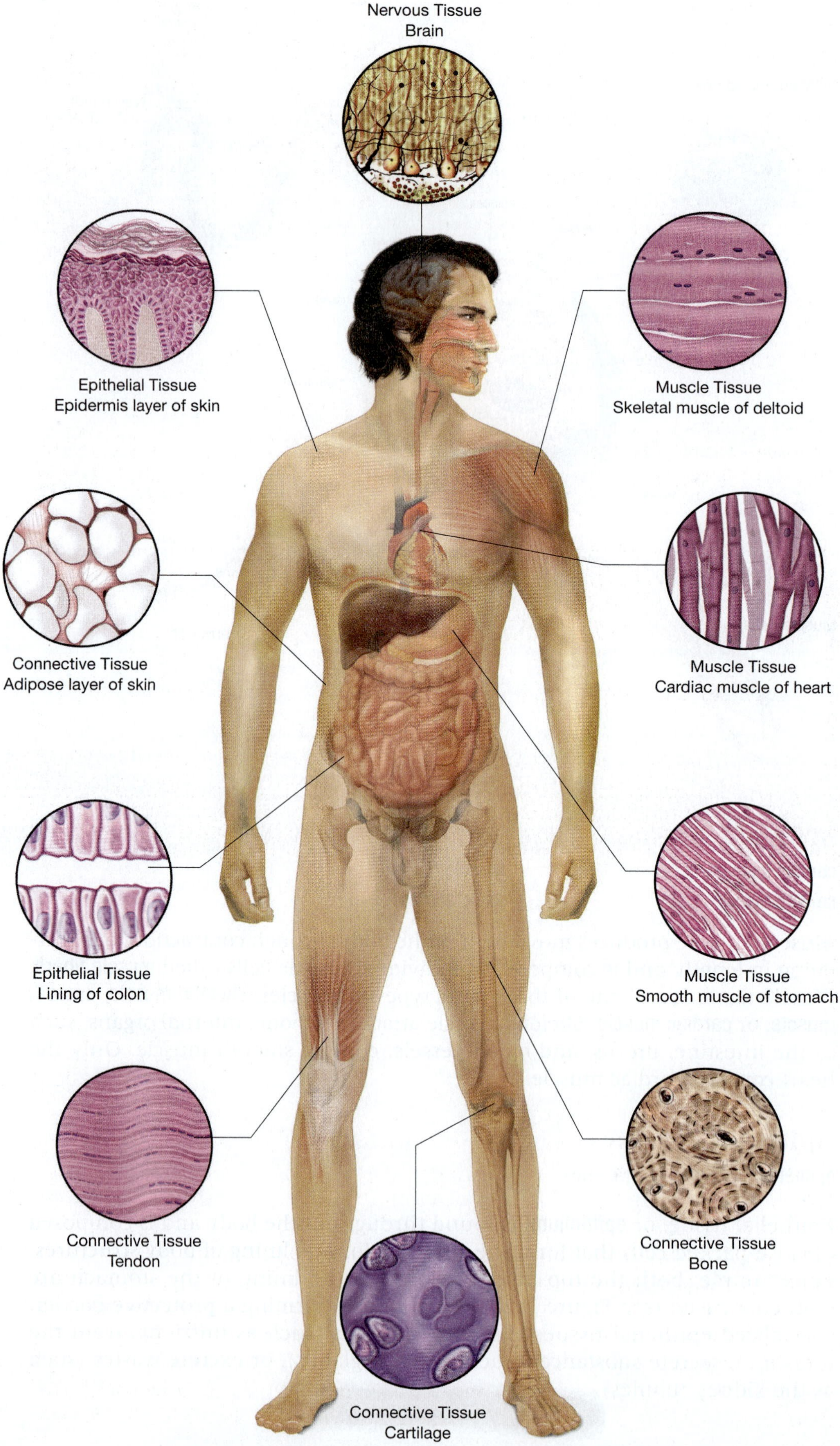

Connective Tissue

adipose (AD-ih-pohs)
bone
cartilage (KAR-tih-lij)
tendons

Connective tissue is the supporting and protecting tissue in body structures. Because connective tissue performs different functions depending on its location, it appears in several forms so that each is able to perform the task required at that location. For example, **bone** provides structural support for the whole body. **Cartilage** is the shock absorber in joints. **Tendons** tightly connect skeletal muscles to bones. **Adipose** provides protective padding around body structures (see Figure 2-2).

What's In A Name?
Look for these word parts:
adip/o = fat
-ose = pertaining to

Nervous Tissue

brain
nerves
neurons
spinal cord

Nervous tissue is made up of cells called **neurons** (see Figure 2-2). This tissue forms the **brain**, **spinal cord**, and a network of **nerves** throughout the entire body, allowing for the conduction of electrical impulses to send information between the brain and the rest of the body.

What's In A Name?
Look for these word parts:
neur/o = nerve
spin/o = spine
-al = pertaining to

PRACTICE AS YOU GO

A. Complete the Statement

1. The levels of organization of the body in order from smallest to largest are: ______, ______, ______, ______, ______.
2. No matter its shape, all cells have ______, a ______, and a ______.
3. ______ tissue lines internal organs and serves as a covering for the skin.
4. ______ muscle is located in the heart, ______ muscle is attached to bones, and ______ muscle is found in internal organs.
5. Cartilage and tendons are examples of ______ tissue.
6. Nervous tissue is composed of ______.

Organs and Systems

Organs are composed of several different types of tissue that work as a unit to perform special functions. For example, the stomach contains smooth muscle tissue, nervous tissue, and epithelial tissue that allow it to contract to mix food with digestive juices.

Several organs working in a coordinated manner to perform a complex function or functions comprise a system. To continue with our example, the stomach plus the other digestive system organs—the oral cavity, pharynx, esophagus, liver, gallbladder, pancreas, small intestine, and large intestine—work together to ingest, digest, and absorb food.

Table 2-1 ■ presents the organ systems this book discusses, along with the major organs found in each system, the system functions, and the medical specialties that treat conditions of that system.

■ TABLE 2-1 Organ Systems of the Human Body

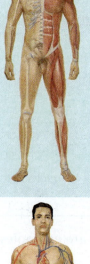

System and Medical Specialty	Word Parts	Structures	Functions
Integumentary System (in-teg-yoo-MEN-tah-ree) **dermatology** (der-mah-TALL-oh-jee) **plastic surgery** (PLAS-tik)	**-ary** = pertaining to **dermat/o** = skin **-logy** = study of	• Skin • Hair • Nails • Sweat glands • Sebaceous glands	Forms protective two-way barrier; aids in temperature regulation
Musculoskeletal System (MS) (mus-kyoo-loh-SKEL-eh-tal) **orthopedics** (or-thoh-PEE-diks) **orthopedic surgery** (or-thoh-PEE-dik) **rheumatology** (roo-mah-TALL-oh-jee)	**muscul/o** = muscle **-al** = pertaining to **orth/o** = straight **ped/o** = foot **-ic** = pertaining to **-logy** = study of	• Bones • Joints • Muscles	Skeleton supports and protects body, forms blood cells, and stores minerals; muscles produce movement
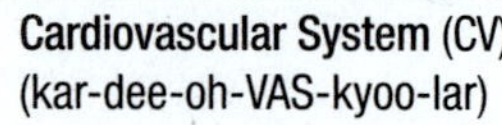 **Cardiovascular System** (CV) (kar-dee-oh-VAS-kyoo-lar) **cardiology** (kar-dee-ALL-oh-jee)	**cardi/o** = heart **vascul/o** = blood vessel **-ar** = pertaining to **-logy** = study of	• Heart • Arteries • Veins 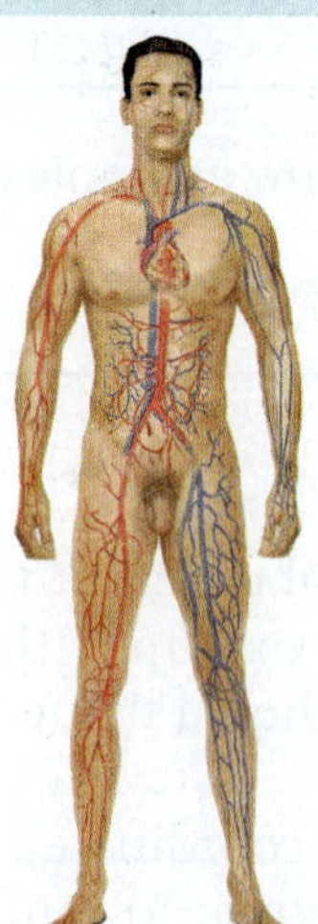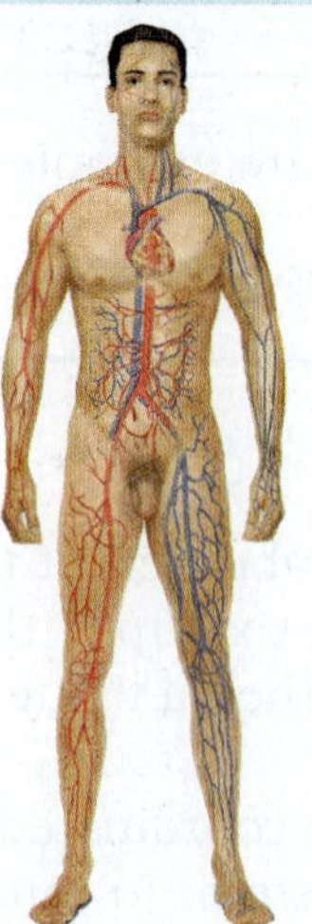	Pumps blood throughout entire body to transport nutrients, oxygen, and wastes

■ **TABLE 2-1** Organ Systems of the Human Body (continued)

System and Medical Specialty	Word Parts	Structures	Functions
Blood (Hematic System) (hee-MAT-ik) **hematology** (hee-mah-TALL-oh-jee)	**hemat/o** = blood **-ic** = pertaining to **-logy** = study of	• Plasma • Erythrocytes • Leukocytes • Platelets	Transports oxygen, protects against pathogens, and controls bleeding
Lymphatic System (lim-FAT-ik) **immunology** (im-yoo-NALL-oh-jee)	**lymph/o** = lymph **-atic** = pertaining to **immun/o** = protection **-logy** = study of	• Lymph nodes • Lymphatic vessels • Spleen • Thymus gland • Tonsils 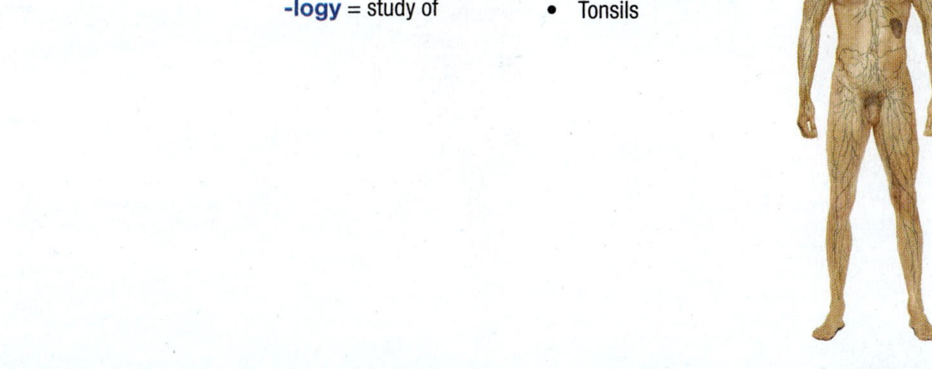	Protects body from disease and invasion from pathogens
Respiratory System **otorhinolaryngology** (ENT) (oh-toh-rye-noh-lair-in-GALL-oh-jee) **pulmonology** (pull-moh-NALL-oh-jee) **thoracic surgery** (tho-RASS-ik)	**-ory** = pertaining to **ot/o** = ear **rhin/o** = nose **laryng/o** = larynx **pulmon/o** = lung **thorac/o** = chest **-ic** = pertaining to **-logy** = study of	• Nasal cavity • Pharynx • Larynx • Trachea • Bronchial tubes • Lungs 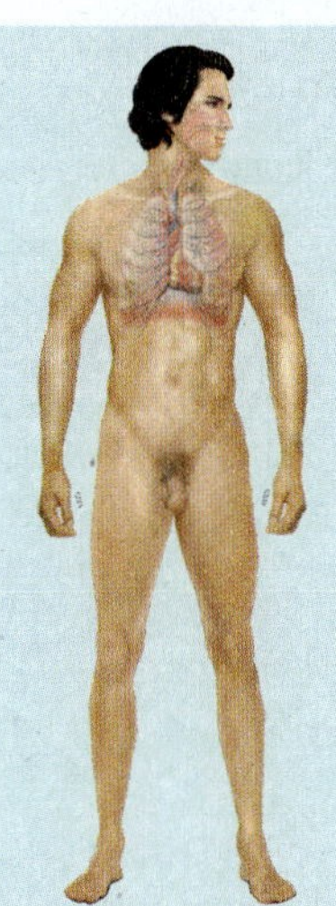	Obtains oxygen from the environment and removes carbon dioxide from the body

■ TABLE 2-1 Organ Systems of the Human Body (continued)

System and Medical Specialty	Word Parts	Structures		Functions
Digestive or Gastrointestinal (GI) System **gastroenterology** (gas-troh-en-ter-ALL-oh-jee) **proctology** (prok-TALL-oh-jee)	**gastr/o** = stomach **enter/o** = small intestine **proct/o** = rectum and anus **-al** = pertaining to **-logy** = study of	• Oral cavity • Pharynx • Esophagus • Stomach • Small intestine • Large intestine • Liver • Gallbladder • Pancreas • Salivary glands		Ingests, digests, and absorbs nutrients for the body
Urinary System (YOO-rih-nair-ee) **nephrology** (neh-FROL-oh-jee) **urology** (yoo-RALL-oh-jee)	**urin/o** = urine **-ary** = pertaining to **nephr/o** = kidney **ur/o** = urine **-logy** = study of	• Kidneys • Ureters • Urinary bladder • Urethra	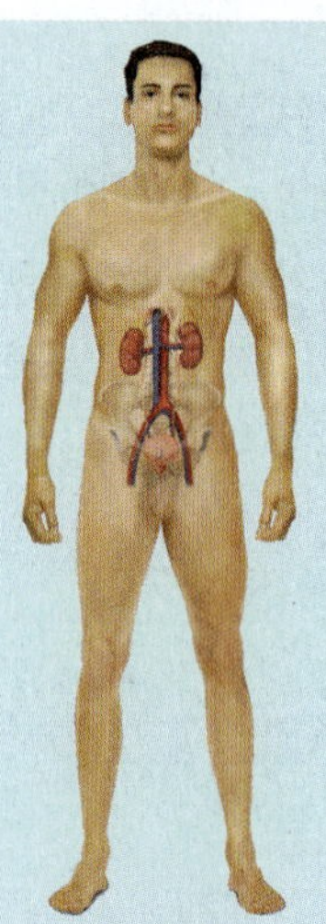	Filters waste products out of blood and removes them from body
Female Reproductive System **gynecology** (GYN) (gigh-neh-KALL-oh-jee) **obstetrics** (OB) (ob-STET-riks)	**gynec/o** = female **-logy** = study of	• Ovaries • Fallopian tubes • Uterus • Vagina • Vulva • Breasts	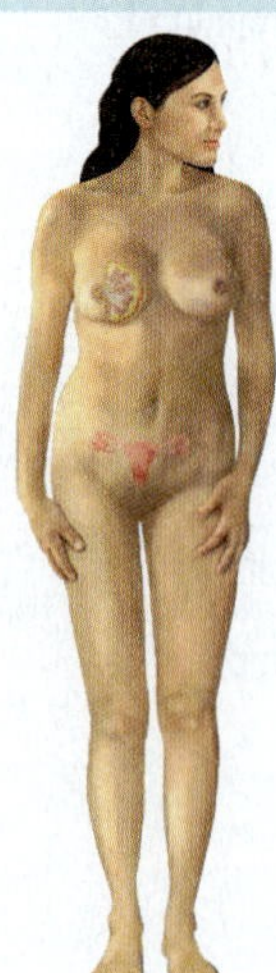	Produces eggs for reproduction, provides place for growing baby, and nourishes infant

■ TABLE 2-1 Organ Systems of the Human Body (continued)

System and Medical Specialty	Word Parts	Structures	Functions
Male Reproductive System **urology** (yoo-RALL-oh-jee)	**ur/o** = urine **-logy** = study of	• Testes • Epididymis • Vas deferens • Penis • Seminal vesicles • Prostate gland • Bulbourethral gland	Produces sperm for reproduction
Endocrine System (EN-doh-krin) **endocrinology** (en-doh-krin-ALL-oh-jee)	**endo-** = within **crin/o** = to secrete **-ine** = pertaining to **-logy** = study of	• Pituitary gland • Pineal gland • Thyroid gland • Parathyroid glands • Thymus gland • Adrenal glands • Pancreas • Ovaries • Testes 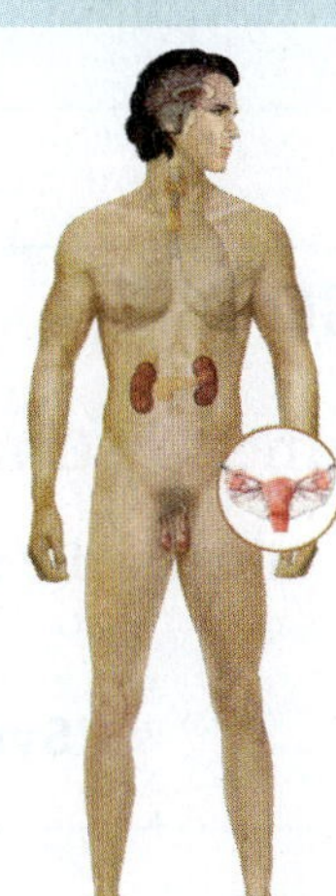	Regulates metabolic activities of the body
Nervous System **neurology** (noo-RALL-oh-jee) **neurosurgery** (noo-roh-SER-jer-ee)	**-ous** = pertaining to **neur/o** = nerve **-logy** = study of	• Brain • Spinal cord • Nerves 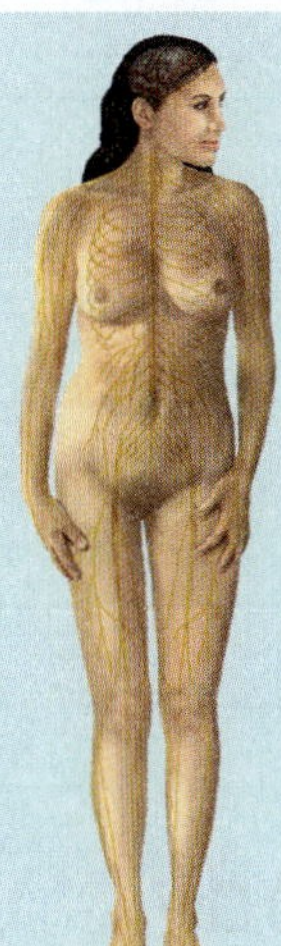	Receives sensory information and coordinates body's response

TABLE 2-1 Organ Systems of the Human Body (continued)

System and Medical Specialty	Word Parts	Structures	Functions
Special Senses ophthalmology (off-thal-MALL-oh-jee)	**ophthalm/o** = eye **-logy** = study of	• Eyes	Sensory organ that converts light into electrical impulses allowing for vision
otorhinolaryngology (ENT) (oh-toh-rye-noh-lair-in-GALL-oh-jee)	**ot/o** = ear **rhin/o** = nose **laryng/o** = larynx **-logy** = study of	• Ears	Sensory organ with dual purpose: converts sound waves into electrical impulses allowing for hearing, and maintains body's sense of balance

PRACTICE AS YOU GO

B. Organ System and Function Challenge

For each organ listed below, identify the name of the system to which it belongs and then match it to its function.

Organ	System	Function
1. ________ skin	____________________	**a.** supports the body
2. ________ heart	____________________	**b.** provides place for growing baby
3. ________ stomach	____________________	**c.** filters waste products from blood
4. ________ uterus	____________________	**d.** provides two-way barrier
5. ________ bones	____________________	**e.** produces movement
6. ________ lungs	____________________	**f.** produces sperm
7. ________ kidney	____________________	**g.** ingests, digests, and absorbs nutrients
8. ________ testes	____________________	**h.** coordinates body's response
9. ________ brain	____________________	**i.** pumps blood through blood vessels
10. ________ muscles	____________________	**j.** obtains oxygen

Body

anatomical position

What's In A Name?

Look for this word part:
-al = pertaining to

As shown in the previous sections, the body is the sum of all its systems, organs, tissues, and cells. It is important to learn the anatomical terminology that applies to the body as a whole in order to correctly identify specific locations and directions when dealing with patients. The **anatomical position** is used when describing the positions and relationships of structures in the human body. A body in the anatomical position is standing erect with the arms at the sides of the body, the palms of the hands facing forward, and the eyes looking straight ahead. In addition, the legs are parallel with the feet, and the toes are pointing forward (see Figure 2-3 ■). For descriptive purposes, the assumption is always that the person is in the anatomical position even if the body or parts of the body are in any other position.

Body Planes

coronal plane (koh-ROH-nal)
coronal section
cross-section
frontal plane
frontal section
horizontal plane
longitudinal section
median plane
midsagittal plane (mid-SAJ-ih-tal)
sagittal plane (SAJ-ih-tal)
sagittal section
transverse plane
transverse section

Use terminology for body planes to assist medical personnel in describing the body and its parts. To understand body planes, imagine cuts slicing through the body at various angles. This imaginary slicing allows for use of more specific language when describing parts of the body. These body planes, illustrated in Figure 2-4 ■, include the following:

1. **Sagittal plane:** This vertical plane runs lengthwise from front to back and divides the body, or any of its parts, into right and left portions. The right and left sides do not have to be equal. If the sagittal plane passes through the middle of the body, thus dividing it into equal right and left halves, it

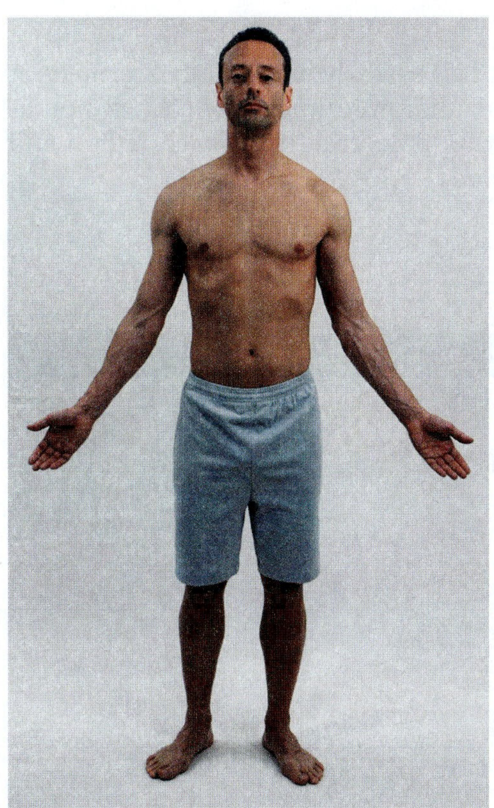

■ **Figure 2-3** The anatomical position: standing erect, gazing straight ahead, arms down at sides, palms facing forward, fingers extended, legs together, and toes pointing forward. *(Patrick Watson/Pearson Education, Inc.)*

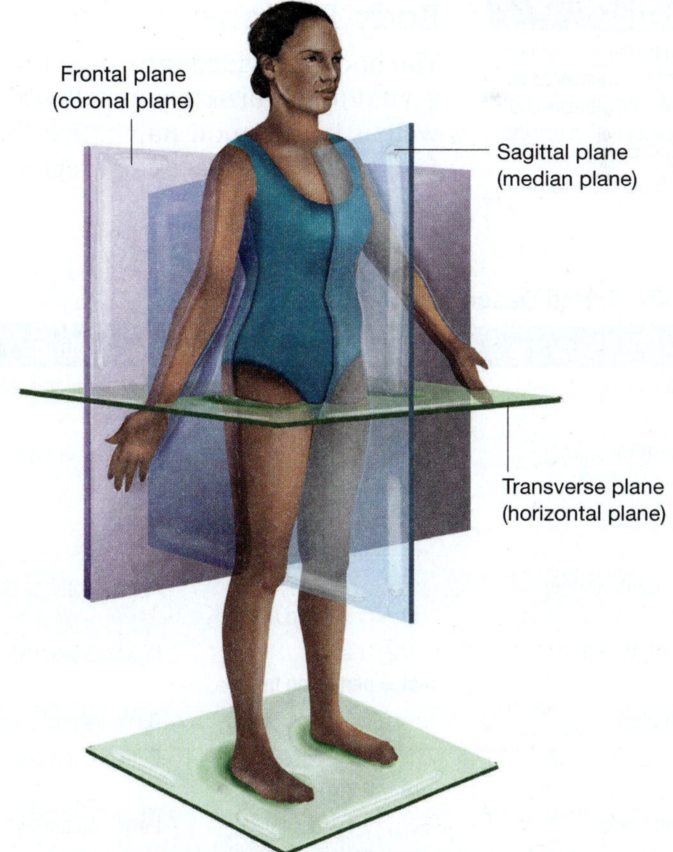

■ **Figure 2-4** The planes of the body. The sagittal plane is vertical from front to back, the frontal plane is vertical from left to right, and the transverse plane is horizontal.

What's In A Name?

Look for these word parts:
medi/o = middle
trans- = across
-al = pertaining to
-an = pertaining to

is called a **midsagittal** or **median plane**. A cut along the sagittal plane yields a **sagittal section** view of the inside of the body.

2. **Frontal plane:** The frontal, or **coronal plane**, divides the body into front and back portions; a vertical, lengthwise plane is running from side to side. A cut along the frontal plane yields a **frontal** or **coronal section** view of the inside of the body.
3. **Transverse plane:** The transverse, or **horizontal plane**, is a crosswise plane that runs parallel to the ground. This imaginary cut would divide the body, or its parts, into upper and lower portions. A cut along the transverse plane yields a **transverse section** view of the inside of the body.

The terms **cross-section** and **longitudinal section** are frequently used to describe internal views of structures. A lengthwise slice along the long axis of a structure produces a longitudinal section. A slice perpendicular to the long axis of a structure produces a cross-section view.

PRACTICE AS YOU GO

C. Body Plane Matching

Match each body plane to its definition.

1. ________ frontal plane
2. ________ sagittal plane
3. ________ transverse plane

a. divides the body into right and left
b. divides the body into upper and lower
c. divides the body into anterior and posterior

Med Term Tip

As you learn medical terminology, it is important to remember to no longer use common phrases and terms. Many people often use the term *stomach* (an organ) when they actually mean *abdomen* (a body region).

Body Regions

The body is divided into large regions that can easily be identified externally. It is vital to familiarize yourself with both the anatomical name of each region as well as its common name. See Table 2-2 ■ for a description of each region and Figure 2-5 ■ to locate each region on the body.

■ TABLE 2-2 Terms Describing Body Regions

Region	Word Parts	Description
abdominal region (ab-DOM-ih-nal)	**abdomin/o** = abdomen **-al** = pertaining to	Abdomen; on anterior side of trunk
brachial region (BRAY-kee-al)	**brachi/o** = arm **-al** = pertaining to	Upper extremities (UE) or arms
cephalic region (seh-FAL-ik)	**cephal/o** = head **-ic** = pertaining to	Head
cervical region (SER-vih-kal)	**cervic/o** = neck **-al** = pertaining to	Neck; connects head to trunk
crural region (KREW-ral)	**crur/o** =leg **-al** = pertaining to	Lower extremities (LE) or legs
dorsum (DOOR-sum)	**dors/o** = back of body	Back; on posterior side of trunk
gluteal region (GLOO-tee-al)	**glute/o** = buttock **-al** = pertaining to	Buttocks; on posterior side of trunk
pelvic region (PEL-vik)	**pelv/o** = pelvis **-ic** = pertaining to	Pelvis; on anterior side of trunk
pubic region (PYOO-bik)	**pub/o** = genital region **-ic** = pertaining to	Region containing external genitals; on anterior side of trunk

TABLE 2-2 Terms Describing Body Regions (continued)

Region	Word Parts	Description
thoracic region (tho-RASS-ik)	**thorac/o** = chest **-ic** = pertaining to	Chest; on anterior side of trunk; also called *thorax*
trunk		Contains all body regions other than head, neck, and extremities; also called *torso*
vertebral region (VER-teh-bral)	**vertebr/o** = vertebra **-al** = pertaining to	Overlies spinal column or vertebrae; on posterior side of trunk

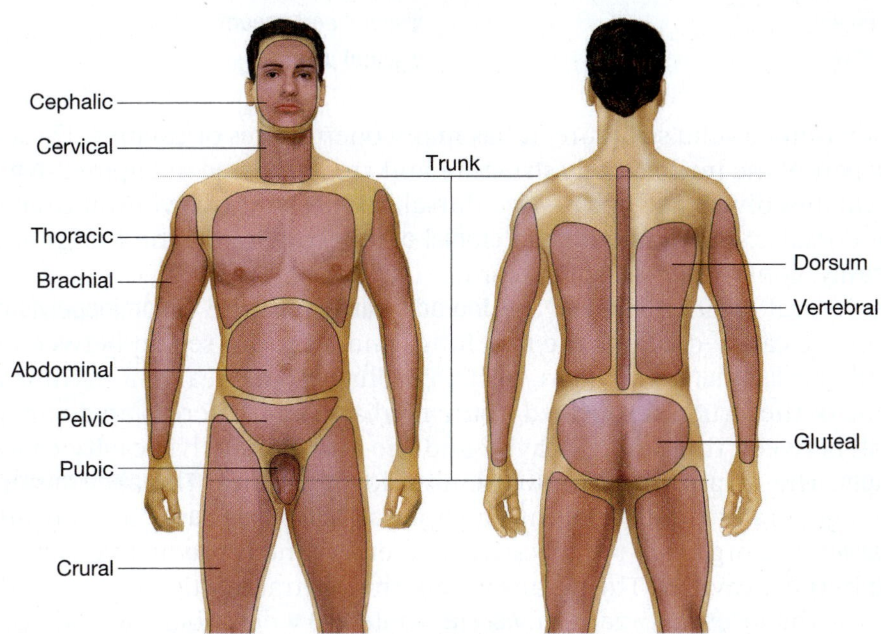

Figure 2-5 Anterior and posterior views of the body illustrating the location of various body regions.

PRACTICE AS YOU GO

D. Body Region Practice

For each term below, write the corresponding body region.

1. head ______
2. genitals ______
3. leg ______
4. buttocks ______
5. neck ______
6. arm ______
7. back ______
8. chest ______

Body Cavities

abdominal cavity
abdominopelvic cavity (ab-dom-ih-noh-PEL-vik)
cranial cavity (KRAY-nee-al)
diaphragm (DYE-ah-fram)
mediastinum (mee-dee-as-TYE-num)
parietal layer (pah-RYE-eh-tal)
parietal peritoneum
parietal pleura
pelvic cavity
pericardial cavity (pair-ih-KAR-dee-al)
peritoneum (pair-ih-toh-NEE-um)
pleura (PLOO-rah)
pleural cavity (PLOO-ral)
spinal cavity
thoracic cavity
viscera (VISS-er-ah)
visceral layer (VISS-er-al)
visceral peritoneum
visceral pleura

What's In A Name?

Look for these word parts:
abdomin/o = abdomen
crani/o = skull
pelv/o = pelvis
pariet/o = cavity wall
pleur/o = pleura
spin/o = spine
thorac/o = chest
viscer/o = internal organ
peri- = around
-al = pertaining to
-ic = pertaining to

The body is not a solid structure; it has many open spaces or cavities. These cavities are part of the normal body structure and are illustrated in Figure 2-6 ■. Four major cavities divide the body—two dorsal cavities and two ventral cavities.

The dorsal cavities include the **cranial cavity**, containing the brain, and the **spinal cavity**, containing the spinal cord.

The ventral cavities include the **thoracic cavity** and the **abdominopelvic cavity**. The thoracic cavity contains the two lungs and a central region between them called the **mediastinum**. The heart, aorta, esophagus, trachea, and thymus gland are some of the structures located in the mediastinum. There is an actual physical wall between the thoracic cavity and the abdominopelvic cavity called the **diaphragm**. The diaphragm is a muscle used for breathing. The abdominopelvic cavity is generally subdivided into a superior **abdominal cavity** and an inferior **pelvic cavity**. The organs of the digestive, excretory, and reproductive systems are located in these cavities. The organs within the ventral cavities are referred to as a group as the internal organs or **viscera**. Table 2-3 ■ describes the body cavities and their major organs.

Med Term Tip

The kidneys are the only major abdominopelvic organ located outside the sac formed by the peritoneum. Because they are found behind this sac, their position is referred to as *retroperitoneal* (**retro-** = behind; **peritone/o** = peritoneum; **-al** = pertaining to).

All of the ventral cavities are lined by, and the viscera are encased in, a two-layer membrane called the **pleura** in the thoracic cavity and the **peritoneum** in the abdominopelvic cavity. The outer layer that lines the cavities is called the **parietal layer** (i.e., **parietal pleura** and **parietal peritoneum**), and the inner layer that encases the viscera is called the **visceral layer** (i.e., **visceral pleura** and **visceral peritoneum**).

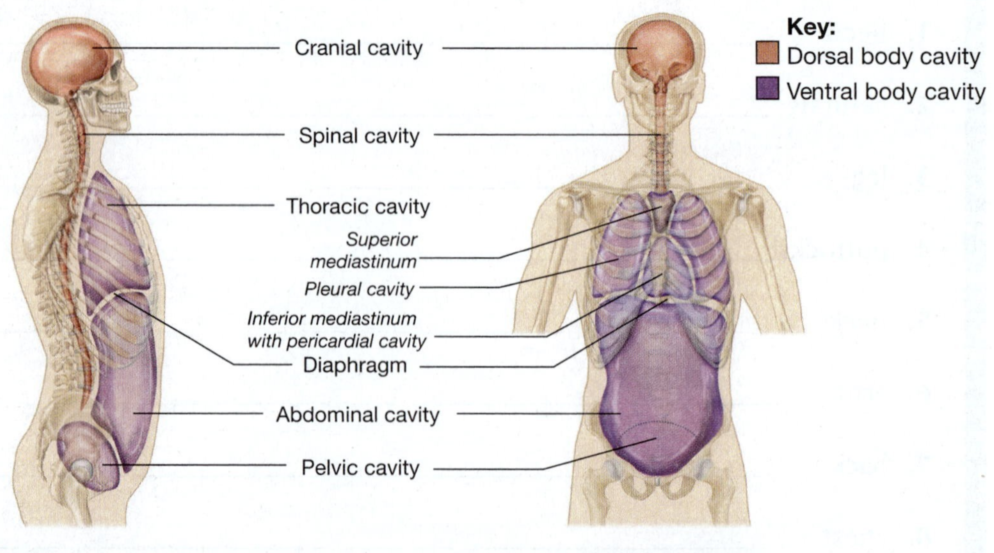

■ **Figure 2-6** The dorsal (red) and ventral (purple) body cavities.

■ **TABLE 2-3** Body Cavities and Their Major Organs

Cavity	Major Organs
Dorsal cavities	
Cranial cavity	Brain
Spinal cavity	Spinal cord
Ventral cavities	
Thoracic cavity	Pleural cavity: lungs
	Pericardial cavity: heart
	Mediastinum: heart, esophagus, trachea, thymus gland, aorta
Abdominopelvic cavities	
Abdominal cavity	Stomach, spleen, liver, gallbladder, pancreas, and portions of the small intestine and colon
Pelvic cavity	Urinary bladder, ureters, urethra, and portions of the small intestine and colon
	Female: uterus, ovaries, fallopian tubes, vagina
	Male: prostate gland, seminal vesicles, portion of vas deferens

Within the thoracic cavity, the pleura is subdivided, forming the **pleural cavity**, containing the lungs, and the **pericardial cavity**, containing the heart. The larger abdominopelvic cavity is usually subdivided into regions in order to precisely refer to different areas. Two different methods of subdividing this cavity are used: the anatomical divisions and the clinical divisions. Choose a method partly on personal preference and partly on which system best describes the patient's condition. See Table 2-4■ for a description of these methods for dividing the abdominopelvic cavity.

■ **TABLE 2-4** Methods of Subdividing the Abdominopelvic Cavity

Anatomical Divisions of the Abdomen

- Right hypochondriac (high-poh-KON-dree-ak): Right lateral region of upper row beneath the lower ribs
- Epigastric (ep-ih-GAS-trik): Middle area of upper row above the stomach
- Left hypochondriac: Left lateral region of the upper row beneath the lower ribs
- Right lumbar: Right lateral region of the middle row at the waist
- Umbilical (um-BIL-ih-kal): Central area over the navel
- Left lumbar: Left lateral region of the middle row at the waist
- Right inguinal (ING-gwih-nal): Right lateral region of the lower row at the groin
- Hypogastric (high-poh-GAS-trik): Middle region of the lower row beneath the navel
- Left inguinal: Left lateral region of the lower row at the groin

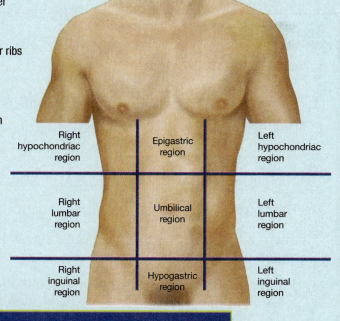

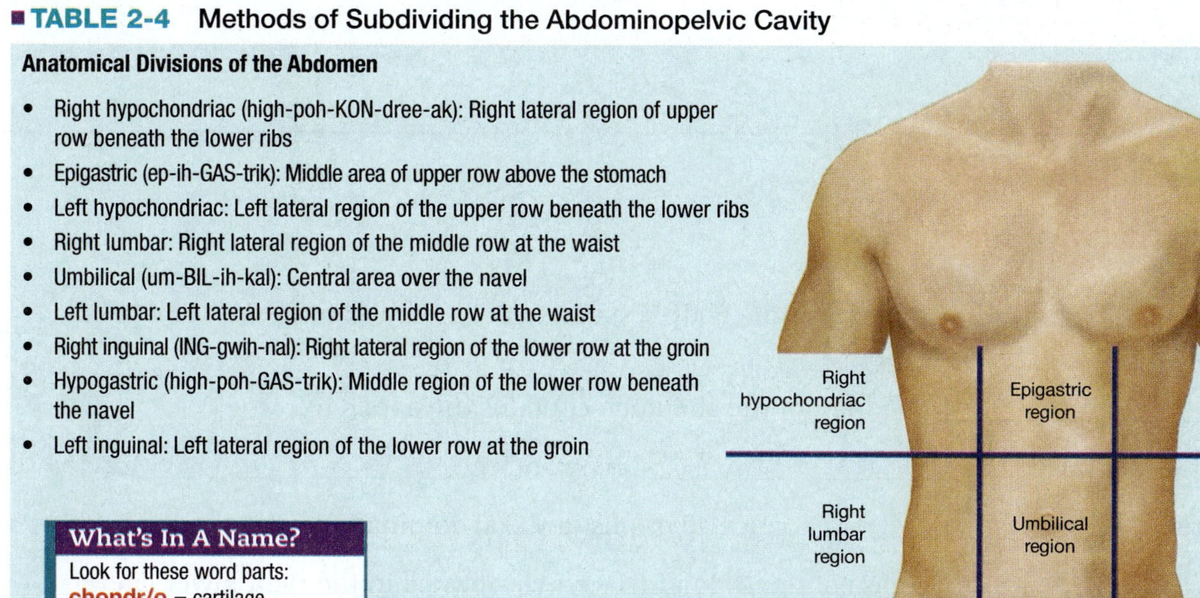

What's In A Name?

Look for these word parts:
chondr/o = cartilage
gastr/o = stomach
inguin/o = groin
lumb/o = loin (low back)
epi- = above
hypo- = below
-al = pertaining to
-ar = pertaining to
-iac = pertaining to
-ic = pertaining to

Med Term Tip

To visualize the nine anatomical divisions, imagine a tic-tac-toe diagram over this region.

Med Term Tip

The term *hypochondriac*, literally meaning *below the cartilage* (of the ribs), has come to refer to a person who believes he or she is sick when there is no obvious cause for illness. These patients commonly complain of aches and pains in the hypochondriac region.

TABLE 2-4 Methods of Subdividing the Abdominopelvic Cavity (continued)

Clinical Divisions of the Abdomen

- Right upper quadrant (RUQ): Contains majority of liver, gallbladder, small portion of pancreas, right kidney, small intestine, and colon
- Right lower quadrant (RLQ): Contains small intestine and colon, right ovary and fallopian tube, appendix, and right ureter
- Left upper quadrant (LUQ): Contains small portion of liver, spleen, stomach, majority of pancreas, left kidney, small intestine, and colon
- Left lower quadrant (LLQ): Contains small intestine and colon, left ovary and fallopian tube, and left ureter
- Midline organs: uterus, bladder, prostate gland

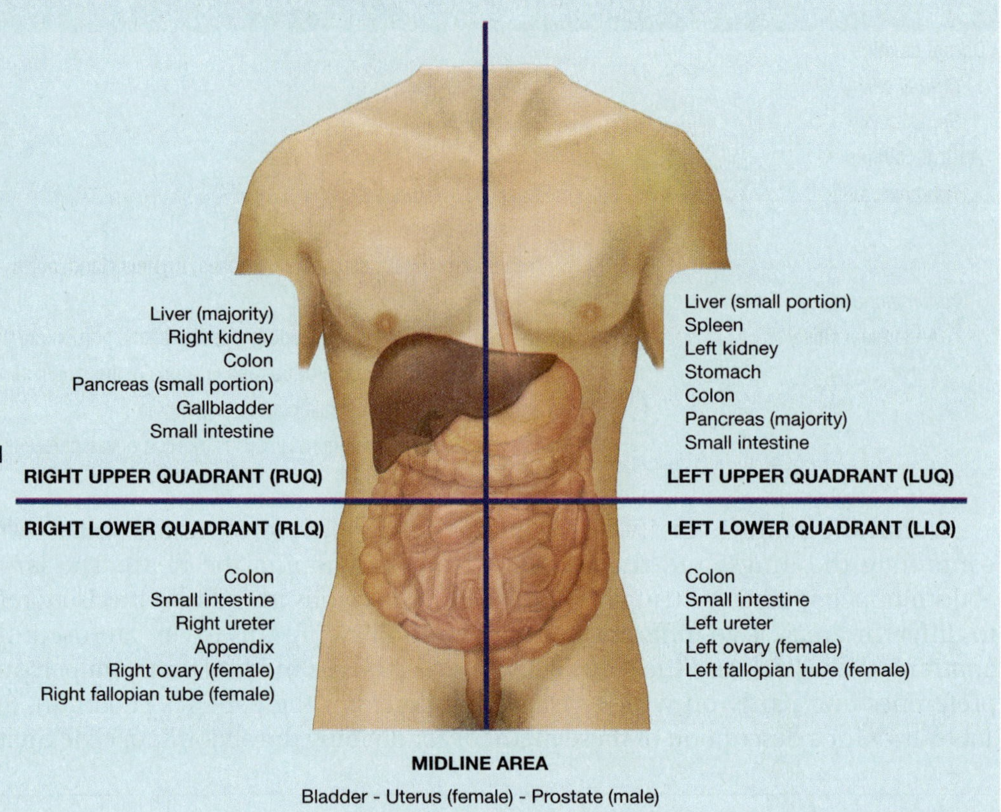

PRACTICE AS YOU GO

E. Complete the Statement

1. In the ____________________ position, the body is standing erect with arms at sides and palms facing forward.
2. The ____________________ quadrant of the abdomen contains the appendix.
3. The dorsal cavities are the ____________________ cavity and the ____________________ cavity.
4. There are ____________________ anatomical divisions in the abdominal cavity.
5. The ____________________ region of the abdominal cavity is located in the right lower lateral region near the groin.
6. Within the thoracic cavity, the lungs are found in the ____________________ cavity and the heart is found in the ____________________ cavity.

Directional Terms

Directional terms describe the positions of structures relative to other structures or locations in the body. Table 2-5 ■ presents commonly used terms for describing the position of the body or its parts. They are listed in pairs that have opposite meanings; for example, superior versus inferior, anterior versus posterior, medial versus lateral, proximal versus distal, superficial versus deep, and supine versus prone. Directional terms are illustrated in Figure 2-7 ■.

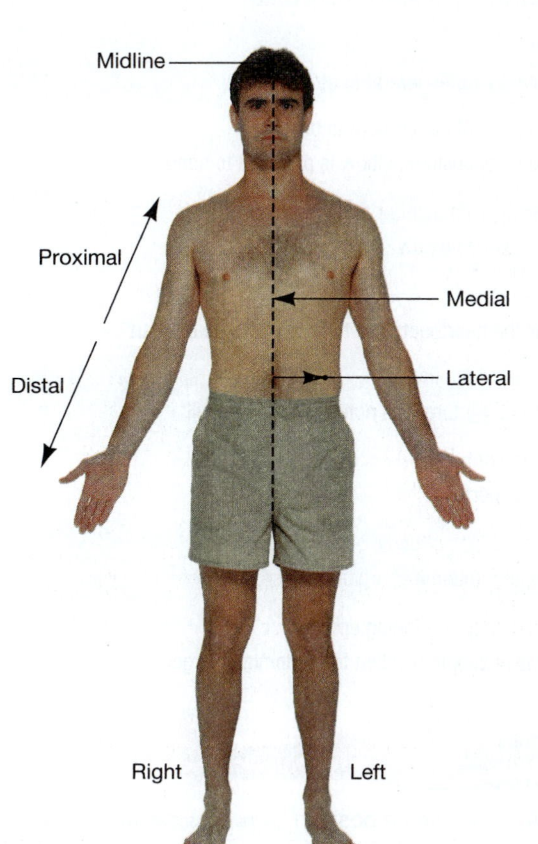

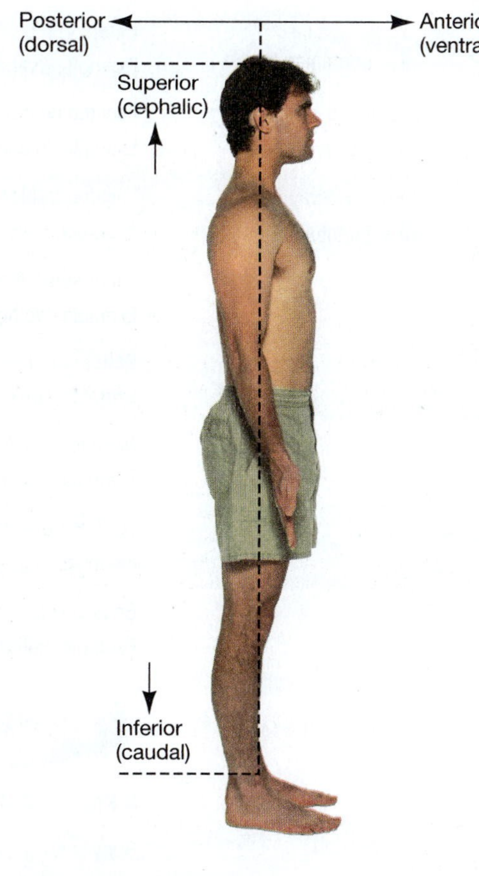

■ **Figure 2-7** Anterior and lateral views of the body illustrating directional terms. *(Michal Heron/Pearson Education, Inc.)*

■ **TABLE 2-5** Terms for Describing Body Position

Term	Word Parts	Description
superior (soo-PEE-ree-or) or **cephalic** (seh-FAL-ik)	**super/o** = above **-ior** = pertaining to **cephal/o** = head **-ic** = pertaining to	More toward head, or above another structure Example: Adrenal glands are superior to the kidneys
inferior (in-FEE-ree-or) or **caudal** (KAWD-al)	**infer/o** = below **-ior** = pertaining to **caud/o** = tail **-al** = pertaining to	More toward feet or tail or below another structure Example: Intestines are inferior to the heart
anterior (an-TEE-ree-or) or **ventral** (VEN-tral)	**anter/o** = front **-ior** = pertaining to **ventr/o** = belly **-al** = pertaining to	More toward front or belly side of body Example: Navel is located on anterior surface of body
posterior (poss-TEE-ree-or) or **dorsal** (DOR-sal)	**poster/o** = back **-ior** = pertaining to **dors/o** = back **-al** = pertaining to	More toward back or spinal cord side of body Example: Posterior wall of right kidney was excised

TABLE 2-5 Terms for Describing Body Position (continued)

Term	Word Parts	Description
medial (MEE-dee-al)	**medi/o** = middle **-al** = pertaining to	Refers to middle or near middle of body or structure Example: Heart is medially located in chest cavity
lateral (LAT-er-al)	**later/o** = side **-al** = pertaining to	Refers to the side Example: Ovaries are located lateral to uterus
proximal (PROK-sim-al)	**proxim/o** = near to **-al** = pertaining to	Located nearer to point of attachment to body Example: In anatomical position, elbow is proximal to hand
distal (DIS-tal)	**dist/o** = away from **-al** = pertaining to	Located farther away from point of attachment to body Example: Hand is distal to elbow
apex (AY-peks)		Tip or summit of an organ Example: We hear the heartbeat by listening over apex of heart
base		Bottom or lower part of organ Example: On X-ray, a fracture was noted at base of skull
superficial		More toward surface of body Example: Cut was superficial
deep		Further away from surface of body Example: Incision into abdominal organ is a deep incision
supine (soo-PINE)		Body is lying horizontally and facing upward Example: Patient is in supine position for abdominal surgery **Figure 2-8A** The supine position. *(Richard Logan/Pearson Education, Inc.)*
prone (PROHN)		Body is lying horizontally and facing downward Example: Patient is placed in prone position for spinal surgery **Figure 2-8B** The prone position. *(Richard Logan/Pearson Education, Inc.)*

PRACTICE AS YOU GO

F. Directional Opposites

For each directional term provided, write the term for the "opposite" direction.

1. superior ______________________
2. prone ______________________
3. medial ______________________
4. dorsal ______________________

5. superficial ____________________

6. base ____________________

7. proximal ____________________

8. anterior ____________________

9. caudal ____________________

Routes and Methods of Drug Administration

aerosol (AIR-oh-sol)
buccal (BUK-al)
eardrops
eyedrops
inhalation (in-hah-LAY-shun)
intracavitary (in-trah-KAV-ih-tair-ee)
intradermal (in-trah-DER-mal)
intramuscular (in-trah-MUS-kyoo-lar)
intrathecal (in-trah-THEE-kal)
intravenous (in-trah-VEE-nus)
oral (OR-al)
parenteral (par-EN-ter-al)
rectal (REK-tal)
subcutaneous (sub-kyoo-TAY-nee-us)
sublingual (sub-LING-gwal)
suppositories (suh-POZ-ih-tor-ees)
topical (TOP-ih-kal)
transdermal (tranz-DER-mal)
vaginal (VAJ-in-al)

The method by which a drug is introduced into the body is referred to as the *route of administration*. To be effective, drugs must be administered by a particular route. In some cases, there may be a variety of routes by which a drug can be given. For instance, the female hormone estrogen can be given orally in pill form or by a patch applied to the skin. The most common routes of administration are described in Table 2-6■.

■ TABLE 2-6 Common Routes of Drug Administration

Method	Word Parts	Description
oral	**or/o** = mouth **-al** = pertaining to	Includes all drugs given by mouth; advantages: ease of administration and slow rate of absorption via the stomach and intestinal wall; disadvantages: slowness of absorption and destruction of some chemical compounds by gastric juices; additionally, some medications, such as aspirin, can have corrosive action on stomach lining
sublingual (sl)	**sub-** = under **lingu/o** = tongue **-al** = pertaining to	Includes drugs held under the tongue and not swallowed; medication is absorbed by blood vessels on underside of the tongue as saliva dissolves it; rate of absorption is quicker than oral route; nitroglycerin to treat angina pectoris (chest pain) is administered by this route

■ Figure 2-9 Sublingual medication administration. A male patient with a nitroglycerin tablet placed under his tongue. *(Michal Heron/ Pearson Education, Inc.)*

TABLE 2-6 Common Routes of Drug Administration (continued)

Method	Word Parts	Description
inhalation	**in-** = inward **hal/o** = to breathe	Includes drugs inhaled directly into nose and mouth; **aerosol** (**aer/o** = air) sprays are administered by this route

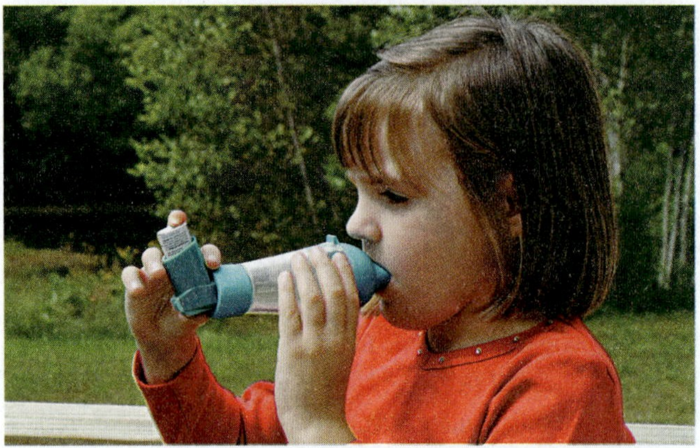

Figure 2-10 Inhalation medication administration. This young girl is using a metered-dose inhaler. *(Michal Heron/Pearson Education, Inc.)*

Method	Word Parts	Description
parenteral	**para-** = beside **enter/o** = intestine **-al** = pertaining to	An invasive method of administering drugs as it requires skin to be punctured by a needle; needle with syringe attached is introduced either under the skin or into a muscle, vein, or body cavity
intracavitary	**intra-** = within **-ary** = pertaining to	Injection into body cavity such as peritoneal cavity or chest cavity; one type of parenteral route of administration
intradermal (ID)	**intra-** = within **derm/o** = skin **-al** = pertaining to	Very shallow injection just under top layer of the skin; commonly used in skin testing for allergies and tuberculosis testing; one type of parenteral route of administration

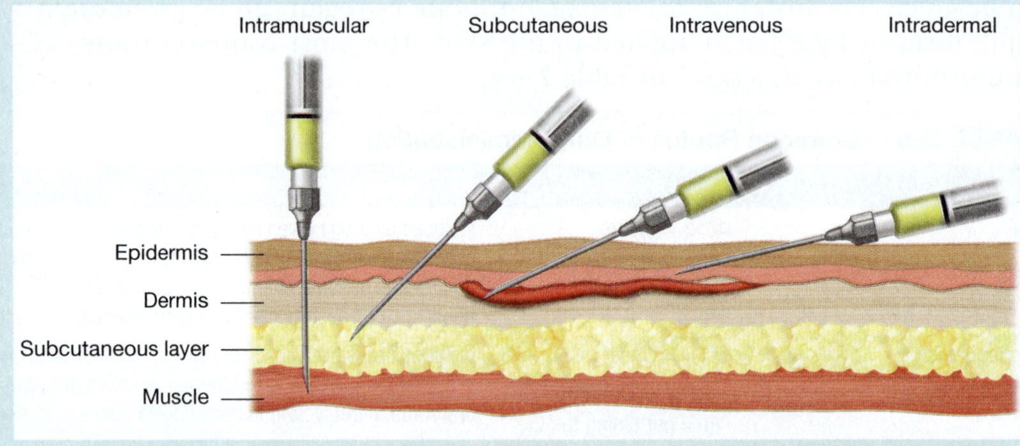

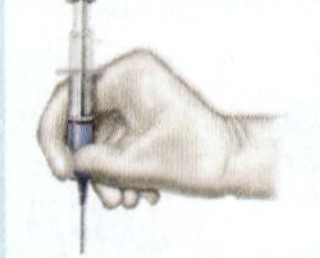
Intramuscular

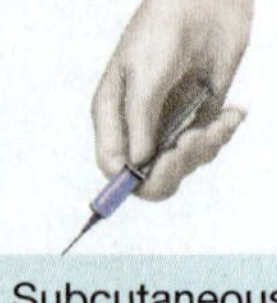
Subcutaneous

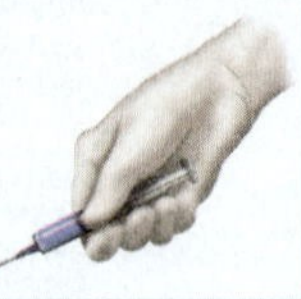
Intravenous

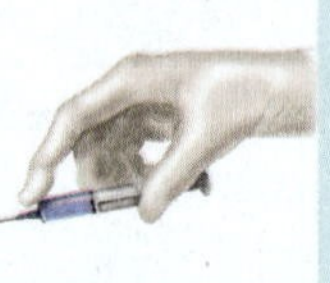
Intradermal

Figure 2-11 Parenteral medication administration. The angle of needle insertion for four different types of parenteral injections.

Method	Word Parts	Description
intramuscular (IM)	**intra-** = within **muscul/o** = muscle **-ar** = pertaining to	Injection directly into muscle of buttocks, thigh, or upper arm; used when there is a large amount of medication or it is irritating (see again Figure 2-11); one type of parenteral route of administration

TABLE 2-6 Common Routes of Drug Administration (continued)

Method	Word Parts	Description
intrathecal	**intra-** = within **thec/o** = sheath (meninges) **-al** = pertaining to	Injection into meningeal space surrounding the brain and spinal cord; one type of parenteral route of administration
intravenous (IV)	**intra-** = within **ven/o** = vein **-ous** = pertaining to	Injection into veins; route may be set up to deliver medication very quickly or to deliver continuous drip of medication (see again Figure 2-11); one type of parenteral route of administration
subcutaneous (subcut)	**sub-** = under **cutane/o** = skin **-ous** = pertaining to	Injection into subcutaneous layer of skin, usually outer part of upper arm, or abdomen (see again Figure 2-11); for example, insulin injection; one type of parenteral route of administration
transdermal	**trans-** = across **derm/o** = skin **-al** = pertaining to	Includes medications that coat underside of a patch, which is applied to skin where it is then absorbed; examples include birth control patches, nicotine patches, and sea sickness patches
rectal	**rect/o** = rectum **-al** = pertaining to	Includes medications introduced directly into rectal cavity in the form of **suppositories** (suppos, supp) or solution; drugs may have to be administered by this route if patient is unable to take them by mouth due to nausea, vomiting, or surgery
topical (top)	**topic/o** = a specific area **-al** = pertaining to	Includes medications applied directly to skin or mucous membranes; distributed in ointment, cream, or lotion form and used to treat skin infections and eruptions
vaginal	**vagin/o** = vagina **-al** = pertaining to	Includes tablets and suppositories that may be inserted vaginally to treat vaginal yeast infections and other irritations
eyedrops		Includes drops used during eye examinations to dilate pupil of eye for better examination of interior of eye; also placed into eye to control eye pressure in glaucoma and treat infections
eardrops		Includes drops placed directly into ear canal for purpose of relieving pain or treating infection
buccal	**bucc/o** = cheek **-al** = pertaining to	Includes drugs placed under lip or between cheek and gum

PRACTICE AS YOU GO

G. Matching Routes of Drug Administration

1. ________ given by mouth — a. inhalation
2. ________ injected into muscle — b. intravenous
3. ________ breathed into nose or mouth — c. topical
4. ________ injected into vein — d. oral
5. ________ applied directly to skin — e. sublingual
6. ________ placed under tongue — f. intramuscular

Abbreviations

AP	anteroposterior	**LUQ**	left upper quadrant
CV	cardiovascular	**MS**	musculoskeletal
ENT	ear, nose, and throat	**OB**	obstetrics
GI	gastrointestinal	**PA**	posteroanterior
GYN	gynecology	**RLQ**	right lower quadrant
ID	intradermal	**RUQ**	right upper quadrant
IM	intramuscular	**sl**	sublingual
IV	intravenous	**subcut**	subcutaneous
lat	lateral	**suppos, supp**	suppository
LE	lower extremity	**top**	apply topically
LLQ	left lower quadrant	**UE**	upper extremity

Chapter Review

Practice Exercises

A. Prefix Practice

Circle the prefixes in the following terms and define in the space provided.

1. epigastric ____________________
2. pericardium ____________________
3. hypochondriac ____________________
4. retroperitoneal ____________________

B. Match Organs and Systems

Match each organ to its body system.

1. _______ heart
2. _______ kidneys
3. _______ joints
4. _______ prostate gland
5. _______ hair
6. _______ thyroid gland
7. _______ uterus
8. _______ stomach
9. _______ lungs
10. _______ spleen
11. _______ brain
12. _______ eye
13. _______ muscles
14. _______ ear
15. _______ blood

a. integumentary system
b. digestive system
c. endocrine system
d. female reproductive system
e. nervous system
f. musculoskeletal system
g. male reproductive system
h. respiratory system
i. urinary system
j. cardiovascular system
k. hematic system
l. lymphatic system
m. special senses

C. What's the Abbreviation?

1. musculoskeletal ______
2. lateral ______
3. right upper quadrant ______
4. cardiovascular ______
5. gastrointestinal ______
6. anteroposterior ______
7. obstetrics ______
8. left lower quadrant ______

D. Fill in the blank with the missing corresponding noun or adjective.

	Noun	Adjective
1.	chest	______
2.	______	cephalic
3.	______	cervical
4.	arm	______
5.	buttocks	______
6.	______	crural
7.	______	spinal
8.	back	______
9.	abdomen	______
10.	______	cranial

E. Writing Directional Terms

For each term defined below, write the correct combining form that goes with the suffix given, and then write the complete term.

	Definition	Combining Form	Term
1.	pertaining to near to	______-al	______
2.	pertaining to above	______-ior	______
3.	pertaining to the middle	______-al	______
4.	pertaining to the belly	______-al	______
5.	pertaining to the tail	______-al	______
6.	pertaining to front	______-ior	______
7.	pertaining to the side	______-al	______
8.	pertaining to back	______-al	______
9.	pertaining to below	______-ior	______
10.	pertaining to back	______-ior	______

F. Terminology Matching

Match each organ to its body cavity.

1. ________ gallbladder	a. right upper quadrant
2. ________ appendix	b. left upper quadrant
3. ________ urinary bladder	c. right lower quadrant
4. ________ small intestine	d. left lower quadrant
5. ________ right kidney	e. all quadrants
6. ________ left ovary	f. midline structure
7. ________ stomach	
8. ________ colon	
9. ________ right ureter	
10. ________ pancreas (majority)	

G. Drug Administration Practice

Name the route of drug administration for the following descriptions.

1. under the tongue ________________
2. into the anus or rectum ________________
3. applied to the skin ________________
4. injected under the first layer of skin ________________
5. injected into a muscle ________________
6. injected into a vein ________________
7. by mouth ________________

H. Spelling Practice

Some of the terms below are misspelled. Identify the incorrect terms and spell them correctly in the blank provided.

1. parenteral ________________
2. hypokondriac ________________
3. integumentery ________________
4. cytology ________________
5. peritoneum ________________
6. inguinal ________________
7. intravenus ________________
8. saggital ________________
9. otorhinolaryngology ________________
10. epitheleum ________________

I. Fill in the Blank

cardiology	otorhinolaryngology	urology	gynecology
ophthalmology	gastroenterology	dermatology	orthopedics

1. John is a musician who plays an electric bass guitar and is experiencing difficulty in hearing soft voices. He would consult a physician in ________________________.
2. Ruth is a stock trader with the Chicago Board of Trade. She has had a pounding and racing heartbeat. She would consult a physician specializing in ________________________.
3. Mary Ann is experiencing excessive bleeding from the uterus. She would consult a ________________________ doctor.
4. José has fractured his wrist in a fall. A physician in ________________________ would see him for an examination.
5. A physician who performs eye exams specializes in the field of ________________________.
6. When her daughter had repeated bladder infections, Mrs. Cortez sought the opinion of a specialist in ________________________.
7. Martha could not get rid of a persistent skin rash with over-the-counter creams. She decided to make an appointment with a specialist in ________________________.
8. After reviewing his X-ray, the specialist in ________________________ informed Mr. Sparks that he had a stomach ulcer.

Labeling Exercises

Image A

Write the labels for this figure on the numbered lines provided.

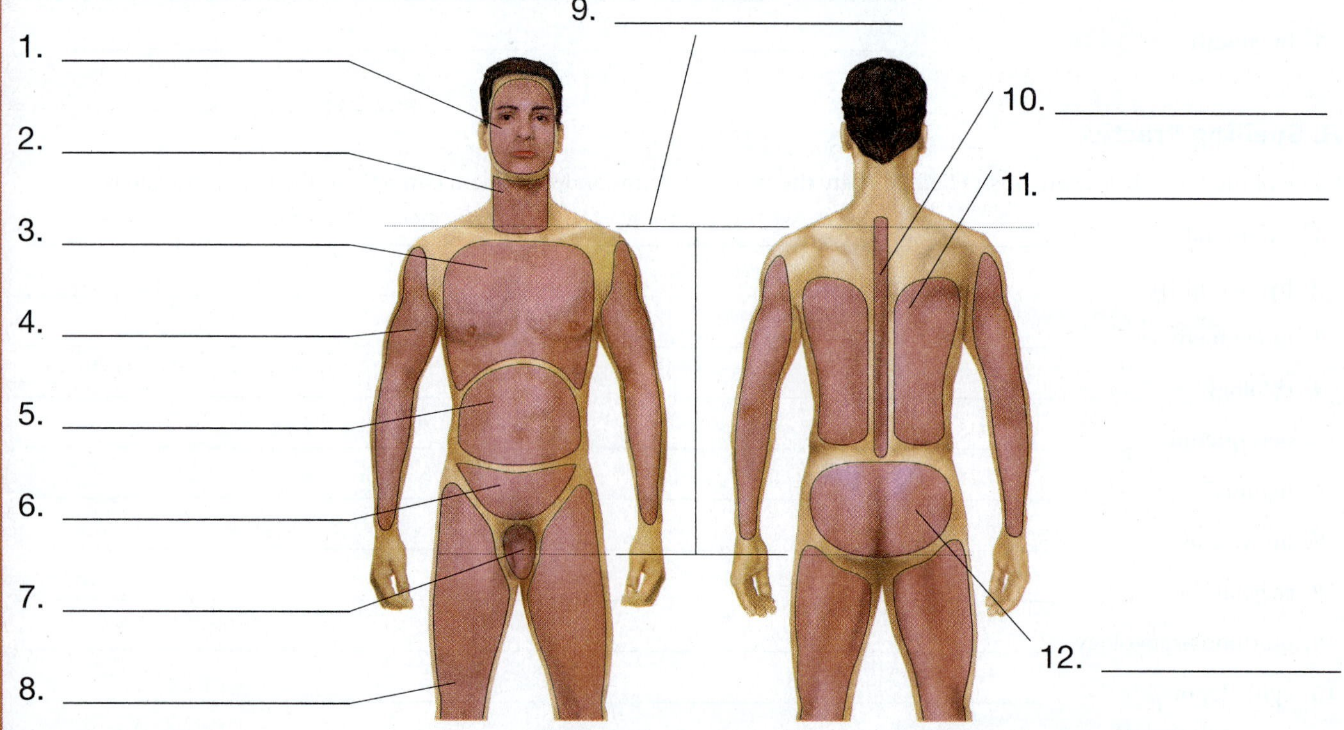

Image B

Write the labels for this figure on the numbered lines provided.

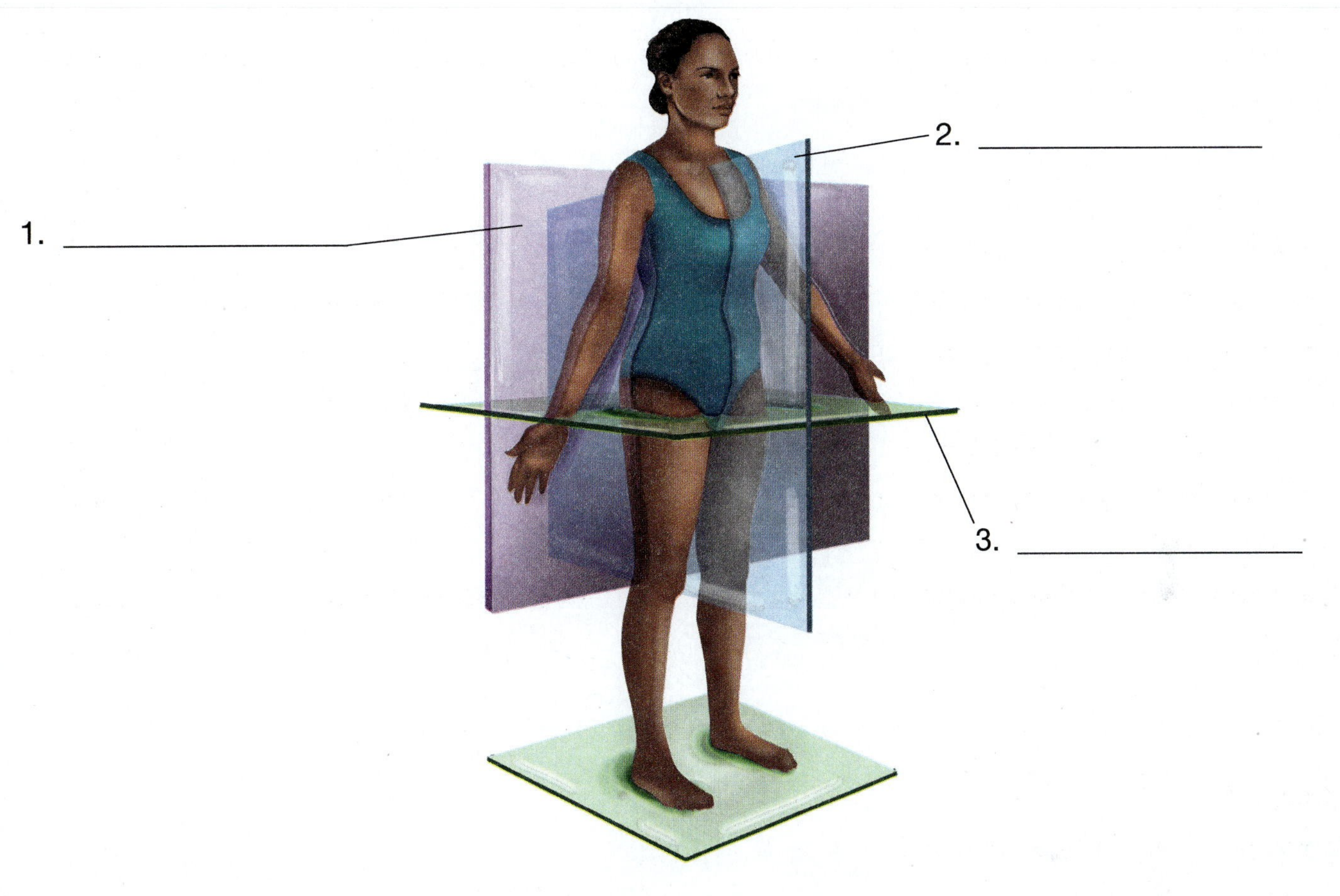

MyLab Medical Terminology™

MyLab Medical Terminology is a premium online homework management system that includes a host of features to help you study. Registered users will find:

- A multitude of activities and assignments built within the MyLab platform
- Powerful tools that track and analyze your results—allowing you to create a personalized learning experience
- Videos and audio pronunciations to help enrich your progress
- Streaming lesson presentations (Guided Lectures) and self-paced learning modules
- A space where you and your instructors can check your progress and manage your assignments

Chapter 3

Integumentary System

Learning Objectives

Upon completion of this chapter, you will be able to

1. Identify and define the combining forms, prefixes, and suffixes introduced in this chapter.
2. Correctly spell and pronounce medical terms and major anatomical structures relating to the integumentary system.
3. List and describe the four purposes of the skin.
4. Describe the layers of the skin and the subcutaneous layer and their functions.
5. List and describe the accessory organs of the skin.
6. Identify and define integumentary system anatomical terms.
7. Identify and define selected integumentary system pathology terms.
8. Identify and define selected integumentary system diagnostic procedures.
9. Identify and define selected integumentary system therapeutic procedures.
10. Identify and define selected medications relating to the integumentary system.
11. Define selected abbreviations associated with the integumentary system.

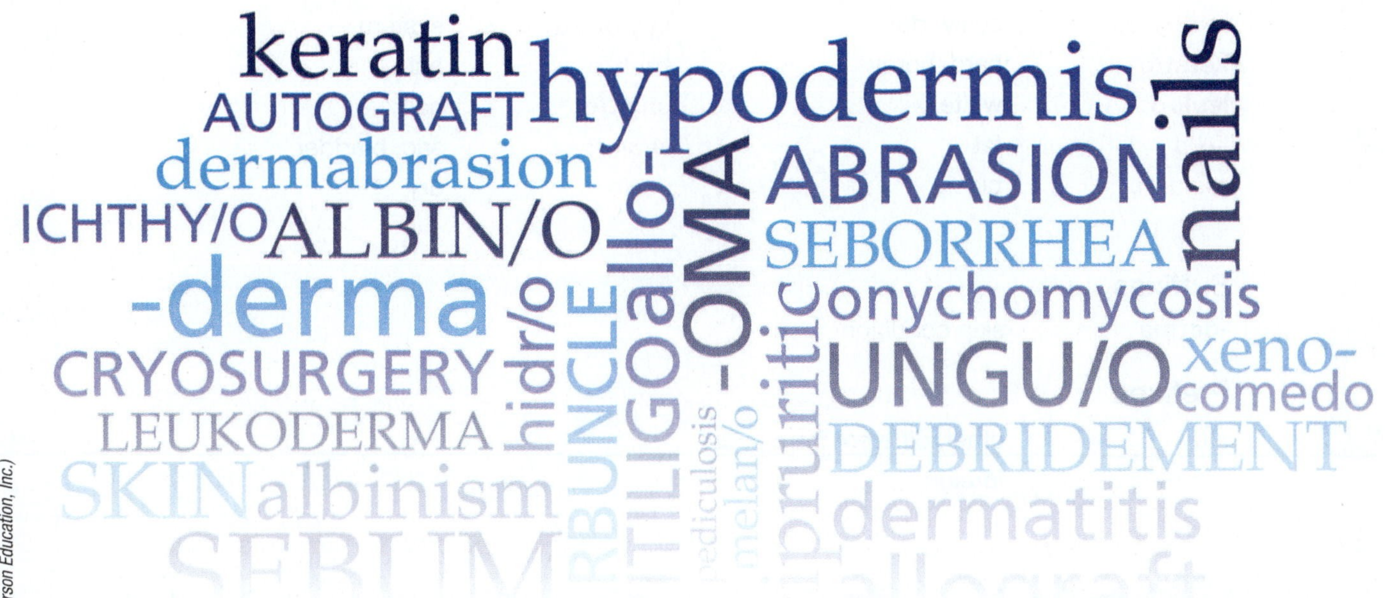

(Pearson Education, Inc.)

INTEGUMENTARY SYSTEM
AT A GLANCE

Function

The skin provides a protective two-way barrier between our internal environment and the outside world. It also plays an important role in temperature regulation, houses sensory receptors to detect the environment around us, and secretes important fluids.

Organs

The primary structures that comprise the integumentary system:

skin
hair
nails
sebaceous glands
sweat glands

Word Parts

Presented here are the most common word parts (with their meanings) used to build integumentary system terms. For a more comprehensive list, refer to the Terminology section of this chapter.

Combining Forms

albin/o	white
cauter/o	to burn
cry/o	cold
cutane/o	skin
derm/o	skin
dermat/o	skin
diaphor/o	profuse sweating
electr/o	electricity
erythr/o	red
hidr/o	sweat
ichthy/o	scaly, dry
kerat/o	hard, horny
leuk/o	white
lip/o	fat
melan/o	black
myc/o	fungus
necr/o	death
onych/o	nail
pedicul/o	lice
phot/o	light
py/o	pus
rhytid/o	wrinkle
sarc/o	flesh
scler/o	hard
seb/o	oil
system/o	system
trich/o	hair
ungu/o	nail
vesic/o	sac, bladder
xer/o	dry

Suffixes

-derma	skin condition

Prefixes

allo-	other, different from usual
xeno-	foreign

Integumentary System Illustrated

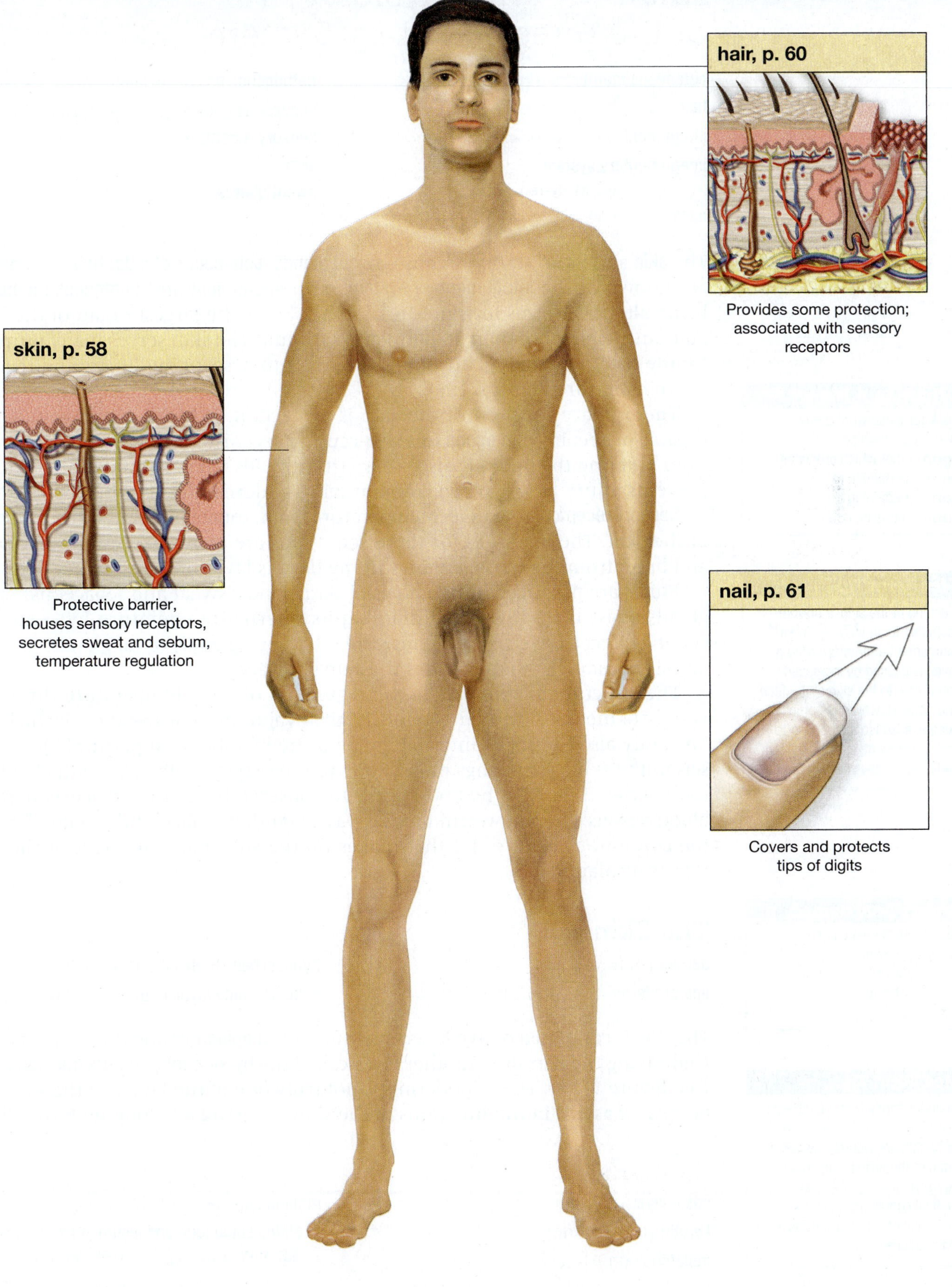

hair, p. 60
Provides some protection; associated with sensory receptors
skin, p. 58
Protective barrier, houses sensory receptors, secretes sweat and sebum, temperature regulation
nail, p. 61
Covers and protects tips of digits

Anatomy and Physiology of the Integumentary System

cutaneous membrane (kyoo-TAY-nee-us)
hair
integument (in-TEG-yoo-ment)
integumentary system (in-teg-yoo-MEN-tah-ree)
nails
pathogens (PATH-oh-jenz)
sebaceous glands (sih-BAY-shus)
sensory receptors
skin
sweat glands

The **skin** and its accessory organs—**sweat glands**, **sebaceous glands**, **hair**, and **nails**—are known as the **integumentary system**, with **integument** and **cutaneous membrane** being alternate terms for skin. In fact, the skin is the largest organ of the body and can weigh more than 20 pounds in an adult. The skin serves many purposes for the body: protecting, housing nerve receptors, secreting fluids, and regulating temperature.

The primary function of the skin is protection. It forms a two-way barrier capable of keeping **pathogens** (disease-causing organisms) and harmful chemicals from entering the body. It also stops critical fluids from escaping the body and prevents injury to the internal organs lying underneath the skin.

Sensory receptors that detect temperature, pain, touch, and pressure are located in the skin. The messages for these sensations are conveyed to the spinal cord and brain from the nerve endings in the dermis layer of the skin.

Fluids are produced in two types of skin glands: sweat and sebaceous. Sweat glands assist the body in maintaining its internal temperature by creating a cooling effect as sweat evaporates. The sebaceous glands, or oil glands, produce an oily substance that lubricates the skin's surface.

The structure of skin aids in the regulation of body temperature through a variety of means. As noted previously, the evaporation of sweat cools the body. The body also lowers its internal temperature by dilating superficial blood vessels in the skin. This brings more blood to the surface of the skin, which allows the release of heat. If the body needs to conserve heat, it constricts superficial blood vessels, keeping warm blood away from the surface of the body. Finally, the continuous layer of fat that makes up the subcutaneous layer of the skin acts as insulation.

What's In A Name?
Look for these word parts:
path/o = disease
-gen = that which produces
-ary = pertaining to
-ory = pertaining to
-ous = pertaining to

Med Term Tip
Flushing of the skin, a normal response to an increase in environmental temperature or to a fever, is caused by increased blood flow to the skin of the face and neck. However, in some people, it is also a response to embarrassment, called blushing, and is not easily controlled.

The Skin

dermis (DER-mis)
epidermis (ep-ih-DER-mis)
hypodermis (high-poh-DER-mis)
subcutaneous layer (sub-kyoo-TAY-nee-us)

The skin is composed of two layers, the superficial **epidermis** and the deeper **dermis**. Underlying the dermis is another layer called the **hypodermis**, or **subcutaneous layer** (see Figure 3-1 ■). The hypodermis is not truly one of the layers of the skin, but because it assists in the functions of the skin, it is studied along with the skin.

What's In A Name?
Look for these word parts:
derm/o = skin
epi- = above
hypo- = below
sub- = under

Med Term Tip
An understanding of the different layers of the skin is important for healthcare workers because much of the terminology relating to types of injections and medical conditions, such as burns, is described using these designations.

Epidermis

basal layer (BAY-sal)
keratin (KAIR-ah-tin)
melanin (MEL-ah-nin)
melanocytes (mel-AN-oh-sights)
stratified squamous epithelium (STRAT-ih-fyde / SKWAY-mus / ep-ih-THEE-lee-um)

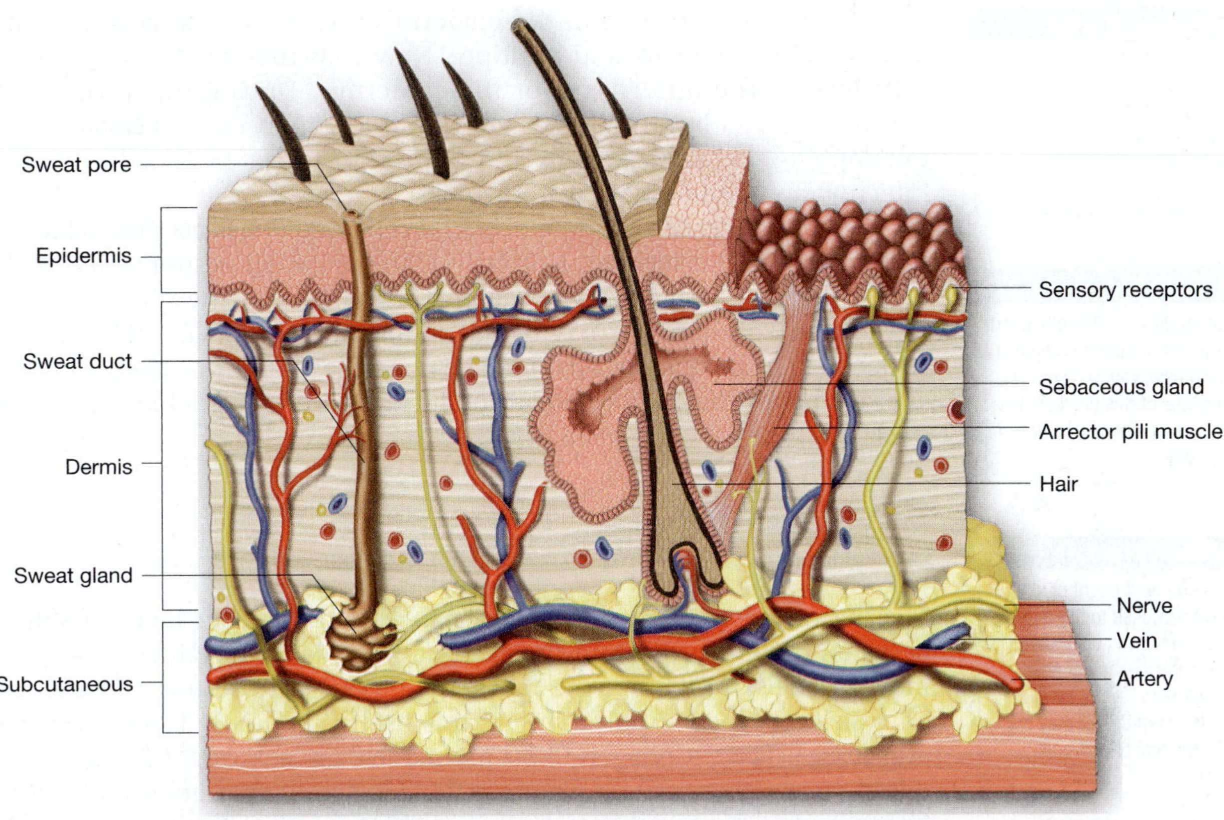

■ **Figure 3-1** Skin structure, including the layers of the skin, the subcutaneous layer, and the accessory organs: sweat gland, sebaceous gland, and hair.

The epidermis is composed of **stratified squamous epithelium** (see Figure 3-2■). This type of epithelial tissue consists of flat, scale-like cells arranged in overlapping layers or strata. The epidermis does not have a blood supply or any connective tissue, so it is dependent for nourishment on the deeper layers of skin.

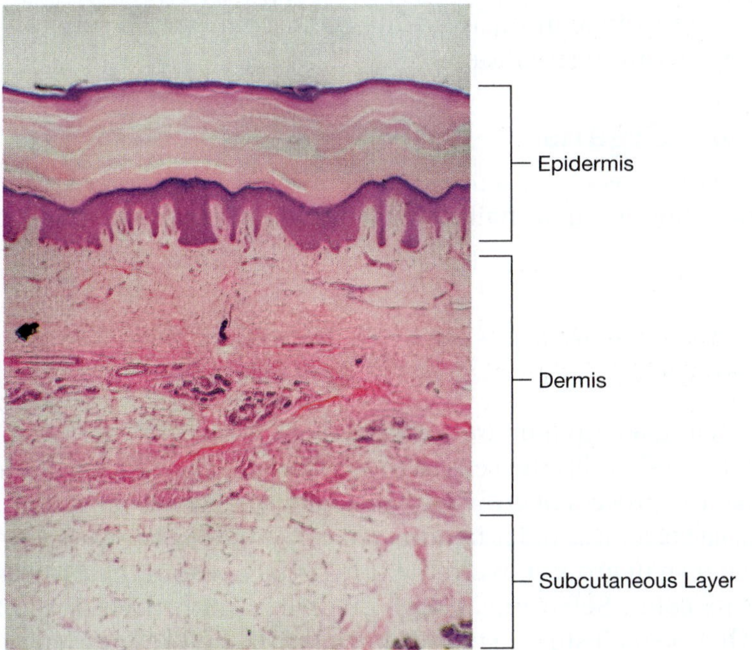

■ **Figure 3-2** Photomicrograph showing the two layers of the skin and the subcutaneous layer. *(Jubal Harshaw/ Shutterstock)*

What's In A Name?

Look for these word parts:
bas/o = base
melan/o = black
-al = pertaining to
-cyte = cell
-ous = pertaining to

Med Term Tip

We lose 30,000–50,000 old, dead skin cells per minute and replace them with new, younger cells. In fact, because of this process, the epidermis is completely replaced every 25 days.

Med Term Tip

A suntan can be thought of as a protective response to the rays of the sun. However, when the melanin in the skin is not able to absorb all the rays of the sun, the skin burns and DNA may be permanently and dangerously damaged.

Med Term Tip

Ridges formed in the dermis of our fingertips are what give each of us unique fingerprints. These do not change during a person's lifetime and so are a reliable means of identification. In fact, fingerprints are still visible on Egyptian mummies.

What's In A Name?

Look for these word parts:
lip/o = fat
-cyte = cell

Med Term Tip

Our hair turns gray as part of the normal aging process as the body produces less melanin (or white if little to no melanin is produced).

The deepest layer within the epidermis is called the **basal layer.** Cells in this layer continually grow and multiply. New cells that are forming push the old cells toward the outer layer of the epidermis. During this process, the cells shrink, die, and become filled with a hard protein called **keratin.** These dead, overlapping, keratinized cells allow the skin to act as an effective barrier to infection and also make it waterproof.

The basal layer also contains special cells called **melanocytes**, which produce the black pigment **melanin.** Not only is this pigment responsible for the color of the skin, but it also protects against damage from the ultraviolet (UV) rays of the sun. This damage may be in the form of leather-like skin and wrinkles, which are not hazardous, or it may be one of several forms of skin cancer. Dark-skinned people have more melanin and are generally less likely to get wrinkles or skin cancer.

Dermis

collagen fibers (KOL-ah-jen)
corium (KOH-ree-um)

The dermis, also referred to as the **corium**, is the deeper layer of skin, located between the epidermis and the subcutaneous layer (see Figure 3-2). Its name means "true skin." Unlike the thinner epidermis, the dermis is living tissue with an excellent blood supply. The dermis itself is composed of connective tissue and **collagen fibers.** Collagen fibers are made from a strong, fibrous protein present in connective tissue, forming a flexible "glue" that gives connective tissue its strength. The dermis houses hair follicles, sweat glands, sebaceous glands, blood vessels, lymph vessels, sensory receptors, nerve fibers, and muscle fibers.

Subcutaneous Layer

lipocytes (LIP-oh-sights)

The subcutaneous layer (or hypodermis) is a continuous layer of fat that separates the dermis from deeper tissues (see Figure 3-2). Composed of fat cells called **lipocytes**, its functions include protecting deeper tissues of the body from trauma, acting as insulation from heat and cold, and serving as a source of energy in a starvation situation.

Accessory Organs

The accessory organs of the skin are the anatomical structures located within the dermis, including the hair, nails, sebaceous glands, and sweat glands.

Hair

arrector pili (ah-REK-tor / pie-lie)
hair follicle (FALL-ih-kl)
hair root
hair shaft

The fibers that make up hair are composed of the protein keratin, the same hard protein material that fills the cells of the epidermis. The process of hair formation is much like the process of growth in the epidermal layer of the skin. The deeper cells in the **hair root** force older keratinized cells to move upward, forming the **hair shaft.** The hair shaft grows toward the skin surface within the **hair follicle.** Melanin gives hair its color. Sebaceous glands release oil directly into the hair follicle. Each hair has a small slip of smooth muscle attached to it called the **arrector pili** muscle (see Figure 3-3 ■). When this muscle contracts, the hair shaft stands up, resulting in "goose bumps."

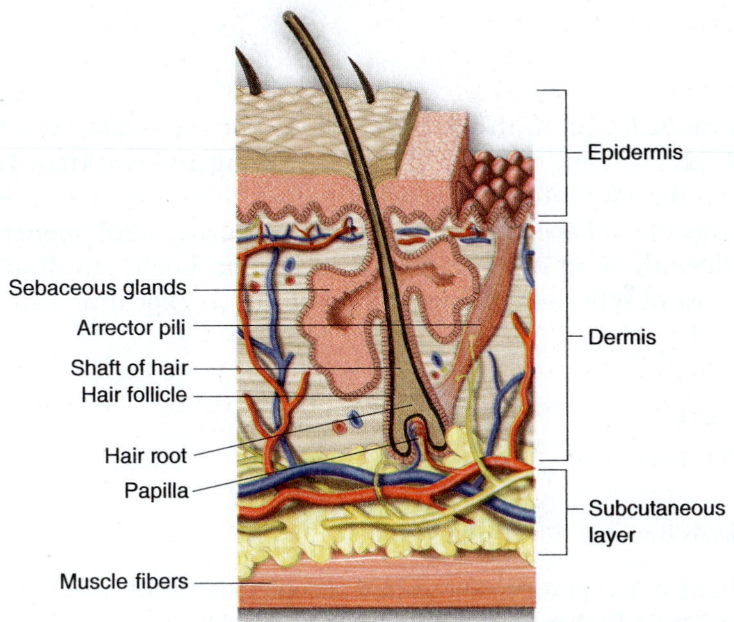

■ **Figure 3-3** Structure of a hair and its associated sebaceous gland.

Nails

cuticle (KYOO-tih-kl)
free edge
lunula (LOO-nyoo-lah)
nail bed
nail body
nail root

Nails are a flat plate of keratin called the **nail body** that covers the top ends of fingers and toes. The nail body is connected to the tissue underneath by the **nail bed**. Nails grow longer from the **nail root**, which is found at the base of the nail and is covered and protected by the soft tissue **cuticle**. The **free edge** is the exposed edge that is trimmed when nails become too long. The light-colored half-moon area at the base of the nail is the **lunula** (see Figure 3-4 ■).

Med Term Tip

Because of its rich blood supply and light color, the nail bed is an excellent place to check patients for low oxygen levels in their blood. Deoxygenated blood is a very dark purple-red and gives skin a bluish tinge called *cyanosis*.

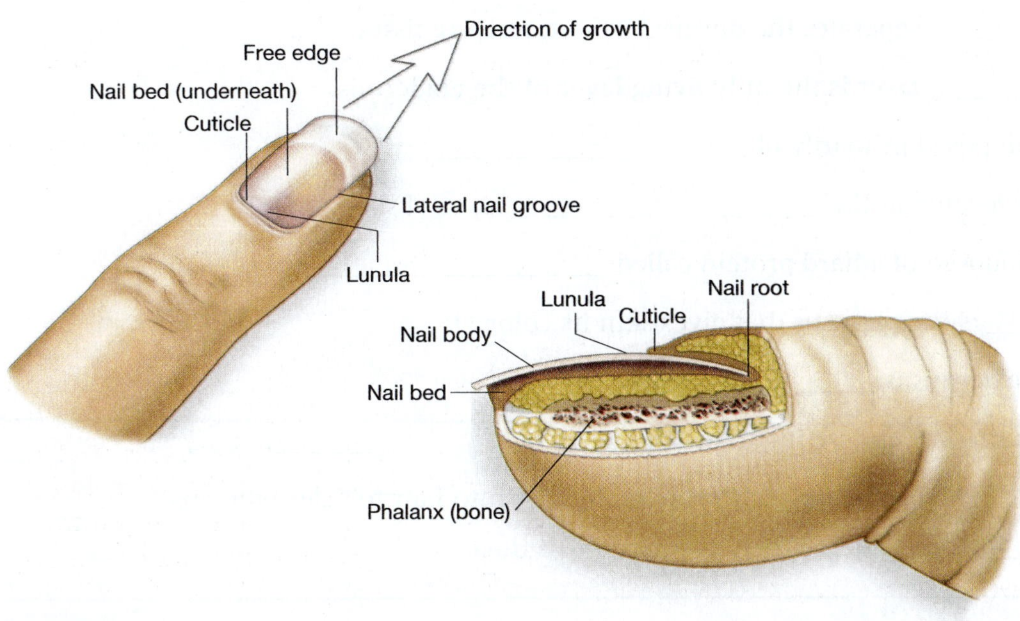

■ **Figure 3-4** External and internal structures of nails.

Sebaceous Glands

sebum

Sebaceous glands, found in the dermis, secrete the oil **sebum**, which lubricates the hair and skin, thereby helping to prevent drying and cracking. These glands secrete sebum directly into hair follicles, rather than a duct (see Figure 3-1). Secretion from the sebaceous glands increases during adolescence, playing a role in the development of acne. Sebum secretion begins to diminish as age increases. A loss of sebum in old age, along with sun exposure, can account for wrinkles and dry skin.

Sweat Glands

apocrine glands (AP-oh-krin)
perspiration
sudoriferous glands (soo-doh-RIF-er-us)
sweat duct
sweat pore

What's In A Name?
Look for these word parts:
crin/o = to secrete
-ous = pertaining to

Word Watch
Be careful when using **hydr/o** meaning *water* and **hidr/o** meaning *sweat.*

About 2 million sweat glands, also called **sudoriferous glands**, are found throughout the body. These highly coiled glands are located in the dermis. Sweat travels to the surface of the skin through a **sweat duct**. The surface opening of a sweat duct is called a **sweat pore** (see Figure 3-1).

Sweat glands function to cool the body as sweat evaporates. Sweat or **perspiration** contains a small amount of waste products but is normally colorless and odorless. However, there are sweat glands called **apocrine glands** in the pubic and underarm areas that secrete a thicker sweat, which can produce an odor when it comes into contact with bacteria on the skin. This is what is recognized as body odor.

PRACTICE AS YOU GO

A. Complete the Statement

1. The two layers of skin are the superficial ____________________ and deeper ____________________.
2. The ____________________ separates the dermis from underlying tissue.
3. The ____________________ layer is the only living layer of the epidermis.
4. The hypodermis is composed primarily of ____________________.
5. Sensory receptors are located in the ____________________ layer of skin.
6. Nails and hair are composed of a hard protein called ____________________.
7. ____________________ is the pigment that gives skin its color.
8. Another name for the dermis is ____________________.
9. The nail body is connected to underlying tissue by the ____________________.
10. ____________________ glands release their product directly into hair follicles whereas ____________________ glands release their product into a duct.

Terminology

Word Parts Used to Build Integumentary System Terms

The following lists contain the combining forms, suffixes, and prefixes used to build terms in the remaining sections of this chapter.

Combining Forms

Combining Form	Meaning
albin/o	white
angi/o (see Chapter 5)	vessel
bas/o	base
bi/o	life
carcin/o	cancer
cauter/o	to burn
chem/o	chemical
cis/o	to cut
cortic/o (see Chapter 4)	outer layer
cry/o	cold
cutane/o	skin
cyt/o	cell
derm/o	skin
dermat/o	skin
diaphor/o	profuse sweating
electr/o	electricity
erythr/o	red
esthesi/o (see Chapter 12)	feeling
hem/o (see Chapter 6)	blood
hidr/o	sweat
ichthy/o	scaly, dry
kerat/o	hard, horny
leuk/o	white
lip/o	fat
melan/o	black
myc/o	fungus
necr/o	death
onych/o	nail
pedicul/o	lice
phot/o	light
py/o	pus
rhytid/o	wrinkle
sarc/o	flesh
scler/o	hard
seb/o	oil
septic/o (see Chapter 6)	infection
system/o	system
trich/o	hair
ungu/o	nail
vesic/o	sac
xer/o	dry

Suffixes

Suffix	Meaning
-al	pertaining to
-derma	skin condition
-ectomy	surgical removal
-emia (see Chapter 6)	blood condition
-ia	state, condition
-iasis	abnormal condition
-ic	pertaining to
-ism	state of
-itis	inflammation
-logy	study of
-malacia	abnormal softening
-oma	mass, tumor
-opsy	view of
-osis	abnormal condition
-ous	pertaining to
-phagia (see Chapter 8)	eat, swallow
-plasty	surgical repair
-rrhea	discharge
-tic	pertaining to
-tome	instrument to cut
-ule	small

Prefixes

Prefix	Meaning
allo-	other
an-	without
anti-	against
auto-	self
de-	without
epi-	above
ex-	outward
hyper-	excessive
hypo-	below
intra-	within
para-	beside
sub-	under
xeno-	foreign

Adjective Forms of Anatomical Terms

Term	Word Parts	Definition
cutaneous (kyoo-TAY-nee-us)	cutane/o = skin -ous = pertaining to	Pertaining to skin
dermal (DER-mal)	derm/o = skin -al = pertaining to	Pertaining to skin
dermic (DER-mik)	derm/o = skin -ic = pertaining to	Pertaining to skin
epidermal (ep-ih-DER-mal)	epi- = above derm/o = skin -al = pertaining to	Pertaining to above [upon] skin
hypodermic (high-poh-DER-mik)	hypo- = below derm/o = skin -ic = pertaining to	Pertaining to below skin
intradermal (ID) (in-trah-DER-mal)	intra- = within derm/o = skin -al = pertaining to	Pertaining to within skin
subcutaneous (subcut) (sub-kyoo-TAY-nee-us)	sub- = under cutane/o = skin -ous = pertaining to	Pertaining to under skin
ungual (UNG-gwal)	ungu/o = nail -al = pertaining to	Pertaining to nails

PRACTICE AS YOU GO

B. Give the adjective form for each anatomical structure.

1. A nail ______________________________

2. The skin ______________ or ______________

3. Above the skin ______________________________

4. Below the skin ______________ or ______________

5. Within the skin ______________________________

Pathology

Term	Word Parts	Definition
Medical Specialties		
dermatology (Derm, derm) (der-mah-TALL-oh-jee)	dermat/o = skin -logy = study of	Branch of medicine involving diagnosis and treatment of conditions and diseases of the integumentary system; physician is a *dermatologist*
plastic surgery		Surgical specialty involved in repair, reconstruction, or improvement of body structures such as damaged, missing, or misshapen skin; physician is a *plastic surgeon*
Signs and Symptoms		
abrasion (ah-BRAY-zhun)		A scraping-away of skin surface by friction
anhidrosis (an-high-DROH-sis)	an- = without hidr/o = sweat -osis = abnormal condition	Abnormal condition of no sweat
bulla (BUL-luh)	*Bulla* is the Latin term for bubble	Large blister; larger than a vesicle
comedo (KOM-ee-doh)		Collection of hardened sebum in hair follicle; also called a *blackhead*
contusion		Injury caused by a blow to the body; causes swelling, pain, and bruising; skin is not broken
cyst (SIST) ■ **Figure 3-5** Cyst.		Fluid-filled sac under the skin
depigmentation (dee-pig-men-TAY-shun)	de- = without	Loss of normal skin color or pigment
diaphoresis (dye-ah-foh-REE-sis)	diaphor/o = profuse sweating	Profuse sweating
ecchymosis (ek-ih-MOH-sis) ■ **Figure 3-6** Male lying supine with large ecchymosis on lateral rib cage and shoulder. *(Michal Heron/Pearson Education, Inc.)*	-osis = abnormal condition	Skin discoloration caused by blood collecting under the skin following blunt trauma to the skin; a bruise

Pathology (continued)

Term	Word Parts	Definition
erythema (air-ih-THEE-mah)	erythr/o = red hem/o = blood	Redness or flushing of skin
erythroderma (eh-rith-roh-DER-mah)	erythr/o = red -derma = skin condition	Condition of having reddened or flushed skin
eschar (ES-kar)		Thick layer of dead tissue and tissue fluid that develops over deep burn area
fissure (FISH-er) ■ **Figure 3-7** Fissure.		Crack-like lesion or groove on skin
hirsutism (HER-soo-tizm)	-ism = state of	Excessive hair growth over body
hyperemia (high-per-EE-mee-ah)	hyper- = excessive -emia = blood condition	Redness of skin due to increased blood flow
hyperhidrosis (high-per-high-DROH-sis)	hyper- = excessive hidr/o = sweat -osis = abnormal condition	Abnormal condition of excessive sweat
hyperpigmentation (high-per-pig-men-TAY-shun)	hyper- = excessive	Abnormal amount of pigmentation in skin
lesion (LEE-zhun)		General term for wound, injury, or abnormality
leukoderma (loo-koh-DER-mah)	leuk/o = white -derma = skin condition	Having skin that appears white because normal skin pigment is absent; may be all of the skin or just in some areas
lipoma (lih-POH-mah)	lip/o = fat -oma = mass	Fatty mass
macule (MAK-yool) ■ **Figure 3-8** Macule.	-ule = small	Flat, discolored area flush with skin surface; example would be freckle or birthmark

Pathology (continued)

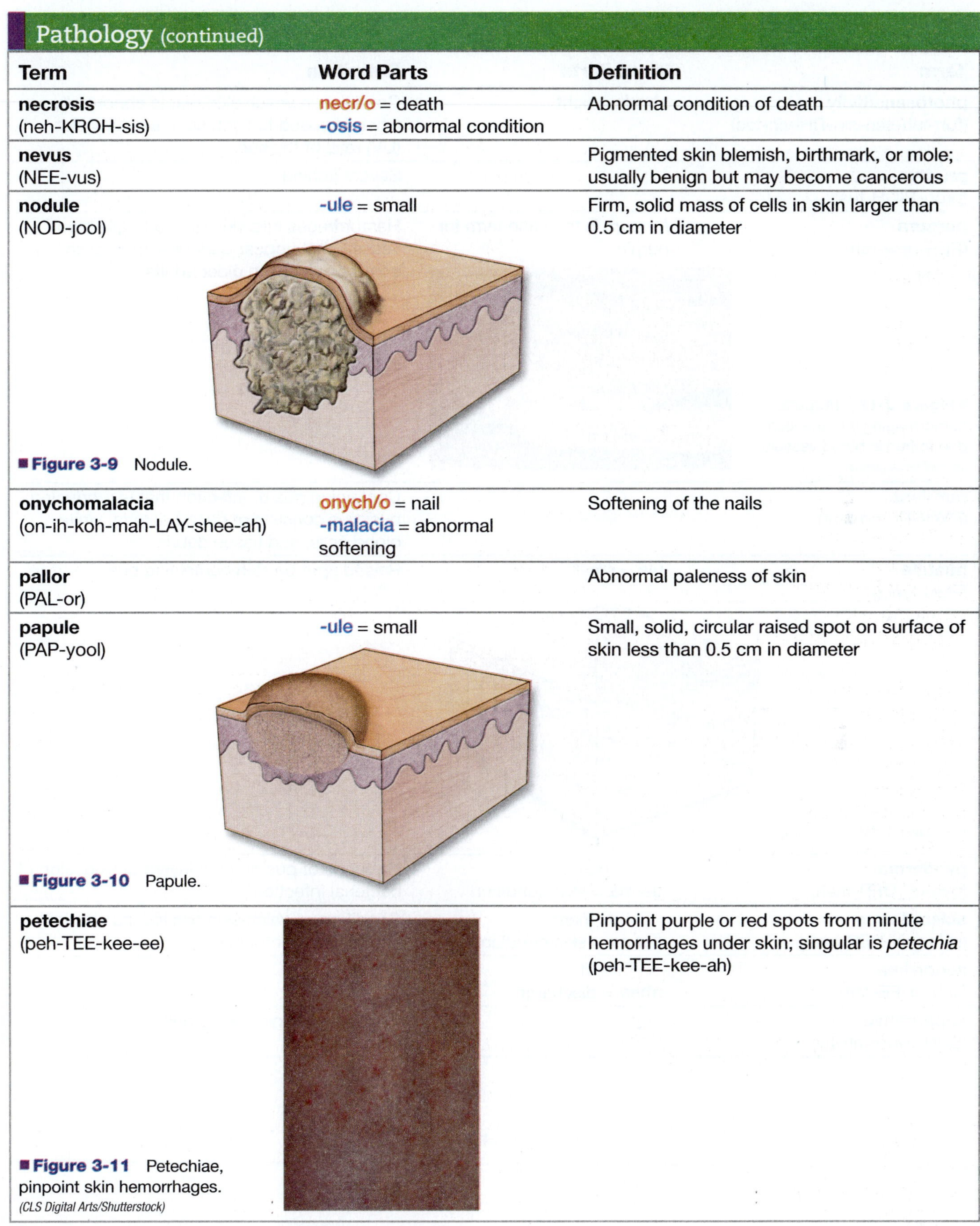

Term	Word Parts	Definition
necrosis (neh-KROH-sis)	necr/o = death -osis = abnormal condition	Abnormal condition of death
nevus (NEE-vus)		Pigmented skin blemish, birthmark, or mole; usually benign but may become cancerous
nodule (NOD-jool) ■ **Figure 3-9** Nodule.	-ule = small	Firm, solid mass of cells in skin larger than 0.5 cm in diameter
onychomalacia (on-ih-koh-mah-LAY-shee-ah)	onych/o = nail -malacia = abnormal softening	Softening of the nails
pallor (PAL-or)		Abnormal paleness of skin
papule (PAP-yool) ■ **Figure 3-10** Papule.	-ule = small	Small, solid, circular raised spot on surface of skin less than 0.5 cm in diameter
petechiae (peh-TEE-kee-ee) ■ **Figure 3-11** Petechiae, pinpoint skin hemorrhages. *(CLS Digital Arts/Shutterstock)*		Pinpoint purple or red spots from minute hemorrhages under skin; singular is *petechia* (peh-TEE-kee-ah)

Pathology (continued)

Term	Word Parts	Definition
photosensitivity (foh-toh-sen-sih-TIH-vih-tee)	**phot/o** = light	Condition in which skin reacts abnormally when exposed to light, such as ultraviolet (UV) rays of the sun
pruritus (proo-RIGH-tus)		Severe itching
purpura (PER-pew-rah)	*Purpura* is the Latin term for purple 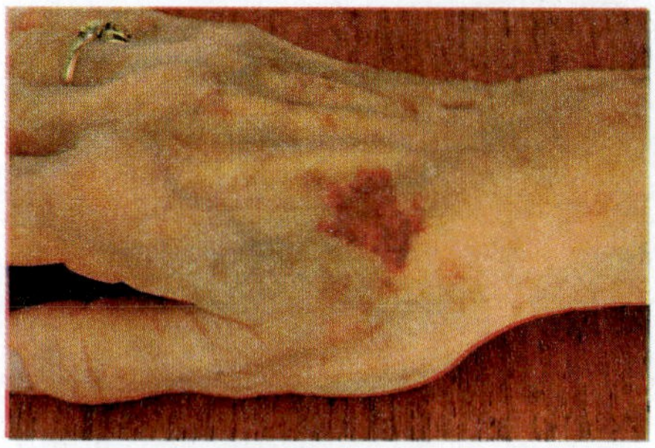	Hemorrhages into skin due to fragile blood vessels that appear dark brown/purplish; commonly seen in older adults
■ **Figure 3-12** Purpura, hemorrhaging into the skin due to fragile blood vessels. *(Scimat/Science Source)*		
purulent (PYOOR-yoo-lent)		Containing pus or infection that is producing pus; pus consists of dead bacteria, white blood cells, and tissue debris
pustule (PUS-tyool)	**-ule** = small 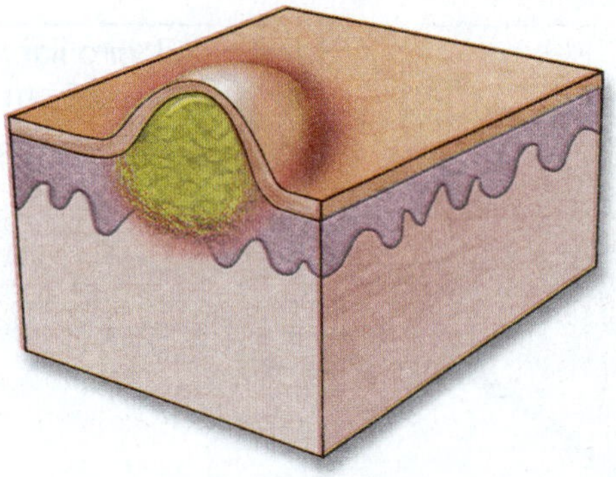	Raised spot on skin containing pus
■ **Figure 3-13** Pustule.		
pyoderma (pye-oh-DER-mah)	**py/o** = pus **-derma** = skin condition	Presence of pus on or in layers of skin; sign of bacterial infection
scleroderma (sklair-ah-DER-mah)	**scler/o** = hard **-derma** = skin condition	Condition in which skin has lost its elasticity and become hardened
seborrhea (seb-or-EE-ah)	**seb/o** = oil **-rrhea** = discharge	Oily discharge
suppurative (SUP-pyoor-ah-tiv)		Containing or producing pus

Pathology (continued)

Term	Word Parts	Definition
ulcer (UL-ser) 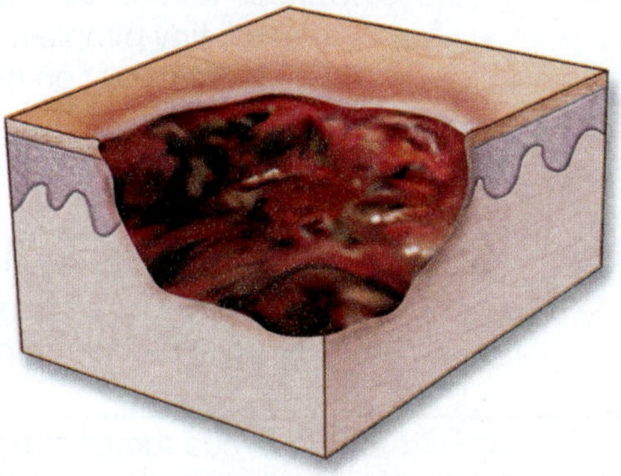 ■ **Figure 3-14** Ulcer.		Open sore or lesion in skin or mucous membrane
urticaria (er-tih-KAIR-ee-ah)	-ia = state, condition	Also called *hives*; skin eruption of pale reddish wheals with severe itching; usually associated with food allergy, stress, or drug reactions
vesicle (VES-ih-kl) 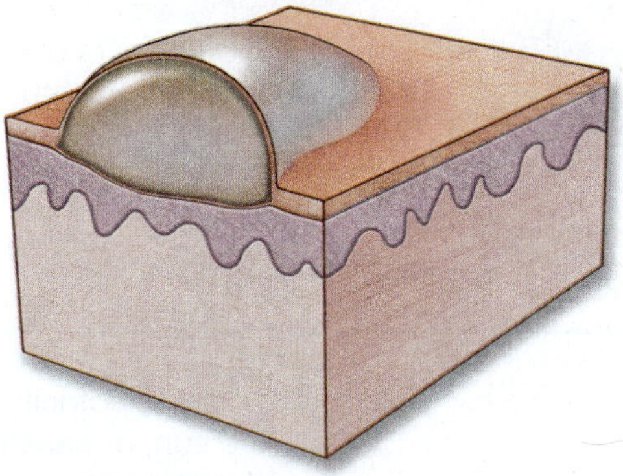 ■ **Figure 3-15** Vesicle.	vesic/o = sac	Blister; small, fluid-filled raised spot on skin
wheal (HWEEL) 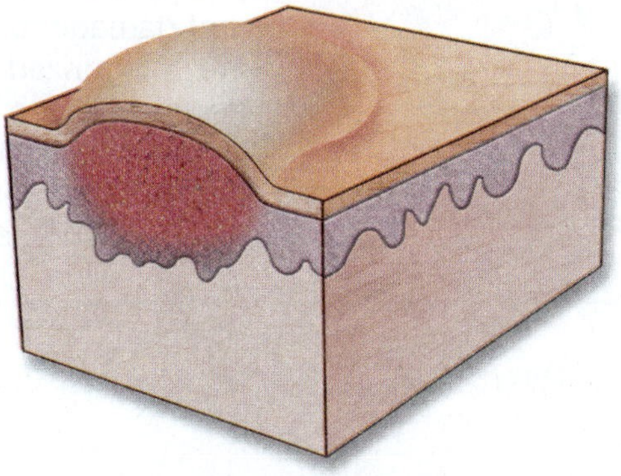 ■ **Figure 3-16** Wheal.		Small, round, swollen area on skin; typically seen in allergic skin reactions such as *hives* and usually accompanied by urticaria
xeroderma (zeer-oh-DER-mah)	xer/o = dry -derma = skin condition	Condition in which skin is abnormally dry
Skin		
abscess (AB-sess)		Collection of pus in skin
acne (AK-nee)		Inflammatory disease of sebaceous glands and hair follicles resulting in papules and pustules

Pathology (continued)

Term	Word Parts	Definition
acne rosacea (AK-nee / roh-ZAY-shee-ah)		Chronic form of acne seen in adults involving redness, tiny pimples, and broken blood vessels, primarily on nose and cheeks
acne vulgaris (AK-nee / vul-GAIR-is)		Common form of acne seen in teenagers; characterized by comedos, papules, and pustules
albinism (AL-bih-nizm)	albin/o = white -ism = state of	Genetic condition in which body is unable to make melanin; characterized by white hair and skin and red pupils due to lack of pigment
basal cell carcinoma (BCC) (BAY-sal / sell / kar-sih-NOH-mah)	bas/o = base -al = pertaining to carcin/o = cancer -oma = tumor	Cancerous tumor of basal cell layer of epidermis; frequent type of skin cancer that rarely metastasizes or spreads; these cancers can arise on sun-exposed skin
■ **Figure 3-17** Basal cell carcinoma. A frequent type of skin cancer that rarely metastasizes. *(Centers for Disease Control and Prevention)*		
burn		Damage to skin that can result from exposure to open fire, electricity, ultraviolet (UV) light from the sun, or caustic chemicals; seriousness depends on amount of body surface involved and depth of burn as determined by amount of damage to each layer; skin and burns are categorized as first-degree (superficial), second-degree (partial thickness), or third-degree (full thickness); see Figure 3-18 ■ for a description of damage associated with each degree of burn; extent of burn is estimated using Rule of Nines (see Figure 3-19 ■)

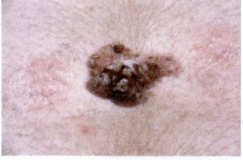

Pathology (continued)

Term	Word Parts	Definition

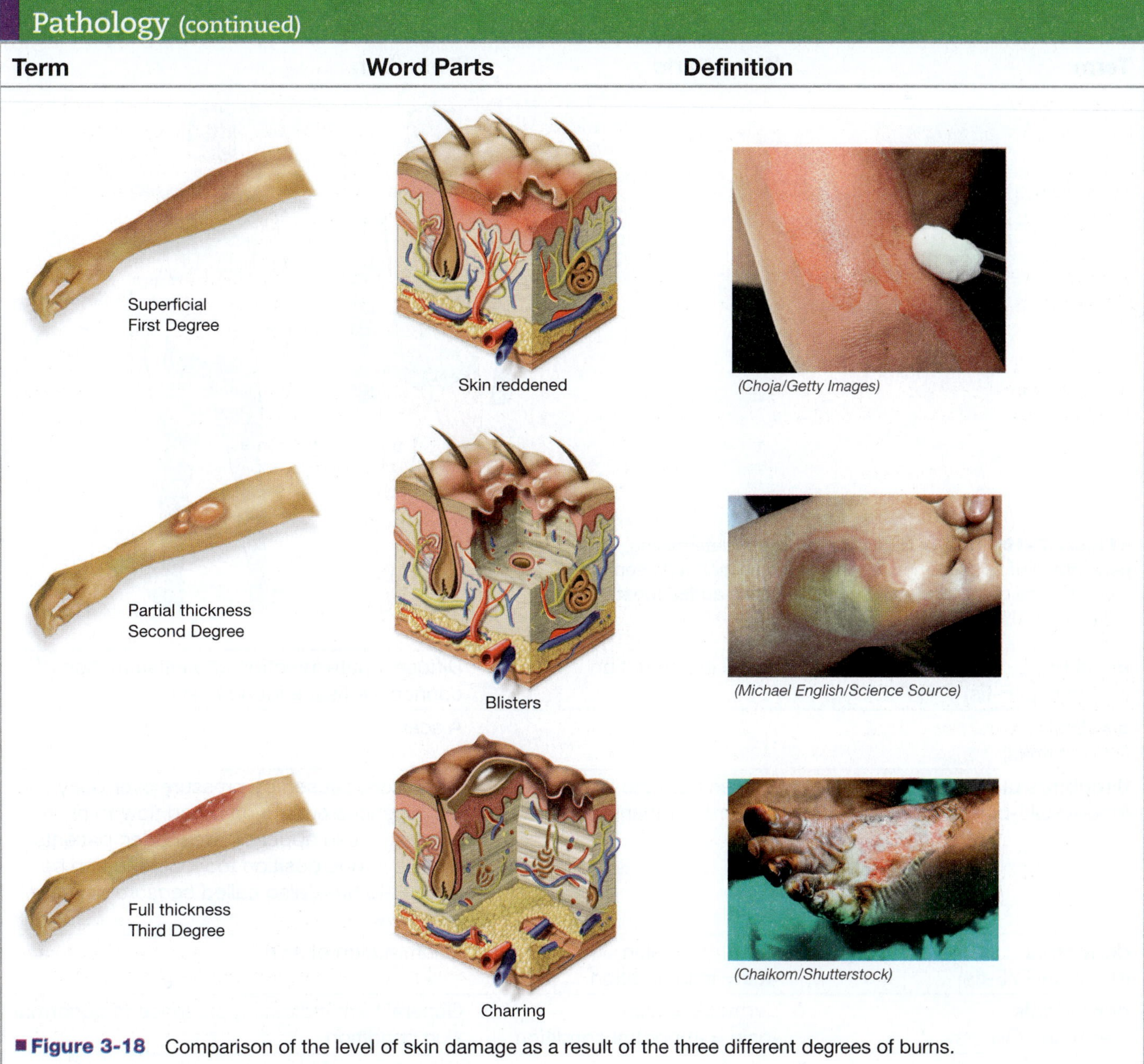

■ **Figure 3-18** Comparison of the level of skin damage as a result of the three different degrees of burns.

Pathology (continued)

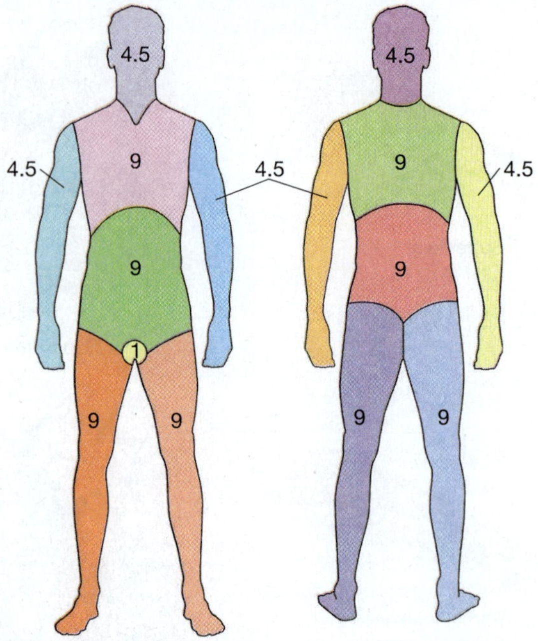

■ **Figure 3-19** Rule of Nines. A method for determining percentage of body burned. Each colored section represents a percentage of the body surface. All sections added together will equal 100%.

Term	Word Parts	Definition
cellulitis (sell-yoo-LYE-tis)	-itis = inflammation	Diffuse, acute infection and inflammation of connective tissue found in skin
cicatrix (SIK-ah-triks)		A scar
decubitus ulcer (decub) (dee-KYOO-bih-tus)	Comes from the Latin word *decumbo*, meaning *lying down*	Open sore caused by pressure over bony prominences cutting off blood flow to overlying skin; can appear in bedridden patients who lie in one position too long and can be difficult to heal; also called *bedsore* or *pressure sore*
dermatitis (der-mah-TYE-tis)	dermat/o = skin -itis = inflammation	Inflammation of skin
dermatosis (der-mah-TOH-sis)	dermat/o = skin -osis = abnormal condition	General term indicating presence of abnormal skin condition
dry gangrene (GANG-green)		Late stages of gangrene characterized by affected area becoming dried, blackened, and shriveled; referred to as *mummified*
eczema (EK-zeh-mah)		Superficial dermatitis of unknown cause accompanied by redness, vesicles, itching, and crusting
gangrene (GANG-green)		Tissue necrosis usually due to deficient blood supply
ichthyosis (ik-thee-OH-sis)	ichthy/o = scaly, dry -osis = abnormal condition	Condition in which skin becomes dry, scaly, and keratinized

Pathology (continued)

Term	Word Parts	Definition
impetigo (im-peh-TYE-goh)		Highly infectious bacterial infection of skin with pustules that rupture and become crusted over
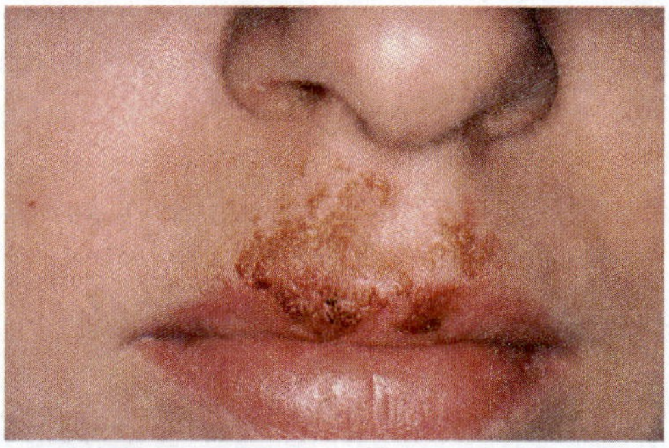 ■ **Figure 3-20** Impetigo, a highly contagious bacterial infection. *(Biophoto Associates/Science Source/Getty Images)*		
Kaposi's sarcoma (KAP-oh-seez / sar-KOH-mah)	sarc/o = flesh -oma = tumor	Form of skin cancer frequently seen in acquired immunodeficiency syndrome (AIDS) patients; consists of brownish-purple papules that spread from skin and metastasize to internal organs
keloid (KEE-loyd)		Formation of raised and thickened hypertrophic scar after injury or surgery
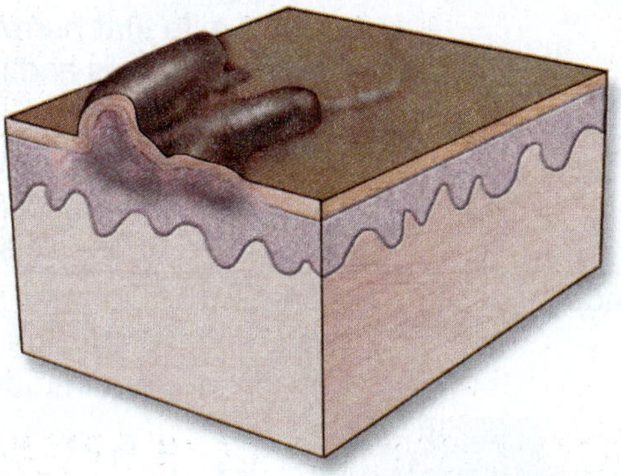 ■ **Figure 3-21** Keloid.		
keratosis (kair-ah-TOH-sis)	kerat/o = hard, horny -osis = abnormal condition	Term for any skin condition involving overgrowth and thickening of epidermis layer
laceration (lass-er-AY-shun)		Torn or jagged wound; incorrectly used to describe a cut
malignant melanoma (MM) (mah-LIG-nant / mel-ah-NOH-mah)	melan/o = black -oma = tumor	Dangerous form of skin cancer caused by uncontrolled growth of melanocytes; may quickly metastasize or spread to internal organs
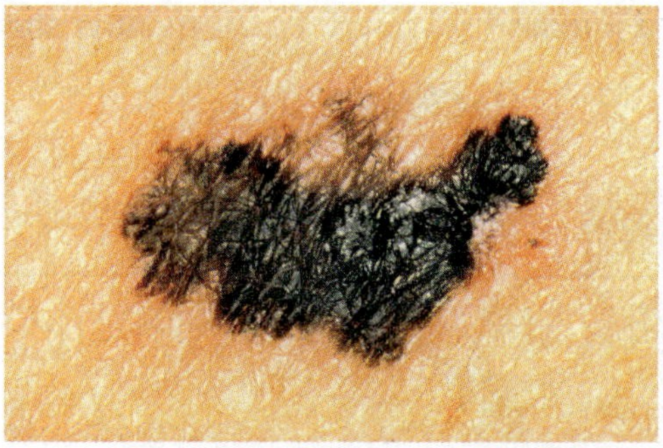 ■ **Figure 3-22** Malignant melanoma. This photograph demonstrates the highly characteristic color of this tumor. *(National Cancer Institute)*		

Pathology (continued)

Term	Word Parts	Definition
pediculosis (peh-dik-yoo-LOH-sis)	pedicul/o = lice -osis = abnormal condition	Infestation with lice; eggs laid by lice are called *nits* and cling tightly to hair
psoriasis (soh-RYE-ah-sis)	-iasis = abnormal condition	Chronic inflammatory condition consisting of papules forming "silvery scale" patches with circular borders
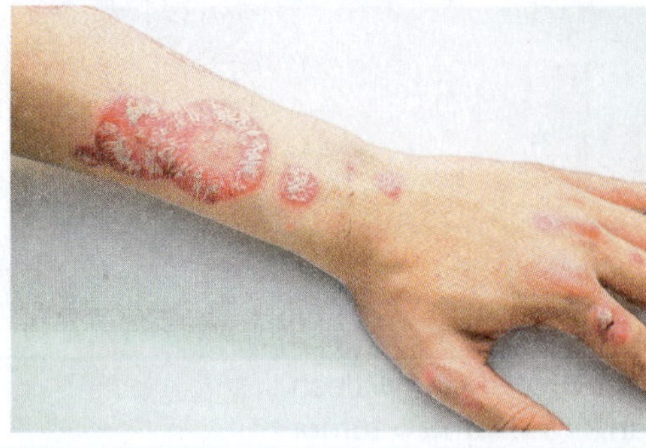 ■ **Figure 3-23** This photograph demonstrates the "silvery scale" circular patches that are characteristic of psoriasis. *(Baworn47/Shutterstock)*		
rubella (roo-BELL-ah)		Contagious viral skin infection; commonly called *German measles*
scabies (SKAY-bees)		Contagious skin disease caused by egg-laying mite that burrows through skin and causes redness and intense itching; often seen in children
sebaceous cyst (sih-BAY-shus / SIST)	seb/o = oil	Sac under skin filled with sebum or oil from sebaceous gland; can grow to large size and may need to be excised
squamous cell carcinoma (SCC) (SKWAY-mus / sell / kar-sih-NOH-mah)	carcin/o = cancer -oma = tumor	Cancer of epidermis layer of skin that may invade deeper tissue and metastasize; often begins as sore that does not heal
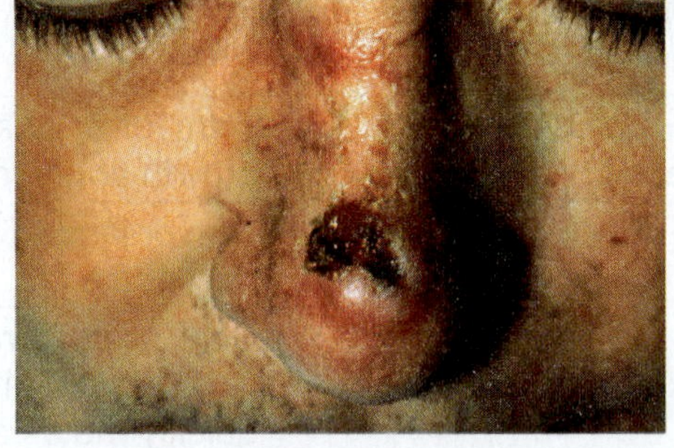 ■ **Figure 3-24** Squamous cell carcinoma. *(National Cancer Institute)*		
strawberry hemangioma (hee-man-jee-OH-mah)	hem/o = blood angi/o = vessel -oma = mass	Congenital collection of dilated blood vessels causing red birthmark that fades a few months after birth
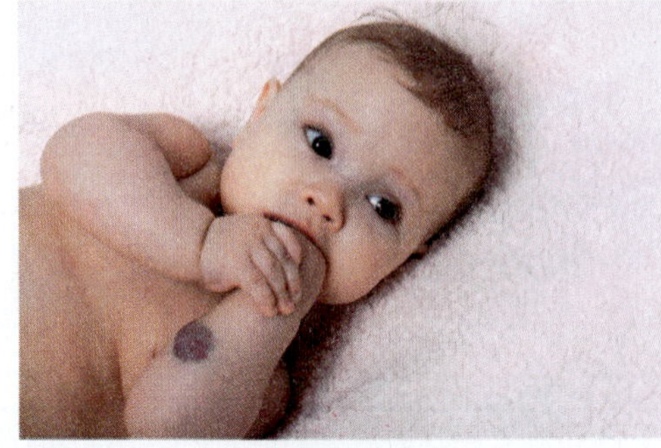 ■ **Figure 3-25** Strawberry hemangioma, a birthmark caused by a collection of blood vessels in the skin. *(Gordana Sermek/Shutterstock)*		

Pathology (continued)

Term	Word Parts	Definition
systemic lupus erythematosus (SLE) (sis-TEM-ik / LOO-pus / air-ih-them-ah-TOH-sus)	system/o = system -ic = pertaining to erythr/o = red	Chronic disease of connective tissue that injures skin, joints, kidneys, nervous system, and mucous membranes; autoimmune condition meaning that body's own immune system attacks normal tissue of body; may produce characteristic red, scaly butterfly rash across cheeks and nose
tinea (TIN-ee-ah)		Fungal skin disease resulting in itching, scaling lesions
tinea capitis (TIN-ee-ah / KAP-ih-tis)	*Capitis* is the Latin term for the head	Fungal infection of scalp; commonly called *ringworm*
tinea pedis (TIN-ee-ah / PEE-dis)	*Pedis* is the Latin term for the foot	Fungal infection of foot; commonly called *athlete's foot*
varicella (vair-ih-SELL-ah)		Contagious viral skin infection; commonly called *chickenpox*
■ **Figure 3-26** Varicella or chickenpox, a viral skin infection. In this photograph, the rash is beginning to form scabs. *(Beneda Miroslav/Shutterstock)*		
verruca (ver-ROO-kah)		Commonly called *warts*; benign growth caused by virus; has rough surface removed by chemicals and/or laser therapy
vitiligo (vit-ill-EYE-goh)		Disappearance of pigment from skin in patches, causing milk-white appearance; also called *leukoderma*
wet gangrene (GANG-green)		Area of gangrene that becomes secondarily infected by pus-producing bacteria
Hair		
alopecia (al-oh-PEE-shee-ah)		Absence or loss of hair, especially of head; commonly called *baldness*
carbuncle (KAR-bung-kl)		Furuncle involving several hair follicles
furuncle (FYOO-rung-kl)		Bacterial infection of hair follicle; characterized by redness, pain, and swelling; also called a *boil*
trichomycosis (trik-oh-my-KOH-sis)	trich/o = hair myc/o = fungus -osis = abnormal condition	Abnormal condition of hair fungus

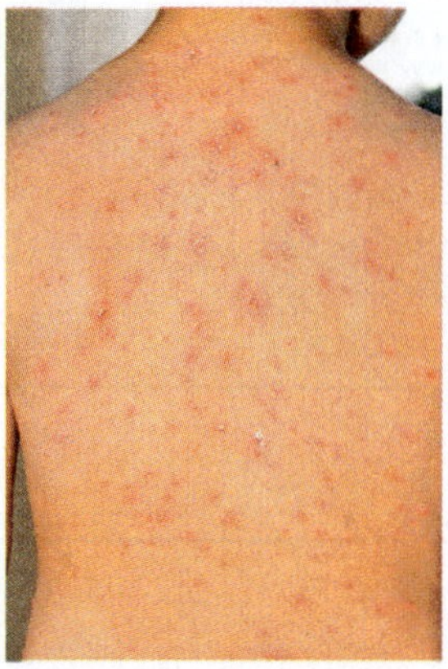

Pathology (continued)

Term	Word Parts	Definition
Nails		
onychia (oh-NIK-ee-ah)	onych/o = nail -ia = state, condition	Infected nail bed
onychomycosis (on-ih-koh-my-KOH-sis)	onych/o = nail myc/o = fungus -osis = abnormal condition	Abnormal condition of nail fungus
onychophagia (on-ih-koh-FAY-jee-ah)	onych/o = nail -phagia = eat, swallow	Nail eating (nail biting)
paronychia (pair-oh-NIK-ee-ah)	para- = beside onych/o = nail -ia = state, condition	Infection of skin fold around a nail

■ **Figure 3-27** Paronychia.
(Zlikovec/Shutterstock)

PRACTICE AS YOU GO

C. Match each pathology term with its definition.

1. ________ eczema
2. ________ nevus
3. ________ lipoma
4. ________ urticaria
5. ________ bedsore
6. ________ acne rosacea
7. ________ acne vulgaris
8. ________ hirsutism
9. ________ alopecia
10. ________ gangrene
11. ________ scleroderma
12. ________ albinism

a. decubitus ulcer
b. lack of skin pigment
c. acne commonly seen in adults
d. hardened skin
e. redness, vesicles, itching, crusts
f. birthmark
g. excessive hair growth
h. caused by deficient blood supply
i. fatty tumor
j. hives
k. baldness
l. acne of adolescence

Diagnostic Procedures

Term	Word Parts	Definition
Clinical Laboratory Tests		
culture and sensitivity (C&S)		Laboratory test that grows a colony of bacteria removed from infected area in order to identify specific infecting bacteria and then determine its sensitivity to a variety of antibiotics
Biopsy Procedures		
biopsy (BX, bx) (BYE-op-see)	bi/o = life -opsy = view of	Piece of tissue removed by syringe and needle, knife, punch, or brush to examine under a microscope; used to aid in diagnosis
excisional biopsy (ek-SIZH-ih-nal)	ex- = outward cis/o = to cut -al = pertaining to	Entire suspicious area of tissue removed for examination
exfoliative cytology (ex-FOH-lee-ah-tiv / sigh-TALL-oh-jee)	ex- = outward cyt/o = cell -logy = study of	Scraping cells from tissue and then examining them under a microscope
frozen section (FS)		Thin piece of tissue cut from frozen specimen for rapid examination under a microscope
fungal scrapings	-al = pertaining to	Scrapings, taken with curette or scraper, of tissue from lesions are placed on growth medium and examined under a microscope to identify fungal growth
punch biopsy		Small cylinder of tissue is removed by an instrument that pierces through tissue like a hole punch
shave biopsy		Using scalpel or razor to remove epidermis or dermis tissue elevated above surface of skin

Word Watch

Be careful when using bi- meaning *two* and bi/o meaning *life*.

Therapeutic Procedures

Term	Word Parts	Definition
Skin Grafting		
allograft (AL-oh-graft)	allo- = other	Skin graft from one person to another; donor is usually a cadaver; also called *homograft* (homo- = same)
autograft (AW-toh-graft)	auto- = self	Skin graft from person's own body

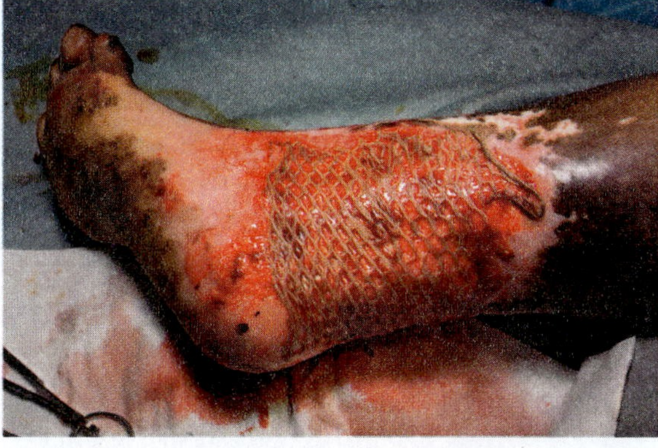

■ **Figure 3-28** A freshly applied autograft. Note that the donor skin has been perforated so that it can be stretched to cover a larger burned area. *(Grandriver/Getty Images)*

Therapeutic Procedures (continued)

Term	Word Parts	Definition
dermatome (DER-mah-tohm)	derm/o = skin -tome = instrument to cut	Instrument for cutting skin or thin transplants of skin
dermatoplasty (DER-mah-toh-plas-tee)	dermat/o = skin -plasty = surgical repair	Skin grafting; transplantation of skin
skin graft (SG)		Transfer of skin from normal area to cover another site; used to treat burn victims and after some surgical procedures; also called *dermatoplasty*
xenograft (ZEN-oh-graft)	xeno- = foreign	Skin graft from animal of another species (usually a pig) to a human; also called *heterograft* (hetero- = different)
Surgical Procedures		
cauterization (kaw-ter-ih-ZAY-shun)	cauter/o = to burn	Destruction of tissue by using caustic chemicals, electric currents, or by heating or freezing
cryosurgery (kry-oh-SER-jer-ee)	cry/o = cold	Use of extreme cold to freeze and destroy tissue
curettage (kyoo-reh-TAZH)		Removal of superficial skin lesions with curette (surgical instrument shaped like a spoon) or scraper
debridement (dih-BREED-mint)		Removal of foreign material and dead or damaged tissue from a wound
electrocautery (ee-lek-troh-KAW-teh-ree)	electr/o = electricity	To destroy tissue with electric current
incision and drainage (I&D)	cis/o = to cut	Making an incision to create an opening for drainage of material such as pus
onychectomy (on-ih-KEK-toh-mee)	onych/o = nail -ectomy = surgical removal	Removal of a nail
Plastic Surgery Procedures		
chemabrasion (kee-mah-BRAY-zhun)	chem/o = chemical	Abrasion using chemicals; also called *chemical peel*
dermabrasion (DERM-ah-bray-zhun)	derm/o = skin	Abrasion or rubbing using wire brushes or sandpaper; performed to remove acne scars, tattoos, and scar tissue
laser therapy		Removal of skin lesions and birthmarks using laser beam that emits intense heat and power at close range; laser converts frequencies of light into one small, powerful beam
liposuction (LIP-oh-suk-shun)	lip/o = fat	Removal of fat beneath skin by means of suction
rhytidectomy (rit-ih-DEK-toh-mee)	rhytid/o = wrinkle -ectomy = surgical removal	Surgical removal of excess skin to eliminate wrinkles; commonly referred to as a *face-lift*

PRACTICE AS YOU GO

D. Procedure Matching

Match each procedure term with its definition.

1. ________ debridement — **a.** surgical removal of wrinkled skin
2. ________ cauterization — **b.** instrument to cut thin slices of skin

3. ________ chemabrasion c. removing a piece of tissue for examination

4. ________ dermatoplasty d. use of extreme cold to destroy tissue

5. ________ biopsy e. skin grafting

6. ________ rhytidectomy f. removal of lesions with scraper

7. ________ curettage g. removal of skin with brushes

8. ________ dermabrasion h. removal of damaged skin

9. ________ dermatome i. destruction of tissue with electric current

10. ________ cryosurgery j. chemical peel

Pharmacology

Vocabulary

Term	Word Parts	Definition
broad spectrum		Ability of drug to be effective against wide range of microorganisms
placebo		Inactive, harmless substance used to satisfy patient's desire for medication; also used in research when given to control group of persons in a study in which another group receives a drug; effect of placebo versus drug is then observed
unit dose		Drug dosage system that provides prepackaged, prelabeled, individual medications that are ready for immediate use by patient

Drugs

Classification	Word Parts	Action	Examples
anesthetic (an-es-THET-ik)	an- = without esthesi/o = feeling -tic = pertaining to	Deadens pain when applied to skin	lidocaine, Xylocaine; procaine, Novocain
antibiotic (an-tye-bye-AW-tik)	anti- = against bi/o = life -tic = pertaining to	Kills bacteria causing skin infections	bacitracin/neomycin/polymixinB, Neosporin ointment
antifungal (an-tye-FUNG-al)	anti- = against -al = pertaining to	Kills fungi infecting skin	miconazole, Monistat; clotrima-zole, Lotrimin
antiparasitic (an-tye-pair-ah-SIT-ik)	anti- = against -ic = pertaining to	Kills mites or lice	lindane, Kwell; permethrin, Nix
antipruritic (an-tye-proo-RIH-tik)	anti- = against -ic = pertaining to	Reduces severe itching	diphenhydramine, Benadryl; camphor/pramoxine/zinc, Caladryl
antiseptic (an-tih-SEP-tik)	anti- = against septic/o = infection -tic = pertaining to	Kills bacteria in skin cuts and wounds or at surgical site	isopropyl alcohol; hydrogen peroxide
corticosteroid cream (kor-tih-koh-STAIR-oyd)	cortic/o = outer layer	Cream containing a hormone produced by adrenal cortex that has very strong anti-inflammatory properties	hydrocortisone, Cortaid; triamcin-olone, Kenalog

Abbreviations

#	number	**īī**	two
BCC	basal cell carcinoma	**īīī**	three
bid	two times a day	**MM**	malignant melanoma
BX, bx	biopsy	**oint**	ointment
C&S	culture and sensitivity	**qid**	four times a day
decub	decubitus ulcer	**SCC**	squamous cell carcinoma
Derm, derm	dermatology	**SG**	skin graft
FS	frozen section	**SLE**	systemic lupus erythematosus
I&D	incision and drainage	**STSG**	split-thickness skin graft
ī	one	**subcut**	subcutaneous
ID	intradermal	**tid**	three times a day
		UV	ultraviolet
		x	times

Word Watch

Be careful when using the abbreviation *ID* meaning *intradermal* and *I&D* meaning *incision and drainage.*

PRACTICE AS YOU GO

E. Give the abbreviation for each term.

1. frozen section ______________________
2. incision and drainage ______________________
3. intradermal ______________________
4. subcutaneous ______________________
5. ultraviolet ______________________
6. biopsy ______________________
7. culture and sensitivity ______________________
8. basal cell carcinoma ______________________
9. decubitus ulcer ______________________
10. dermatology ______________________

Chapter Review

Real-World Applications

Medical Record Analysis

This Dermatology Consultation Report contains 11 medical terms. Underline each term and write it in the list below the report. Then explain each term as you would for a nonmedical person.

Dermatology Consultation Report

Reason for Consultation:	Possible recurrence of basal cell carcinoma, left cheek
History of Present Illness:	Patient is a 74-year-old male first seen by his regular physician five years ago for persistent facial lesions. Biopsies revealed basal cell carcinoma in two lesions, one on the nasal tip and the other on the left cheek. These were successfully excised. The patient noted that the left cheek lesion returned approximately one year ago. Patient reports pruritus and states the lesion is growing larger.
Results of Physical Exam:	Examination revealed a 10 × 14 mm lesion on left cheek 20 mm anterior to the ear. The lesion displays marked erythema and poorly defined borders. The area immediately around the lesion shows depigmentation with vesicles.
Assessment:	Recurrence of basal cell carcinoma
Recommendations:	Due to the lesion's size, shape, and recurrence, deep excision of the carcinoma through the epidermis and dermis layers followed by dermatoplasty is recommended.

Term	Explanation
1. ______	______
2. ______	______
3. ______	______
4. ______	______
5. ______	______
6. ______	______
7. ______	______
8. ______	______
9. ______	______
10. ______	______
11. ______	______

Chart Note Transcription

The chart note below contains 10 phrases that can be reworded with a medical term presented in this chapter. Each phrase is identified with an underline. Determine the medical term and write your answers in the spaces provided.

Pearson General Hospital Consultation Report

Task Edit View Time Scale Options Help Download Archive Date: 17 May 2017

Current Complaint:	A 64-year-old female with an open sore **1** on her right leg is seen by the specialist in treating diseases of the skin. **2**
Past History:	Patient states she first noticed an area of pain, severe itching, **3** and redness of the skin **4** just below her right knee about six weeks ago. One week later, raised spots containing pus **5** appeared. Patient states the raised spots containing pus ruptured and the open sore appeared.
Signs and Symptoms:	Patient has a deep open sore 5 × 3 cm. It is 4 cm distal to the knee on the lateral aspect of the right leg. It appears to extend into the deeper skin layer, **6** and the edges show signs of tissue death. **7** The open sore has a small amount of drainage but there is no odor. A sample of the drainage that was grown in the lab to identify the microorganism and determine the best antibiotic **8** of the drainage revealed *Staphylococcus* bacteria in the open sore.
Diagnosis:	Inflammation of connective tissue in the skin **9**
Treatment:	Removal of damaged tissue **10** of the open sore followed by application of an antibiotic cream. Patient was instructed to return to the skin disease specialist's office in two weeks, or sooner if the open sore does not heal or if it begins draining pus.

1. ______________________________
2. ______________________________
3. ______________________________
4. ______________________________
5. ______________________________
6. ______________________________
7. ______________________________
8. ______________________________
9. ______________________________
10. ______________________________

Case Study

Below is a case study presentation of a patient with a condition discussed in this chapter. Read the case study and answer the questions below. Some questions will ask for information not included within this chapter. Use your text, a medical dictionary, or any other reference material you choose to answer these questions.

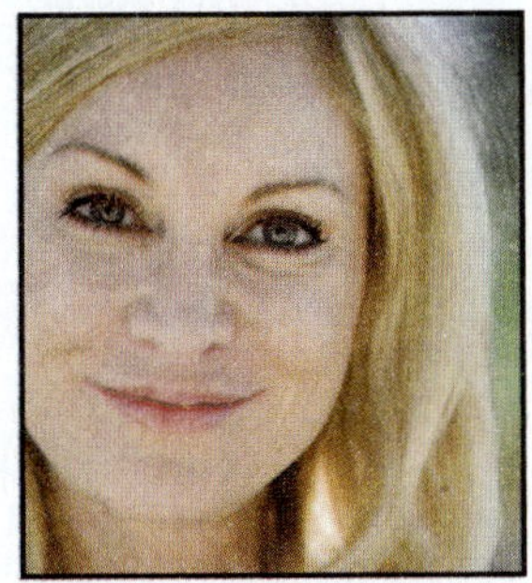

(Monkey Business Images/Shutterstock)

A 40-year-old female is seen in the dermatologist's office, upon the recommendation of her internist, for a workup for suspected SLE. Her presenting symptoms include erythema rash across her cheeks and nose, photosensitivity resulting in raised rash in sun-exposed areas, patches of alopecia, and pain and stiffness in her joints. The dermatologist examines the patient and orders exfoliative cytology and fungal scrapings to rule out other sources of the rash. Her internist had already placed the patient on oral anti-inflammatory medication for joint pain. The dermatologist orders corticosteroid cream for the rash. The patient is advised to use a sunscreen and make a follow-up appointment for results of the biopsy.

Questions

1. What pathological condition does the internist think this patient might have? Look this condition up in a reference source, and include a short description of it. SLE is an autoimmune disease. Use a reference source to look up the name of another autoimmune disease.

____

____

2. List and define each of the patient's presenting symptoms in your own words.

____

____

3. What diagnostic tests did the dermatologist perform? Describe them in your own words. Why were they important in helping the dermatologist make a diagnosis?

____

____

4. Each physician initiated a treatment. Describe them in your own words.

____

____

5. What do you think the term *workup* means?

____

____

Practice Exercises

A. Complete the Term

For each definition given below, fill in the blank with the word part that completes the term.

Definition	Term
1. use of cold to destroy tissue	________surgery
2. abnormal softening of the nail	________malacia
3. skin graft from one person to another	________graft
4. abnormal condition of death	________osis
5. profuse sweating	________esis
6. skin graft from another species to a human	________graft
7. abnormal condition of not sweating	an________osis
8. oily discharge	________rrhea
9. abnormal condition of lice	________osis
10. using suction to remove fat from under skin	________suction
11. study of the skin	________logy
12. abnormal condition of hair fungus	________mycosis
13. scaly skin	________osis
14. surgical removal of wrinkles	________ectomy
15. dry skin condition	________derma

B. Describe the Type of Burn

1. first-degree ____________________
2. second-degree ____________________
3. third-degree ____________________

C. Define the Term

1. macule ____________________
2. papule ____________________
3. cyst ____________________
4. fissure ____________________
5. pustule ____________________
6. wheal ____________________
7. vesicle ____________________
8. ulcer ____________________
9. nodule ____________________
10. laceration ____________________

D. Word Building Practice

The combining form **dermat/o** refers to the skin. Use it to write a term that means:

1. inflammation of the skin __________
2. any abnormal skin condition __________
3. an instrument for cutting the skin __________
4. specialist in skin __________
5. surgical repair of the skin __________
6. study of the skin __________

The combining form **melan/o** means *black*. Use it to write a term that means:

7. black tumor __________
8. black cell __________

The suffix **-derma** means *skin*. Use it to write a term that means:

9. hardened skin __________
10. white skin __________
11. red skin __________

The combining form **onych/o** refers to the nail. Use it to write a term that means:

12. abnormal softening of the nails __________
13. infection around the nail __________
14. nail eating (biting) __________
15. removal of the nail __________

E. Using Abbreviations

Fill in each blank with the appropriate abbreviation.

1. Mrs. Brown developed a(n) __________ from laying supine too long.
2. __________ is an autoimmune disease attacking connective tissue.
3. The __________ test identified a bacterial infection.
4. The black mole tumor turned out be __________.
5. A(n) __________ was necessary to cover the burn.
6. A(n) __________ was performed to drain the pus from the abscess.
7. __________ often begins as a sore that does not heal, while a __________ tumor forms in the basal layer of the epidermis.
8. __________ treats conditions of the integumentary system.

F. Fill in the Blank

impetigo	tinea	keloid	exfoliative cytology	xeroderma
petechiae	frozen section	paronychia	scabies	Kaposi's sarcoma

1. The winter climates can cause dry skin. The medical term for this is ______________________.
2. Kim has experienced small, pinpoint, purplish spots caused by bleeding under the skin. This is called ______________.
3. Janet has a fungal skin disease. This is called ______________________.
4. A contagious skin disease caused by a mite is ______________________.
5. An infection around the entire nail is called ______________________.
6. A form of skin cancer affecting AIDS patients is called ______________________.
7. Latrivia has a bacterial skin infection that results in pustules crusting and rupturing. It is called ______________.
8. James's burn scar became a hypertrophic ______________________.
9. For a(n) ______________________ test, cells scraped off the skin are examined under a microscope.
10. During surgery, a(n) ______________________ was ordered for a rapid exam of tissue cut from a tumor.

G. Pharmacology Challenge

Fill in the classification for each drug description, then match the brand name.

	Drug Description	Classification	Brand Name
1.	________ kills fungi	______________	a. Kwell
2.	________ reduces severe itching	______________	b. Cortaid
3.	________ kills mites and lice	______________	c. Benadryl
4.	________ powerful anti-inflammatory	______________	d. Neosporin
5.	________ deadens pain	______________	e. Monistat
6.	________ kills bacteria	______________	f. Xylocaine

H. Spelling Practice

Some of the following terms are misspelled. Identify the incorrect terms and spell them correctly in the blank provided.

1. anesthetic ______________________
2. chemobrasion ______________________
3. rytidectomy ______________________
4. urticaria ______________________
5. hyperhydrosis ______________________
6. peronychia ______________________
7. varicella ______________________
8. sebaceous ______________________
9. decubitis ______________________
10. purulent ______________________

I. Complete the Statement

1. The accessory organs of the skin include the _____________, _____________, _____________, and _____________.
2. The deepest (living) layer of the epidermis is the _____________.
3. _____________ is the pigment responsible for skin color.
4. The dermis is composed of connective tissue and _____________ fibers.
5. The subcutaneous layer is a continuous layer of _____________ that separates the skin from deeper tissues.
6. Hair and nails are composed of the hard protein _____________.
7. _____________ is responsible for lubricating the hair and skin.
8. Most of the sweat glands in the body are _____________ glands.

Labeling Exercises

Image A

Write the labels for this figure on the numbered lines provided.

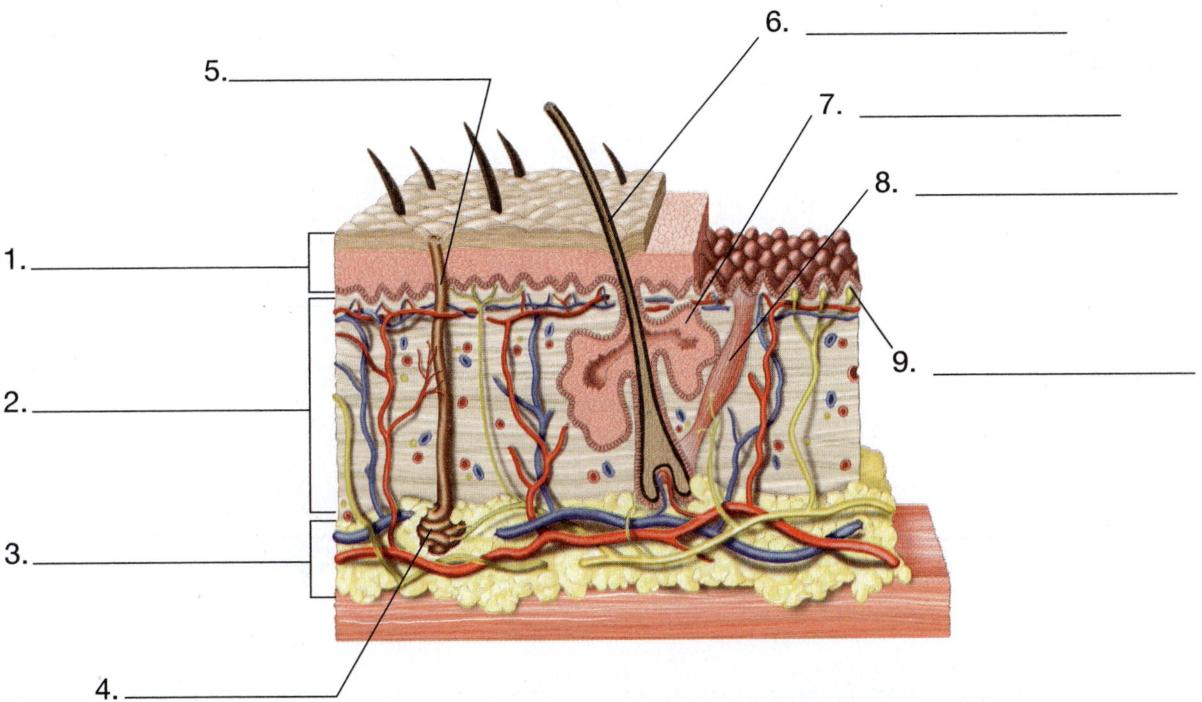

Image B

Write the labels for this figure on the numbered lines provided.

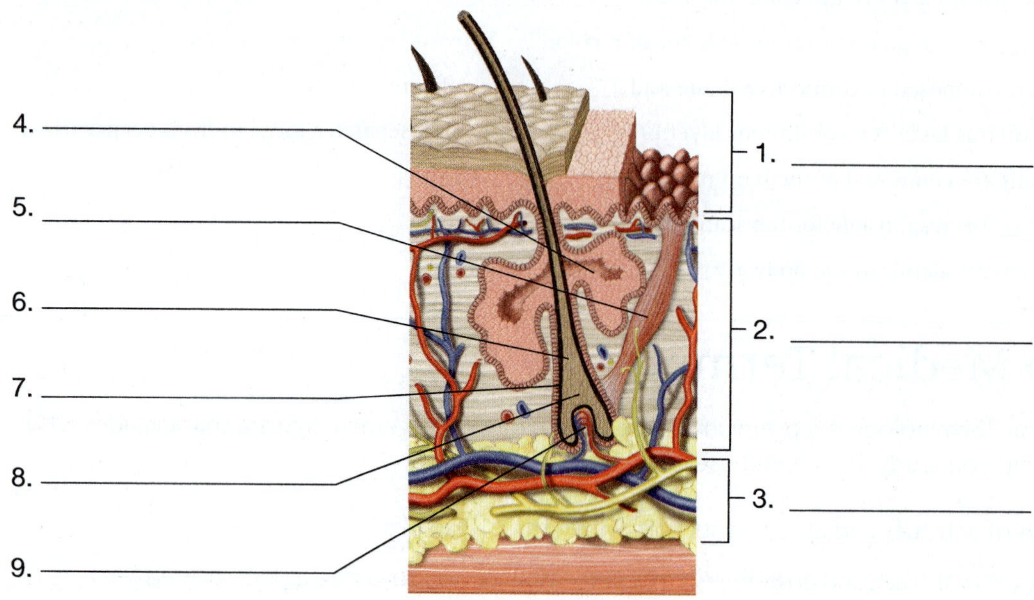

Image C

Write the labels for this figure on the numbered lines provided.

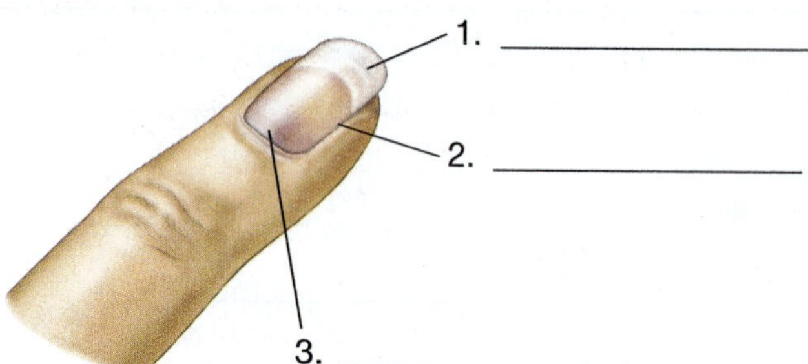

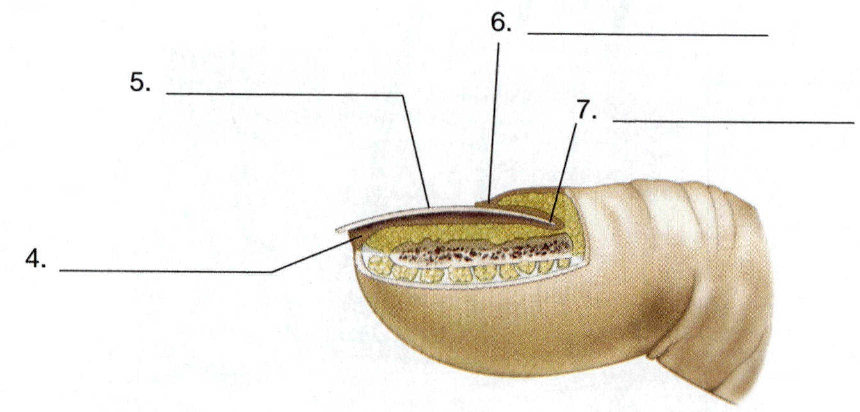

Chapter 4

Musculoskeletal System

Learning Objectives

Upon completion of this chapter, you will be able to

1. Identify and define the combining forms, suffixes, and prefixes introduced in this chapter.
2. Correctly spell and pronounce medical terms and major anatomical structures relating to the musculoskeletal system.
3. Locate and describe the major organs of the musculoskeletal system and their functions.
4. Correctly place bones in either the axial or the appendicular skeleton.
5. List and describe the components of a long bone.
6. Identify bony projections and depressions.
7. Identify the parts of a synovial joint.
8. Describe the characteristics of the three types of muscle tissue.
9. Use movement terminology correctly.
10. Identify and define musculoskeletal system anatomical terms.
11. Identify and define selected musculoskeletal system pathology terms.
12. Identify and define selected musculoskeletal system diagnostic procedures.
13. Identify and define selected musculoskeletal system therapeutic procedures.
14. Identify and define selected medications relating to the musculoskeletal system.
15. Define selected abbreviations associated with the musculoskeletal system.

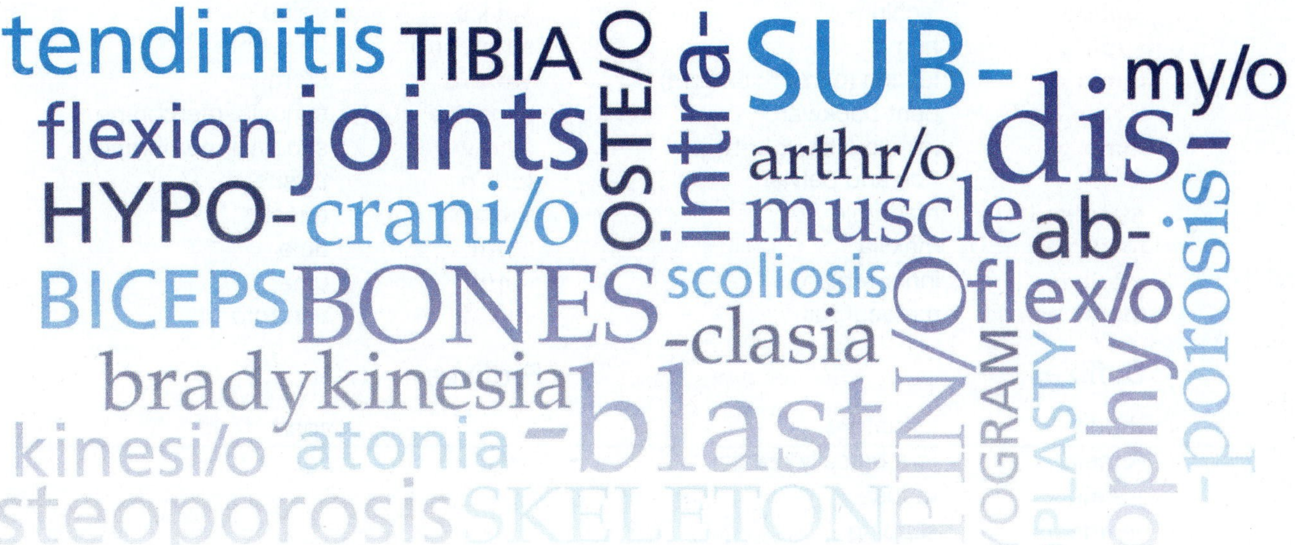

(Pearson Education, Inc.)

SECTION I: SKELETAL SYSTEM

AT A GLANCE

Function

The skeletal system consists of 206 bones that make up the internal framework of the body, called the skeleton. The skeleton supports the body, protects internal organs, serves as a point of attachment for skeletal muscles for body movement, produces blood cells, and stores minerals.

Organs

The primary structures that comprise the skeletal system:

bones **joints**

Word Parts

Presented here are the most common word parts (with their meanings) used to build skeletal system terms. For a more comprehensive list, refer to the Terminology section of this chapter.

Combining Forms

ankyl/o	stiff joint
arthr/o	joint
articul/o	joint
burs/o	sac
carp/o	carpus
cervic/o	neck
chondr/o	cartilage
clavicul/o	clavicle
coccyg/o	coccyx
cortic/o	outer layer
cost/o	rib
crani/o	skull
femor/o	femur
fibul/o	fibula
humer/o	humerus
ili/o	ilium
ischi/o	ischium
kyph/o	hump
lamin/o	lamina (part of vertebra)
lord/o	bent backward
lumb/o	loin (low back between ribs and pelvis)
mandibul/o	mandible
maxill/o	maxilla
medull/o	inner region
metacarp/o	metacarpus
metatars/o	metatarsus
myel/o	bone marrow, spinal cord
orth/o	straight
oste/o	bone
patell/o	patella
pector/o	chest
ped/o	child; foot
pelv/o	pelvis
phalang/o	phalanges
pod/o	foot
prosthet/o	addition
pub/o	pubis
radi/o	radius; ray (X-ray)
sacr/o	sacrum
scapul/o	scapula
scoli/o	crooked
spin/o	spine
spondyl/o	vertebrae
stern/o	sternum
synovi/o	synovial membrane
synov/o	synovial membrane
tars/o	tarsus
thorac/o	chest
tibi/o	tibia
uln/o	ulna
vertebr/o	vertebra

Suffixes

-blast	immature
-clasia	to surgically break
-desis	to fuse
-listhesis	slipping
-logic	pertaining to study of
-porosis	porous

Prefixes

dis-	apart
non-	not

Skeletal System Illustrated

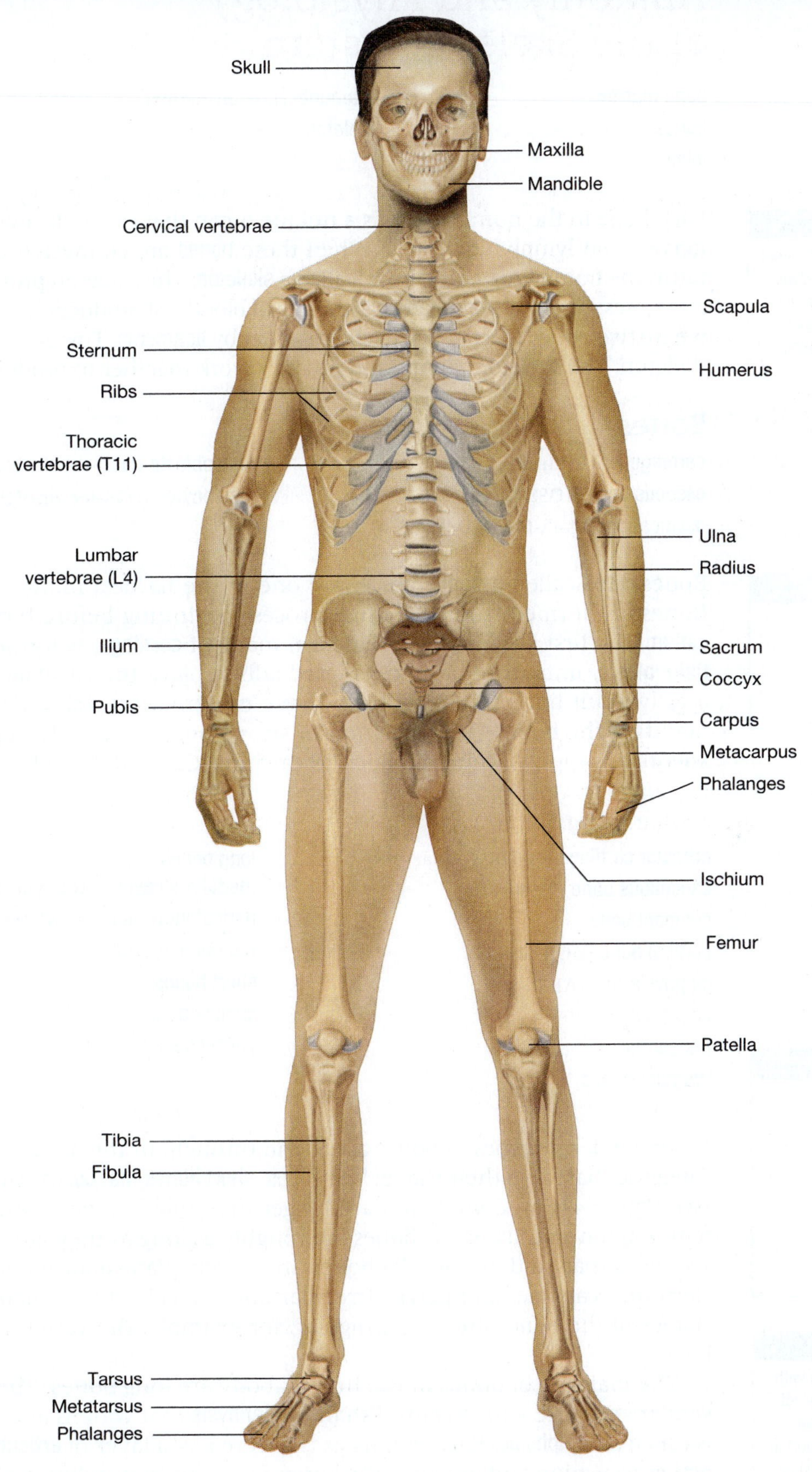

Anatomy and Physiology of the Skeletal System

bone marrow
bones
joints
ligaments (LIG-ah-ments)
skeleton

Med Term Tip

The term *skeleton*, from the Greek word *skeltos* meaning *dried up*, was originally used in reference to a dried-up mummified body, but over time came to be used for bones.

Each bone in the human body is a unique organ that carries its own blood supply, nerves, and lymphatic vessels. When these **bones** are connected to each other, it forms the framework of the body called a **skeleton**. The skeleton protects vital organs and stores minerals. **Bone marrow** is the site of blood cell production. A **joint** is the place where two bones meet and are held together by **ligaments**. This gives flexibility to the skeleton. The skeleton, joints, and muscles work together to produce movement.

Bones

cartilage (KAR-tih-lij)
osseous tissue (OSS-ee-us)
ossification (oss-ih-fih-KAY-shun)
osteoblasts (OSS-tee-oh-blasts)
osteocytes (OSS-tee-oh-sights)

What's In A Name?

Look for these word parts:
oste/o = bone
-blast = immature
-cyte = cell
-ous = pertaining to

Bones, also called **osseous tissue**, are one of the hardest materials in the body. Bones are formed from a gradual process beginning before birth called **ossification**. The first model of the skeleton, made of **cartilage**, is formed in the fetus. **Osteoblasts**, immature bone cells, gradually replace the cartilage with bone. In a fully adult bone, the osteoblasts have matured into **osteocytes** that work to maintain the bone. The formation of strong bones is greatly dependent on an adequate supply of minerals such as calcium (Ca) and phosphorus (P).

Bone Structure

articular cartilage (ar-TIK-yoo-lar)
cancellous bone (KAN-sel-us)
compact bone
cortical bone (KOR-tih-kal)
diaphysis (dye-AF-ih-sis)
epiphysis (eh-PIF-ih-sis)
flat bones
irregular bones
long bones
medullary cavity (MED-yoo-lair-ee)
periosteum (pair-ee-OSS-tee-um)
red bone marrow
short bones
spongy bone
yellow bone marrow

What's In A Name?

Look for these word parts:
articul/o = joint
cortic/o = outer layer
medull/o = inner region
oste/o = bone
peri- = around
-al = pertaining to
-ar = pertaining to
-ary = pertaining to

Several different types of bones are found throughout the body and fall into four categories based on their shape: **long bones**, **short bones**, **flat bones**, and **irregular bones** (see Figure 4-1 ■). Long bones are longer than they are wide; examples are the femur and humerus. Short bones are roughly as long as they are wide; examples are the carpals and tarsals. Flat bones are usually plate-shaped bones such as the sternum, scapulae, and pelvis. Irregular bones received their name because the shapes of the bones are very irregular; for example, the vertebrae are irregular bones.

Med Term Tip

Do not confuse a long bone with a large bone. A long bone is not necessarily a large bone. The bones of your fingers are short in length, but since they are longer than they are wide, they are classified as long bones.

The majority of bones in the human body are long bones. These bones have similar structure with a central shaft or **diaphysis** that widens at each end, which is called an **epiphysis**. Each epiphysis is covered by a layer of **articular cartilage** that acts as a cushion and prevents the bones in a joint from rubbing directly on each other. The remaining surface of each bone is covered with a thin connective tissue membrane called the **periosteum**, which contains numerous blood vessels,

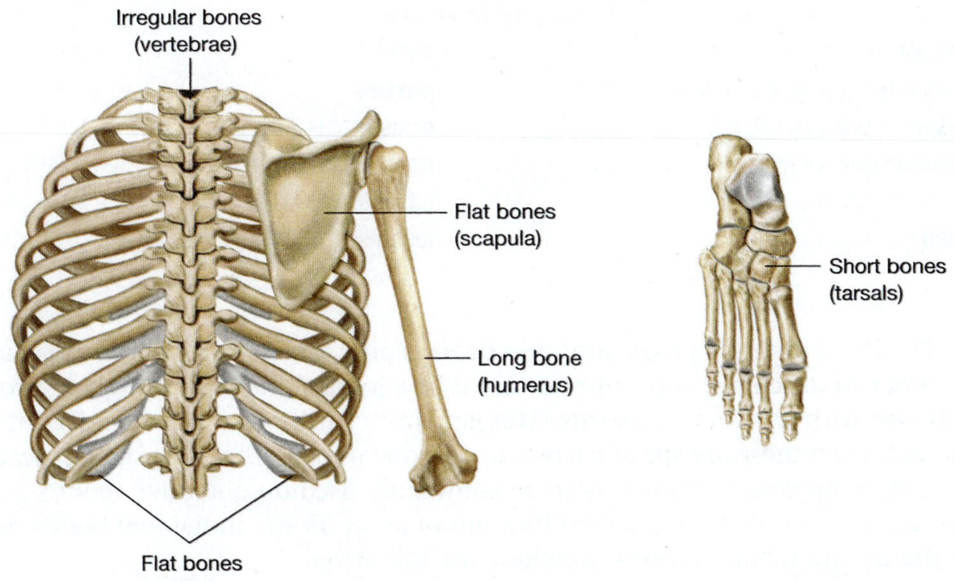

Figure 4-1 Classification of bones by shape.

nerves, and lymphatic vessels. The dense and hard exterior surface bone is called **cortical** or **compact bone**. **Cancellous** or **spongy bone** is found inside the bone. As its name indicates, spongy bone has spaces in it, giving it a spongelike appearance. These spaces contain **red bone marrow,** which manufactures most of the blood cells and is found in some parts of all bones.

Med Term Tip

The term *diaphysis* comes from the Greek term meaning *to grow between.*

The center of the diaphysis contains an open canal called the **medullary cavity**. Early in life, this cavity also contains red bone marrow, but as a person ages, the red bone marrow of the medullary cavity gradually converts to **yellow bone marrow**, which consists primarily of fat cells. Figure 4-2 ■ contains an illustration of the structure of long bones.

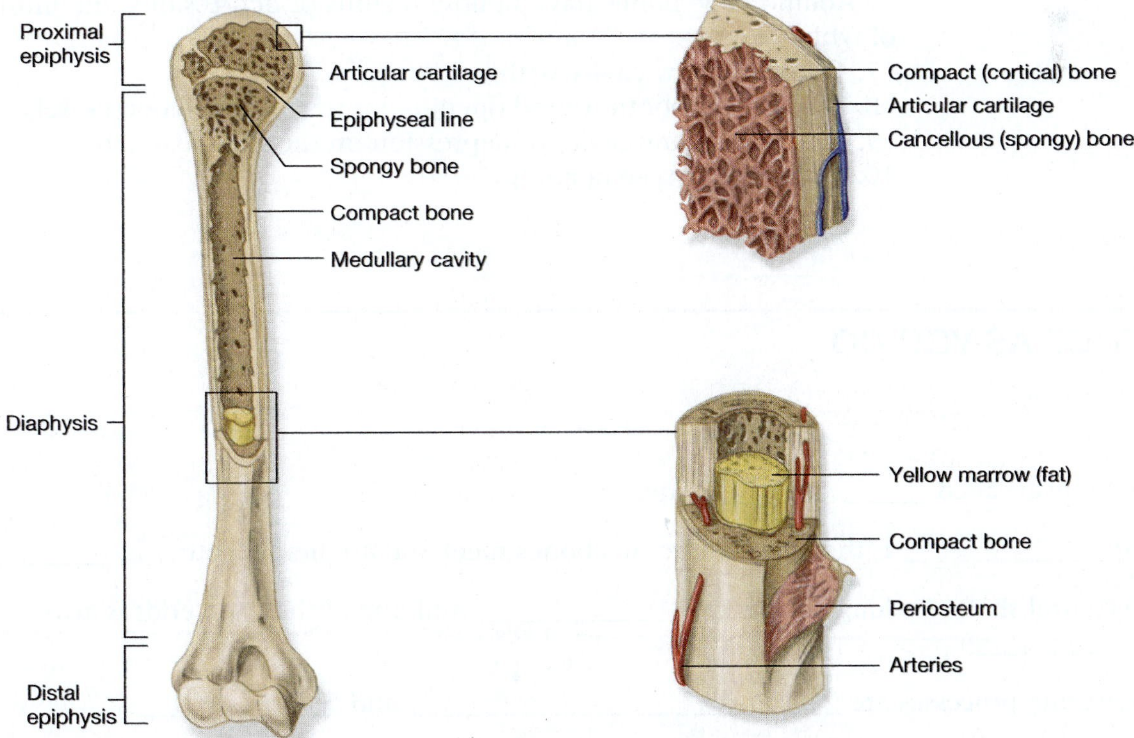

Figure 4-2 Components of a long bone. The entire long bone is on the left side, accompanied by a blow-up of the proximal epiphysis and a section of the diaphysis.

Bone Projections and Depressions

condyle (KON-dile)
epicondyle (ep-ih-KON-dile)
fissure (FISH-er)
foramen (for-AY-men)
fossa (FOSS-ah)
head
neck
process
sinus (SIGH-nus)
trochanter (troh-KAN-ter)
tubercle (TOO-ber-kl)
tuberosity (too-ber-OSS-ih-tee)

Med Term Tip

The elbow, commonly referred to as the *funny bone*, is actually a projection of the ulna called the *olecranon process.*

Bones have many projections and depressions; some are rounded and smooth in order to articulate with another bone in a joint. Others are rough to provide muscles with attachment points. The general term for any bony projection is a **process**. Then there are specific terms to describe the different shapes and locations of various processes. These terms are commonly used on operative reports and in physicians' records for clear identification of areas on the individual bones. Some of the common bony processes include the following:

1. The **head** is a large, smooth, ball-shaped end on a long bone. It may be separated from the body or shaft of the bone by a narrow area called the **neck**.
2. A **condyle** refers to a smooth, rounded portion at the end of a bone.
3. The **epicondyle** is a projection located above or on a condyle.
4. The **trochanter** refers to a large rough process for the attachment of a muscle.
5. A **tubercle** is a small, rough process that provides the attachment for tendons and muscles.
6. The **tuberosity** is a large, rough process that provides the attachment for tendons and muscles.

What's In A Name?

Look for this word part:
epi- = above

See Figure 4-3 ■ for an illustration of the processes found on the femur.

Additionally, bones have hollow regions or depressions, the most common of which are the:

7. **Sinus**: a hollow cavity within a bone.
8. **Foramen**: a smooth, round opening for nerves and blood vessels.
9. **Fossa**: a shallow cavity or depression on the surface of a bone.
10. **Fissure**: a slit-type opening.

PRACTICE AS YOU GO

A. Complete the Statement

1. Bone is also called _______________ tissue.
2. A(n) _______________ is the place where two bones meet and are held together by _______________.
3. The central shaft of a long bone is the _______________ and one of the wide ends is a(n) _______________.
4. Three bony processes are _______________, _______________, and _______________.
5. Two bony depressions are _______________ and _______________.

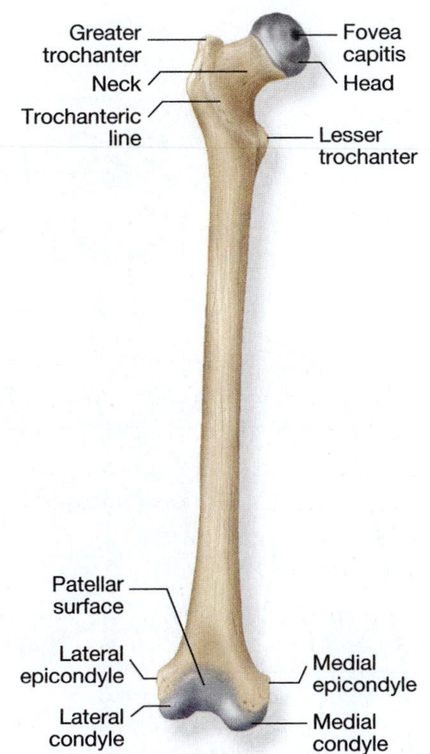

Figure 4-3 Bony processes found on the femur.

Skeleton

appendicular skeleton (ap-en-DIK-yoo-lar)
axial skeleton (AK-see-al)

The human skeleton has two divisions: the **axial skeleton** and the **appendicular skeleton**. Figures 4-4 ■ and 4-8 illustrate these two skeletons.

What's In A Name?
Look for these word parts:
-al = pertaining to
-ar = pertaining to

Axial Skeleton

cervical vertebrae
coccyx (KOK-siks)
cranium (KRAY-nee-um)
ethmoid bone (ETH-moyd)
facial bones
frontal bone
hyoid bone (HIGH-oyd)
intervertebral disk (in-ter-VER-teh-bral)
lacrimal bone (LAK-rim-al)
lumbar vertebrae
mandible (MAN-dih-bl)
maxilla (mak-SIL-ah)
nasal bone
occipital bone (ok-SIP-ih-tal)
palatine bone (PAL-ah-tyne)
parietal bone (pah-RYE-eh-tal)
rib cage
sacrum (SAY-krum)
sphenoid bone (SFEE-noyd)
sternum (STER-num)
temporal bone (TEM-por-al)
thoracic vertebrae
vertebral column (VER-teh-bral)
vomer bone (VOH-mer)
zygomatic bone (zye-goh-MAT-ik)

Med Term Tip
Newborn infants have about 300 bones at birth that will fuse into 206 bones as an adult.

The axial skeleton includes the bones of the head, neck, spine, chest, and trunk of the body (see Figure 4-4). These bones form the central axis for the whole body and protect many of the internal organs such as the brain, lungs, and heart.

The head or skull is divided into two parts consisting of the **cranium** and **facial bones**. These bones surround and protect the brain, eyes, ears, nasal cavity, and oral cavity from injury. The muscles for chewing and moving the head are attached to the cranial bones. The cranium encases the brain and consists

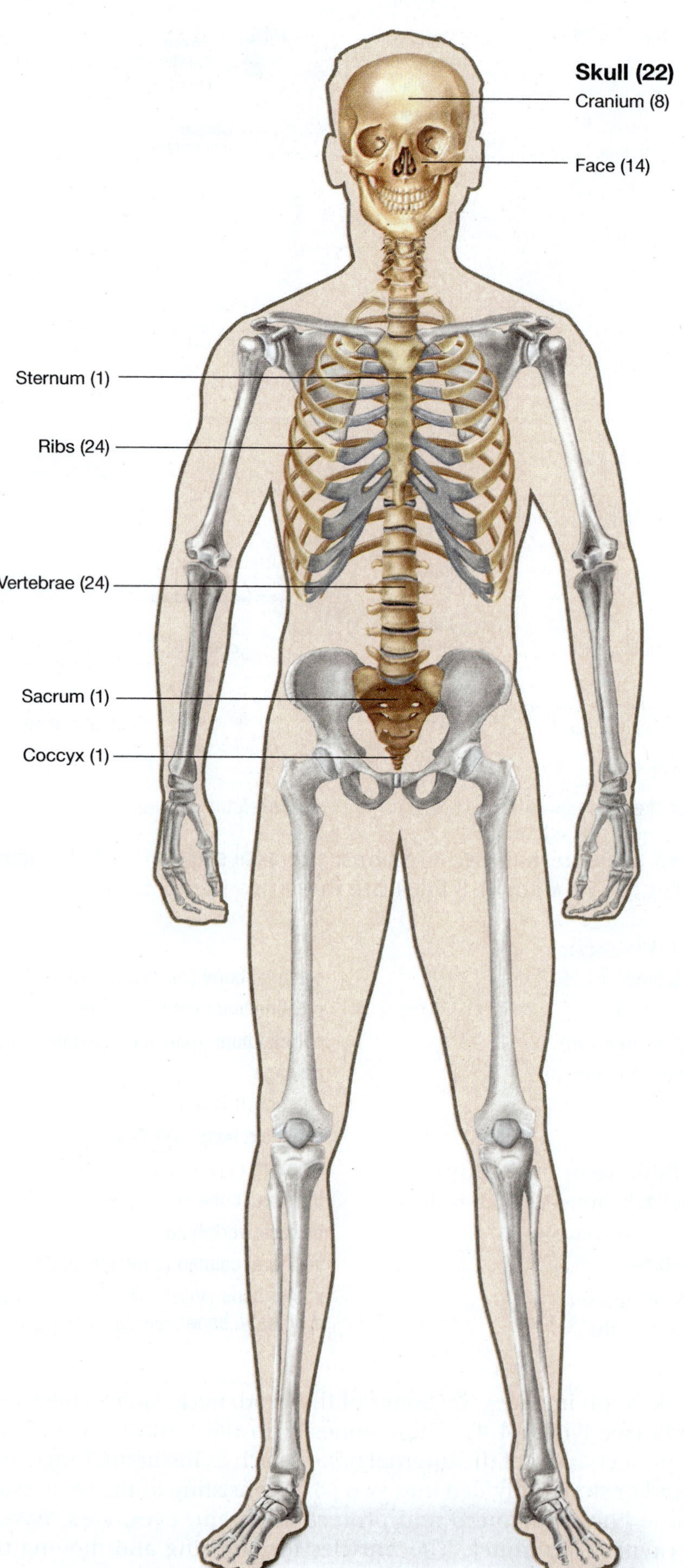

■ **Figure 4-4** Bones of the axial skeleton. Number of bones in each section of the axial skeleton is indicated in parentheses.

of the **frontal**, **parietal**, **temporal**, **ethmoid**, **sphenoid**, and **occipital bones**. The facial bones surround the mouth, nose, and eyes, and include the **mandible**, **maxilla**, **zygomatic**, **vomer**, **palatine**, **nasal**, and **lacrimal bones**. The cranial and facial bones are illustrated in Figure 4-5 ■ and described in Table 4-1 ■.

The **hyoid bone** is a single U-shaped bone suspended in the neck between the mandible and larynx. It is a point of attachment for swallowing and speech muscles.

The trunk of the body consists of the **vertebral column**, **sternum**, and **rib cage**. The vertebral or spinal column is divided into five sections: **cervical vertebrae**, **thoracic vertebrae**, **lumbar vertebrae**, **sacrum**, and **coccyx** (see Figure 4-6 ■ and Table 4-2 ■). Located between each pair of vertebrae, from the cervical through the lumbar regions, is an **intervertebral disk**. Each disk is composed of fibrocartilage to provide a cushion between the vertebrae. The rib cage has 12 pairs of ribs attached at the back to the vertebral column. Ten of the pairs are also attached to the sternum in the front (see Figure 4-7 ■). The lowest two pairs are called *floating ribs* and

Med Term Tip

The hyoid bone is the only bone in the human skeleton that does not interact directly (articulate) with another bone.

Med Term Tip

The term *coccyx* comes from the Greek word for the cuckoo because the shape of these small bones extending off the sacrum resembles this bird's bill.

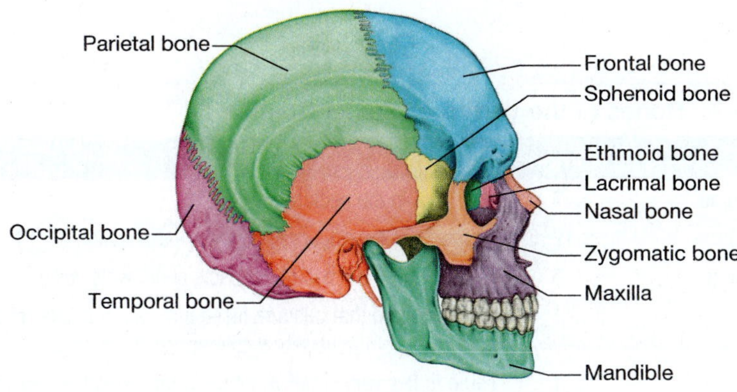

■ **Figure 4-5** Bones of the skull. Note: the palatine and vomer bones are not visible in sagittal view. *(Stihii/Shutterstock)*

■ **TABLE 4-1** Bones of the Skull

Name	Number	Description
Cranial Bones		
Frontal bone	1	Forehead
Parietal bones	2	Upper sides of cranium and roof of skull
Occipital bone	1	Back and base of skull
Temporal bones	2	Sides and base of cranium
Sphenoid bone	1	Bat-shaped bone that forms part of base of skull and floor and sides of eye orbit
Ethmoid bone	1	Forms part of eye orbit, nose, and floor of cranium
Facial Bones		
Lacrimal bones	2	Inner corner of each eye
Nasal bones	2	Form part of nasal septum and support bridge of nose
Maxilla	1	Upper jaw
Mandible	1	Lower jawbone; only movable bone of the skull
Zygomatic bones	2	Cheekbones
Vomer bone	1	Base of nasal septum
Palatine bone	1	Hard palate (PAL-et) roof of oral cavity and floor of nasal cavity

What's In A Name?

Look for these word parts:
-al = pertaining to
-ar = pertaining to
-oid = resembling
-tic = pertaining to

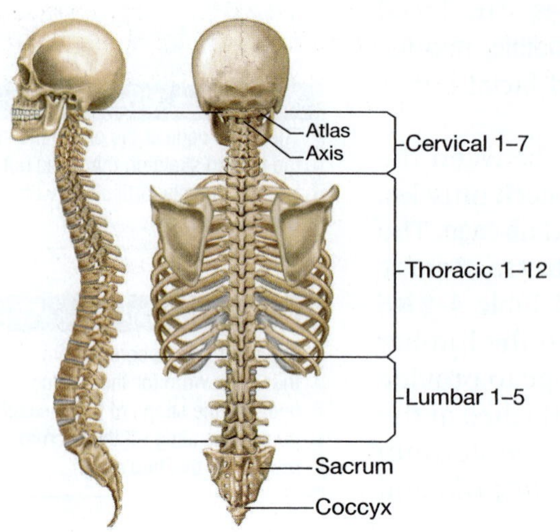

■ **Figure 4-6** Divisions of the vertebral column.

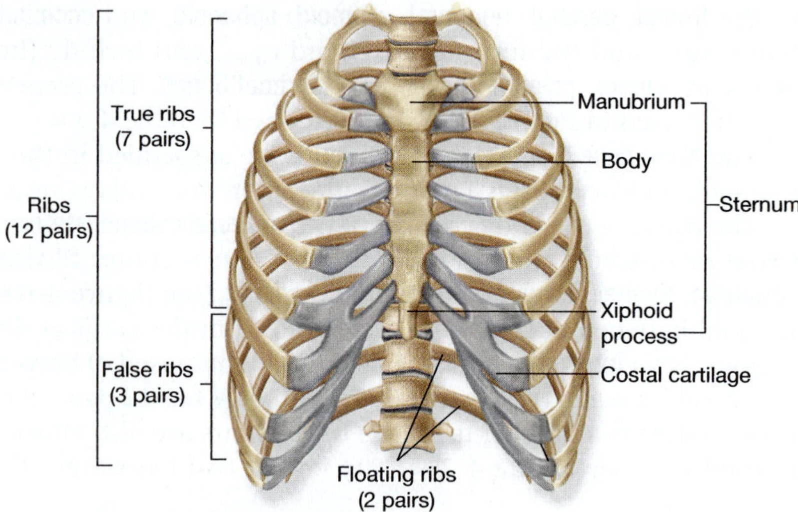

■ **Figure 4-7** The structure of the rib cage.

■ **TABLE 4-2** Bones of the Vertebral/Spinal Column

Name	Number	Description
Cervical vertebrae	7	Vertebrae in the neck region
Thoracic vertebrae	12	Vertebrae in the chest region with ribs attached
Lumbar vertebrae	5	Vertebrae in the small of the back, about waist level
Sacrum	1	Five vertebrae that become fused into one triangular-shaped flat bone at the base of the vertebral column
Coccyx	1	Three to five very small vertebrae attached to the sacrum; often become fused

are attached only to the vertebral column. The rib cage serves to provide support for organs, such as the heart and lungs.

Appendicular Skeleton

carpus (KAR-pus)
clavicle (KLAV-ih-kl)
femur (FEE-mer)
fibula (FIB-yoo-lah)
humerus (HYOO-mer-us)
ilium (IL-ee-um)
innominate bone (ih-NOM-ih-nit)
ischium (ISS-kee-um)
lower extremities
metacarpus (met-ah-KAR-pus)
metatarsus (met-ah-TAR-sus)
os coxae (OSS / KOK-see)
patella (pah-TEL-ah)
pectoral girdle (PEK-toh-ral)
pelvic girdle (PEL-vik)
phalanges (fah-LAN-jeez)
pubis (PYOO-bis)
radius (RAY-dee-us)
scapula (SKAP-yoo-lah)
tarsus (TAR-sus)
tibia (TIB-ee-ah)
ulna (UL-nah)
upper extremities

The appendicular skeleton consists of the **pectoral girdle**, **upper extremities (UE)**, **pelvic girdle**, and **lower extremities (LE)** (see Figure 4-8 ■). These are the bones for the appendages or limbs and, along with the muscles attached to them, are responsible for body movement.

What's In A Name?

Look for these word parts:
pector/o = chest
pelv/o = pelvis
-al = pertaining to
-ic = pertaining to

Med Term Tip

The term *girdle*, meaning *something that encircles or confines*, refers to the entire bony structure of the shoulder and the pelvis. If just one bone from these areas is being discussed, like the ilium of the pelvis, it would be named as such. If, however, the entire pelvis is being discussed, it would be called the *pelvic girdle*.

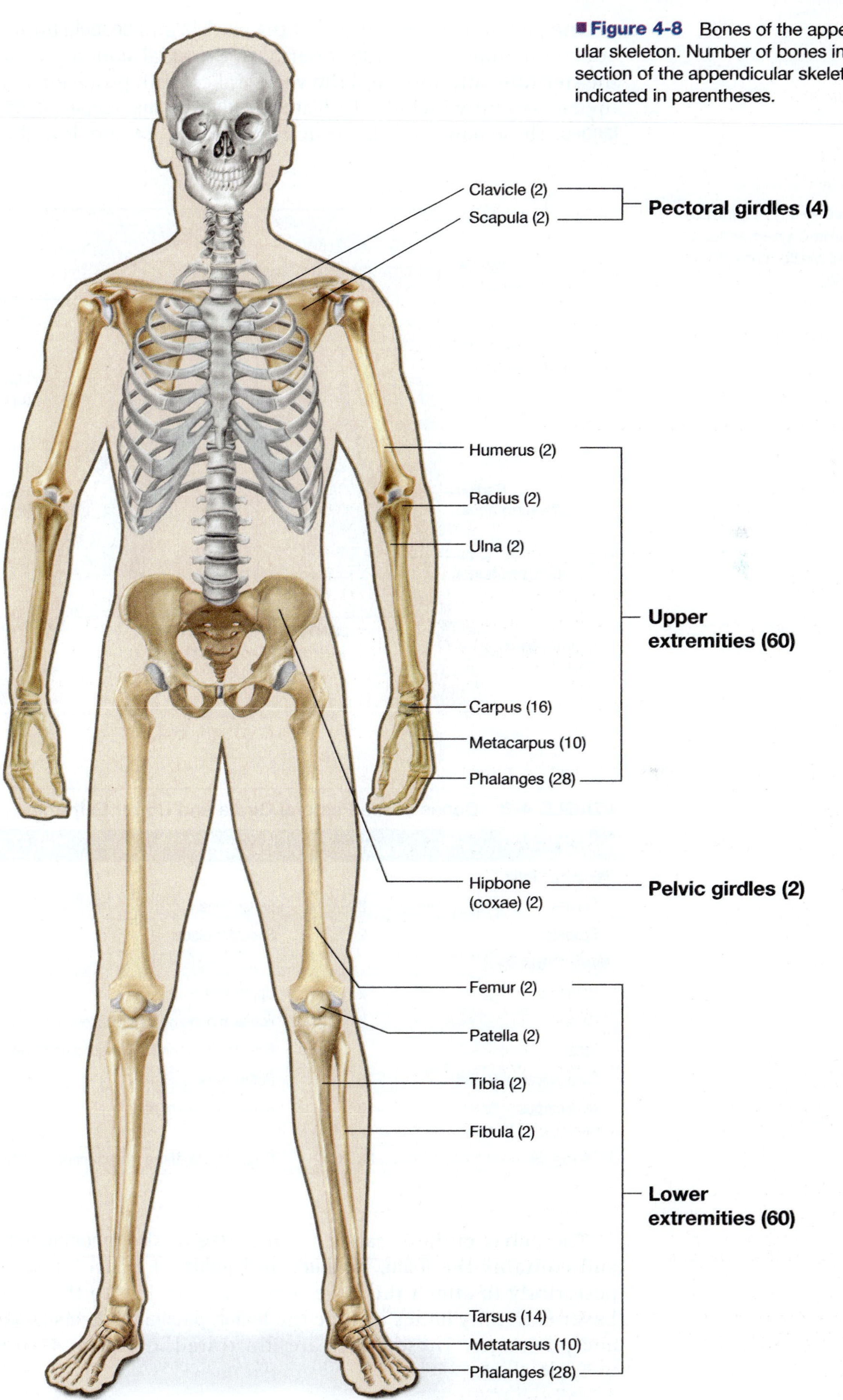

Figure 4-8 Bones of the appendicular skeleton. Number of bones in each section of the appendicular skeleton is indicated in parentheses.

The pectoral girdle consists of the **clavicle** and **scapula** bones. It functions to attach the upper extremity, or arm, to the axial skeleton by articulating with the sternum anteriorly and the vertebral column posteriorly. The bones of the upper extremity include the **humerus, ulna, radius, carpus, metacarpus,** and **phalanges.** These bones are illustrated in Figure 4-9■ and described in Table 4-3■.

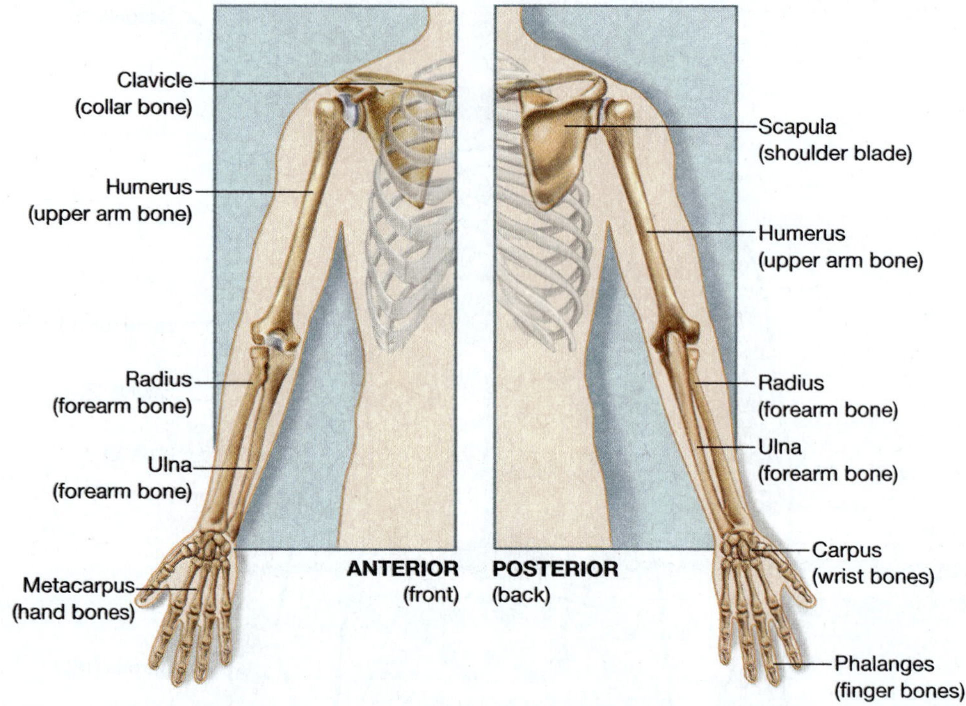

■ **Figure 4-9** Anatomical and common names for the pectoral girdle and upper extremity.

■ **TABLE 4-3 Bones of the Pectoral Girdle and Upper Extremity**

Name	Number	Description
Pectoral Girdle		
Clavicle	2	Collar bone
Scapula	2	Shoulder blade
Upper Extremity		
Humerus	2	Upper arm bone
Radius	2	Forearm bone on thumb side of lower arm
Ulna	2	Forearm bone on little finger side of lower arm
Carpus (carpal bones)	16	Bones of wrist
Metacarpus (metacarpal bones)	10	Bones in palm of hand
Phalanges	28	Finger bones; three in each finger and two in each thumb

The pelvic girdle is called the **os coxae** or the **innominate bone** or hipbone and contains the **ilium, ischium,** and **pubis.** It articulates with the sacrum posteriorly to attach the lower extremity, or leg, to the axial skeleton. The lower extremity bones include the **femur, patella, tibia, fibula, tarsus, metatarsus,** and phalanges. These bones are illustrated in Figure 4-10■ and described in Table 4-4■.

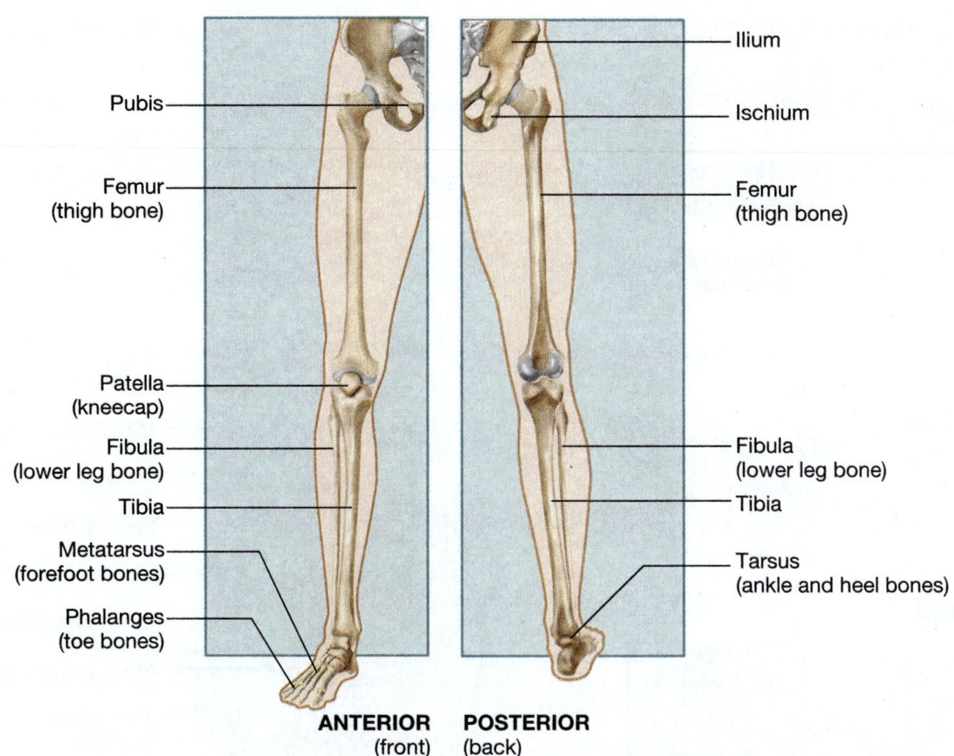

■ **Figure 4-10** Anatomical and common names for the pelvic girdle and lower extremity.

■ **TABLE 4-4** Bones of the Pelvic Girdle and Lower Extremity

Name	Number	Description
Pelvic Girdle/Os Coxae		
Ilium	2	Part of the hipbone
Ischium	2	Part of the hipbone
Pubis	2	Part of the hipbone
Lower Extremity		
Femur	2	Upper leg bone; thigh bone
Patella	2	Kneecap
Tibia	2	Shin bone; thicker lower leg bone
Fibula	2	Thinner long bone in lateral side of lower leg
Tarsus (tarsal bones)	14	Ankle and heel bones
Metatarsus (metatarsal bones)	10	Forefoot bones
Phalanges	28	Toe bones; three in each toe and two in each great toe

Joints

articulation (ar-tik-yoo-LAY-shun)
bursa (BER-sah)
cartilaginous joints (kar-tih-LAJ-ih-nus)
fibrous joints (FYE-bruss)
joint capsule
range of motion
synovial fluid
synovial joint (sin-OH-vee-al)
synovial membrane

What's In A Name?
Look for these word parts:
articul/o = joint
fibr/o = fibers
synovi/o = synovial membrane
-al = pertaining to
-ous = pertaining to

Joints are formed when two or more bones meet. This is also referred to as an **articulation**. There are three types of joints determined by the amount of movement allowed between the bones: **synovial joints**, **cartilaginous joints**, and **fibrous joints** (see Figure 4-11 ■).

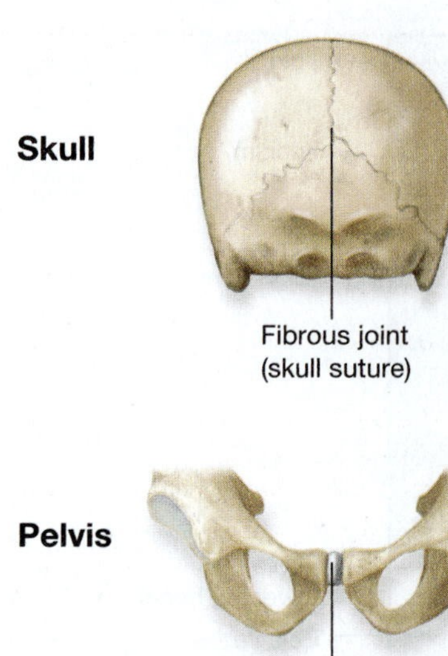

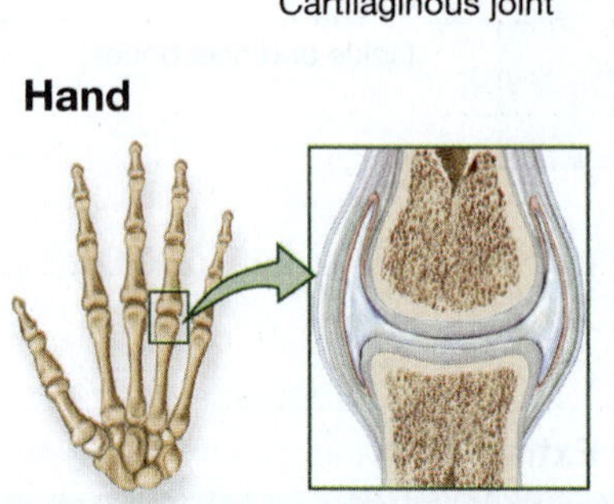

■ **Figure 4-11** Examples of three types of joints found in the body.

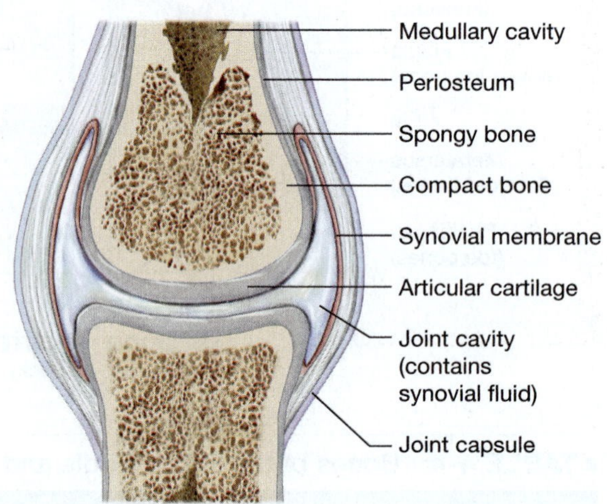

■ **Figure 4-12** Structure of a generalized synovial joint.

Most joints are freely moving synovial joints (see Figure 4-12 ■), which are enclosed by an elastic **joint capsule**. The joint capsule is lined with **synovial membrane**, which secretes **synovial fluid** to lubricate the joint. As noted earlier, the ends of bones in a synovial joint are covered by a layer of articular cartilage. Cartilage is very tough, but still flexible. It withstands high levels of stress to act as a shock absorber for the joint and prevents bone from rubbing against bone. Cartilage is found in several other areas of the body, such as the nasal septum, external ear, eustachian tube, larynx, trachea, bronchi, and intervertebral disks. One example of a synovial joint is the ball-and-socket joint found at the shoulder or hip. The ball rotating in the socket allows for a wide range of motion. Bands of strong connective tissue called ligaments bind bones together at the joint. The maximum amount of movement allowed at a joint is referred to as its **range of motion** (ROM). Range of motion is measured in degrees of a circle.

Some synovial joints contain a saclike structure called a **bursa**, which is composed of connective tissue and lined with synovial membrane. Most commonly found between bones and ligaments or tendons, bursas function to reduce friction. Some common bursa locations are the elbow, knee, and shoulder joints.

Not all joints are freely moving. Fibrous joints allow almost no movement since the ends of the bones are joined by thick fibrous tissue, which may even fuse into solid bone. The sutures of the skull are an example of a fibrous joint. Cartilaginous joints allow for slight movement but hold bones firmly in place by a solid piece of cartilage. An example of this type of joint is the pubic symphysis, the point at which the left and right pubic bones meet in the front of the lower abdomen.

Med Term Tip

Bursitis is an inflammation of the bursa located between bony prominences such as at the shoulder. *Housemaid's knee*, a term thought to have originated from the damage to the knees that occurred when maids knelt to scrub floors, is a form of bursitis and carries the medical name *prepatellar bursitis*.

PRACTICE AS YOU GO

B. Give the Anatomical Name

1. kneecap ______
2. ankle bones ______
3. collar bone ______
4. thigh bone ______
5. toe bones ______
6. wrist bones ______
7. shin bone ______
8. shoulder blade ______
9. finger bones ______

Terminology

Word Parts Used to Build Skeletal System Terms

The following lists contain the combining forms, suffixes, and prefixes used to build terms in the remaining sections of this chapter.

Combining Forms

ankyl/o	stiff joint	**kyph/o**	hump	**prosthet/o**	addition
arthr/o	joint	**lamin/o**	lamina	**pub/o**	pubis
burs/o	bursa	**lord/o**	bent backward	**radi/o**	radius, ray (X-ray)
carp/o	carpus	**lumb/o**	loin	**sacr/o**	sacrum
cervic/o	neck	**mandibul/o**	mandible	**sarc/o**	flesh
chondr/o	cartilage	**maxill/o**	maxilla	**scapul/o**	scapula
clavicul/o	clavicle	**medull/o**	inner region	**scoli/o**	crooked
coccyg/o	coccyx	**metacarp/o**	metacarpus	**spin/o**	spine
cortic/o	outer layer	**metatars/o**	metatarsus	**spondyl/o**	vertebra
cost/o	rib	**myel/o**	bone marrow, spinal cord	**stern/o**	sternum
crani/o	skull	**orth/o**	straight	**synov/o**	synovial membrane
cutane/o	skin	**oste/o**	bone	**system/o**	system
erythr/o	red	**patell/o**	patella	**tars/o**	tarsus
femor/o	femur	**path/o**	disease	**thorac/o**	chest
fibul/o	fibula	**ped/o**	child; foot	**tibi/o**	tibia
humer/o	humerus	**phalang/o**	phalanges	**uln/o**	ulna
ili/o	ilium	**pod/o**	foot	**vertebr/o**	vertebra
ischi/o	ischium				

Suffixes

-ac	pertaining to	**-iatry**	medical treatment	**-ous**	pertaining to
-al	pertaining to	**-ic**	pertaining to	**-pathy**	disease
-algia	pain	**-itis**	inflammation	**-plasty**	surgical repair
-ar	pertaining to	**-listhesis**	slipping	**-porosis**	porous
-ary	pertaining to	**-logic**	pertaining to study of	**-scope**	instrument for viewing
-centesis	puncture to withdraw fluid	**-logy**	study of	**-scopic**	pertaining to visually examining
-clasia	surgically break	**-malacia**	abnormal softening	**-scopy**	process of visually examining
-desis	to fuse	**-metry**	process of measuring	**-stenosis**	narrowing
-eal	pertaining to	**-oma**	tumor	**-tic**	pertaining to
-ectomy	surgical removal	**-ory**	pertaining to	**-tome**	instrument to cut
-genic	producing	**-osis**	abnormal condition		
-gram	record	**-otomy**	cutting into		
-graph	to record				
-graphy	process of recording				

Prefixes

anti-	against	**inter-**	between	**per-**	through
bi-	two	**intra-**	within	**pre-**	before
dis-	apart	**non-**	not	**sub-**	under
ex-	outward				

Adjective Forms of Anatomical Terms

Term	Word Parts	Definition
carpal (KAR-pal)	**carp/o** = carpus **-al** = pertaining to	Pertaining to carpus
cervical (SER-vih-kal)	**cervic/o** = neck **-al** = pertaining to	Pertaining to neck
clavicular (klah-VIK-yoo-lar)	**clavicul/o** = clavicle **-ar** = pertaining to	Pertaining to clavicle
coccygeal (kok-SIH-jee-al)	**coccyg/o** = coccyx **-eal** = pertaining to	Pertaining to coccyx
cortical (KOR-tih-kal)	**cortic/o** = outer layer **-al** = pertaining to	Pertaining to outer layer
costal (KOS-tal)	**cost/o** = rib **-al** = pertaining to	Pertaining to rib
cranial (KRAY-nee-al)	**crani/o** = skull **-al** = pertaining to	Pertaining to skull
femoral (FEM-or-al)	**femor/o** = femur **-al** = pertaining to	Pertaining to femur

Adjective Forms of Anatomical Terms (continued)

Term	Word Parts	Definition
fibular (FIB-yoo-lar)	**fibul/o** = fibula **-ar** = pertaining to	Pertaining to fibula
humeral (HYOO-mer-al)	**humer/o** = humerus **-al** = pertaining to	Pertaining to humerus
iliac (IL-ee-ak)	**ili/o** = ilium **-ac** = pertaining to	Pertaining to ilium
intervertebral (in-ter-VER-teh-bral)	**inter-** = between **vertebr/o** = vertebra **-al** = pertaining to	Pertaining to between vertebrae
intracranial (in-trah-KRAY-nee-al)	**intra-** = within **crani/o** = skull **-al** = pertaining to	Pertaining to within skull
ischial (ISS-kee-al)	**ischi/o** = ischium **-al** = pertaining to	Pertaining to ischium
lumbar (LUM-bar)	**lumb/o** = low back **-ar** = pertaining to	Pertaining to low back
mandibular (man-DIB-yoo-lar)	**mandibul/o** = mandible **-ar** = pertaining to	Pertaining to mandible
maxillary (MAK-sih-lair-ee)	**maxill/o** = maxilla **-ary** = pertaining to	Pertaining to maxilla
medullary (MED-yoo-lair-ee)	**medull/o** = inner region **-ary** = pertaining to	Pertaining to inner region
metacarpal (met-ah-KAR-pal)	**metacarp/o** = metacarpus **-al** = pertaining to	Pertaining to metacarpus
metatarsal (met-ah-TAR-sal)	**metatars/o** = metatarsus **-al** = pertaining to	Pertaining to metatarsus
patellar (pah-TEL-ar)	**patell/o** = patella **-ar** = pertaining to	Pertaining to patella
phalangeal (fah-LAN-jee-al)	**phalang/o** = phalanges **-eal** = pertaining to	Pertaining to phalanges
pubic (PYOO-bik)	**pub/o** = pubis **-ic** = pertaining to	Pertaining to pubis
radial (RAY-dee-al)	**radi/o** = radius **-al** = pertaining to	Pertaining to radius
sacral (SAY-kral)	**sacr/o** = sacrum **-al** = pertaining to	Pertaining to sacrum
scapular (SKAP-yoo-lar)	**scapul/o** = scapula **-ar** = pertaining to	Pertaining to scapula
spinal (SPY-nal)	**spin/o** = spine **-al** = pertaining to	Pertaining to spine
sternal (STER-nal)	**stern/o** = sternum **-al** = pertaining to	Pertaining to sternum
tarsal (TAR-sal)	**tars/o** = tarsus **-al** = pertaining to	Pertaining to tarsus

Adjective Forms of Anatomical Terms (continued)

Term	Word Parts	Definition
thoracic (tho-RASS-ik)	thorac/o = thorax -ic = pertaining to	Pertaining to thorax
tibial (TIB-ee-al)	tibi/o = tibia -al = pertaining to	Pertaining to tibia
ulnar (UL-nar)	uln/o = ulna -ar = pertaining to	Pertaining to ulna
vertebral (VER-teh-bral)	vertebr/o = vertebra -al = pertaining to	Pertaining to a vertebra

PRACTICE AS YOU GO

C. Adjective Form Practice

Give the adjective form for the following bones.

1. femur ______________________
2. sternum ______________________
3. clavicle ______________________
4. coccyx ______________________
5. maxilla ______________________
6. tibia ______________________
7. patella ______________________
8. phalanges ______________________
9. humerus ______________________
10. pubis ______________________

Pathology

Term	Word Parts	Definition
Medical Specialties		
chiropractic (kye-roh-PRAK-tik)	-tic = pertaining to	Healthcare profession concerned with diagnosis and treatment of malalignment conditions of spine and musculoskeletal system with intention of affecting nervous system and improving health; healthcare professional is a *chiropractor*

Pathology (continued)

Term	Word Parts	Definition
orthopedics (Orth, Ortho) (or-thoh-PEE-diks)	**orth/o** = straight **ped/o** = child, foot **-ic** = pertaining to	Branch of medicine specializing in diagnosis and treatment of conditions of musculoskeletal system; also called *orthopedic surgery*; physician is an *orthopedist* or *orthopedic surgeon*; name derived from straightening **(orth/o)** deformities in children **(ped/o)**
orthotics (or-THOT-iks)	**orth/o** = straight **-tic** = pertaining to	Healthcare profession specializing in making orthopedic appliances such as braces and splints; person skilled in making and adjusting these appliances is an *orthotist*; *orthotic* is the appliance
podiatry (poh-DYE-ah-tree)	**pod/o** = foot **-iatry** = medical treatment	Healthcare profession specializing in diagnosis and treatment of disorders of feet and lower legs; healthcare professional is a *podiatrist*
prosthetics (pross-THET-iks)	**prosthet/o** = addition **-ic** = pertaining to	Healthcare profession specializing in making artificial body parts; person skilled in making and adjusting prostheses is a *prosthetist*; *prosthesis* is a manufactured substitute for any missing body part, such as an artificial leg
rheumatology (roo-mah-TALL-oh-jee)	**-logy** = study of	Branch of medicine (subspecialty of internal medicine) specializing in diagnosis and treatment of musculoskeletal and autoimmune conditions affecting joints, muscles, and bones; physician is a *rheumatologist*
Signs and Symptoms		
arthralgia (ar-THRAL-jee-ah)	**arthr/o** = joint **-algia** = pain	Joint pain
bursitis (ber-SIGH-tis)	**burs/o** = bursa **-itis** = inflammation	Inflammation of a bursa
callus (KAL-us)		Mass of bone tissue that forms at fracture site during its healing
chondromalacia (kon-droh-mah-LAY-shee-ah)	**chondr/o** = cartilage **-malacia** = abnormal softening	Softening of cartilage
crepitation (krep-ih-TAY-shun)		Noise produced by bones or cartilage rubbing together in conditions such as arthritis; also called *crepitus*
ostealgia (oss-tee-AL-jee-ah)	**oste/o** = bone **-algia** = pain	Bone pain
synovitis (sin-oh-VIGH-tis)	**synov/o** = synovial membrane **-itis** = inflammation	Inflammation of synovial membrane

Pathology (continued)

Term	Word Parts	Definition
Fractures		
closed fracture		Fracture in which there is no open skin wound; also called a *simple fracture*

■ **Figure 4-13** A) Closed (or simple) fracture and B) open (or compound) fracture.

Term	Word Parts	Definition
Colles' fracture (KAW-leez)		Common type of wrist fracture

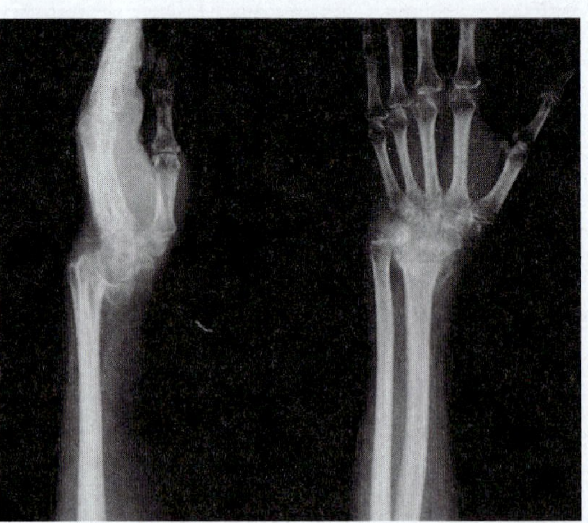

■ **Figure 4-14** Colles' fracture.
(Akawath/Shutterstock)

Term	Word Parts	Definition
comminuted fracture (kom-ih-NYOOT-ed)		Fracture in which bone is shattered, splintered, or crushed into many small pieces or fragments
compound fracture		Fracture in which bone has broken through skin; also called an *open fracture* (see Figure 4-13B)

Pathology (continued)

Term	Word Parts	Definition
compression fracture		Fracture involving loss of height of a vertebral body; may be result of trauma, but in older people, especially women, may be caused by conditions like osteoporosis
fracture (FX, Fx) ■ **Figure 4-15** Figure illustrating the fracture lines seen in different types of fractures. *(Alila Medical Media/Shutterstock)*	Transverse Oblique Spiral Greenstick Comminuted	Broken bone
greenstick fracture		Fracture in which there is an incomplete break; one side of bone is broken and other side is bent; fracture type commonly found in children due to their softer and more pliable bone structure
impacted fracture		Fracture in which bone fragments are pushed into each other
oblique fracture (oh-BLEEK) ■ **Figure 4-16** X-ray showing oblique fracture of the tibia. *(Puwadol Jaturawutthichai/Shutterstock)*		Fracture at an angle to bone
pathologic fracture (path-oh-LOJ-ik)	path/o = disease -logic = pertaining to study of	Fracture caused by diseased or weakened bone
spiral fracture	-al = pertaining to	Fracture in which fracture line spirals around shaft of bone; can be caused by twisting injury and is often slower to heal than other types of fractures
stress fracture		Slight fracture caused by repetitive, low-impact forces, like running, rather than single, forceful impact

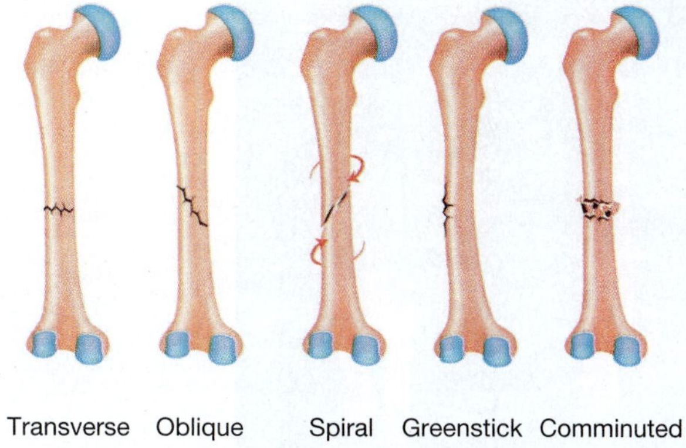

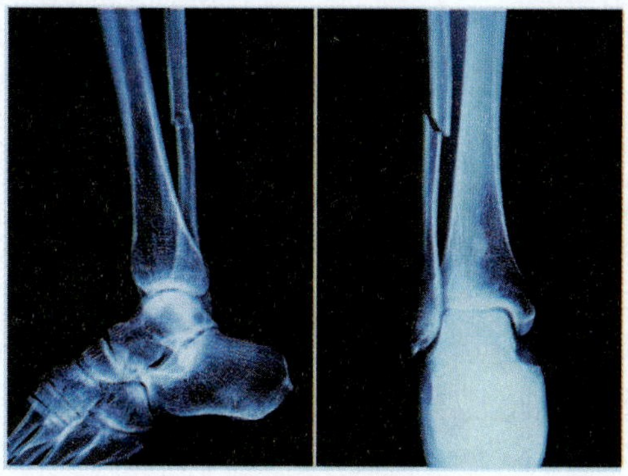

Pathology (continued)

Term	Word Parts	Definition
transverse fracture		Complete fracture that is straight across bone at right angles to long axis of bone
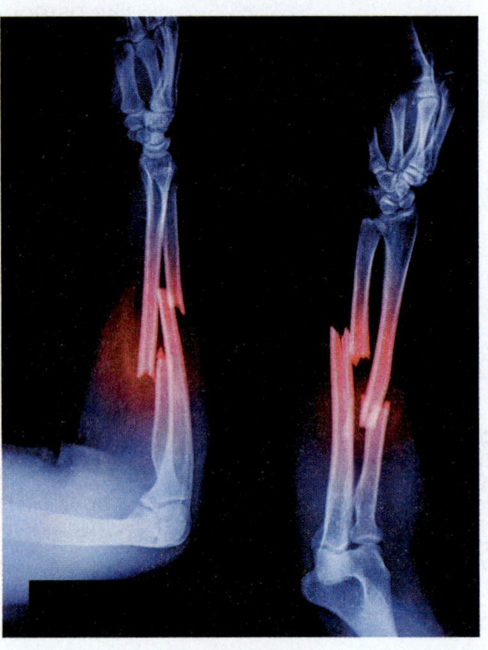 ■ **Figure 4-17** X-ray showing transverse fracture of radius and ulna. *(Puwadol Jaturawutthichai/Shutterstock)*		
Bones		
chondroma (kon-DROH-mah)	chondr/o = cartilage -oma = tumor	Tumor, usually benign, that forms in cartilage
Ewing's sarcoma (YOO-ingz / sar-KOH-mah)	sarc/o = flesh -oma = tumor	Malignant growth found in shaft of long bones that spreads through periosteum; removal is treatment of choice because tumor will metastasize or spread to other organs
exostosis (eks-oss-TOH-sis)	ex- = outward oste/o = bone -osis = abnormal condition	Bony, outward projection from surface of a bone; also called *bone spur*
myeloma (my-eh-LOH-mah)	myel/o = bone marrow -oma = tumor	Tumor that forms in bone marrow tissue
osteochondroma (oss-tee-oh-kon-DROH-mah)	oste/o = bone chondr/o = cartilage -oma = tumor	Tumor, usually benign, that consists of both bone and cartilage tissue
osteogenic sarcoma (oss-tee-oh-JEN-ik / sar-KOH-mah)	oste/o = bone -genic = producing sarc/o = flesh -oma = tumor	Most common type of bone cancer; usually begins in osteocytes found at ends of long bones; also called *osteosarcoma*
osteoma (OSS-tee-oh-mah)	oste/o = bone -oma = tumor	Tumor found in bone tissue
osteomalacia (oss-tee-oh-mah-LAY-shee-ah)	oste/o = bone -malacia = abnormal softening	Softening of bones caused by deficiency of calcium; thought to be caused by insufficient sunlight and vitamin D in children

Pathology (continued)

Term	Word Parts	Definition
osteomyelitis (oss-tee-oh-my-eh-LYE-tis)	oste/o = bone myel/o = bone marrow -itis = inflammation	Inflammation of bone and bone marrow
osteopathy (oss-tee-OP-ah-thee)	oste/o = bone -pathy = disease	General term for bone disease
osteoporosis (oss-tee-oh-poh-ROH-sis)	oste/o = bone -porosis = porous	Decrease in bone mass producing a thinning and weakening of bone with resulting fractures; bone becomes more porous, especially in spine and pelvis
Paget's disease (PAH-jets)		Fairly common metabolic disease of bone from unknown causes; usually attacks middle-aged and older adults and is characterized by bone destruction and deformity; named for Sir James Paget, a British surgeon
rickets (RIK-ets)		Deficiency in calcium and vitamin D found in early childhood that results in bone deformities, especially bowed legs
Spinal Column		
ankylosing spondylitis (ang-kih-LOH-sing / spon-dih-LYE-tis)	ankyl/o = stiff joint spondyl/o = vertebra -itis = inflammation	Inflammatory spinal condition resembling rheumatoid arthritis and results in gradual stiffening and fusion of vertebrae; more common in men than in women
herniated nucleus pulposus (HNP) (HER-nee-ay-ted / NOO-klee-us / pul-POH-sus)		Herniation or protrusion of intervertebral disk; also called *herniated disk* or *ruptured disk*; may require surgery
■ **Figure 4-18** Magnetic resonance imaging (MRI) image demonstrating a back herniated disk. *(Michelle Milano/ Shutterstock)*		
kyphosis (kye-FOH-sis)	kyph/o = hump -osis = abnormal condition	Abnormal increase in outward curvature of thoracic spine; also known as *hunchback* or *humpback*; see Figure 4-19 ■ for illustration of abnormal spine curvatures

Pathology (continued)

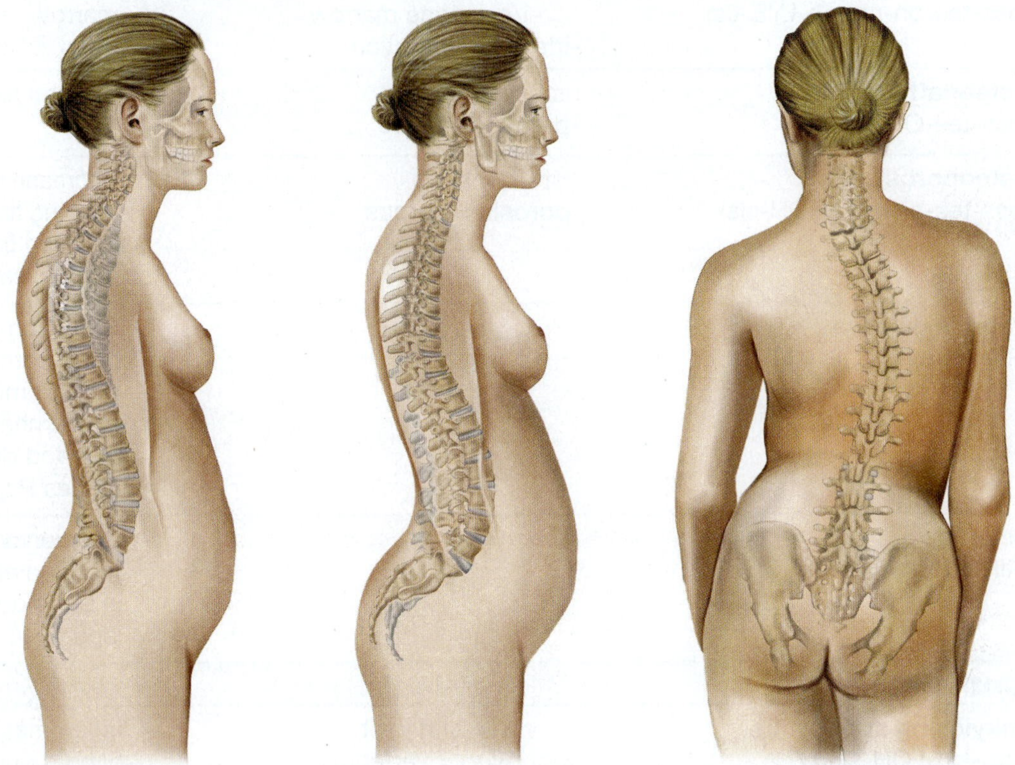

Term	Word Parts	Definition
■ **Figure 4-19** Abnormal spinal curvatures: kyphosis, lordosis, and scoliosis. **Kyphosis** (excessive posterior thoracic curvature - hunchback) **Lordosis** (excessive anterior lumbar curvature - swayback) **Scoliosis** (lateral curvature)		
lordosis (lor-DOH-sis)	lord/o = bent backward -osis = abnormal condition	Abnormal increase in forward curvature of lumbar spine; also known as *swayback*
scoliosis (skoh-lee-OH-sis)	scoli/o = crooked -osis = abnormal condition	Abnormal lateral curvature of spine; see again Figure 4-19 for illustration of abnormal spine curvatures
spina bifida (SPY-nah / BIF-ih-dah)	spin/o = spine bi- = two	Congenital anomaly occurring when vertebra fails to fully form around spinal cord; see also Figure 12-12C
spinal stenosis (steh-NOH-sis)	spin/o = spine -al = pertaining to **Word Watch** Watch how the term *stenosis* is used in this condition. It most often appears as the suffix **-stenosis**. However, in this case, it is used as a freestanding word.	Narrowing of spinal canal causing pressure on cord and nerves
spondylolisthesis (spon-dih-loh-liss-THEE-sis)	spondyl/o = vertebra -listhesis = slipping	Forward sliding of lumbar vertebra over vertebra below it
spondylosis (spon-dih-LOH-sis)	spondyl/o = vertebra -osis = abnormal condition	Specifically refers to ankylosing of spine, but commonly used in reference to any degenerative condition of vertebral column

Pathology (continued)

Term	Word Parts	Definition
whiplash		Cervical muscle and ligament sprain or strain as a result of sudden movement forward and backward of head and neck; can occur as a result of rear-end auto collision
Joints		
bunion (BUN-yun)		Inflammation of bursa of first metatarsophalangeal joint (base of big toe)
dislocation	dis- = apart	Occurs when bones in a joint are displaced from normal alignment and ends of bones are no longer in contact
gout (GOWT)		Type of arthritis presenting as pain and swelling usually in first metatarsophalangeal joint; caused by high uric acid blood level resulting in uric acid crystals being deposited in soft tissue; more common in men
osteoarthritis (OA) (oss-tee-oh-ar-THRY-tis)	oste/o = bone arthr/o = joint -itis = inflammation	Arthritis resulting in degeneration of bones and joints, especially those bearing weight; results in bone rubbing against bone; also called *degenerative joint disease (DJD)*
prepatellar bursitis (pree-pah-TELL-ar / ber-SIGH-tis)	pre- = before patell/o = patella -ar = pertaining to burs/o = bursa -itis = inflammation	Pain and swelling in bursa located between patella and skin; seen often in persons who kneel frequently; commonly called *housemaid's knee*
rheumatoid arthritis (RA) (ROO-mah-toyd / ar-THRY-tis)	arthr/o = joint -itis = inflammation	Chronic form of arthritis with inflammation of joints, swelling, stiffness, pain, and changes in cartilage that can result in crippling deformities; considered to be autoimmune disease

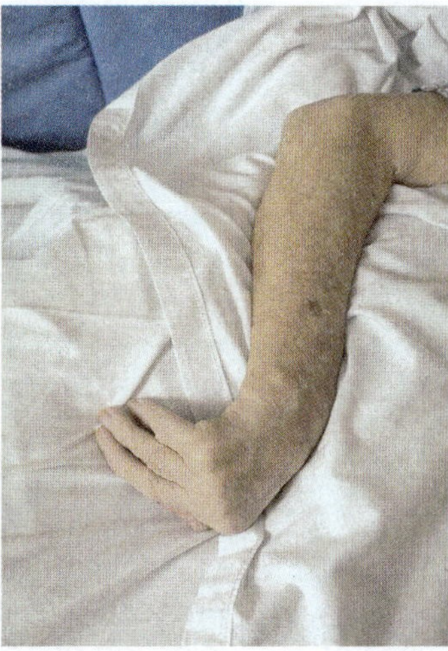

■ **Figure 4-20** Patient with typical rheumatoid arthritis contractures. *(Michal Heron/Pearson Education, Inc.)*

Pathology (continued)

Term	Word Parts	Definition
sprain		Damage to ligaments surrounding a joint due to overstretching, but no dislocation of joint or fracture of bone
subluxation (sub-luks-AY-shun)	sub- = under	Incomplete dislocation; joint alignment is disrupted, but ends of bones remain in contact
systemic lupus erythematosus (SLE) (sis-TEM-ik / LOO-pus / air-ih-them-ah-TOH-sus)	system/o = system -ic = pertaining to erythr/o = red	Chronic inflammatory autoimmune disease of connective tissue affecting many systems that may include joint pain and arthritis; may be mistaken for rheumatoid arthritis
talipes (TAL-ih-peez)		Congenital deformity causing misalignment of ankle joint and foot; also referred to as *clubfoot*

PRACTICE AS YOU GO

D. Pathology Matching

Match each term to its definition.

_____ **1.** chondromalacia — **a.** abnormal outward curvature of thoracic spine

_____ **2.** exostosis — **b.** an incomplete dislocation

_____ **3.** rheumatoid arthritis — **c.** thinning and weakening of the bone

_____ **4.** subluxation — **d.** bone spur

_____ **5.** bunion — **e.** softening of cartilage

_____ **6.** spina bifida — **f.** braces and splints

_____ **7.** kyphosis — **g.** inflammation at base of big toe

_____ **8.** osteoporosis — **h.** shattered fracture

_____ **9.** orthotics — **i.** a congenital anomaly

_____ **10.** comminuted — **j.** considered to be an autoimmune disease

Diagnostic Procedures

Term	Word Part	Definition
Diagnostic Imaging		
arthrogram (AR-throh-gram)	arthr/o = joint -gram = record	X-ray record of a joint, usually taken after joint has been injected by contrast medium
arthrography (ar-THROG-rah-fee)	arthr/o = joint -graphy = process of recording	Process of X-raying a joint, usually after injection of contrast medium into joint space

Diagnostic Procedures (continued)

Term	Word Part	Definition
bone scan 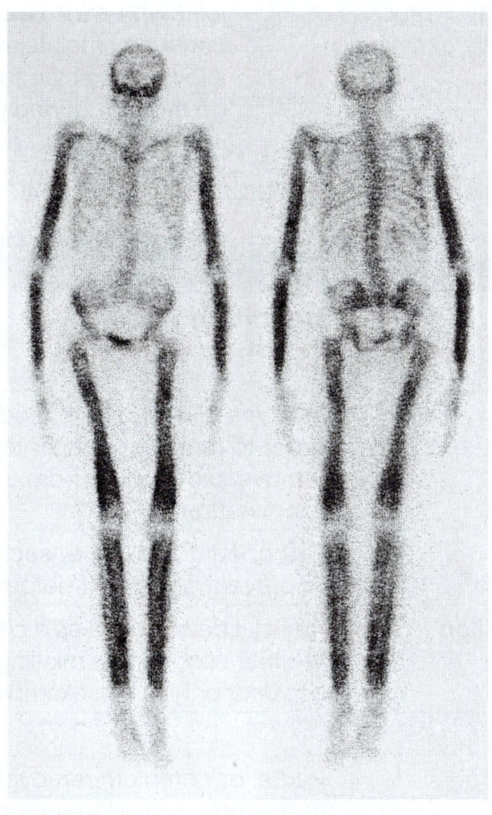 ■ **Figure 4-21** Photograph illustrating the appearance of a bone scan. The darker regions are produced by bone areas that take up more of the radioactive dye. *(Susan Law Cain/Shutterstock)*		Nuclear medicine procedure in which patient is given radioactive dye and then scanning equipment is used to visualize bones; especially useful in identifying stress fractures, observing progress of treatment for osteomyelitis, and locating cancer metastases to bone
dual-energy X-ray absorptiometry (DXA, DEXA) (ab-sorp-shee-AHM-eh-tree)	**-metry** = process of measuring	Measurement of bone density using low-dose X-ray for purpose of detecting osteoporosis
myelogram (MY-eh-loh-gram)	**myel/o** = spinal cord **-gram** = record	X-ray record of spinal column after injection of opaque dye
myelography (my-eh-LOG-rah-fee)	**myel/o** = spinal cord **-graphy** = process of recording	Study of spinal column after injecting opaque contrast material; particularly useful in identifying herniated nucleus pulposus pinching a spinal nerve **Med Term Tip** The combining form **myel/o** means *marrow* and is used for both the spinal cord and bone marrow. To the ancient Greek philosophers and physicians, the spinal cord appeared to be much like the marrow found in the medullary cavity of a long bone.
radiograph (RAY-dee-oh-graf)	**radi/o** = ray **-graph** = record	Image produced by X-rays striking photographic film; commonly referred to as an *X-ray*
radiography (ray-dee-OG-rah-fee)	**radi/o** = ray **-graphy** = process of recording	Diagnostic imaging procedure using X-rays to study internal structure of body; especially useful for visualizing bones and joints
Endoscopic Procedures		
arthroscope (AR-throh-skohp)	**arthr/o** = joint **-scope** = instrument for viewing	Instrument used to view inside a joint

Diagnostic Procedures (continued)

Term	Word Part	Definition
arthroscopy (ar-THROS-koh-pee)	arthr/o = joint -scopy = process of visually examining	Examination of interior of a joint by entering joint with *arthroscope*; arthroscope contains small television camera that allows physician to view interior of joint on monitor during procedure; some joint conditions can be repaired during arthroscopy

Therapeutic Procedures

Term	Word Part	Definition
Medical Treatments		
arthrocentesis (ar-throh-sen-TEE-sis)	arthr/o = joint -centesis = puncture to withdraw fluid	Involves insertion of a needle into joint cavity in order to remove or aspirate fluid; may be done to remove excess fluid from a joint or to obtain fluid for examination
orthotic (or-THOT-ik)	orth/o = straight -tic = pertaining to	Orthopedic appliance, such as brace or splint, used to prevent or correct deformities
prosthesis (pross-THEE-sis)	prosthet/o = addition	Artificial device used as a substitute for body part that is either congenitally missing or absent as a result of accident or disease; example would be an artificial leg
Surgical Procedures		
amputation (am-pyoo-TAY-shun)		Partial or complete removal of a limb for a variety of reasons, including tumors, gangrene, intractable pain, crushing injury, or uncontrollable infection
arthroclasia (ar-throh-KLAY-zee-ah)	arthr/o = joint -clasia = surgically break	To forcibly break loose a fused joint while patient is under anesthetic; fusion usually caused by buildup of scar tissue or adhesions
arthrodesis (ar-throh-DEE-sis)	arthr/o = joint -desis = to fuse	Procedure to stabilize a joint by fusing bones together
arthroscopic surgery (ar-throh-SKOP-ik)	arthr/o = joint -scopic = pertaining to visually examining	Performing a surgical procedure while using arthroscope to view internal structure, such as a joint
arthrotomy (ar-THROT-oh-mee)	arthr/o = joint -otomy = cutting into	Surgical procedure that cuts into a joint capsule
bone graft		Piece of bone taken from patient used to take the place of removed bone or bony defect at another site
bunionectomy (bun-yun-EK-toh-mee)	-ectomy = surgical removal	Removal of bursa at joint of great toe
bursectomy (ber-SEK-toh-mee)	burs/o = bursa -ectomy = surgical removal	Surgical removal of a bursa
chondrectomy (kon-DREK-toh-mee)	chondr/o = cartilage -ectomy = surgical removal	Surgical removal of cartilage
chondroplasty (KON-droh-plas-tee)	chondr/o = cartilage -plasty = surgical repair	Surgical repair of cartilage
craniotomy (kray-nee-OT-oh-mee)	crani/o = skull -otomy = cutting into	Surgical procedure that cuts into skull

Therapeutic Procedures (continued)

Term	Word Part	Definition
laminectomy (lam-ih-NEK-toh-mee)	**lamin/o** = lamina **-ectomy** = surgical removal	Removal of vertebral posterior arch to correct severe back problems and pain caused by compression of spinal nerve
osteoclasia (oss-tee-oh-KLAY-zee-ah)	**oste/o** = bone **-clasia** = surgically break	Surgical procedure involving intentional breaking of bone to correct a deformity
osteotome (OSS-tee-oh-tohm)	**oste/o** = bone **-tome** = instrument to cut	Instrument used to cut bone
osteotomy (oss-tee-OT-ah-mee)	**oste/o** = bone **-otomy** = cutting into	Surgical procedure that cuts into a bone
percutaneous diskectomy (per-kyoo-TAY-nee-us / dis-KEK-toh-mee)	**per-** = through **cutane/o** = skin **-ous** = pertaining to **-ectomy** = surgical removal	Thin catheter tube is inserted into intervertebral disk through skin and herniated or ruptured disk material is sucked out or a laser is used to vaporize it
spinal fusion	**spin/o** = spine **-al** = pertaining to	Surgical immobilization of adjacent vertebrae; may be done for several reasons, including correction for herniated disk
synovectomy (sin-oh-VEK-toh-mee)	**synov/o** = synovial membrane **-ectomy** = surgical removal	Surgical removal of synovial membrane
total hip arthroplasty (THA) (AR-throh-plas-tee)	**arthr/o** = joint **-plasty** = surgical repair	Surgical reconstruction of hip by implanting prosthetic or artificial hip joint; also called *total hip replacement (THR)*
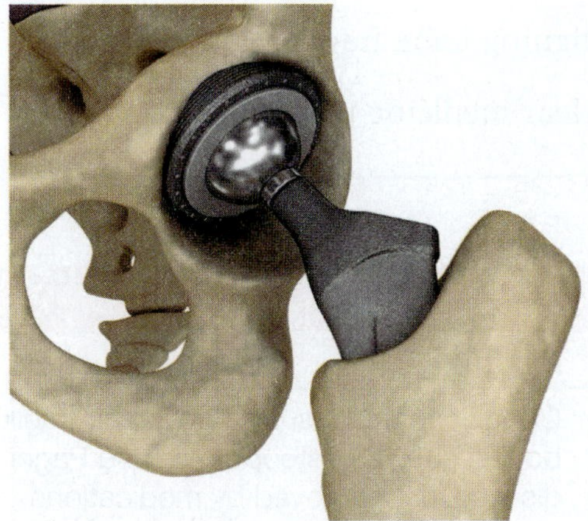 ■ **Figure 4-22** Prosthetic hip joint. *(Alex Mit/Shutterstock)*		
total knee arthroplasty (TKA) (AR-throh-plas-tee)	**arthr/o** = joint **-plasty** = surgical repair	Surgical reconstruction of knee joint by implanting prosthetic knee joint; also called *total knee replacement (TKR)*
Fracture Care		
cast		Application of solid material to immobilize extremity or portion of body as a result of fracture, dislocation, or severe injury; may be made of plaster of Paris or fiberglass
fixation		Procedure to stabilize fractured bone while it heals; *external fixation* includes casts, splints, and pins inserted through skin; *internal fixation* includes pins, plates, rods, screws, and wires that are applied during *open reduction*

Therapeutic Procedures (continued)

Term	Word Part	Definition
reduction		Correcting fracture by realigning bone fragments; *closed reduction* is doing manipulation without entering body; *open reduction* is process of making surgical incision at site of fracture to do reduction; necessary when bony fragments need to be removed or *internal fixation*, such as plates or pins, is required
traction		Applying a pulling force on fractured or dislocated limb or vertebral column in order to restore normal alignment

PRACTICE AS YOU GO

E. Procedure Matching

Match each term to its definition.

_____ **1.** reduction	**a.** an X-ray
_____ **2.** osteoclasia	**b.** fusing bones to stabilize a joint
_____ **3.** bone scan	**c.** intentional breaking of a bone
_____ **4.** radiograph	**d.** replacement body part
_____ **5.** prosthesis	**e.** realigning bone fragments
_____ **6.** arthrodesis	**f.** nuclear medicine procedure

Pharmacology

Classification	Word Parts	Action	Examples
bone reabsorption inhibitors		Conditions that result in weak and fragile bones, such as osteoporosis and Paget's disease, are improved by medications that inhibit reabsorption of bones	alendronate, Fosamax; ibandronate, Boniva
calcium supplements and vitamin D therapy		Maintaining high blood levels of calcium in association with vitamin D helps maintain bone density; used to treat osteomalacia, osteoporosis, and rickets	calcium carbonate, Oystercal, Tums; calcium citrate, Cal-Citrate, Citracal
corticosteroids	**cortic/o** = outer layer	Natural or synthetic adrenal cortex hormone; has very strong anti-inflammatory properties; particularly useful in treating rheumatoid arthritis	prednisone; methylprednisolone, Medrol; dexamethasone, Decadron
nonsteroidal anti-inflammatory drugs (NSAIDs)	**non-** = not **-al** = pertaining to **anti-** = against **-ory** = pertaining to	Large group of drugs (other than corticosteroids) that provide mild pain relief and anti-inflammatory benefits for conditions such as arthritis	ibuprofen, Advil, Motrin; naproxen, Aleve, Naprosyn; aspirin, Bayer's, Bufferin

Abbreviations

AE	above elbow	**NSAID**	nonsteroidal anti-inflammatory drug
AK	above knee	**OA**	osteoarthritis
BDT	bone density testing	**ORIF**	open reduction–internal fixation
BE	below elbow	**Orth, Ortho**	orthopedics
BK	below knee	**P**	phosphorus
C1, C2, etc.	first cervical vertebra, second cervical vertebra, etc.	**RA**	rheumatoid arthritis
Ca	calcium	**RLE**	right lower extremity
DJD	degenerative joint disease	**ROM**	range of motion
DXA, DEXA	dual-energy X-ray absorptiometry	**RUE**	right upper extremity
FX, Fx	fracture	**SLE**	systemic lupus erythematosus
HNP	herniated nucleus pulposus	**T1, T2, etc.**	first thoracic vertebra, second thoracic vertebra, etc.
JRA	juvenile rheumatoid arthritis	**THA**	total hip arthroplasty
L1, L2, etc.	first lumbar vertebra, second lumbar vertebra, etc.	**THR**	total hip replacement
LE	lower extremity	**TKA**	total knee arthroplasty
LLE	left lower extremity	**TKR**	total knee replacement
LUE	left upper extremity	**UE**	upper extremity

PRACTICE AS YOU GO

F. What's the Abbreviation?

1. total knee replacement ______________________
2. herniated nucleus pulposus ______________________
3. upper extremity ______________________
4. fifth lumbar vertebra ______________________
5. above the knee ______________________
6. fracture ______________________
7. nonsteroidal anti-inflammatory drug ______________________

SECTION II: MUSCULAR SYSTEM

AT A GLANCE

Function

Muscles are bundles, sheets, or rings of tissue that produce movement by contracting and pulling on the structures to which they are attached.

Organs

The primary structure that comprises the muscular system:

muscles

Word Parts

Presented here are the most common word parts (with their meanings) used to build muscular system terms. For a more comprehensive list, refer to the Terminology section of this chapter.

Combining Forms

duct/o	to bring
extens/o	to stretch out
fasci/o	fibrous band
fibr/o	fibers
flex/o	to bend
habilitat/o	ability
hydr/o	water
kinesi/o	movement
muscul/o	muscle
my/o	muscle
myos/o	muscle
phon/o	sound
physic/o	body
plant/o	sole of foot
rotat/o	to revolve
ten/o	tendon
tend/o	tendon
tendin/o	tendon
therm/o	heat
vers/o	to turn

Suffixes

-asthenia	weakness
-ion	action
-kinesia	movement
-phoresis	carrying
-tonia	tone
-trophic	pertaining to development

Prefixes

ab-	away from
ad-	toward
circum-	around
e-	outward

Muscular System Illustrated

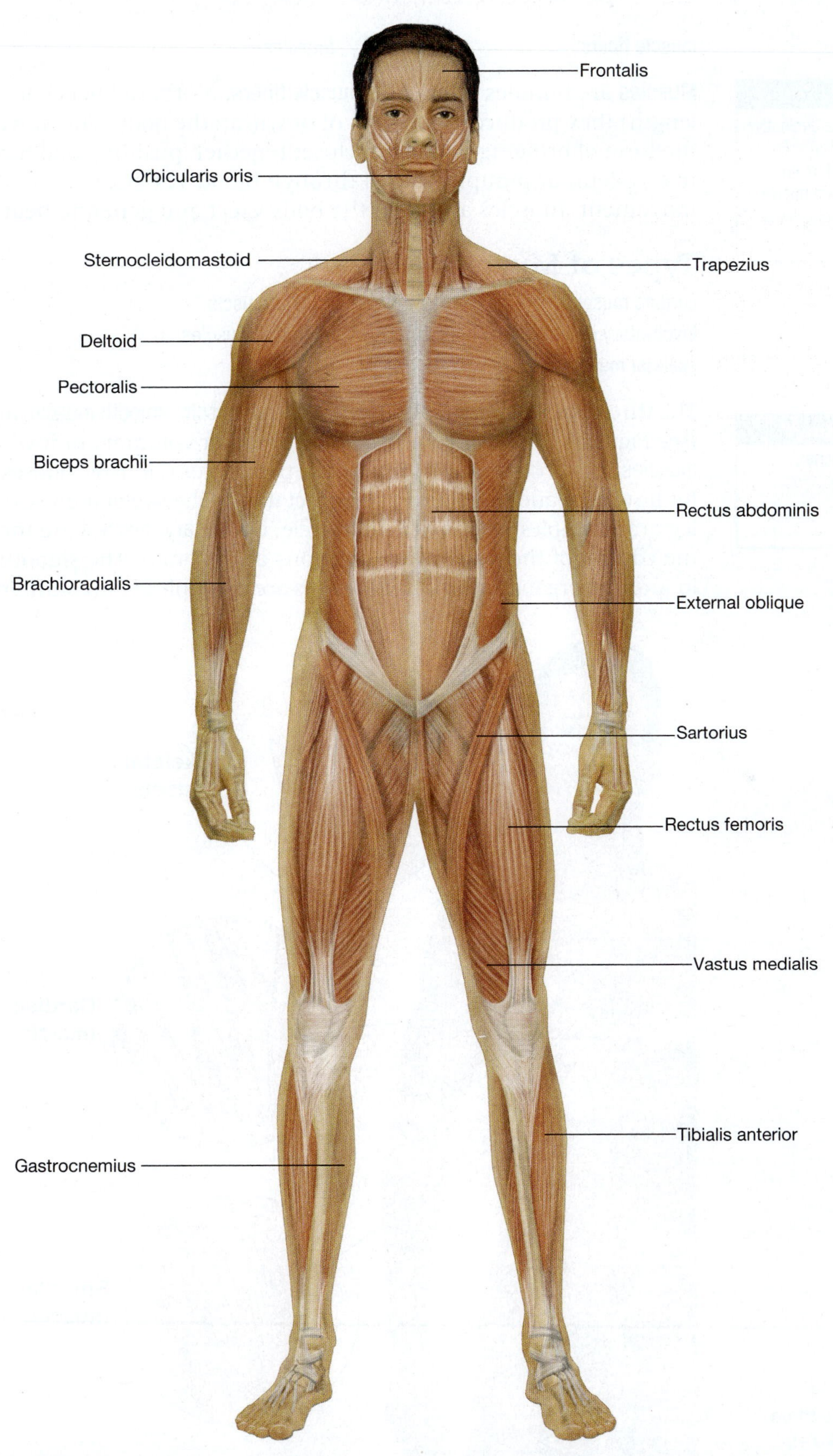

Anatomy and Physiology of the Muscular System

muscle fibers **muscles**

Med Term Tip

The term *muscle* is the diminutive form of the Latin word *mus* or "little mouse." This is thought to describe how the skin ripples when a muscle contracts, like a little mouse running.

Muscles are bundles of parallel **muscle fibers**. As these fibers contract (shorten in length) they produce movement of or within the body. The movement may take the form of bringing two bones closer together, pushing food through the digestive system, or pumping blood through blood vessels. In addition to producing movement, muscles also hold the body erect and generate heat.

Types of Muscles

cardiac muscle
involuntary muscles
skeletal muscle
smooth muscle
voluntary muscles

What's In A Name?

Look for these word parts:
cardi/o = heart
-ac = pertaining to
in- = not

The three types of muscle tissue are **skeletal muscle**, **smooth muscle**, and **cardiac muscle** (see Figure 4-23 ■). Muscle tissue may be either voluntary or involuntary. **Voluntary muscles** are those muscles for which a person consciously chooses to contract and for how long and how hard to contract them. The skeletal muscles of the arm and leg are examples of this type of muscle. **Involuntary muscles** are the muscles under the control of the subconscious regions of the brain. The smooth muscles found in internal organs and cardiac muscles are examples of involuntary muscle tissue.

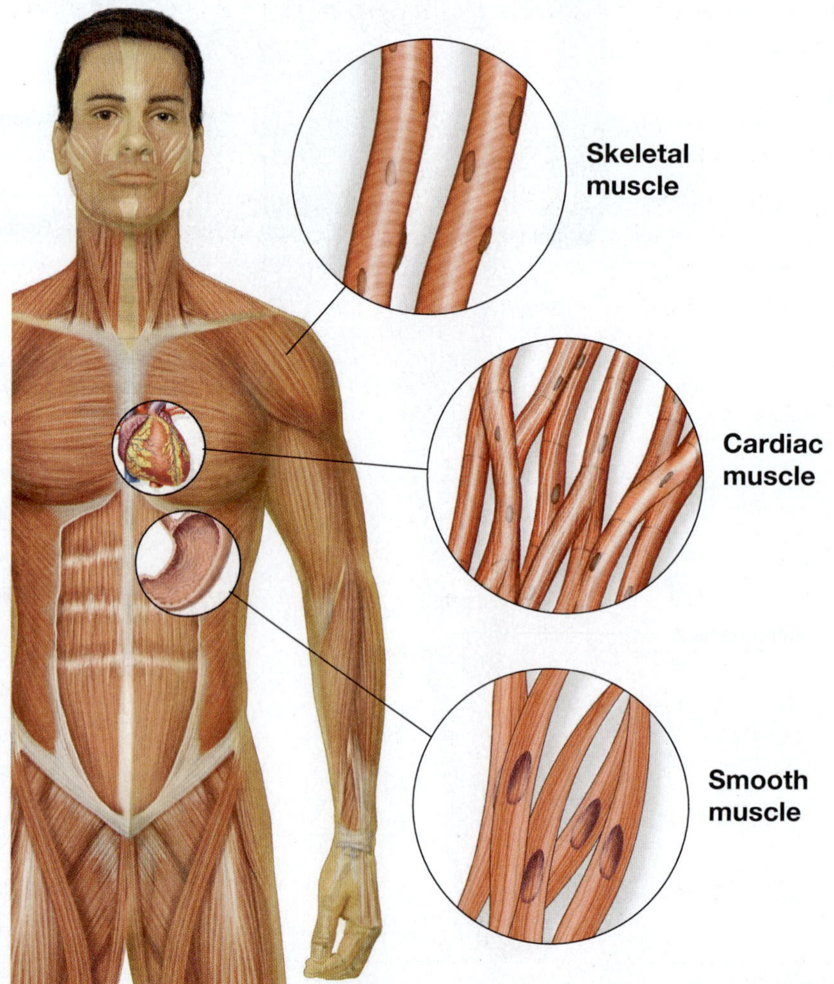

■ **Figure 4-23** The three types of muscles: skeletal, smooth, and cardiac.

Skeletal Muscle

fascia (FASH-ee-ah)
motor neurons
myoneural junction (my-oh-NOO-ral)
neuromuscular junction (noo-roh-MUS-kyoo-lar)
striated muscles (STRY-ay-ted)
tendon (TEN-dun)

A skeletal muscle is directly or indirectly attached to a bone and produces voluntary movement of the skeleton. It is also referred to as a **striated muscle** because of its striped appearance under a microscope (see Figure 4-24 ■). Each muscle is wrapped in layers of fibrous connective tissue called **fascia**. The fascia tapers at each end of a skeletal muscle to form a very strong **tendon**. The tendon then inserts into the periosteum covering a bone to anchor the muscle to the bone. Skeletal muscles are stimulated by **motor neurons** of the nervous system. The point at which the motor nerve contacts a muscle fiber is called the **myoneural junction** or the **neuromuscular junction**.

Med Term Tip

The human body has more than 400 skeletal muscles, which account for almost 50% of the body's weight.

Smooth Muscle

visceral muscle (VISS-er-ral)

Smooth muscle tissue is found in association with internal organs. For this reason, it is also referred to as **visceral muscle**. The name *smooth muscle* refers to the muscle's microscopic appearance; it lacks the striations of skeletal muscle (see again Figure 4-24). Smooth muscle is found in the walls of hollow organs, such as the stomach; tube-shaped organs, such as the respiratory airways; and blood vessels. It is responsible for the involuntary muscle action associated with movement of the internal organs, such as churning food, constricting a blood vessel, and uterine contractions.

What's In A Name?

Look for these word parts:
cardi/o = heart
muscul/o = muscle
my/o = muscle
neur/o = nerve
viscer/o = internal organ
-al = pertaining to
-ar = pertaining to

Cardiac Muscle

myocardium (my-oh-KAR-dee-um)

Cardiac muscle, or **myocardium**, makes up the wall of the heart (see again Figure 4-24). With each involuntary contraction, the heart squeezes to pump blood out of its chambers and through the blood vessels. This muscle is more thoroughly described in Chapter 5, Cardiovascular System.

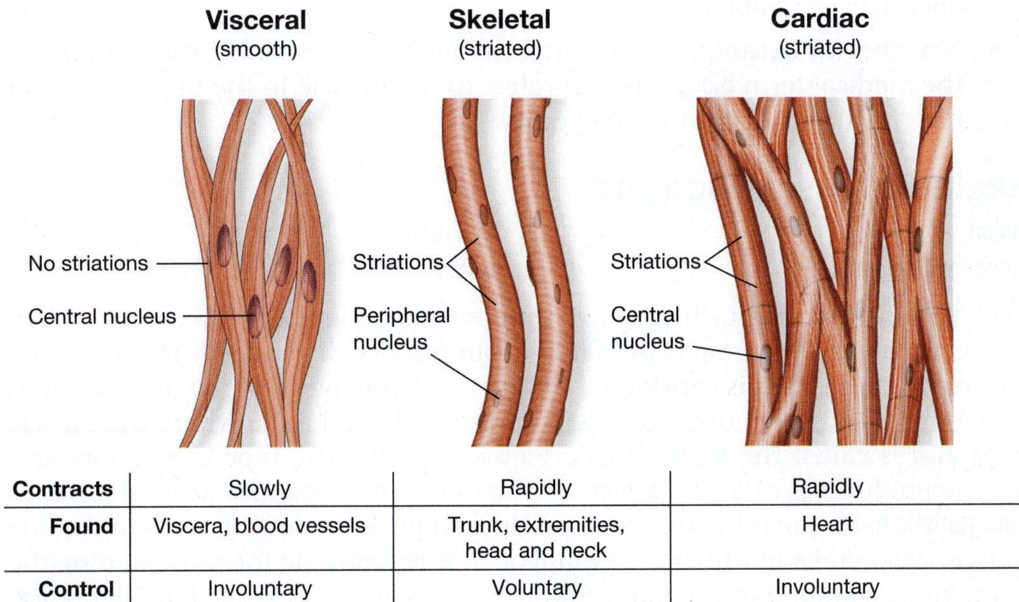

	Visceral (smooth)	Skeletal (striated)	Cardiac (striated)
Contracts	Slowly	Rapidly	Rapidly
Found	Viscera, blood vessels	Trunk, extremities, head and neck	Heart
Control	Involuntary	Voluntary	Involuntary

■ **Figure 4-24** Characteristics of the three types of muscles.

PRACTICE AS YOU GO

G. Complete the Statement

1. Another name for visceral muscle is ________________ muscle.
2. Nerves contact skeletal muscle fibers at the ________________ junction.
3. The three types of muscle are ________________, ________________, and ________________.

Naming Skeletal Muscles

biceps (BYE-seps)
extensor carpi
external oblique
flexor carpi
gluteus maximus (GLOO-tee-us / MAKS-ih-mus)
rectus abdominis (REK-tus / ab-DOM-ih-nis)
sternocleidomastoid (ster-noh-kly-doh-MAS-toyd)

The name of a muscle often reflects its location, origin and insertion, size, action, fiber direction, or number of attachment points, as illustrated by the following examples:

- **Location:** the term **rectus abdominis** means *straight* (rectus) abdominal muscle.
- **Origin and insertion:** the **sternocleidomastoid** is named for its two origins (**stern/o** for sternum and **cleid/o** for clavicle) and single insertion (mastoid process).
- **Size:** when gluteus, meaning rump area, is combined with maximus, meaning large, we have the term **gluteus maximus**.
- **Action:** the **flexor carpi** and **extensor carpi** muscles are named as such because they produce flexion and extension at the wrist.
- **Fiber direction:** the **external oblique** muscle is an abdominal muscle whose fibers run at an oblique angle.
- **Number of attachment points:** the prefix **bi-**, meaning two, can form the medical term **biceps**, which refers to the muscle in the upper arm that has two heads or connecting points.

What's In A Name?

Look for these word parts:
cleid/o = clavicle
extens/o = to stretch out
flex/o = to bend
stern/o = sternum
-al = pertaining to
bi- = two
ex- = outward

Skeletal Muscle Actions

action
antagonistic pairs
insertion
origin

Skeletal muscles are attached to two different bones and overlap a joint. When a muscle contracts, the two bones move, but not usually equally. The less movable of the two bones is considered to be the starting point of the muscle and is called the **origin**. The more movable bone is considered to be where the muscle ends and is called the **insertion** (see Figure 4-25 ■). The type of movement a muscle produces is called its **action**. Muscles are often arranged around joints in **antagonistic pairs**, meaning that they produce opposite actions. For example, one muscle will bend a joint while its antagonist is responsible for straightening the joint. Some common terminology for muscle actions are described in Table 4-5 ■.

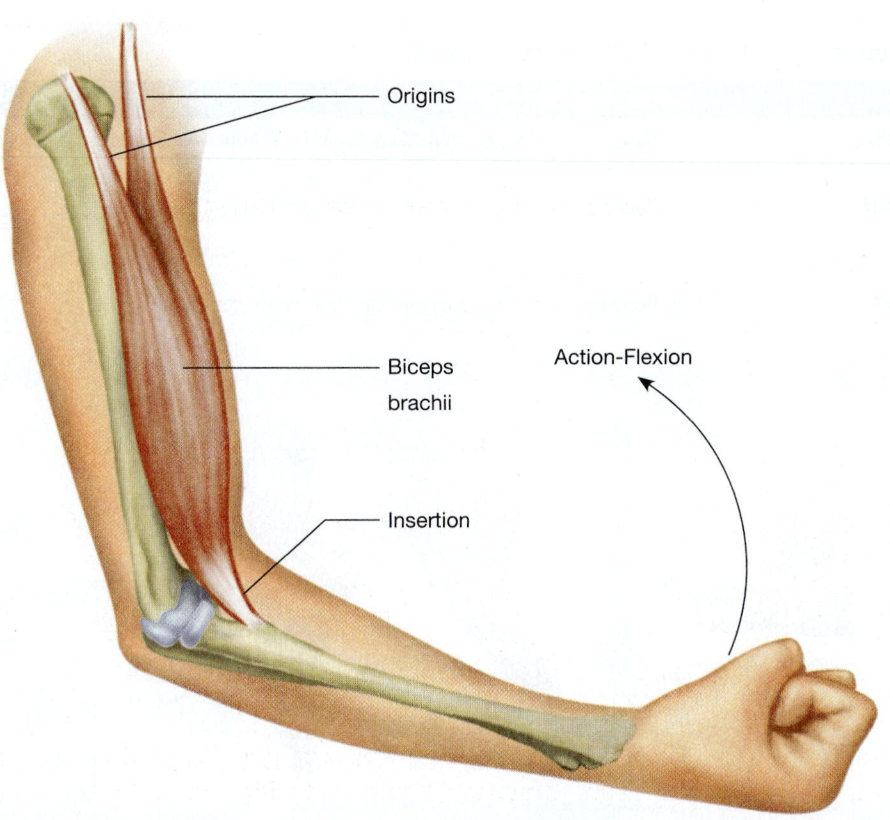

Figure 4-25 Origin and insertion of a muscle

TABLE 4-5 Muscle Actions Grouped by Antagonistic Pairs

Action	Word Parts	Description
abduction (ab-DUK-shun)	**ab-** = away from **duct/o** = to bring **-ion** = action	Movement away from midline of the body (see Figure 4-26 ■)
adduction (ah-DUK-shun)	**ad-** = toward **duct/o** = to bring **-ion** = action	Movement toward midline of the body (see again Figure 4-26)
flexion (FLEK-shun)	**flex/o** = to bend **-ion** = action	Act of bending or being bent (see Figure 4-27 ■)

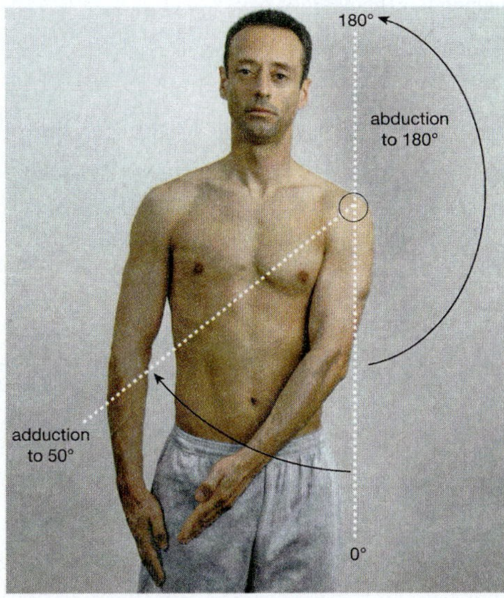

Figure 4-26 Abduction and adduction of the shoulder joint. *(Patrick Watson/Pearson Education, Inc.)*

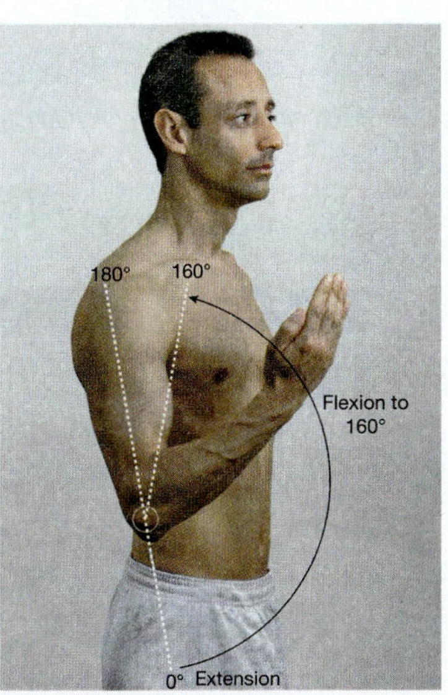

Figure 4-27 Flexion and extension of the elbow joint. *(Patrick Watson/Pearson Education, Inc.)*

■ **TABLE 4-5** Muscle Actions Grouped by Antagonistic Pairs (continued)

Action	Word Parts	Description
extension (eks-TEN-shun)	**extens/o** = to stretch out **-ion** = action	Movement that brings limb into or toward a straight condition (see again Figure 4-27)
dorsiflexion (dor-sih-FLEK-shun)	**dors/o** = back of body **flex/o** = to bend **-ion** = action	Backward bending, as of hand or foot (see Figure 4-28A ■)
plantar flexion (PLAN-tar / FLEK-shun)	**plant/o** = sole of foot **-ar** = pertaining to **flex/o** = to bend **-ion** = action	Bending sole of foot; pointing toes downward (see Figure 4-28B ■)

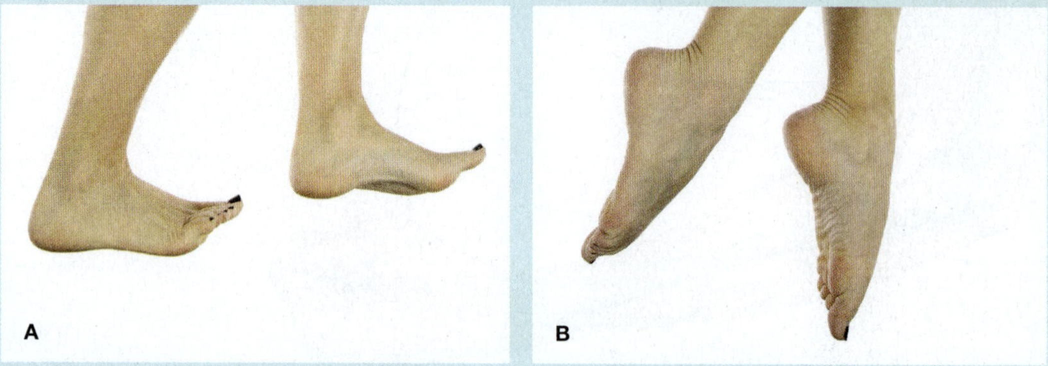

A B

■ **Figure 4-28** Dorsiflexion (A) and plantar flexion (B) of the ankle joint. *(Alan Poulsons Photography/Shutterstock)*

Action	Word Parts	Description
eversion (ee-VER-zhun)	**e-** = outward **vers/o** = to turn **-ion** = action	Turning outward (see Figure 4-29 ■)
inversion (in-VER-zhun)	**in-** = inward **vers/o** = to turn **-ion** = action	Turning inward (see again Figure 4-29)
pronation (proh-NAY-shun)		To turn downward or backward as with the hand or foot (see Figure 4-30 ■)
supination (soo-pih-NAY-shun)		Turning the palm or foot upward (see again Figure 4-30)
elevation		To raise a body part, as in shrugging the shoulders
depression		A downward movement, as in dropping the shoulders
The circular actions described below are an exception to the antagonistic pair arrangement.		
circumduction (ser-kum-DUK-shun)	**circum-** = around **duct/o** = to bring **-ion** = action	Movement in a circular direction from a central point as if drawing a large, imaginary circle in the air
opposition	**Med Term Tip** Primates are the only animals with opposable thumbs.	Moving thumb away from palm; the ability to move the thumb into contact with the other fingers
rotation	**rotat/o** = to revolve **-ion** = action	Moving around a central axis

TABLE 4-5 Muscle Actions Grouped by Antagonistic Pairs (continued)

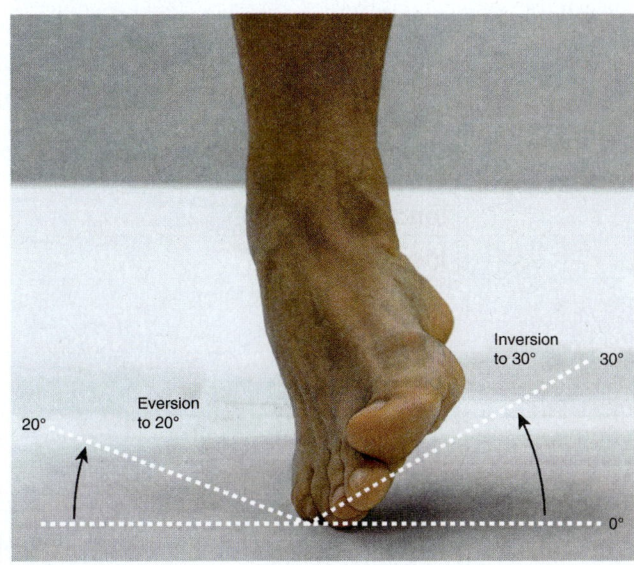

Figure 4-29 Eversion and inversion of the foot.
(Patrick Watson/Pearson Education, Inc.)

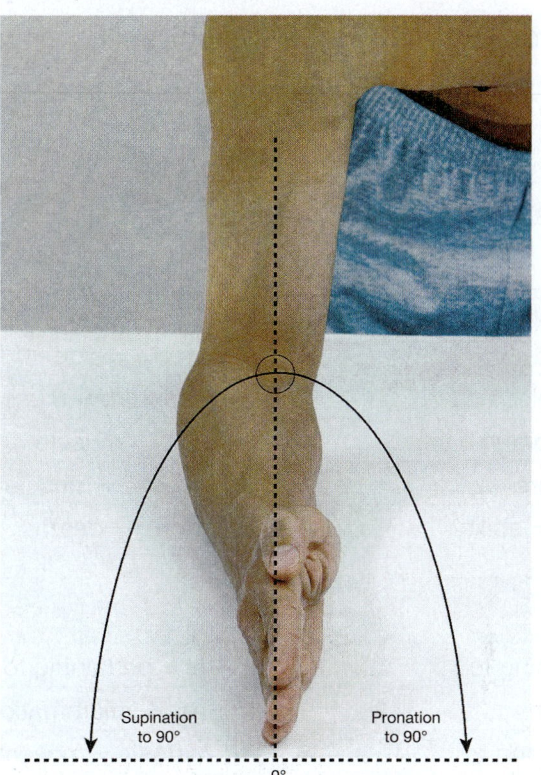

Figure 4-30 Pronation and supination of the forearm.
(Patrick Watson/Pearson Education, Inc.)

PRACTICE AS YOU GO

H. Terminology Matching

Match each term to its definition.

1. ________ abduction	**a.** backward bending of the foot
2. ________ rotation	**b.** bending the foot to point toes toward the ground
3. ________ plantar flexion	**c.** straightening motion
4. ________ extension	**d.** motion around a central axis
5. ________ dorsiflexion	**e.** motion away from the body
6. ________ flexion	**f.** moving the thumb away from the palm
7. ________ adduction	**g.** motion toward the body
8. ________ opposition	**h.** bending motion

Terminology

Word Parts Used to Build Muscular System Terms

The following lists contain the combining forms, suffixes, and prefixes used to build terms in the remaining sections of this chapter.

Combining Forms		
bi/o = life	**hydr/o** = water	**phon/o** = sound
carp/o = carpus	**kinesi/o** = movement	**physic/o** = body
cry/o = cold	**later/o** = side	**ten/o** = tendon
electr/o = electricity	**muscul/o** = muscle	**tend/o** = tendon
fasci/o = fibrous band	**my/o** = muscle	**tendin/o** = tendon
fibr/o = fibers	**myos/o** = muscle	**therm/o** = heat
habilitat/o = ability	**necr/o** = death	

Suffixes		
-al = pertaining to	**-ic** = pertaining to	**-phoresis** = carrying
-algia = pain	**-itis** = inflammation	**-plasty** = surgical repair
-ar = pertaining to	**-kinesia** = movement	**-rrhaphy** = suture
-asthenia = weakness	**-logy** = study of	**-rrhexis** = rupture
-desis = to fuse	**-opsy** = view of	**-therapy** = treatment
-dynia = pain	**-otomy** = cutting into	**-tonia** = tone
-gram = record	**-ous** = pertaining to	**-trophic** = pertaining to development
-graphy = process of recording	**-pathy** = disease	**-trophy** = development

Prefixes		
a- = without	**hyper-** = excessive	**re-** = again
brady- = slow	**hypo-** = insufficient	**ultra-** = beyond
dys- = abnormal; difficult	**poly-** = many	
epi- = above	**pseudo-** = false	

Adjective Forms of Anatomical Terms

Term	Word Parts	Definition
fascial (FASH-ee-al)	**fasci/o** = fibrous band **-al** = pertaining to	Pertaining to fascia
muscular (MUS-kyoo-lar)	**muscul/o** = muscle **-ar** = pertaining to	Pertaining to muscles
musculoskeletal (mus-kyoo-loh-SKEL-eh-tal)	**muscul/o** = muscle **-al** = pertaining to	Pertaining to muscles and skeleton
tendinous (TEN-dih-nus)	**tendin/o** = tendon **-ous** = pertaining to	Pertaining to tendons

Pathology

Term	Word Parts	Definition
Medical Specialties		
kinesiology (kih-nee-see-ALL-oh-jee)	kinesi/o = movement -logy = study of	Science that studies movement, how it is produced, and muscles involved
occupational therapy (OT)	-al = pertaining to	Assists persons to regain, develop, and improve skills important for independent functioning (activities of daily living); specialist is *occupational therapist*
physical medicine	physic/o = body -al = pertaining to	Branch of medicine focused on restoring function; primarily cares for patients with musculoskeletal and nervous system disorders; physician is *physiatrist*
physical therapy (PT)	physic/o = body -al = pertaining to	Evaluation and treatment of disorders and rehabilitation of people using physical methods such as heat, cold, massage, and exercise; specialist is *physical therapist*
Signs and Symptoms		
adhesion		Scar tissue forming in fascia surrounding muscle, making it difficult to stretch muscle
atonia	a- = without -tonia = tone	Lack of muscle tone
atrophy (AT-rah-fee)	a- = without -trophy = development	Poor muscle development as a result of muscle disease, nervous system disease, or lack of use; commonly referred to as *muscle wasting*
bradykinesia (brad-ee-kih-NEE-zee-ah)	brady- = slow -kinesia = movement	Having slow movements
contracture (kon-TRAK-chur)		Abnormal shortening of muscle fibers, tendons, or fascia, making it difficult to stretch muscle
dyskinesia (dis-kih-NEE-zee-ah)	dys- = difficult, abnormal -kinesia = movement	Having difficult or abnormal movement
dystonia	dys- = abnormal -tonia = tone	Having abnormal muscle tone
hyperkinesia (high-per-kih-NEE-zee-ah)	hyper- = excessive -kinesia = movement	Having excessive amount of movement
hypertonia	hyper- = excessive -tonia = tone	Having excessive muscle tone
hypertrophy (high-PER-troh-fee)	hyper- = excessive -trophy = development	Increase in muscle bulk as a result of use, as with lifting weights
hypokinesia (high-poh-kih-NEE-zee-ah)	hypo- = insufficient -kinesia = movement	Having insufficient amount of movement
hypotonia	hypo- = insufficient -tonia = tone	Having insufficient muscle tone
intermittent claudication (klaw-dih-KAY-shun)		Attacks of severe pain and lameness caused by ischemia of muscles, typically calf muscles; brought on by walking even very short distances

Pathology (continued)

Term	Word Parts	Definition
myalgia (my-AL-jee-ah)	**my/o** = muscle **-algia** = pain	Muscle pain
myasthenia (my-as-THEE-nee-ah)	**my/o** = muscle **-asthenia** = weakness	Muscle weakness
myotonia	**my/o** = muscle **-tonia** = tone	Muscle tone
spasm		Sudden, involuntary, strong muscle contraction
tenodynia (ten-oh-DIN-ee-ah)	**ten/o** = tendon **-dynia** = pain	Tendon pain
Muscles		
fibromyalgia (figh-broh-my-AL-jee-ah)	**fibr/o** = fibers **my/o** = muscle **-algia** = pain	Condition with widespread aching and pain in muscles and soft tissue
lateral epicondylitis (ep-ih-kon-dih-LYE-tis)	**later/o** = side **-al** = pertaining to **epi-** = above **-itis** = inflammation	Inflammation of muscle attachment to lateral epicondyle of elbow; often caused by strongly gripping; commonly called *tennis elbow*
muscular dystrophy (MD) (MUS-kyoo-lar / DIS-troh-fee)	**muscul/o** = muscle **-ar** = pertaining to **dys-** = abnormal **-trophy** = development	Inherited disease causing progressive muscle degeneration, weakness, and atrophy
myopathy (my-OP-ah-thee)	**my/o** = muscle **-pathy** = disease	General term for muscle disease
myorrhexis (my-oh-REK-sis)	**my/o** = muscle **-rrhexis** = rupture	Tearing a muscle
necrotizing fasciitis (NF) (NEK-ruh-tye-zing / fash-ee-EYE-tis)	**necr/o** = death **fasci/o** = fibrous band **-itis** = inflammation	Infection, usually bacterial, that results in death of body's soft tissue (skin, fat, and fascia); commonly called *flesh-eating disease*
polymyositis (pol-ee-my-oh-SIGH-tis)	**poly-** = many **myos/o** = muscle **-itis** = inflammation	Simultaneous inflammation of two or more muscles
pseudohypertrophic muscular dystrophy (soo-doh-high-per-TROH-fik)	**pseudo-** = false **hyper-** = excessive **-trophic** = pertaining to development **muscul/o** = muscle **-ar** = pertaining to **dys-** = abnormal **-trophy** = development	Type of inherited muscular dystrophy in which muscle tissue is gradually replaced by fatty tissue, giving appearance of a healthy and strong muscle; also called *Duchenne's muscular dystrophy*
torticollis (tor-tih-KALL-iss)		Severe neck spasms pulling head to one side; commonly called *wryneck* or a *crick in the neck*
Tendons, Muscles, and/or Ligaments		
carpal tunnel syndrome (CTS)	**carp/o** = carpus **-al** = pertaining to	Repetitive motion disorder with pain caused by compression of finger flexor tendons and median nerve as they pass through carpal tunnel of wrist

Pathology (continued)

Term	Word Parts	Definition
ganglion cyst (GANG-lee-on)		Cyst that forms on tendon sheath, usually on hand, wrist, or ankle
repetitive motion disorder		Group of chronic disorders involving tendon, muscle, joint, and nerve damage, resulting from tissue being subjected to pressure, vibration, or repetitive movements for prolonged periods
rotator cuff injury		Rotator cuff consists of joint capsule of shoulder joint reinforced by tendons from several shoulder muscles; high degree of flexibility at shoulder joint puts rotator cuff at risk for strain and tearing
strain		Damage to muscle, tendons, or ligaments due to overuse or overstretching
tendinitis (ten-dih-NIGH-tis)	tendin/o = tendon -itis = inflammation	Inflammation of a tendon

PRACTICE AS YOU GO

I. Terminology Matching

Match each term to its definition.

_____ **1.** adhesion
_____ **2.** lateral epicondylitis
_____ **3.** carpal tunnel syndrome
_____ **4.** myasthenia
_____ **5.** spasm
_____ **6.** muscular dystrophy
_____ **7.** dyskinesia
_____ **8.** intermittent claudication

a. repetitive motion disorder
b. typically occurs in the calf muscles
c. inherited condition
d. scar tissue
e. sudden, involuntary muscle contraction
f. difficult or abnormal movement
g. *tennis elbow*
h. muscle weakness

Diagnostic Procedures

Term	Word Parts	Definition
Clinical Laboratory Test		
creatine kinase (CK) (KREE-ah-teen / KYE-nase)		Muscle enzyme found in skeletal muscle and cardiac muscle; blood levels become elevated in disorders such as heart attack, muscular dystrophy, and other skeletal muscle pathologies; also known as *creatine phosphokinase (CPK)*

Diagnostic Procedures (continued)

Term	Word Parts	Definition
Additional Diagnostic Procedures		
deep tendon reflexes (DTR)		Muscle contraction in response to a stretch caused by striking muscle tendon with a reflex hammer; test used to determine if muscles are responding properly
electromyogram (EMG) (ee-lek-troh-MY-oh-gram)	**electr/o** = electricity **my/o** = muscle **-gram** = record	Hardcopy record produced by electromyography
electromyography (EMG) (ee-lek-troh-my-OG-rah-fee)	**electr/o** = electricity **my/o** = muscle **-graphy** = process of recording	Study and record of strength and quality of muscle contractions as a result of electrical stimulation
muscle biopsy (BYE-op-see)	**bi/o** = life **-opsy** = view of	Removal of muscle tissue for pathological examination

Therapeutic Procedures

Term	Word Parts	Definition
Rehabilitation Procedures		
activities of daily living (ADLs) **Figure 4-31** An occupational therapist assisting a patient with learning independence in activities of daily living *(Lisa S./Shutterstock)*		Activities usually performed during a normal day, such as eating, dressing, and washing
cryotherapy (kry-oh-THAIR-ah-pee)	**cry/o** = cold **-therapy** = treatment	Use of cold in a treatment
gait training		Assisting patient to learn to walk again or how to use assistive device (such as crutches or walker) to walk
hydrotherapy (high-droh-THAIR-ah-pee)	**hydr/o** = water **-therapy** = treatment	Application of warm water as a treatment; can be done in baths, swimming pools, and whirlpools
massage		Kneading or applying pressure by hands to part of body to promote muscle relaxation and reduce tension
mobilization		Treatments such as exercise, massage, and physical manipulation to restore movement to joints and soft tissue
passive range of motion (PROM)		Putting a joint through available range of motion without assistance from patient
phonophoresis (foh-noh-foh-REE-sis)	**phon/o** = sound **-phoresis** = carrying	Use of ultrasound waves to introduce medication across skin and into subcutaneous tissues
rehabilitation	**re-** = again **habilitat/o** = ability	Process of treatment and exercise that can help person with disability attain maximum function and well-being

Therapeutic Procedures (continued)

Term	Word Parts	Definition
therapeutic exercise (thair-ah-PYOO-tik)	-ic = pertaining to	Exercise planned and carried out to achieve specific physical benefit, such as improved range of motion, muscle strengthening, or cardiovascular function
thermotherapy (ther-moh-THAIR-ah-pee)	therm/o = heat -therapy = treatment	Applying heat—often in form of moist, hot packs—to body for therapeutic purposes
ultrasound (US)	ultra- = beyond	Use of high-frequency sound waves to create heat in soft tissues under skin; particularly useful for treating injuries to muscles, tendons, and ligaments, as well as muscle spasms

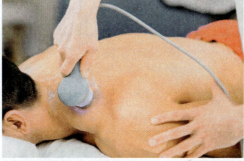

Figure 4-32 Ultrasound treatment to thoracic (neck and upper back) region. *(Microgen/Shutterstock)*

Med Term Tip

Ultrasound waves serve two very different purposes, one of which is for diagnostic imaging. The echoes of these high-frequency waves bouncing off internal structures are captured by a computer and used to generate an image. The other purpose is for the therapeutic treatment of muscle pain and spasms. The same high-frequency sound waves cause the molecules they strike to vibrate, thereby generating heat deep in the muscle tissue.

Surgical Procedures		
carpal tunnel release	carp/o = carpus -al = pertaining to	Surgical cutting of ligament in wrist to relieve nerve pressure caused by carpal tunnel syndrome, which can result from repetitive motion such as typing
fasciotomy (fash-ee-OT-oh-mee)	fasci/o = fibrous band -otomy = cutting into	Surgical procedure that cuts into fascia
myoplasty (MY-oh-plas-tee)	my/o = muscle -plasty = surgical repair	Surgical procedure to repair a muscle
myorrhaphy (my-OR-ah-fee)	my/o = muscle -rrhaphy = suture	To suture a muscle
tendoplasty (TEN-doh-plas-tee)	tend/o = tendon -plasty = surgical repair	Surgical procedure to repair a tendon
tendotomy (ten-DOT-oh-mee)	tend/o = tendon -otomy = cutting into	Surgical procedure that cuts into a tendon
tenodesis (ten-oh-DEE-sis)	ten/o = tendon -desis = fuse	Surgical procedure to stabilize a joint by anchoring down tendons of muscles that move joint
tenoplasty (TEN-oh-plas-tee)	ten/o = tendon -plasty = surgical repair	Surgical procedure to repair a tendon
tenorrhaphy (teh-NOR-ah-fee)	ten/o = tendon -rrhaphy = suture	To suture a tendon

Pharmacology

Classification	Word Parts	Action	Examples
skeletal muscle relaxants	-al = pertaining to	Medication to relax skeletal muscles in order to reduce muscle spasms; also called *antispasmodics*	cyclobenzaprine, Flexeril; carisoprodol, Soma

Abbreviations

ADLs	activities of daily living	**MD**	muscular dystrophy
CK	creatine kinase	**NF**	necrotizing fasciitis
CPK	creatine phosphokinase	**OT**	occupational therapy
CTS	carpal tunnel syndrome	**PROM**	passive range of motion
DTR	deep tendon reflex	**PT**	physical therapy
EMG	electromyogram	**US**	ultrasound
IM	intramuscular		

PRACTICE AS YOU GO

J. What's the Abbreviation?

1. intramuscular ______________________
2. deep tendon reflex ______________________
3. muscular dystrophy ______________________
4. electromyogram ______________________
5. carpal tunnel syndrome ______________________

Chapter Review

Real-World Applications

Medical Record Analysis

This Discharge Summary contains 10 medical terms. Underline each term and write it in the list below the report. Then explain each term as you would to a nonmedical person.

Discharge Summary

Admitting Diagnosis:	Osteoarthritis bilateral knees
Final Diagnosis:	Osteoarthritis bilateral knees with right TKA
History of Present Illness:	Patient is a 68-year-old male. He reports experiencing occasional knee pain and swelling since he injured his knees playing football in high school. These symptoms became worse while he was in his 50s and working on a concrete surface. The right knee has always been more painful than the left. He saw his orthopedic surgeon six months ago because of constant knee pain and swelling severe enough to interfere with sleep and all activities. He required a cane to walk. Radiographs indicated severe bilateral osteoarthritis. He is admitted to the hospital at this time for TKR right knee.
Summary of Hospital Course:	Patient tolerated the surgical procedure well. He began intensive physical therapy for lower-extremity therapeutic exercise and gait training with a walker. He received occupational therapy instruction in ADLs, especially dressing and personal care. He was able to transfer himself out of bed by the third post-op day and was able to ambulate 150 ft with a walker and dress himself on the fifth post-op day.
Discharge Plans:	Patient was discharged home with his wife one week post-op. He will continue rehabilitation as an outpatient. Return to office for post-op checkup in one week.

	Term	Explanation
1.	______________________	______________________________________
2.	______________________	______________________________________
3.	______________________	______________________________________
4.	______________________	______________________________________
5.	______________________	______________________________________
6.	______________________	______________________________________
7.	______________________	______________________________________
8.	______________________	______________________________________
9.	______________________	______________________________________
10.	______________________	______________________________________

Chart Note Transcription

The chart note below contains 11 phrases that can be reworded with a medical term presented in this chapter. Each phrase is identified with an underline. Determine the medical term and write your answers in the space provided.

Pearson General Hospital Consultation Report

Task Edit View Time Scale Options Help Download Archive Date: 17 May 2017

Current Complaint:	An 82-year-old female was transported to the Emergency Room via ambulance with severe left hip pain following a fall on the ice.
Past History:	Patient suffered a broken wrist bone **1** two years earlier that required immobilization by solid material. **2** Following this broken bone, **3** her physician who specializes in treatment of bone conditions **4** diagnosed her with moderate porous bones **5** on the basis of a low-dose X-ray for bone density. **6**
Signs and Symptoms:	Patient reported severe left hip pain, rating it as 8 on a scale of 1 to 10. She held her hip in a bent position **7** and could not tolerate movement toward a straight position. **8** X-rays of the left hip and leg were taken.
Diagnosis:	Shattered broken bone **9** in the neck of the left thigh bone. **10**
Treatment:	Implantation of an artificial hip joint **11** on the left.

1. ______________________________

2. ______________________________

3. ______________________________

4. ______________________________

5. ______________________________

6. ______________________________

7. ______________________________

8. ______________________________

9. ______________________________

10. ______________________________

11. ______________________________

Case Study

Below is a case study presentation of a patient with a condition discussed in this chapter. Read the case study and answer the questions below. Some questions will ask for information not included within this chapter. Use your text, a medical dictionary, or any other reference material you choose to answer these questions.

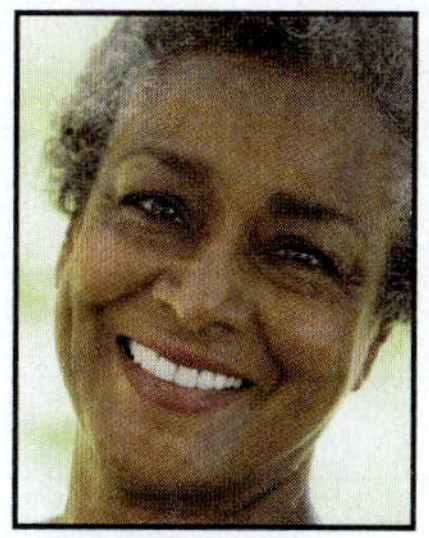

(Monkey Business Images/ Shutterstock)

Mary Pearl, age 60, has come into the physician's office complaining of swelling, stiffness, and arthralgia, especially in her elbows, wrists, and hands. A bone scan revealed acute inflammation in multiple joints with damaged articular cartilage, and an erythrocyte sedimentation rate blood test indicated a significant level of acute inflammation in the body. A diagnosis of acute episode of rheumatoid arthritis was made. The physician ordered nonsteroidal anti-inflammatory medication and physical therapy. The therapist initiated a treatment program of hydrotherapy and therapeutic exercises.

Questions

1. What pathological condition does this patient have? Look this condition up in a reference source and include a short description of it.

   ____

   ____

2. What type of long-term damage may occur in a patient with rheumatoid arthritis?

   ____

   ____

3. Describe the other major type of arthritis mentioned in this textbook.

   ____

   ____

4. What two diagnostic procedures did the physician order? Describe them in your own words. What were the results? (One of these procedures is described in Chapter 6 of this text.)

   ____

   ____

5. What treatments were ordered? Explain what the physical therapy procedures involve.

   ____

   ____

6. This patient is experiencing an acute episode. Explain what this phrase means and contrast it with chronic.

   ____

   ____

Practice Exercises

A. Word Building Practice

The combining form **oste/o** refers to *bone*. Use it to write a term that means:

1. bone cell ____________________
2. immature bone cell ____________________
3. porous bone ____________________
4. disease of the bone ____________________
5. cutting into a bone ____________________
6. instrument to cut bone ____________________
7. inflammation of the bone and bone marrow ____________________
8. abnormal softening of bone ____________________
9. bone and cartilage tumor ____________________

The combining form **my/o** refers to *muscle*. Use it to write a term that means:

10. muscle disease ____________________
11. surgical repair of muscle ____________________
12. suture of muscle ____________________
13. record of muscle electricity ____________________
14. muscle weakness ____________________

The combining form **ten/o** refers to *tendons*. Use it to write a term that means:

15. tendon pain ____________________
16. tendon suture ____________________

The combining form **arthr/o** refers to the *joints*. Use it to write a term that means:

17. to fuse a joint ____________________
18. surgical repair of a joint ____________________
19. cutting into a joint ____________________
20. inflammation of a joint ____________________
21. puncture to withdraw fluid from a joint ____________________
22. pain in the joints ____________________

The combining form **chondr/o** refers to *cartilage*. Use it to write a term that means:

23. surgical removal of cartilage ____________________
24. cartilage tumor ____________________
25. abnormal softening of cartilage ____________________

B. Spinal Column Practice

Name the five regions of the spinal column and indicate the number of bones in each area.

	Name	Number of Bones
1.	____________________	____________________
2.	____________________	____________________
3.	____________________	____________________
4.	____________________	____________________
5.	____________________	____________________

C. Complete the Term

For each definition given below, fill in the blank with the word part that completes the term.

Definition	Term
1. porous bone	osteo____________________
2. a ruptured muscle	____________________rrhexis
3. crooked (lateral curvature of) spine	____________________osis
4. abnormal muscle tone	dys____________________
5. the study of movement	____________________logy
6. abnormal forward curvature of lumbar spine	____________________osis
7. forward slipping of a vertebra	spondylo____________________
8. withdrawing fluid from a joint	____________________centesis
9. movement away from body	____________________duction
10. bone and joint inflammation	____________________arthritis
11. to surgically break a bone	osteo____________________
12. abnormal softening of cartilage	____________________malacia
13. pertaining to muscles	____________________ar
14. muscle weakness	my____________________
15. inflammation of a tendon	____________________itis
16. inflammation of a bursa	____________________itis
17. bone marrow tumor	____________________oma
18. to fuse a joint	arthro____________________

D. Fill in the Blank

carpal tunnel syndrome	rickets	spondylolisthesis	systemic lupus erythematosus
scoliosis	osteogenic sarcoma	lateral epicondylitis	
herniated nucleus pulposus	osteoporosis	pseudohypertrophic muscular dystrophy	

1. Mrs. Lewis, age 84, broke her hip. Her physician will be running tests for what potential ailment? ________________
2. Jamie, age six months, is being given orange juice and vitamin supplements to avoid what condition? ________________
3. George has severe elbow pain after playing tennis four days in a row. He may have ________________.
4. Marshall's doctor told him that he had a ruptured disk. The medical term for this is ________________.
5. Mr. Jefferson's physician has discovered a tumor at the end of his femur. He has been admitted to the hospital for a biopsy to rule out what type of bone cancer? ________________
6. The school nurse has asked Janelle to bend over so that she may examine her back to see if she is developing a lateral curve. What is the nurse looking for? ________________
7. Gerald has experienced a gradual loss of muscle strength over the past five years even though his muscles look large and healthy. The doctors believe he has an inherited muscle disease. What is that disease? ________________
8. Roberta has suddenly developed arthritis in her hands and knees. Rheumatoid arthritis had been ruled out, but what other autoimmune disease might Roberta have? ________________
9. Mark's X-ray demonstrated forward sliding of a lumbar vertebra; the radiologist diagnosed ________________.
10. The orthopedist determined that Marcia's repetitive wrist movements at work caused her to develop ________________.

E. Know Your Bones

For each bone listed below, give its division of the skeleton (axial or appendicular), the total number in the body, and its common name.

	Division	Number	Common Name
1. maxilla	________	________	________
2. carpus	________	________	________
3. scapula	________	________	________
4. patella	________	________	________
5. sternum	________	________	________
6. femur	________	________	________
7. metatarsus	________	________	________
8. tibia	________	________	________
9. clavicle	________	________	________
10. zygomatic bone	________	________	________

F. Using Abbreviations

Fill in the blank with the appropriate abbreviation.

1. The pain in her wrist and hand was determined to be __________.
2. The __________ showed clear evidence of osteoporosis.

3. __________ is an inherited disease with progressive muscle degeneration.
4. Mrs. Mendez underwent a(n) __________ after breaking her hip.
5. He had a(n) __________ to study the strength and quality of muscle contractions.
6. __________ is an arthritis resulting from an autoimmune condition.
7. The young boy fell from the tree and has a greenstick __________.
8. The physician recommended a(n) __________ like ibuprofen for her mild pain.

G. Define the Term

1. chondroplasty ____________________
2. bradykinesia ____________________
3. osteoporosis ____________________
4. lordosis ____________________
5. atrophy ____________________
6. myeloma ____________________
7. prosthesis ____________________
8. craniotomy ____________________
9. arthrocentesis ____________________
10. bursitis ____________________

H. Pharmacology Challenge

Fill in the classification for each drug description, then match the brand name.

	Drug Description	Classification	Brand Name
1. ________	Treats mild pain and is an anti-inflammatory	____________	a. Flexeril
2. ________	Hormone with anti-inflammatory properties	____________	b. Aleve
3. ________	Reduces muscle spasms	____________	c. Fosamax
4. ________	Treats conditions of weakened bones	____________	d. Oystercal
5. ________	Maintains blood calcium levels	____________	e. Medrol

I. Identify the rehabilitation procedure described by each phrase.

1. kneading or applying pressure by hands ____________________
2. treatment to restore movement ____________________
3. using water for treatment purposes ____________________
4. high-frequency sound waves to create heat ____________________
5. use of heat for treatment purposes ____________________
6. medication introduced by ultrasound waves ____________________
7. use of cold for treatment purposes ____________________
8. learning to walk again ____________________

J. Fracture Type Matching

1. ________ comminuted
2. ________ greenstick
3. ________ compound
4. ________ simple
5. ________ impacted
6. ________ transverse
7. ________ oblique
8. ________ spiral

a. fracture line is at an angle
b. fracture line curves around the bone
c. bone is splintered or crushed
d. bone is pressed into itself
e. fracture line is straight across bone
f. skin has been broken
g. no open wound
h. bone only partially broken

K. Spelling Practice

Some of the following terms are misspelled. Identify the incorrect terms and spell them correctly in the blank provided.

1. tendinous ____________________
2. psudohypertrophic ____________________
3. polymyocitis ____________________
4. electromyography ____________________
5. ankylosing ____________________
6. osteocondroma ____________________
7. spondilosis ____________________
8. laminectomy ____________________
9. corticosteroid ____________________
10. exosstosis ____________________

Labeling Exercises

Image A

Write the labels for this figure on the numbered lines provided.

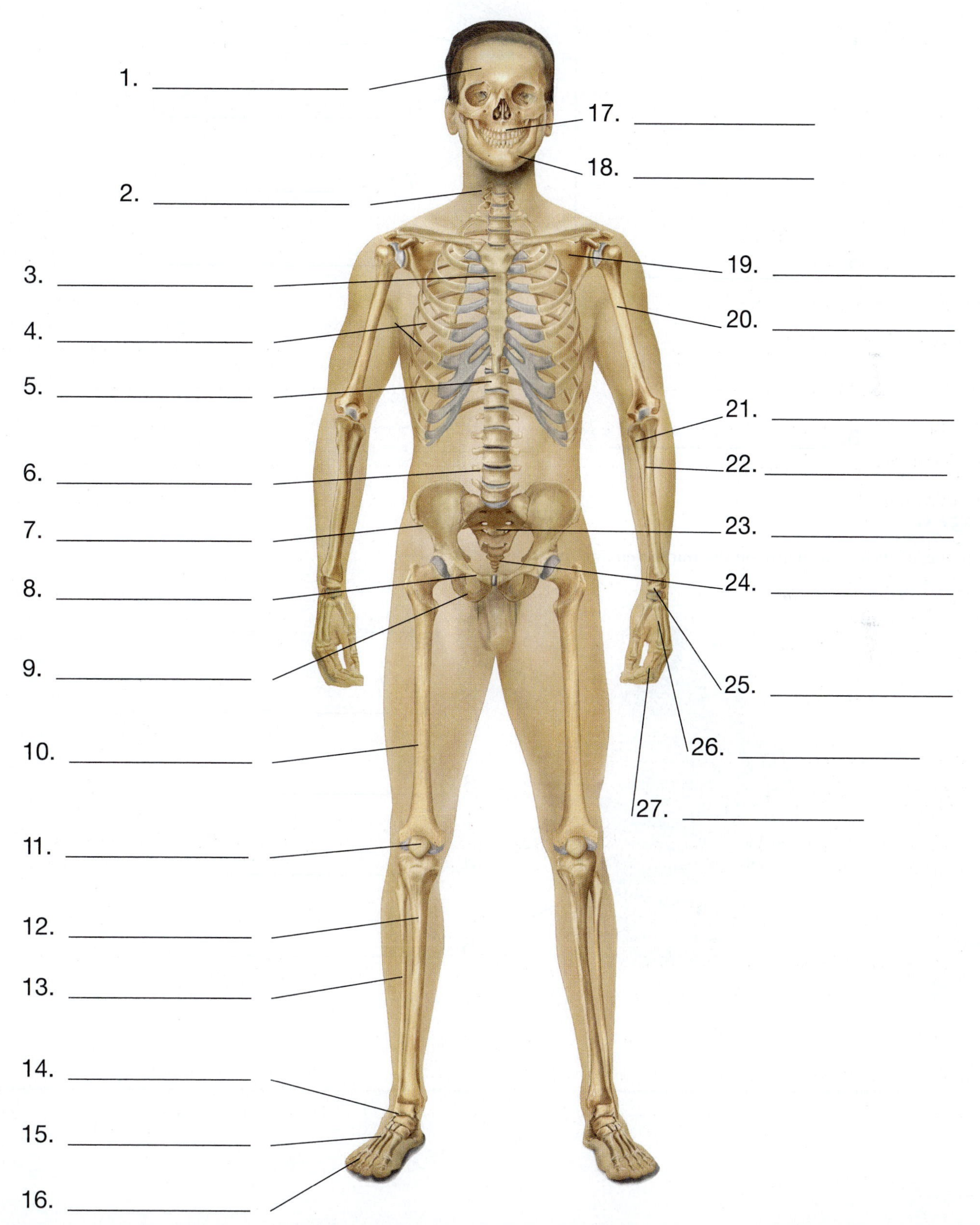

Image B

Write the labels for this figure on the numbered lines provided.

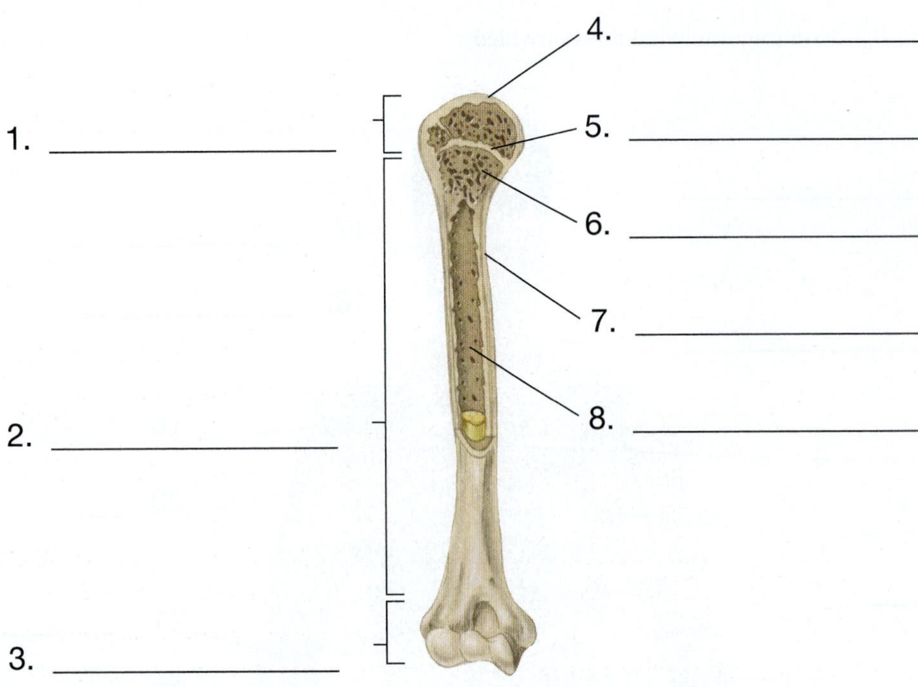

Image C

Write the labels for this figure on the numbered lines provided.

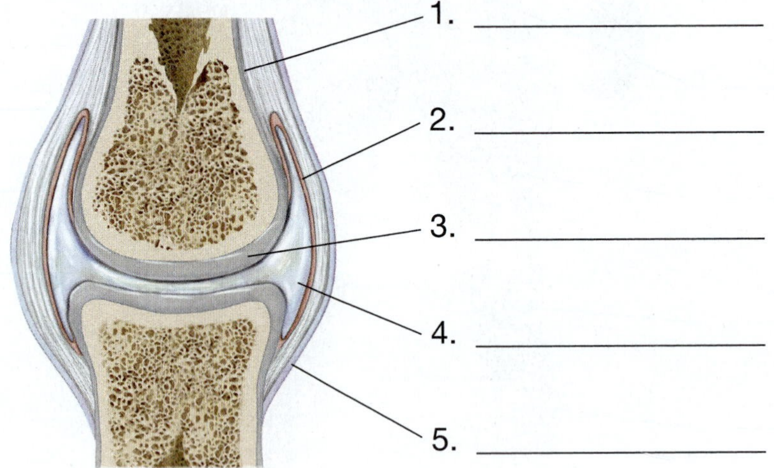

Chapter 5

Cardiovascular System

Learning Objectives

Upon completion of this chapter, you will be able to

1. Identify and define the combining forms, suffixes, and prefixes introduced in this chapter.
2. Correctly spell and pronounce medical terms and major anatomical structures relating to the cardiovascular system.
3. Describe the major organs of the cardiovascular system and their functions.
4. Describe the anatomy of the heart.
5. Describe the flow of blood through the heart.
6. Explain how the electrical conduction system controls the heartbeat.
7. List and describe the characteristics of the three types of blood vessels.
8. Define *pulse* and *blood pressure*.
9. Identify and define cardiovascular system anatomical terms.
10. Identify and define selected cardiovascular system pathology terms.
11. Identify and define selected cardiovascular system diagnostic procedures.
12. Identify and define selected cardiovascular system therapeutic procedures.
13. Identify and define selected medications relating to the cardiovascular system.
14. Define selected abbreviations associated with the cardiovascular system.

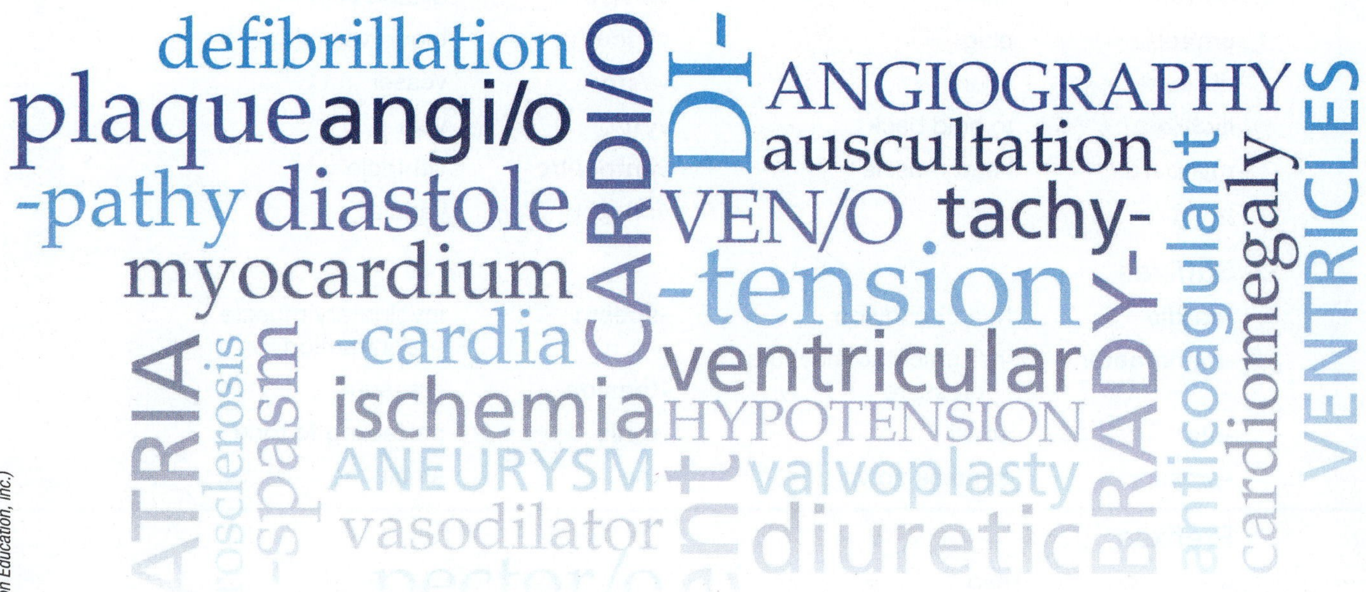

(Pearson Education, Inc.)

CARDIOVASCULAR SYSTEM

AT A GLANCE

Function

The cardiovascular system consists of the pump and vessels that distribute blood to all areas of the body. This system allows for the delivery of needed substances to the cells of the body as well as for the removal of wastes.

Organs

The primary structures that comprise the cardiovascular system:

blood vessels

- **arteries**
- **capillaries**
- **veins**

heart

Word Parts

Presented here are the most common word parts (with their meanings) used to build cardiovascular system terms. For a more comprehensive list, refer to the Terminology section of this chapter.

Combining Forms

angi/o	vessel
aort/o	aorta
arteri/o	artery
arteriol/o	arteriole
ather/o	fatty substance
atri/o	atrium
cardi/o	heart
coron/o	heart
embol/o	plug
fibrin/o	fibers
isch/o	to hold back
myocardi/o	heart muscle
phleb/o	vein
sept/o	wall
son/o	sound
sphygm/o	pulse
steth/o	chest
thromb/o	clot
valv/o	valve
valvul/o	valve
varic/o	dilated vein
vascul/o	blood vessel
vas/o	vessel
ven/o	vein
ventricul/o	ventricle
venul/o	venule

Suffixes

-cardia	heart condition
-manometer	instrument to measure pressure
-ole	small
-pressor	to press down
-spasm	involuntary muscle contraction
-tension	pressure
-tonic	pertaining to tone
-ule	small

Prefixes

di-	two

Cardiovascular System Illustrated

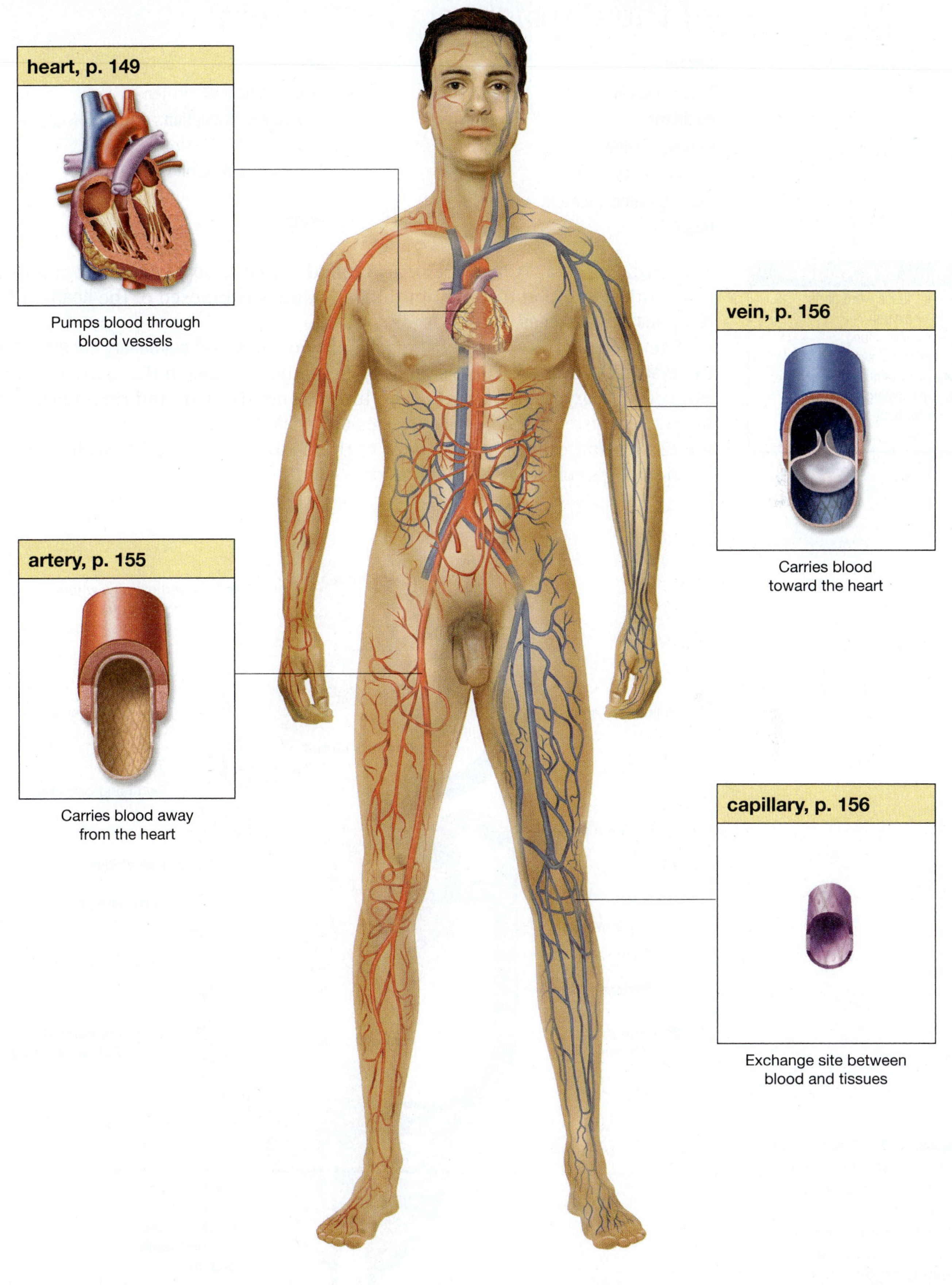

heart, p. 149
Pumps blood through blood vessels
vein, p. 156
Carries blood toward the heart
artery, p. 155
Carries blood away from the heart
capillary, p. 156
Exchange site between blood and tissues

Anatomy and Physiology of the Cardiovascular System

arteries
blood vessels
capillaries
carbon dioxide
circulatory system
deoxygenated (dee-OK-sih-jen-ay-ted)
heart
oxygen
oxygenated (OK-sih-jen-ay-ted)
pulmonary circulation (PULL-mon-air-ee / ser-kyoo-LAY-shun)
systemic circulation (sis-TEM-ik / ser-kyoo-LAY-shun)
veins

What's In A Name?

Look for these word parts:
ox/o = oxygen
pulmon/o = lung
system/o = system
-ary = pertaining to
-ic = pertaining to
de- = without
di- = two

The cardiovascular (CV) system, also called the **circulatory system**, maintains the distribution of blood throughout the body and is composed of the **heart** and the **blood vessels—arteries**, **capillaries**, and **veins**.

The circulatory system is composed of two parts: the **pulmonary circulation** and the **systemic circulation**. The pulmonary circulation, between the heart and lungs, transports **deoxygenated** blood to the lungs to get oxygen, and then back to the heart. The systemic circulation carries **oxygenated** blood away from the heart to the tissues and cells, and then back to the heart (see Figure 5-1 ■). In this way, all the body's cells receive blood and oxygen.

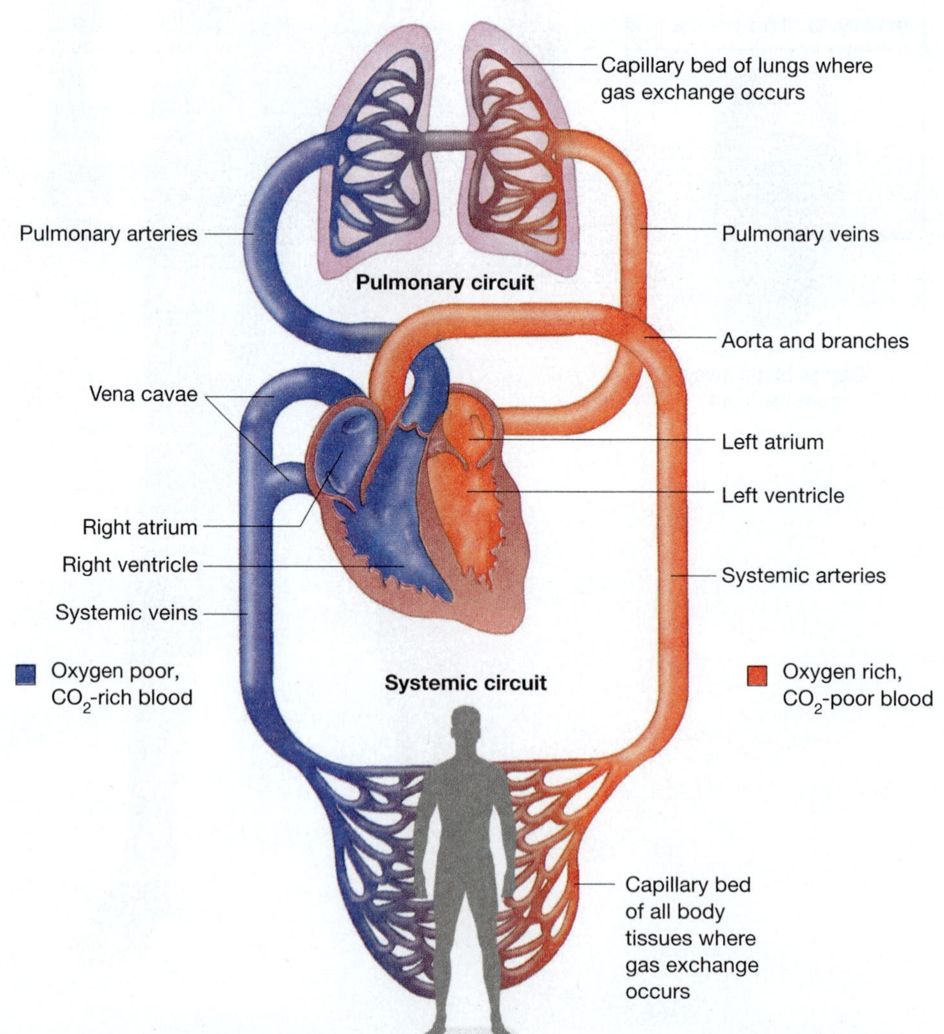

■ **Figure 5-1** A schematic of the circulatory system illustrating the pulmonary circulation picking up oxygen from the lungs and the systemic circulation delivering oxygen to the body.

In addition to distributing **oxygen** and other nutrients, such as glucose and amino acids, the cardiovascular system also collects the waste products from the body's cells. **Carbon dioxide** and other waste products produced by metabolic reaction are transported by the cardiovascular system to the lungs, liver, and kidneys, where they are eliminated from the body.

Heart

apex (AY-peks) **cardiac muscle** (KAR-dee-ak)

The heart, a muscular pump made up of **cardiac muscle** fibers, could be considered a muscle rather than an organ. It has four chambers, or cavities, and beats an average of 60–100 beats per minute (bpm) or about 100,000 times in one day. Each time the cardiac muscle contracts, blood is ejected from the heart and pushed throughout the body within the blood vessels.

The heart is located in the mediastinum in the center of the chest cavity; however, it is not exactly centered; more of the heart is on the left side of the mediastinum than the right (see Figure 5-2 ■). At about the size of a fist and shaped like an upside-down pear, the heart lies directly behind the sternum. The tip of the heart at the lower edge is called the **apex**.

Med Term Tip

Your heart is approximately the size of your clenched fist and pumps 4,000 gallons of blood each day. It will beat at least three billion times during your lifetime.

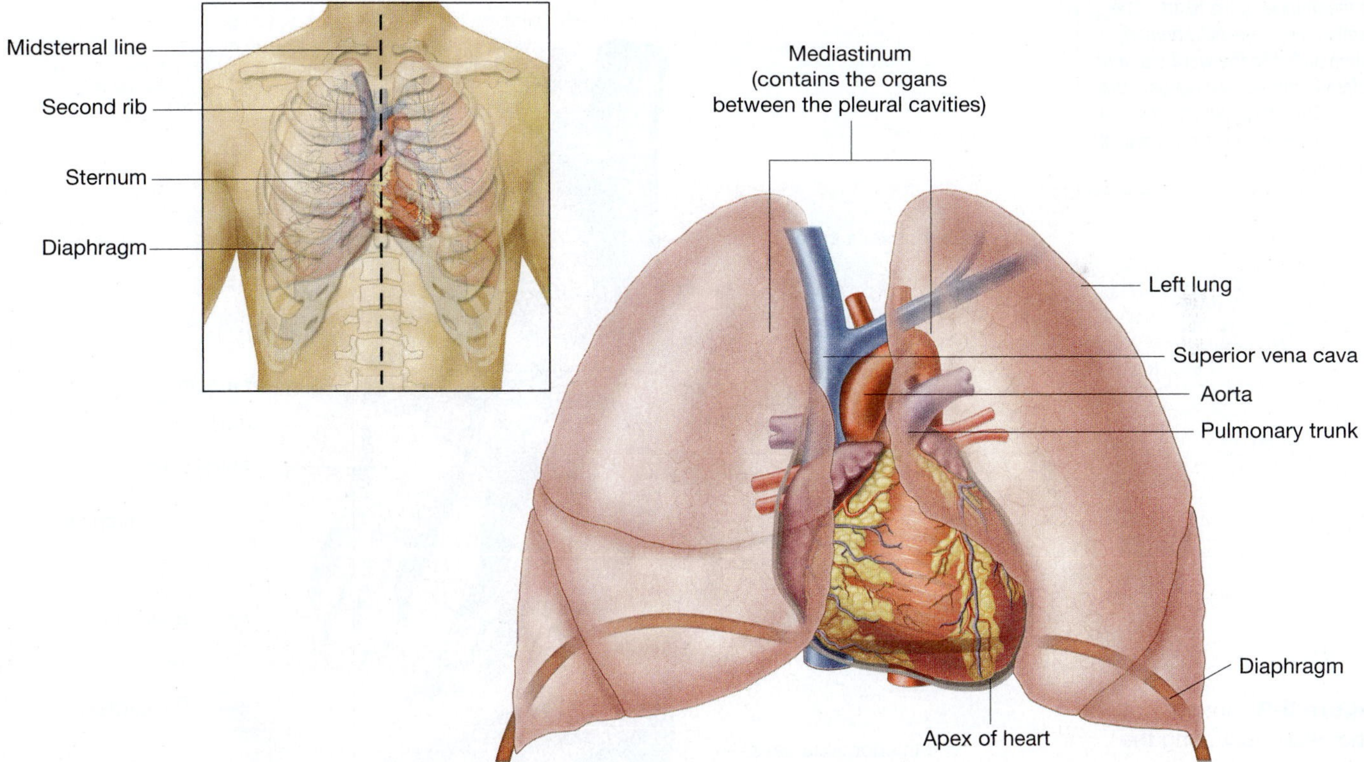

■ **Figure 5-2** Location of the heart within the mediastinum of the thoracic cavity.

What's In A Name?

Look for these word parts:
cardi/o = heart
pariet/o = cavity wall
viscer/o = internal organ
-al = pertaining to
epi- = above

Heart Layers

endocardium (en-doh-KAR-dee-um)
epicardium (ep-ih-KAR-dee-um)
myocardium (my-oh-KAR-dee-um)
parietal pericardium (pah-RYE-eh-tal / pair-ih-KAR-dee-um)
pericardium (pair-ih-KAR-dee-um)
visceral pericardium (VISS-er-al / pair-ih-KAR-dee-um)

Med Term Tip

The layers of the heart become important when studying the disease conditions affecting the heart. For instance, when the prefix **endo-** is added to *carditis*, forming *endocarditis*, we know that the inflammation is within the "inner layer of the heart." In discussing the muscular action of the heart, the combining form **my/o**, meaning *muscle*, is added to *cardium* to form the word *myocardium*. The diagnosis *myocardial infarction* (MI), or heart attack, means that the patient has an infarct or "dead tissue in the muscle of the heart." The prefix **peri-**, meaning *around*, when added to the word *cardium* refers to the sac surrounding the heart. Therefore, *pericarditis* is an "inflammation of the outer sac of the heart."

The wall of the heart is quite thick and is composed of three layers (see Figure 5-3 ■):

1. The **endocardium** is the inner layer of the heart lining the heart chambers. It is a very smooth, thin layer that serves to reduce friction as the blood passes through the heart chambers.
2. The **myocardium** is the thick, muscular middle layer of the heart. Contraction of this muscle layer develops the pressure required to pump blood through the blood vessels.
3. The **epicardium** is the outer layer of the heart. The heart is enclosed within a double-layered pleural sac, called the **pericardium**. The epicardium is the **visceral pericardium**, or inner layer of the sac. The outer layer of the sac is the **parietal pericardium**. Fluid between the two layers of the sac reduces friction as the heart beats.

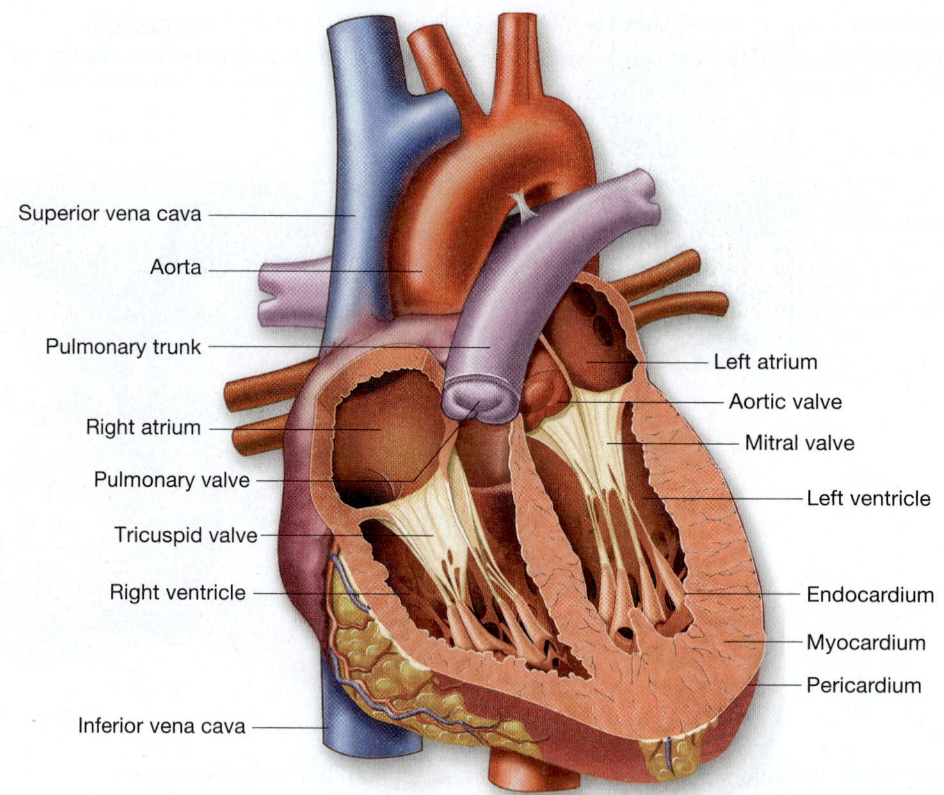

■ **Figure 5-3** Internal view of the heart illustrating the heart chambers, heart layers, and major blood vessels associated with the heart.

Heart Chambers

atria (AY-tree-ah)
interatrial septum (in-ter-AY-tree-al / SEP-tum)
interventricular septum (in-ter-ven-TRIK-yoo-lar / SEP-tum)
ventricles (VEN-trih-kulz)

The heart is divided into four chambers or cavities (see again Figure 5-3). There are two **atria**, or upper chambers, and two **ventricles**, or lower chambers. These chambers are divided into right and left sides by walls called the **interatrial septum** and the **interventricular septum**. The atria are the receiving chambers of the heart. Blood returning to the heart via veins first collects in the atria. The ventricles are the pumping chambers. They have a much thicker myocardium and their contraction ejects blood out of the heart and into the great arteries.

Med Term Tip

The term *ventricle* comes from the Latin term *venter*, which means *little belly*. Although it originally referred to the abdomen and then the stomach, it came to stand for any hollow region inside an organ.

Heart Valves

aortic valve (ay-OR-tik)
atrioventricular valve (ay-tree-oh-ven-TRIK-yoo-lar)
bicuspid valve (bye-KUSS-pid)
cusps
mitral valve (MY-tral)
pulmonary valve (PULL-mon-air-ee)
semilunar valve (sem-ee-LOO-nar)
tricuspid valve (trye-KUSS-pid)

Four valves act as restraining gates to control the direction of blood flow. They are situated at the entrances and exits to the ventricles (see Figure 5-4 ■). Properly functioning valves allow blood to flow only in a forward direction by blocking it from returning to the previous chamber.

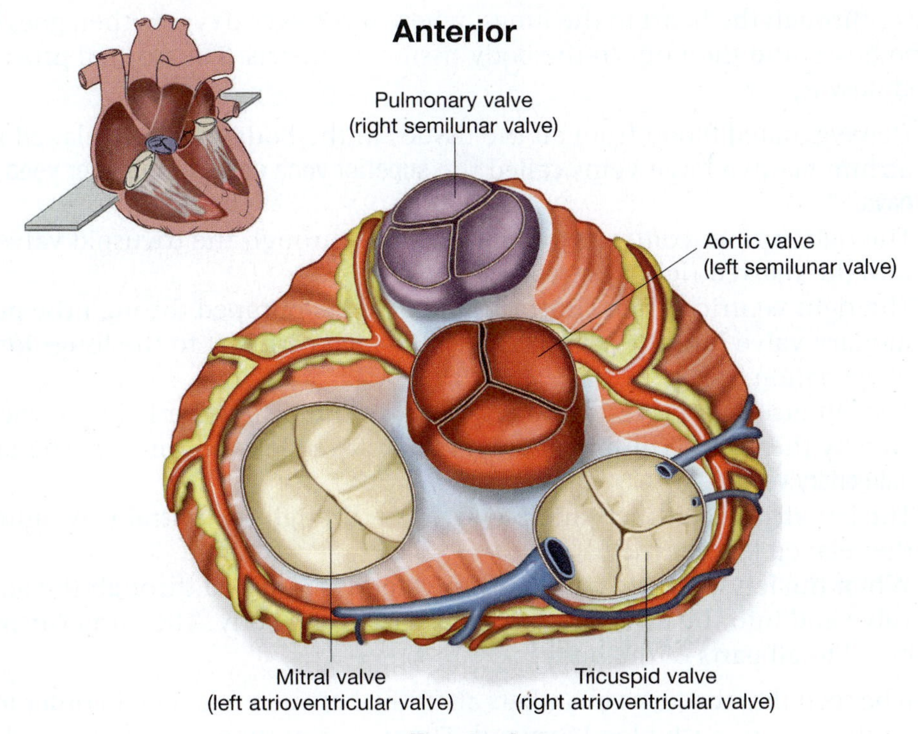

■ **Figure 5-4** Superior view of heart valves illustrating position, size, and shape of each valve.

What's In A Name?

Look for these word parts:
pulmon/o = lung
-al = pertaining to
-ar = pertaining to
bi- = two
semi- = partial
tri- = three

Med Term Tip

The heart makes two distinct sounds, referred to as *lub-dupp*. These sounds are produced by the forceful snapping shut of the heart valves. *Lub* is the closing of the atrioventricular valves. *Dupp* is the closing of the semilunar valves.

The four valves are:

1. **Tricuspid valve:** an **atrioventricular valve** (AV), meaning that it controls the opening between the right atrium and the right ventricle. Once the blood enters the right ventricle, it cannot go back up into the atrium again. The prefix **tri-**, meaning three, indicates that this valve has three leaflets or **cusps**.
2. **Pulmonary valve:** a **semilunar valve**, with the prefix **semi-** meaning *half* and the term **lunar** meaning *moon,* indicate that this valve looks like a half moon. Located between the right ventricle and the pulmonary artery, this valve prevents blood that has been ejected into the pulmonary artery from returning to the right ventricle as it relaxes.
3. **Mitral valve:** also called the **bicuspid valve**, indicating that it has two cusps. Blood flows through this atrioventricular valve to the left ventricle and cannot go back up into the left atrium.
4. **Aortic valve:** a semilunar valve located between the left ventricle and the aorta. Blood leaves the left ventricle through this valve and cannot return to the left ventricle.

Blood Flow Through the Heart

aorta (ay-OR-tah)
diastole (dye-ASS-toh-lee)
inferior vena cava (VEE-nah / KAY-vah)
pulmonary artery (PULL-mon-air-ee)
pulmonary veins
superior vena cava
systole (SIS-toh-lee)

The flow of blood through the heart is very orderly (see Figure 5-5 ■). It progresses through the heart to the lungs, where it receives oxygen; then goes back to the heart; and then out to the body tissues and parts. The normal process of blood flow is:

What's In A Name?

Look for these word parts:
infer/o = below
pulmon/o = lung
super/o = above
-ary = pertaining to
-ior = pertaining to

1. Deoxygenated blood from all the tissues in the body enters a relaxed right atrium via two large veins called the **superior vena cava** and **inferior vena cava**.
2. The right atrium contracts and blood flows through the tricuspid valve into the relaxed right ventricle.
3. The right ventricle then contracts and blood is pumped through the pulmonary valve into the **pulmonary artery**, which carries it to the lungs for oxygenation.
4. The left atrium receives blood returning to the heart after being oxygenated by the lungs. This blood enters the relaxed left atrium from the four **pulmonary veins.**
5. The left atrium contracts and blood flows through the mitral valve into the relaxed left ventricle.
6. When the left ventricle contracts, the blood is pumped through the aortic valve and into the **aorta**, the largest artery in the body. The aorta carries blood to all parts of the body.

It can be seen that the heart chambers alternate between relaxing, in order to fill, and contracting to push blood forward. The period of time a chamber is relaxed is **diastole**. The contraction phase is **systole**.

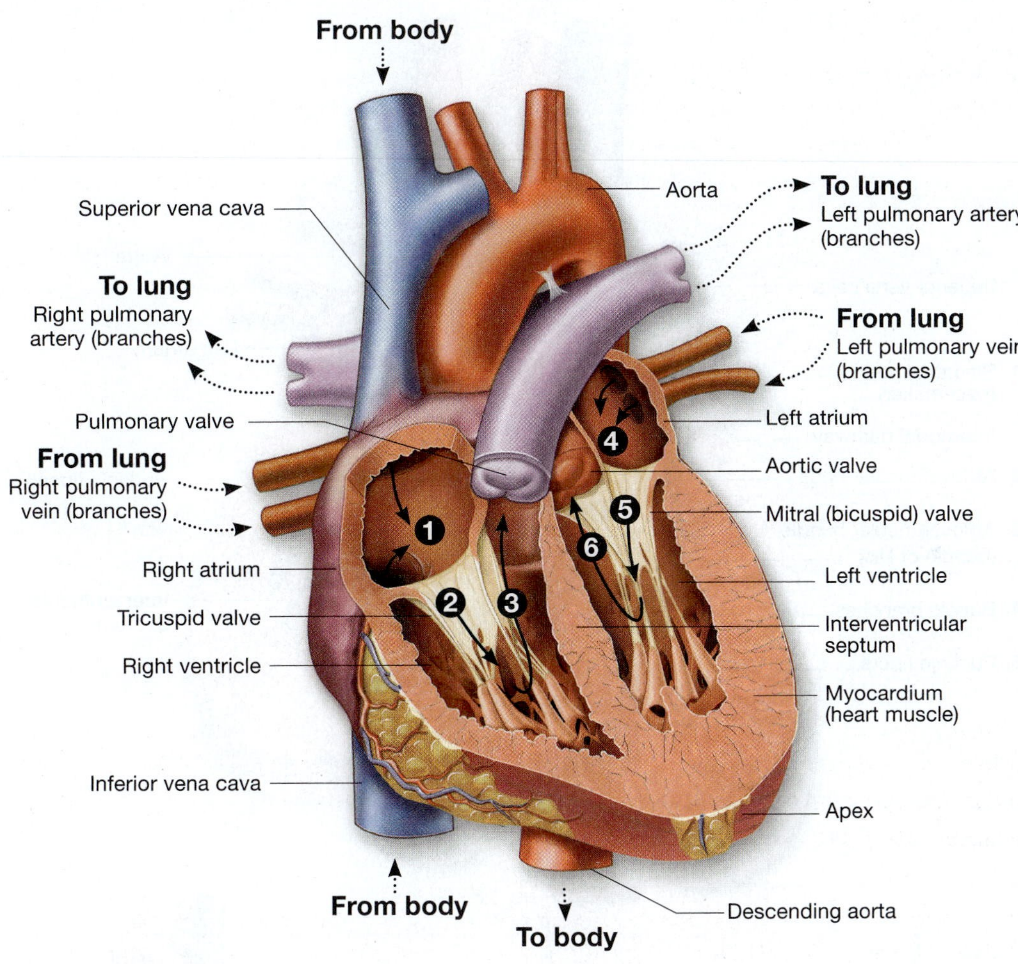

■ **Figure 5-5** The path of blood flow through the chambers of the left and right side of the heart, including the veins delivering blood to the heart and arteries receiving blood ejected from the heart.

Conduction System of the Heart

atrioventricular bundle
atrioventricular node
autonomic nervous system (aw-toh-NOM-ik / NER-vus / SIS-tem)
bundle branches
bundle of His
pacemaker
Purkinje fibers (per-KIN-jee)
sinoatrial node (sigh-noh-AY-tree-al)

The heart rate is regulated by the **autonomic nervous system**; therefore, there is no voluntary control over the beating of the heart. Special tissue within the heart is responsible for conducting an electrical impulse stimulating the different chambers to contract in the correct order.

The path that the impulses travel is as follows (see Figure 5-6 ■):

1. The **sinoatrial (SA, S-A) node**, or **pacemaker**, is where the electrical impulses begin. From the sinoatrial node, a wave of electricity travels through the atria, causing them to contract, or go into systole.
2. The **atrioventricular node** is stimulated.
3. This node transfers the stimulation wave to the **atrioventricular bundle** (formerly called **bundle of His**).
4. The electrical signal next travels down the **bundle branches** within the interventricular septum.
5. The **Purkinje fibers** out in the ventricular myocardium are stimulated, resulting in ventricular systole.

What's In A Name?

Look for these word parts:
atri/o = atrium
-al = pertaining to
-ic = pertaining to
auto- = self

Med Term Tip

The atrioventricular bundle was originally named the *bundle of His* in recognition of the Swiss cardiologist who first discovered these fibers. Current medical terminology usage has moved away from eponyms and toward anatomically descriptive terms for naming structures.

■ **Figure 5-6** The conduction system of the heart; traces the path of the electrical impulse that stimulates the heart chambers to contract in the correct sequence.

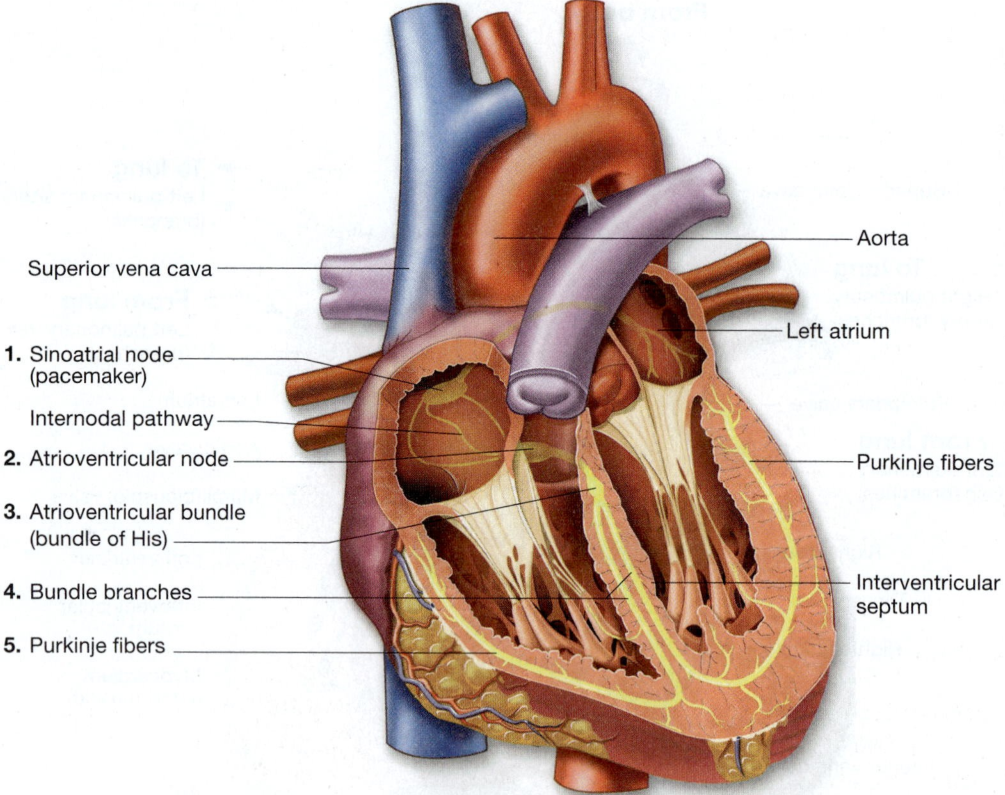

Med Term Tip

The electrocardiogram, referred to as an EKG or ECG, is a measurement of the electrical activity of the heart (see Figure 5-7 ■). This can give the physician information about the health of the heart, especially the myocardium.

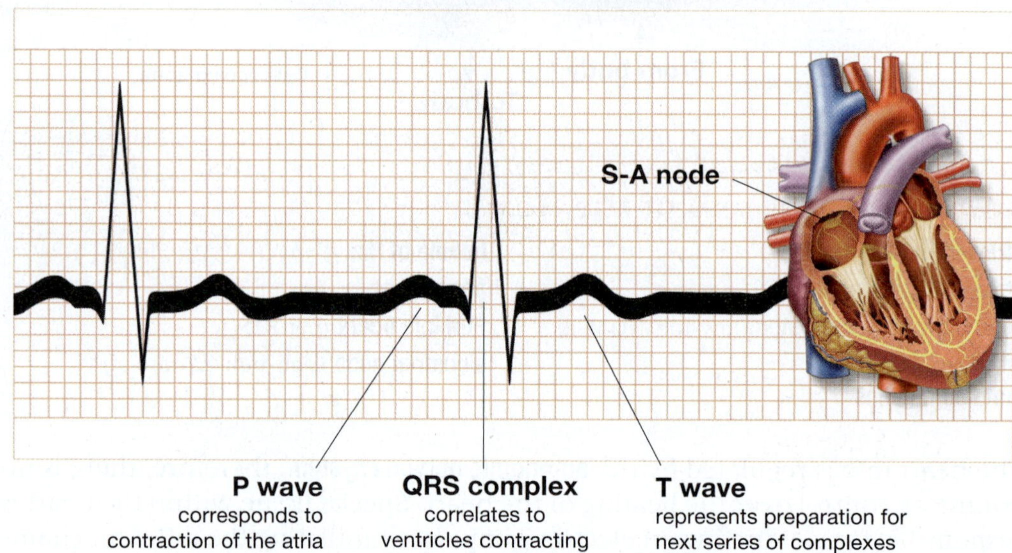

■ **Figure 5-7** An electrocardiogram (EKG or ECG) wave record of the electrical signal as it moves through the conduction system of the heart. This signal stimulates the chambers of the heart to contract and relax in the proper sequence.

PRACTICE AS YOU GO

A. Complete the Statement

1. The study of the heart is called ____________________.
2. The three layers of the heart are ____________________, ____________________, and ____________________.
3. The impulse for the heartbeat (the pacemaker) originates in the ____________________.

4. Arteries carry blood ____________________ the heart.

5. The four heart valves are ____________________, ____________________, ____________________, and ____________________.

6. The ____________________ are the receiving chambers of the heart and the ____________________ are the pumping chambers.

7. The ____________________ circulation carries blood to and from the lungs.

8. The pointed tip of the heart is called the ____________________.

9. The ____________________ divides the heart into left and right halves.

10. ____________________ is the contraction phase of the heartbeat and ____________________ is the relaxation phase.

Blood Vessels

lumen (LOO-men)

There are three types of blood vessels: arteries, capillaries, and veins (see Figure 5-8 ■). These are the pipes that circulate blood throughout the body. The **lumen** is the channel within these vessels through which blood flows.

Arteries

arterioles (ar-TEER-ee-ohlz)

coronary arteries (KOR-ah-nair-ee / AR-ter-eez)

The arteries are the large, thick-walled vessels that carry the blood away from the heart. The walls of arteries contain a thick layer of smooth muscle that can contract or relax to change the size of the arterial lumen. The pulmonary artery carries deoxygenated blood from the right ventricle to the lungs. The largest

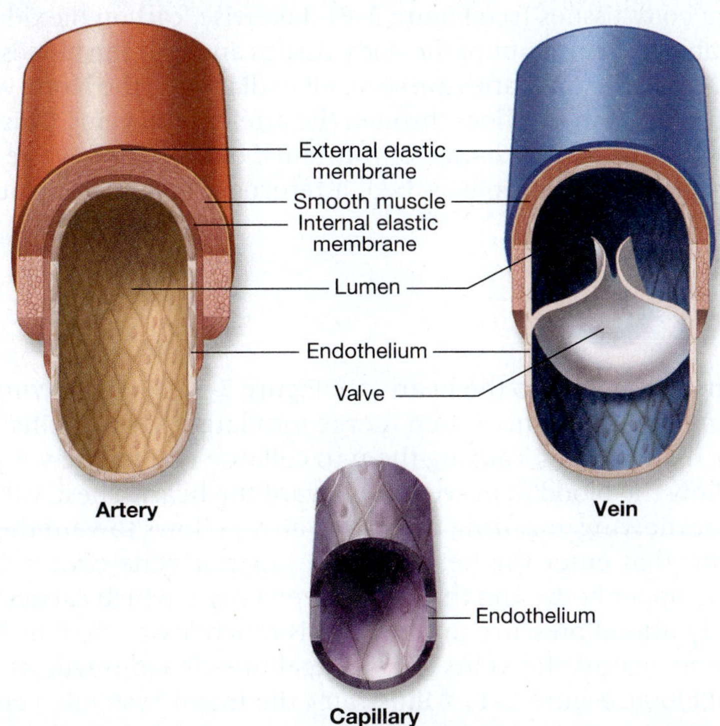

■ **Figure 5-8** Comparative structure of arteries, capillaries, and veins.

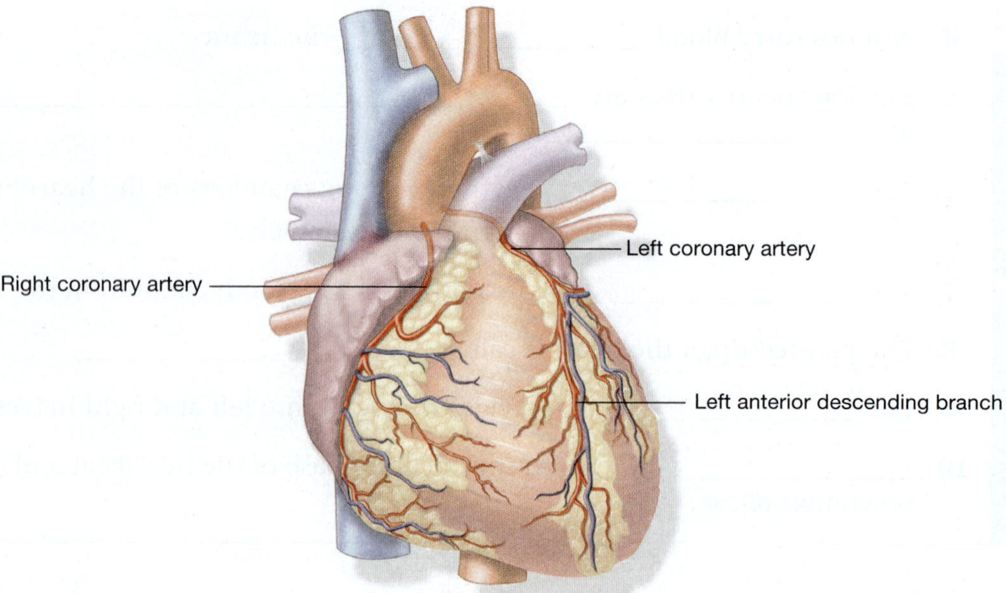

■ **Figure 5-9** The coronary arteries.

Med Term Tip

The term *coronary*, from the Latin word for crown, describes how the great vessels encircle the heart as they emerge from the top of the heart.

artery, the aorta, begins from the left ventricle of the heart and carries oxygenated blood to all the body systems. The **coronary arteries** then branch from the aorta and provide blood to the myocardium (see Figure 5-9 ■). As they travel through the body, the arteries branch into progressively smaller-sized arteries. The smallest of the arteries, called **arterioles**, deliver blood to the capillaries. Figure 5-10 ■ illustrates the major systemic arteries.

Capillaries

capillary bed

Capillaries are a network of tiny blood vessels referred to as a **capillary bed**. Arterial blood flows into a capillary bed, and venous blood flows back out. Capillaries are very thin walled, allowing for the diffusion of the oxygen and nutrients from the blood into the body tissues (see Figure 5-8). Likewise, carbon dioxide and waste products are able to diffuse out of the body tissues and into the bloodstream to be carried away. Since the capillaries are so small in diameter, the blood will not flow as quickly through them as it does through the arteries and veins. This means that the blood has time for an exchange of nutrients, oxygen, and waste material to take place. As blood exits a capillary bed, it returns to the heart through a vein.

Veins

venules (VEN-yools)

The veins carry blood back to the heart (see Figure 5-8). Blood leaving capillaries first enters small **venules**, which then merge into larger veins. Veins have much thinner walls than arteries, causing them to collapse easily. The veins also have valves that allow the blood to move only toward the heart. These valves prevent blood from backflowing, ensuring that blood always flows toward the heart. The two large veins that enter the heart are the superior vena cava, which carries blood from the upper body, and the inferior vena cava, which carries blood from the lower body. Blood pressure in the veins is much lower than in the arteries. Muscular action against the veins and skeletal muscle contractions help in the movement of blood. Figure 5-11 ■ illustrates the major systemic veins.

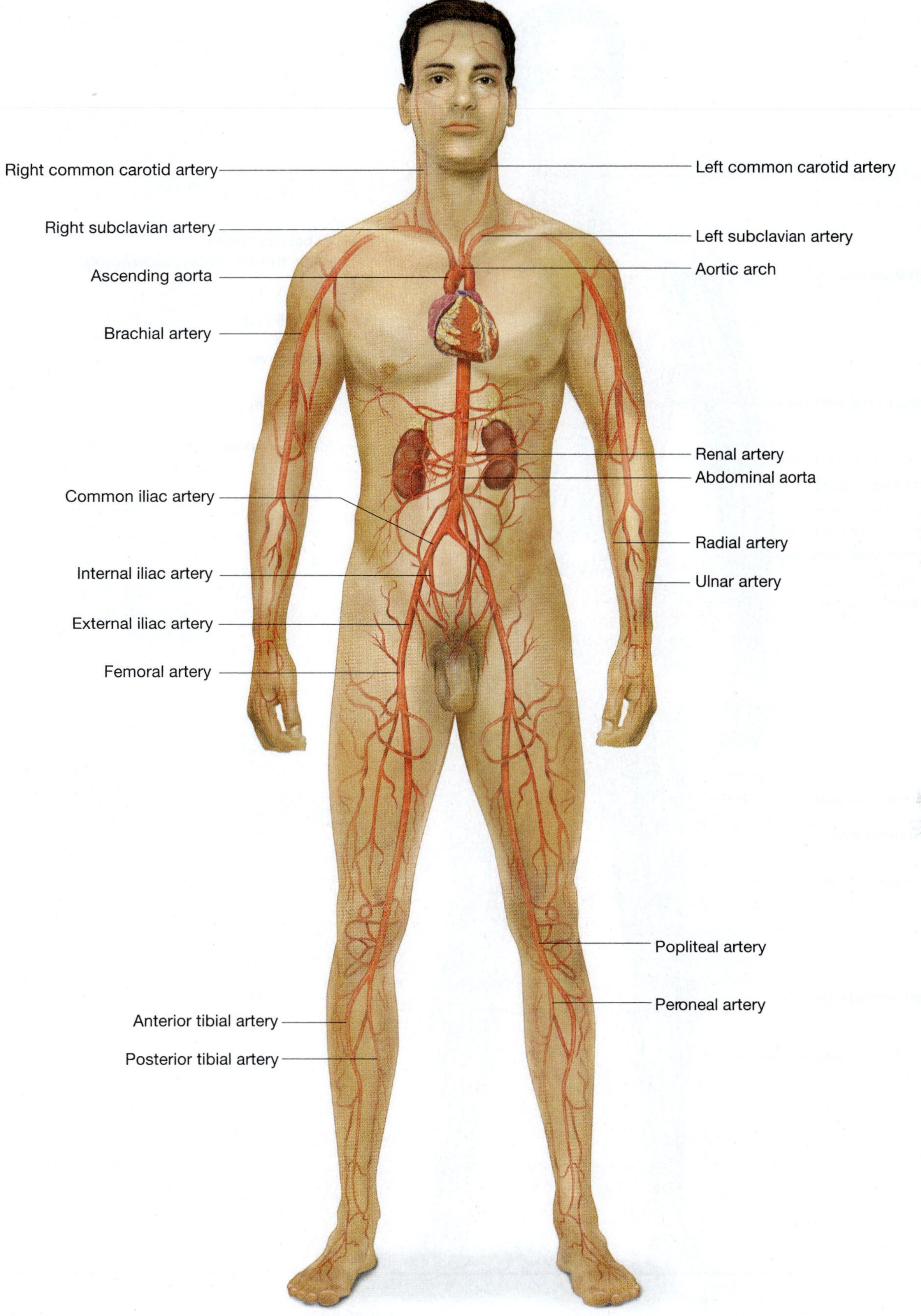
Right common carotid artery
Right subclavian artery
Ascending aorta
Brachial artery
Common iliac artery
Internal iliac artery
External iliac artery
Femoral artery
Anterior tibial artery
Posterior tibial artery
Left common carotid artery
Left subclavian artery
Aortic arch
Renal artery
Abdominal aorta
Radial artery
Ulnar artery
Popliteal artery
Peroneal artery

Figure 5-10 The major arteries of the body.

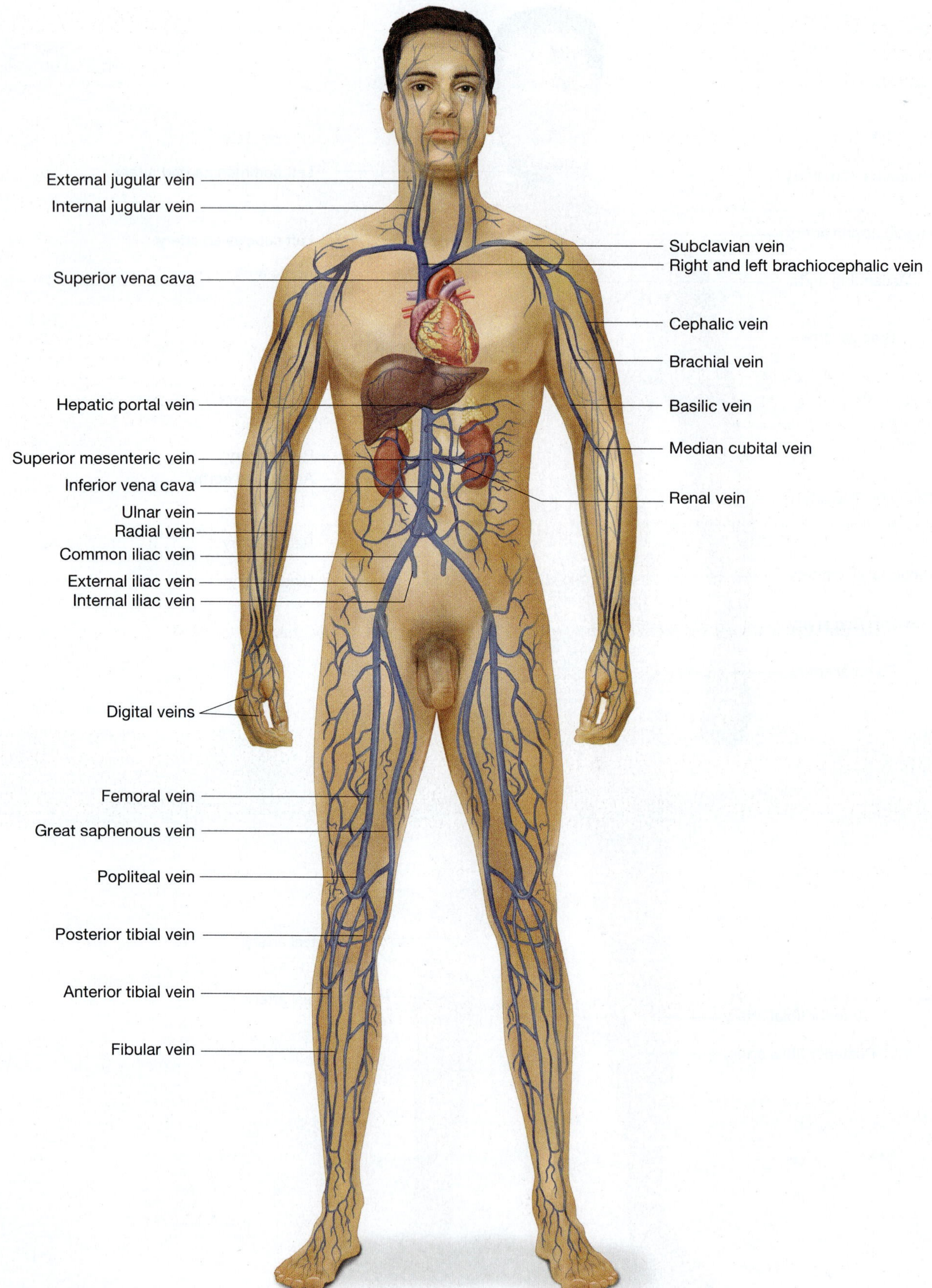
External jugular vein
Internal jugular vein
Superior vena cava
Hepatic portal vein
Superior mesenteric vein
Inferior vena cava
Ulnar vein
Radial vein
Common iliac vein
External iliac vein
Internal iliac vein
Digital veins
Femoral vein
Great saphenous vein
Popliteal vein
Posterior tibial vein
Anterior tibial vein
Fibular vein
Subclavian vein
Right and left brachiocephalic vein
Cephalic vein
Brachial vein
Basilic vein
Median cubital vein
Renal vein

Figure 5-11 The major veins of the body.

Pulse and Blood Pressure

blood pressure	**pulse**
diastolic pressure (dye-ah-STOL-ik)	**systolic pressure** (sis-TOL-ik)

What's In A Name?

Look for this word part:
-ic = pertaining to

Blood pressure (BP) is a measurement of the force exerted by blood against the wall of a blood vessel. During ventricular systole, blood is under a lot of pressure from the ventricular contraction, giving the highest blood pressure reading—the **systolic pressure.** The **pulse**(P) felt at the wrist or throat is the surge of blood caused by the heart contraction. This is why pulse rate is normally equal to heart rate. During ventricular diastole, blood is not being pushed by the heart at all and the blood pressure reading drops to its lowest point—the **diastolic pressure**. Therefore, to see the full range of what is occurring with blood pressure, both numbers are required. Blood pressure is also affected by several other characteristics of the blood and the blood vessels. These include the elasticity of the arteries, the diameter of the blood vessels, the viscosity of the blood, the volume of blood flowing through the vessels, and the amount of resistance to blood flow.

Med Term Tip

The instrument used to measure blood pressure is called a *sphygmomanometer.* The combining form **sphygm/o** means *pulse* and the suffix **-manometer** means *instrument to measure pressure.* A blood pressure reading is reported as two numbers, for example, 120/80. The 120 is the systolic pressure and the 80 is the diastolic pressure. There is no one "normal" blood pressure number. The normal blood pressure for an adult is a systolic pressure less than 120 and diastolic pressure less than 80.

PRACTICE AS YOU GO

B. Complete the Statement

1. The three types of blood vessels are ______________, ______________, and ______________.
2. ______________ carry blood toward the heart.
3. ______________ carry blood away from the heart.
4. Diffusion of oxygen and nutrients from blood into body tissues occurs in the ______________.
5. The highest blood pressure is the ______________ pressure and the lowest blood pressure is the ______________ pressure.

Terminology

Word Parts Used to Build Cardiovascular System Terms

The following lists contain the combining forms, suffixes, and prefixes used to build terms in the remaining sections of this chapter.

Combining Forms

angi/o	vessel	**cardi/o**	heart	**fibrin/o**	fibers
aort/o	aorta	**coron/o**	heart	**hem/o** (see Chapter 6)	blood
arteri/o	artery	**corpor/o**	body	**isch/o**	to hold back
arteriol/o	arteriole	**cutane/o**	skin	**lip/o**	fat
ather/o	fatty substance	**duct/o**	to bring	**my/o**	muscle
atri/o	atrium	**electr/o**	electricity	**myocardi/o**	heart muscle
bi/o	life	**embol/o**	plug		

Combining Forms (continued)

orth/o	straight	**sept/o**	a wall	**varic/o**	dilated vein
pector/o	chest	**son/o**	sound	**vas/o**	vessel
peripher/o (see Chapter 12)	away from center	**sphygm/o**	pulse	**vascul/o**	blood vessel
phleb/o	vein	**steth/o**	chest	**ven/o**	vein
pulmon/o	lung	**thromb/o**	clot	**ventricul/o**	ventricle
scler/o	hard	**valv/o**	valve	**venul/o**	venule
		valvul/o	valve		

Suffixes

-ac	pertaining to	**-logy**	study of	**-rrhexis**	rupture
-al	pertaining to	**-lytic**	destruction	**-sclerosis**	hardening
-ar	pertaining to	**-manometer**	instrument to measure pressure	**-scope**	instrument for viewing
-ary	pertaining to	**-megaly**	enlarged	**-spasm**	involuntary muscle contraction
-cardia	heart condition	**-ole**	small	**-stenosis**	narrowing
-eal	pertaining to	**-oma**	mass	**-tension**	pressure
-ectomy	surgical removal	**-ose**	pertaining to	**-therapy**	treatment
-gram	record	**-ous**	pertaining to	**-tic**	pertaining to
-graphy	process of recording	**-pathy**	disease	**-tonic**	pertaining to tone
-ia	condition	**-plasty**	surgical repair	**-ule**	small
-ic	pertaining to	**-pressor**	to press down		
-itis	inflammation				

Prefixes

a-	without	**hypo-**	insufficient	**re-**	again
anti-	against	**inter-**	between	**tachy-**	fast
brady-	slow	**intra-**	within	**tetra-**	four
de-	without	**per-**	through	**trans-**	across
endo-	inner	**peri-**	around	**ultra-**	beyond
extra-	outside of	**poly-**	many		
hyper-	excessive	**pre-**	before		

Adjective Forms of Anatomical Terms

Term	Word Parts	Definition
aortic (ay-OR-tik)	aort/o = aorta -ic = pertaining to	Pertaining to aorta
arterial (ar-TEE-ree-al)	arteri/o = artery -al = pertaining to	Pertaining to artery

Adjective Forms of Anatomical Terms (continued)

Term	Word Parts	Definition
arteriolar (ar-teer-ee-OH-lar)	**arteriol/o** = arteriole **-ar** = pertaining to	Pertaining to arteriole
atrial (AY-tree-al)	**atri/o** = atrium **-al** = pertaining to	Pertaining to atrium
atrioventricular (AV, A-V) (ay-tree-oh-ven-TRIK-yoo-lar)	**atri/o** = atrium **ventricul/o** = ventricle **-ar** = pertaining to	Pertaining to atrium and ventricle
cardiac (KAR-dee-ak)	**cardi/o** = heart **-ac** = pertaining to	Pertaining to heart
coronary (KOR-ah-nair-ee)	**coron/o** = heart **-ary** = pertaining to	Pertaining to heart
corporeal (kor-POH-ree-al)	**corpor/o** = body **-eal** = pertaining to	Pertaining to body
interatrial (in-ter-AY-tree-al)	**inter-** = between **atri/o** = atrium **-al** = pertaining to	Pertaining to between the atria
interventricular (in-ter-ven-TRIK-yoo-lar)	**inter-** = between **ventricul/o** = ventricle **-ar** = pertaining to	Pertaining to between the ventricles
myocardial (my-oh-KAR-dee-al)	**myocardi/o** = heart muscle **-al** = pertaining to	Pertaining to heart muscle
valvular (VAL-vyoo-lar)	**valvul/o** = valve **-ar** = pertaining to	Pertaining to a valve
vascular (VAS-kyoo-lar)	**vascul/o** = blood vessel **-ar** = pertaining to	Pertaining to a blood vessel
venous (VEE-nus)	**ven/o** = vein **-ous** = pertaining to	Pertaining to a vein
ventricular (ven-TRIK-yoo-lar)	**ventricul/o** = ventricle **-ar** = pertaining to	Pertaining to a ventricle
venular (VEN-yoo-lar)	**venul/o** = venule **-ar** = pertaining to	Pertaining to venule

PRACTICE AS YOU GO

C. Give the adjective form for each anatomical structure/location.

1. The heart ______________________
2. Between the ventricles ______________________
3. An artery ______________________
4. A small vein ______________________
5. The heart muscle ______________________
6. An atrium ______________________

Pathology

Term	Word Parts	Definition
Medical Specialties		
cardiology (kar-dee-ALL-oh-jee)	cardi/o = heart -logy = study of	Branch of medicine involving diagnosis and treatment of conditions and diseases of cardiovascular system; physician is a *cardiologist*
cardiovascular technologist/ technician	cardi/o = heart vascul/o = blood vessel -ar = pertaining to	Healthcare professional trained to perform variety of diagnostic and therapeutic procedures including electrocardiography, echocardiography, and exercise stress tests
Signs and Symptoms		
angiitis (an-jee-EYE-tis)	angi/o = vessel -itis = inflammation	Inflammation of a vessel
angiospasm (AN-jee-oh-spazm)	angi/o = vessel -spasm = involuntary muscle contraction	Involuntary muscle contraction of smooth muscle in wall of a vessel; narrows vessel
angiostenosis (an-jee-oh-steh-NOH-sis)	angi/o = vessel -stenosis = narrowing	Narrowing of a vessel
embolus (EM-boh-lus)	embol/o = plug	Obstruction of blood vessel by blood clot that has broken off from thrombus somewhere else in body and traveled to point of obstruction; if it occurs in coronary artery, may result in myocardial infarction
infarct (IN-farkt)		Area of tissue within organ or part that undergoes necrosis (death) following loss of its blood supply
ischemia (iss-KEE-mee-ah)	isch/o = to hold back hem/o = blood -ia = condition	Localized and temporary deficiency of blood supply due to obstruction to circulation
murmur (MUR-mur)		A sound, in addition to normal heart sounds, arising from blood flowing through heart; extra sound may or may not indicate a heart abnormality
orthostatic hypotension (or-thoh-STAT-ik)	orth/o = straight hypo- = insufficient -tension = pressure	Sudden drop in blood pressure a person experiences when standing straight up suddenly
palpitations (pal-pih-TAY-shunz)		Pounding, racing heartbeats
plaque (PLAK)		Yellow, fatty deposit of lipids in artery that is hallmark of atherosclerosis; also called an *atheroma*

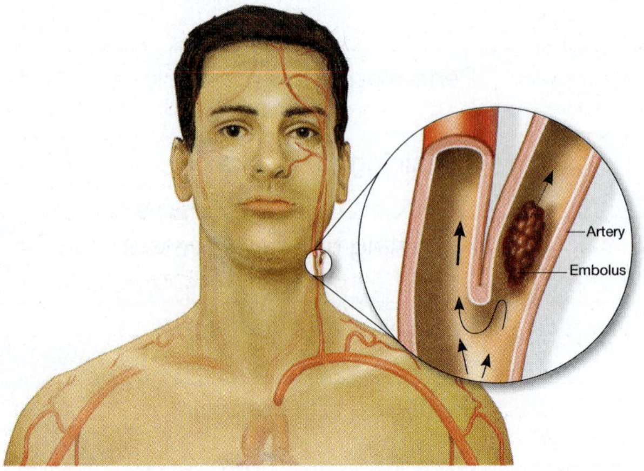

Figure 5-12 Illustration of an embolus floating in an artery. The embolus will become lodged in a blood vessel that is smaller than it is, resulting in occlusion of that artery.

Pathology (continued)

Term	Word Parts	Definition
regurgitation (ree-ger-jih-TAY-shun)	re- = again	To flow backward; in cardiovascular system this refers to backflow of blood through a valve
thrombus (THROM-bus)	thromb/o = clot	Blood clot forming within blood vessel; may partially or completely occlude blood vessel

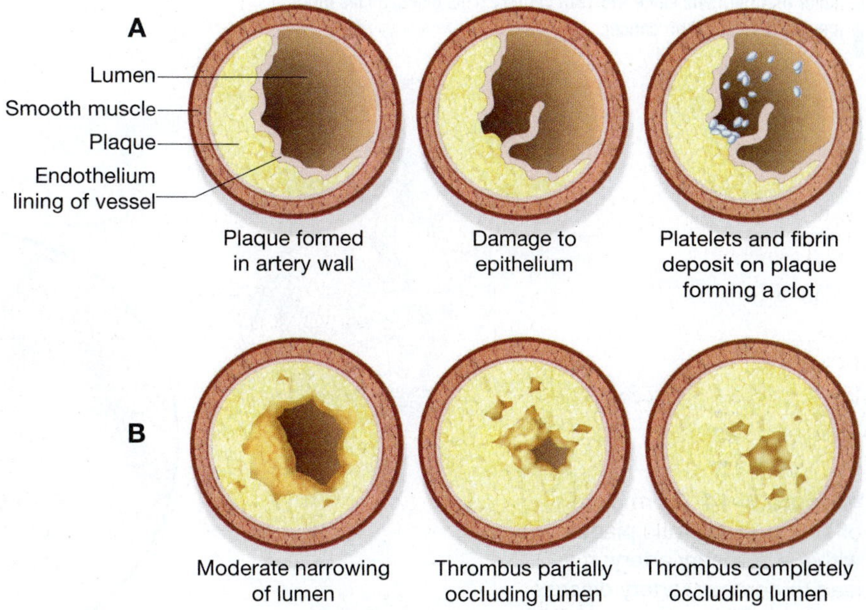

A

Lumen

Smooth muscle

Plaque

Endothelium lining of vessel

Plaque formed in artery wall

Damage to epithelium

Platelets and fibrin deposit on plaque forming a clot

B

Moderate narrowing of lumen

Thrombus partially occluding lumen

Thrombus completely occluding lumen

■ **Figure 5-13** Development of an atherosclerotic plaque that progressively narrows the lumen of an artery.

Term	Word Parts	Definition
Heart		
angina pectoris (an-JYE-nah / PEK-tor-is)	pector/o = chest	Condition in which there is severe pain with sensation of constriction around heart; caused by deficiency of oxygen to heart muscle; commonly called *chest pain* (CP)
cardiac arrest	cardi/o = heart -ac = pertaining to	Complete stopping of heart activity
cardiac tamponade (KAR-dee-ak / tam-poh-NADE)	cardi/o = heart -ac = pertaining to	Pressure on heart as a result of fluid buildup around heart inside pericardial sac; heart becomes unable to pump blood effectively
cardiomegaly (kar-dee-oh-MEG-ah-lee)	cardi/o = heart -megaly = enlarged	Enlarged heart
cardiomyopathy (kar-dee-oh-my-OP-ah-thee)	cardi/o = heart my/o = muscle -pathy = disease	General term for disease of myocardium; can be caused by alcohol abuse, parasites, viral infection, and congestive heart failure; one of most common reasons a patient may require heart transplant
congenital septal defect (CSD)	sept/o = a wall -al = pertaining to	Hole, present at birth, in septum between two heart chambers; results in mixture of oxygenated and deoxygenated blood; can be an *atrial septal defect* (ASD) and a *ventricular septal defect* (VSD)
congestive heart failure (CHF) (kon-JESS-tiv)		Pathological condition of heart in which there is reduced outflow of blood from left side of heart because left ventricle myocardium has become too weak to efficiently pump blood; results in weakness, breathlessness, and edema

Pathology (continued)

Term	Word Parts	Definition
coronary artery disease (CAD) (KOR-ah-nair-ee)	coron/o = heart -ary = pertaining to	Insufficient blood supply to heart muscle due to obstruction of one or more coronary arteries; may be caused by atherosclerosis and may cause angina pectoris and myocardial infarction

Med Term Tip

All types of cardiovascular disease have been the number one killer of Americans since the 19th century. This disease kills more people annually than cancer.

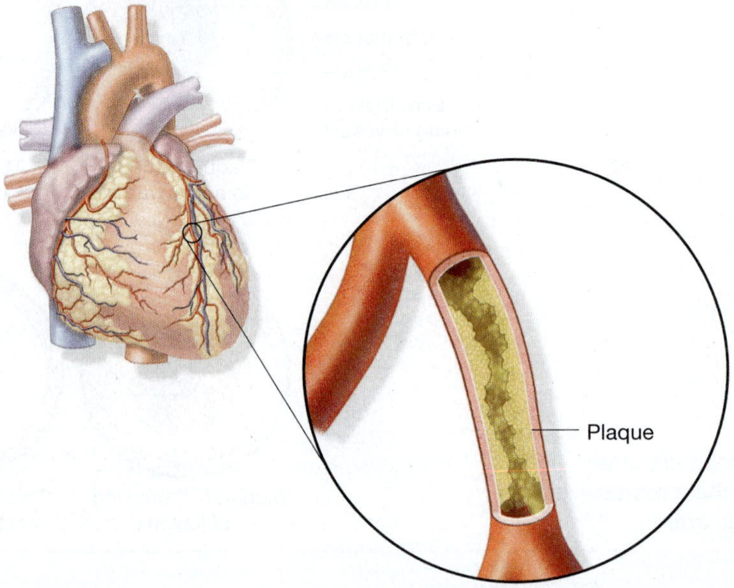

Plaque

■ **Figure 5-14** Formation of an atherosclerotic plaque within a coronary artery; may lead to coronary artery disease, angina pectoris, and myocardial infarction.

Term	Word Parts	Definition
endocarditis (en-doh-kar-DYE-tis)	endo- = inner cardi/o = heart -itis = inflammation	Inflammation of lining membranes of heart; may be due to bacteria or to abnormal immunological response; in bacterial endocarditis, mass of bacteria that forms is referred to as *vegetation*
heart valve prolapse (PROH-laps)		Condition in which cusps or flaps of heart valve are too loose and fail to shut tightly, allowing blood to flow backward through valve when heart chamber contracts; most commonly occurs in mitral valve, but may affect any of heart valves; also called *heart valve incompetence* or *heart valve insufficiency*
heart valve stenosis (steh-NOH-sis)	-stenosis = narrowing	Condition in which cusps or flaps of heart valve are too stiff and are unable to open fully (making it difficult for blood to flow through) or shut tightly (allowing blood to flow backward); condition may affect any of heart valves
myocardial infarction (MI) (my-oh-KAR-dee-al / in-FARK-shun)	myocardi/o = heart muscle -al = pertaining to	Condition caused by partial or complete occlusion or closing of one or more of coronary arteries; symptoms include squeezing pain or heavy pressure in middle of chest (angina pectoris); delay in treatment could result in death; also referred to as a *heart attack*; see Figure 5-15 ■

Pathology (continued)

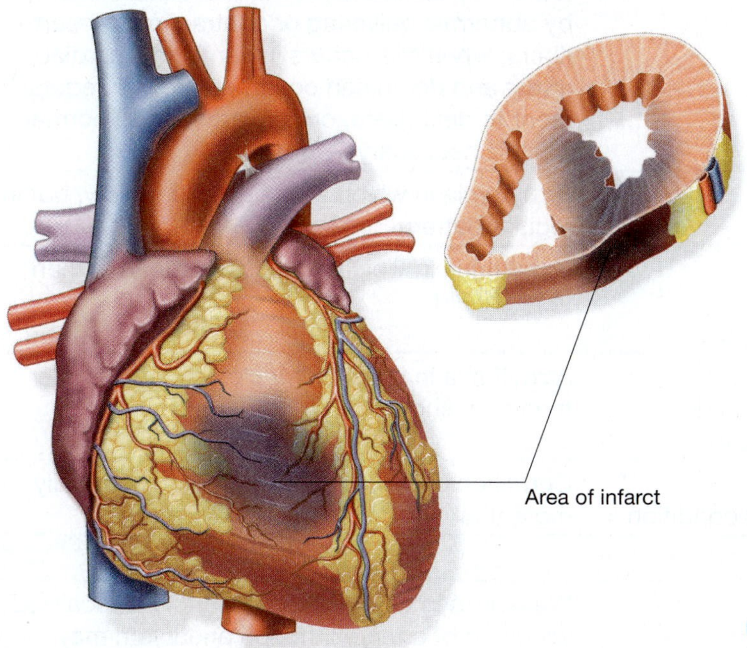

■ **Figure 5-15** External and cross-sectional view of an infarct caused by a myocardial infarction.

Term	Word Parts	Definition
myocarditis (my-oh-kar-DYE-tis)	myocardi/o = heart muscle -itis = inflammation	Inflammation of muscle layer of heart wall
pericarditis (pair-ih-kar-DYE-tis)	peri- = around cardi/o = heart -itis = inflammation	Inflammation of pericardial sac around heart
tetralogy of Fallot (teh-TRALL-oh-jee / fal-LOH)	tetra- = four -logy = study of	Combination of four congenital anomalies: pulmonary stenosis, interventricular septal defect, improper placement of aorta, and hypertrophy of right ventricle; needs immediate surgery to correct
valvulitis (val-vyoo-LYE-tis)	valvul/o = valve -itis = inflammation	Inflammation of a heart valve
Arrhythmias		
arrhythmia (ah-RITH-mee-ah)	a- = without -ia = condition	Irregularity in heartbeat or action; comes in many different forms; may be too fast, too slow, or irregular pattern; some are not serious, while others are life-threatening
bradycardia (brad-ee-KAR-dee-ah)	brady- = slow -cardia = heart condition	Condition of having a slow heart rate, typically less than 60 beats/minute; highly trained aerobic persons may normally have a slow heart rate
bundle branch block (BBB)		Occurs when electrical impulse is blocked from traveling down bundle of His or bundle branches; results in ventricles beating at different rate than atria; also called a *heart block*

Pathology (continued)

Term	Word Parts	Definition
fibrillation (fib) (fih-brill-AY-shun)		Extremely serious arrhythmia characterized by abnormal quivering or contraction of heart fibers; when this occurs in ventricles, cardiac arrest and death can occur; emergency equipment to defibrillate, or convert heart to normal beat, is necessary
flutter		Arrhythmia in which atria beat too rapidly, but in regular pattern
premature atrial contraction (PAC) (AY-tree-al)	pre- = before atri/o = atrium -al = pertaining to	Arrhythmia in which atria contract earlier than they should
premature ventricular contraction (PVC) (ven-TRIK-yoo-lar)	pre- = before ventricul/o = ventricle -ar = pertaining to	Arrhythmia in which ventricles contract earlier than they should
tachycardia (tak-ee-KAR-dee-ah)	tachy- = fast -cardia = heart condition	Condition of having a fast heart rate, typically more than 100 beats/minute while at rest
Blood Vessels		
aneurysm (AN-yoo-rizm)		Weakness in wall of artery resulting in localized widening of artery; although aneurysm may develop in any artery, common sites include aorta in abdomen and cerebral arteries in brain

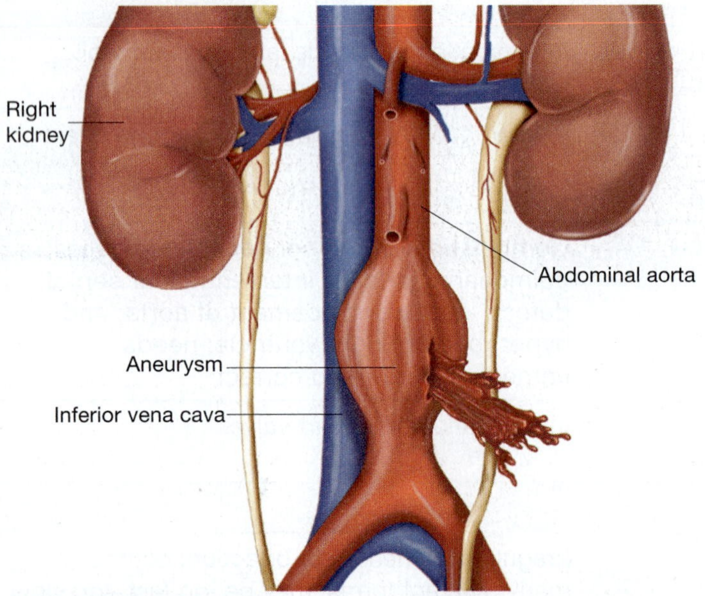

■ **Figure 5-16** Illustration of a large aneurysm in the abdominal aorta that has ruptured.

Term	Word Parts	Definition
arteriorrhexis (ar-tee-ree-oh-REK-sis)	arteri/o = artery -rrhexis = rupture	Ruptured artery; may occur if aneurysm ruptures arterial wall
arteriosclerosis (AS) (ar-tee-ree-oh-skleh-ROH-sis)	arteri/o = artery -sclerosis = hardening	Thickening, hardening, and loss of elasticity of walls of arteries; most often due to atherosclerosis
atheroma (ath-er-OH-mah)	ather/o = fatty substance -oma = mass	Deposit of fatty substance in wall of artery that bulges into and narrows lumen of artery; characteristic of atherosclerosis; also called a *plaque*

Pathology (continued)

Term	Word Parts	Definition
atherosclerosis (ath-er-oh-skleh-ROH-sis)	ather/o = fatty substance -sclerosis = hardening	Most common form of arteriosclerosis; caused by formation of yellowish plaques of cholesterol on inner walls of arteries (see again Figures 5-13 and 5-14)
coarctation of the aorta (CoA) (koh-ark-TAY-shun)		Severe congenital narrowing of aorta
deep vein thrombosis (DVT) (throm-BOH-sis)	thromb/o = clot	Formation of blood clot in a vein deep in the body, most commonly the legs; embolus breaking off from this thrombosis would travel to lungs and block blood flow through lungs
hemorrhoid (HEM-oh-royd)	hem/o = blood	Varicose veins in anal region
hypertension (HTN) (high-per-TEN-shun)	hyper- = excessive -tension = pressure	Blood pressure (BP) above normal range; *essential* or *primary hypertension* occurs directly from cardiovascular disease; *secondary hypertension* refers to high blood pressure resulting from another disease such as kidney disease
hypotension (high-poh-TEN-shun)	hypo- = insufficient -tension = pressure	Decrease in blood pressure (BP); can occur in shock, infection, cancer, anemia, or as death approaches
patent ductus arteriosus (PDA) (PAY-tent / DUK-tus / ar-tee-ree-OH-sis)	duct/o = to bring arteri/o = artery	Congenital heart anomaly in which fetal connection between pulmonary artery and aorta fails to close at birth; condition may be treated with medication and resolve with time; however, in some cases, surgery is required
peripheral vascular disease (PVD)	peripher/o = away from center -al = pertaining to vascul/o = blood vessel -ar = pertaining to	Any abnormal condition affecting blood vessels outside heart; symptoms may include pain, pallor, numbness, and loss of circulation and pulse
phlebitis (fleh-BYE-tis)	phleb/o = vein -itis = inflammation	Inflammation of a vein
polyarteritis (pol-ee-ar-ter-EYE-tis)	poly- = many arteri/o = artery -itis = inflammation	Inflammation of several arteries
Raynaud's phenomenon (ray-NOZ)		Periodic ischemic attacks affecting extremities of body, especially fingers, toes, ears, and nose; affected extremities become cyanotic and very painful; attacks are brought on by arterial constriction due to extreme cold or emotional stress
thrombophlebitis (throm-boh-fleh-BYE-tis)	thromb/o = clot phleb/o = vein -itis = inflammation	Inflammation of vein resulting in formation of blood clots within vein
varicose veins (VAIR-ih-kohs)	varic/o = dilated vein -ose = pertaining to	Swollen and distended veins, usually in legs

PRACTICE AS YOU GO

D. Terminology Matching

Match each term to its definition.

1. ________ arrhythmia	**a.** swollen, distended veins
2. ________ thrombus	**b.** inflammation of vein
3. ________ bradycardia	**c.** serious congenital anomaly
4. ________ murmur	**d.** slow heart rate
5. ________ phlebitis	**e.** cusps are too loose
6. ________ hypotension	**f.** irregular heartbeat
7. ________ varicose veins	**g.** an extra heart sound
8. ________ tetralogy of Fallot	**h.** clot in blood vessel
9. ________ valve prolapse	**i.** low blood pressure
10. ________ plaque	**j.** fatty deposit in artery

Diagnostic Procedures

Term	Word Parts	Definition
Medical Procedures		
auscultation (oss-kul-TAY-shun)		Process of listening to sounds within body by using a stethoscope
sphygmomanometer (sfig-moh-mah-NOM-eh-ter)	sphygm/o = pulse -manometer = instrument to measure pressure	Instrument for measuring blood pressure (BP); also referred to as *blood pressure cuff*
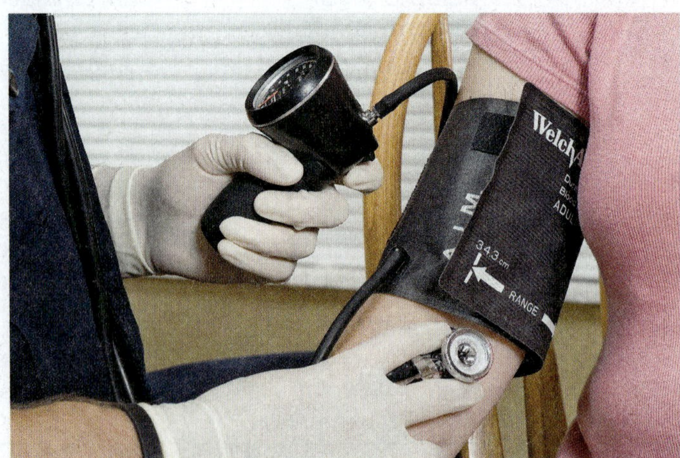 ■ **Figure 5-17** Using a sphygmomanometer to measure blood pressure. *(Michal Heron/Pearson Education, Inc.)*		
stethoscope (STETH-oh-skohp)	steth/o = chest -scope = instrument for viewing	Instrument for listening to body sounds (auscultation), such as chest, heart, or intestines

Diagnostic Procedures (continued)

Term	Word Parts	Definition
Clinical Laboratory Tests		
cardiac biomarkers (KAR-dee-ak)	cardi/o = heart -ac = pertaining to bi/o = life	Blood test to determine level of proteins specific to heart muscle in blood; increase in these proteins may indicate heart muscle damage such as myocardial infarction; proteins include creatine kinase (CK) and troponin
serum lipoprotein level (SEER-um / lip-oh-PROH-teen)	lip/o = fat	Blood test to measure amount of cholesterol and triglycerides in blood; indicator of atherosclerosis risk
Diagnostic Imaging		
angiogram (AN-jee-oh-gram)	angi/o = vessel -gram = record	X-ray record of vessel taken during angiography
angiography (an-jee-OG-rah-fee)	angi/o = vessel -graphy = process of recording	X-rays taken after injection of opaque material into blood vessel; can be performed on aorta as aortic angiography, on heart as angiocardiography, and on brain as cerebral angiography
cardiac scan	cardi/o = heart -ac = pertaining to	Patient is given radioactive thallium intravenously and then scanning equipment is used to visualize heart; especially useful in determining myocardial damage
Doppler ultrasonography (DOP-ler / ul-trah-son-OG-rah-fee)	ultra- = beyond son/o = sound -graphy = process of recording	Measurement of sound-wave echoes as they bounce off tissues and organs to produce an image; procedure is used to measure velocity of blood moving through blood vessels to look for blood clots or deep vein thromboses
echocardiography (ECHO) (ek-oh-kar-dee-OG-rah-fee)	cardi/o = artery -graphy = process of recording	Noninvasive diagnostic procedure using ultrasound to visualize internal cardiac structures; cardiac valve activity can be evaluated using this method
Cardiac Function Tests		
cardiac catheterization (heart cath) (KAR-dee-ak / kath-eh-ter-ih-ZAY-shun)	cardi/o = heart -ac = pertaining to	Passage of thin-tube catheter through blood vessel leading to heart; done to detect abnormalities, to collect cardiac blood samples, and to determine blood pressure within heart
catheter (KATH-eh-ter)		Flexible tube inserted into body for purpose of moving fluids into or out of body; in the cardiovascular system, a catheter is used to place dye into blood vessels so they may be visualized on X-rays
electrocardiogram (ECG, EKG) (ee-lek-troh-KAR-dee-oh-gram)	electr/o = electricity cardi/o = heart -gram = record	Hardcopy record produced by electrocardiography
electrocardiography (ee-lek-troh-kar-dee-OG-rah-fee)	electr/o = electricity cardi/o = heart -graphy = process of recording	Process of recording electrical activity of heart; useful in diagnosis of abnormal cardiac rhythm and heart muscle (myocardium) damage

Diagnostic Procedures (continued)

Term	Word Parts	Definition
Holter monitor		Portable ECG monitor worn by patient for a period of a few hours to a few days to assess heart and pulse activity as person goes through activities of daily living; used to assess patient who experiences chest pain and unusual heart activity during exercise and normal activities
stress testing		Method for evaluating cardiovascular fitness; patient is placed on treadmill or bicycle and then subjected to steadily increasing levels of work; EKG and oxygen levels are taken while patient exercises; test is stopped if abnormalities occur on EKG; also called *exercise test* or *treadmill test*

■ **Figure 5-18** Man undergoing a stress test on a treadmill while physician monitors his condition. *(Serafino Mozzo/Shutterstock)*

Therapeutic Procedures

Term	Word Parts	Definition
Medical Procedures		
cardiopulmonary resuscitation (CPR) (kar-dee-oh-PULL-mon-air-ee / ree-suss-ih-TAY-shun)	cardi/o = heart pulmon/o = lung -ary = pertaining to	Procedure to restore cardiac output and oxygenated air to lungs for person in cardiac arrest; combination of chest compressions (to push blood out of heart) and artificial respiration (to blow air into lungs) is performed by one or two CPR-trained rescuers
defibrillation (dee-fib-rih-LAY-shun)	de- = without	Procedure that converts serious irregular heartbeats, such as fibrillation, by giving electric shocks to heart using instrument called defibrillator; also called *cardioversion*; automated external defibrillators (AEDs) are portable devices that automatically detect life-threatening arrhythmias and deliver appropriate electrical shock; designed to be used by nonmedical personnel and found in public places such as shopping malls and schools

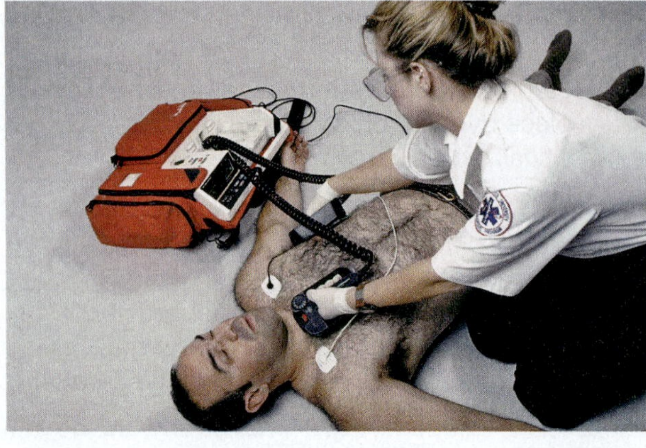

■ **Figure 5-19** An emergency medical technician positions defibrillator paddles on the chest of a supine male patient. *(Floyd Jackson/Pearson Education, Inc.)*

Therapeutic Procedures (continued)

Term	Word Parts	Definition
extracorporeal circulation (ECC) (eks-trah-kor-POR-ee-al)	extra- = outside of corpor/o = body -eal = pertaining to	During open-heart surgery, routing of blood to heart-lung machine so it can be oxygenated and pumped to rest of body
implantable cardioverter-defibrillator (ICD) (KAR-dee-oh-ver-ter / dee-FIB-rih-lay-ter)	cardi/o = heart de- = without	Device implanted in heart that delivers electrical shock to restore normal heart rhythm; particularly useful for persons who experience ventricular fibrillation
pacemaker implantation		Electrical device that substitutes for natural pacemaker of heart; controls beating of heart by series of rhythmic electrical impulses; external pacemaker has electrodes on outside of body; internal pacemaker has electrodes surgically implanted within chest wall ■ **Figure 5-20** X-ray showing a pacemaker implanted in the left side of the chest and the electrode wires running to the heart muscle. *(Chaikom/Shutterstock)*
sclerotherapy (SKLAIR-oh-thair-ah-pee)	scler/o = hard -therapy = treatment	Medical treatment for varicose veins; injection of solution (usually salt solution) directly into varicose vein; irritates lining of vessel, causing it to collapse and stick together
thrombolytic therapy (throm-boh-LIT-ik / THAIR-ah-pee)	thromb/o = clot -lytic = destruction	Process in which drugs, such as streptokinase (SK) or tissue plasminogen activator (tPA), are injected into a blood vessel to dissolve clots and restore blood flow
Surgical Procedures		
aneurysmectomy (an-yoo-riz-MEK-toh-mee)	-ectomy = surgical removal	Surgical removal of sac of an aneurysm
arterial anastomosis (ar-TEE-ree-al / ah-nas-toh-MOH-sis)	arteri/o = artery -al = pertaining to	Surgical joining together of two arteries; performed if artery is severed or if damaged section of artery is removed
atherectomy (ath-er-EK-toh-mee)	ather/o = fatty substance -ectomy = surgical removal	Surgical procedure to remove deposit of fatty substance, atheroma, from artery
coronary artery bypass graft (CABG) (KOR-ah-nair-ee)	coron/o = heart -ary = pertaining to	Open-heart surgery in which blood vessel from another location in body (often a leg vein) is grafted to route blood around blocked coronary artery
embolectomy (em-boh-LEK-toh-mee)	embol/o = plug -ectomy = surgical removal	Removal of embolus or clot from blood vessel
endarterectomy (end-ar-teh-REK-toh-mee)	endo- = inner arteri/o = artery -ectomy = surgical removal	Removal of diseased or damaged inner lining of artery; usually performed to remove atherosclerotic plaques
heart transplantation		Replacement of diseased or malfunctioning heart with donor's heart

Therapeutic Procedures (continued)

Term	Word Parts	Definition
intracoronary artery stent (in-trah-KOR-ah-nair-ee / AR-ter-ee)	**intra-** = within **coron/o** = heart **-ary** = pertaining to	Placement of stent within coronary artery to treat coronary ischemia due to atherosclerosis

A B C

■ **Figure 5-21** The process of placing a stent in a blood vessel. A) A catheter is used to place a collapsed stent next to an atherosclerotic plaque; B) stent is expanded; C) catheter is removed, leaving the expanded stent behind.

Term	Word Parts	Definition
ligation and stripping (lye-GAY-shun)		Surgical treatment for varicose veins; damaged vein is tied off (ligation) and removed (stripping)
percutaneous transluminal coronary angioplasty (PTCA) (per-kyoo-TAY-nee-us / trans-LOO-mih-nal / KOR-ah-nair-ee / AN-jee-oh-plas-tee)	**per-** = through **cutane/o** = skin **-ous** = pertaining to **trans-** = across **-al** = pertaining to **angi/o** = vessel **-plasty** = surgical repair	Method for treating localized coronary artery narrowing; balloon catheter is inserted through skin into coronary artery and inflated to dilate narrow blood vessel

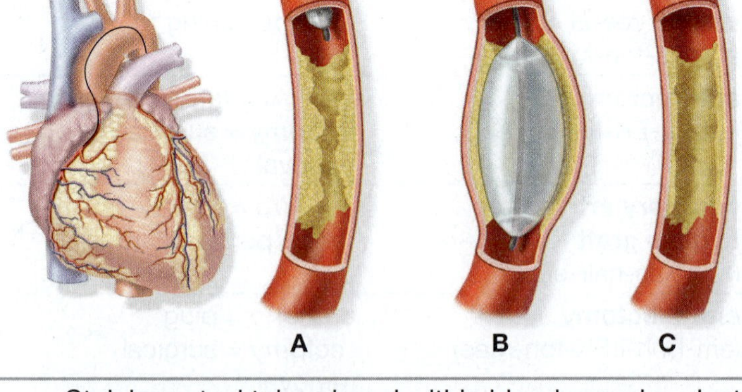

■ **Figure 5-22** Balloon angioplasty: A) deflated balloon catheter is approaching an atherosclerotic plaque; B) plaque is compressed by inflated balloon; C) plaque remains compressed after balloon catheter is removed.

Term	Word Parts	Definition
stent		Stainless steel tube placed within blood vessel or duct to widen lumen (see again Figure 5-21 ■)
valve replacement		Removal of diseased heart valve and replacement with artificial valve
valvoplasty (VAL-voh-plas-tee)	**valv/o** = valve **-plasty** = surgical repair	Surgical procedure to repair a heart valve

Pharmacology

Classification	Word Parts	Action	Examples
ACE inhibitor drugs		Produce vasodilation and decrease blood pressure	benazepril, Lotensin; catopril, Capoten
antiarrhythmic (an-tye-ah-RHYTH-mik)	anti- = against a- = without -ic = pertaining to	Reduces or prevents cardiac arrhythmias	flecainide, Tambocor; ibutilide, Corvert
anticoagulant (an-tye-koh-AG-yoo-lant)	anti- = against	Prevents blood clot formation	heparin; warfarin, Coumadin
antilipidemic (an-tye-lip-ih-DEEM-ik)	anti- = against lip/o = fat -ic = pertaining to	Reduces amount of cholesterol and lipids in bloodstream; treats hyperlipidemia	atorvastatin, Lipitor; simvastatin, Zocor
antiplatelet agents	anti- = against	Inhibit ability of platelets to clump together as part of blood clot	clopidogrel, Plavix; aspirin; ticlopidine, Ticlid
beta-blocker drugs		Treat hypertension and angina pectoris by lowering heart rate	metoprolol, Lopressor; propranolol, Inderal
calcium channel blocker drugs		Treat hypertension, angina pectoris, and congestive heart failure by causing heart to beat less forcefully and less often	diltiazem, Cardizem; nifedipine, Procardia
cardiotonic (kar-dee-oh-TAHN-ik)	cardi/o = heart -tonic = pertaining to tone	Increases force of cardiac muscle contraction; treats congestive heart failure	digoxin, Lanoxin
diuretic (dye-yoo-RET-ik)	-tic = pertaining to	Increases urine production by kidneys, which works to reduce plasma and therefore blood volume, resulting in lower blood pressure	furosemide, Lasix
fibrinolytic (fye-brin-oh-LIT-ik)	fibrin/o = fibers -lytic = destruction	Dissolves existing blood clots	tissue plasminogen activator (tPA); alteplase, Activase
vasodilator (vay-zoh-DYE-lay-ter)	vas/o = vessel	Relaxes smooth muscle in walls of arteries, thereby increasing diameter of blood vessel; used for two main purposes: increasing circulation to ischemic area and reducing blood pressure	nitroglycerin, Nitro-Dur; hydralazine, Apresoline
vasopressor (vay-zoh-PRESS-or)	vas/o = vessel -pressor = to press down	Contracts smooth muscle in walls of blood vessels; raises blood pressure	dopamine, Myocard-DX; vasopressin, Vasostrict

PRACTICE AS YOU GO

E. Procedure Matching

Match each procedure to its definition.

1. ________ cardiac biomarkers
2. ________ Doppler ultrasound
3. ________ Holter monitor
4. ________ cardiac scan
5. ________ stress testing
6. ________ echocardiography
7. ________ extracorporeal circulation
8. ________ ligation and stripping
9. ________ thrombolytic therapy
10. ________ PTCA

a. visualizes heart after patient is given radioactive thallium
b. uses ultrasound to visualize heart beating
c. blood test that indicates heart muscle damage
d. uses treadmill to evaluate cardiac fitness
e. removes varicose veins
f. clot-dissolving drugs
g. measures velocity of blood moving through blood vessels
h. balloon angioplasty
i. use of a heart-lung machine
j. portable EKG monitor

Abbreviations

AED	automated external defibrillator	**CP**	chest pain
AF, A-fib	atrial fibrillation	**CPR**	cardiopulmonary resuscitation
AMI	acute myocardial infarction	**CSD**	congenital septal defect
AS	arteriosclerosis	**CV**	cardiovascular
ASD	atrial septal defect	**DVT**	deep vein thrombosis
ASHD	arteriosclerotic heart disease	**ECC**	extracorporeal circulation
AV, A-V	atrioventricular	**ECG, EKG**	electrocardiogram
BBB	bundle branch block (L for left; R for right)	**ECHO**	echocardiography
BP	blood pressure	**fib**	fibrillation
bpm	beats per minute	**heart cath**	cardiac catheterization
CABG	coronary artery bypass graft	**HTN**	hypertension
CAD	coronary artery disease	**ICD**	implantable cardioverter-defibrillator
cath	catheterization	**ICU**	intensive care unit
CCU	coronary care unit	**IV**	intravenous
CHF	congestive heart failure	**LVH**	left-ventricular hypertrophy
CK	creatine kinase	**MI**	myocardial infarction, mitral insufficiency
CoA	coarctation of the aorta	**mm Hg**	millimeters of mercury

Abbreviations (continued)

MR	mitral regurgitation	**S1**	first heart sound
MS	mitral stenosis **Word Watch** Be careful using the abbreviation *MS*, which can mean either *mitral stenosis* or *multiple sclerosis*.	**S2**	second heart sound
MVP	mitral valve prolapse	**SA, S-A**	sinoatrial
P	pulse	**SK**	streptokinase
PAC	premature atrial contraction	**tPA**	tissue plasminogen activator
PDA	patent ductus arteriosus	**VF, V-fib**	ventricular fibrillation
PTCA	percutaneous transluminal coronary angioplasty	**VSD**	ventricular septal defect
PVC	premature ventricular contraction	**VT, V-tach**	ventricular tachycardia
PVD	peripheral vascular disease		

PRACTICE AS YOU GO

F. What's the Abbreviation?

1. mitral valve prolapse ____________________
2. ventricular septal defect ____________________
3. percutaneous transluminal coronary angioplasty ____________________
4. ventricular fibrillation ____________________
5. deep vein thrombosis ____________________
6. arteriosclerotic heart disease ____________________
7. coarctation of the aorta ____________________
8. tissue plasminogen activator ____________________
9. cardiovascular ____________________
10. extracorporeal circulation ____________________

Chapter Review

Real-World Applications

Medical Record Analysis

This Discharge Summary contains 13 medical terms. Underline each term and write it in the list below the report. Then explain each term as you would to a nonmedical person.

Date: 6/1/2017
Patient: Juanita Johnson
Patient complaint: Severe pain in the right ankle with any movement of lower limb.

Discharge Summary

Admitting Diagnosis:	Difficulty breathing, hypertension, tachycardia
Final Diagnosis:	CHF secondary to mitral valve prolapse
History of Present Illness:	Patient was brought to the Emergency Room by her family because of difficulty breathing and palpitations. Patient reports having experienced these symptoms for the past six months, but this episode is more severe than any previous. Upon admission in the ER, heart rate was 120 beats per minute and blood pressure was 180/110. The results of an EKG and cardiac biomarkers were normal. She was admitted for a complete workup for tachycardia and hypertension.
Summary of Hospital Course:	Patient underwent a full battery of diagnostic tests. A prolapsed mitral valve was observed by echocardiography. A stress test had to be stopped early due to onset of severe difficulty in breathing. Angiocardiography failed to demonstrate significant CAD. Blood pressure and tachycardia were controlled with medications. At discharge, HR was 88 beats per minute and blood pressure was 165/98.
Discharge Plans:	There was no evidence of a myocardial infarction or significant CAD. Patient was placed on a low-salt and low-cholesterol diet. She received instructions on beginning a carefully graded exercise program. She is to continue her medications. If symptoms are not controlled by these measures, a mitral valvoplasty will be considered.

	Term	Explanation
1.	______	______
2.	______	______
3.	______	______
4.	______	______
5.	______	______
6.	______	______
7.	______	______
8.	______	______
9.	______	______
10.	______	______
11.	______	______
12.	______	______
13.	______	______

Chart Note Transcription

The chart note below contains 11 phrases that can be reworded with a medical term presented in this chapter. Each phrase is identified with an underline. Determine the medical term and write your answers in the space provided.

Pearson General Hospital Coronary Care Unit

Task Edit View Time Scale Options Help Download Archive Date: 17 May 2017

Current Complaint:	A 56-year-old male was admitted to the Cardiac Care Unit from the Emergency Room with left arm pain, severe pain around the heart, **1** an abnormally slow heartbeat, **2** and nausea and vomiting.
Past History:	Patient reports no heart problems prior to this episode. He has taken medication for high blood pressure **3** for the past five years. His family history is significant for a father and brother who both died in their 50s from death of heart muscle. **4**
Signs and Symptoms:	Patient reports severe pain around the heart that radiates into his left jaw and arm. A record of the heart's electrical activity **5** and a blood test to determine the amount of heart damage **6** were abnormal.
Diagnosis:	An acute death of heart muscle **4** resulting from insufficient blood flow to heart muscle due to obstruction of coronary artery. **7**
Treatment:	First, provide supportive care during the acute phase. Second, evaluate heart damage by passing a thin tube through a blood vessel into the heart to detect abnormalities **8** and evaluate heart fitness by having patient exercise on a treadmill. **9** Finally, perform surgical intervention by either inflating a balloon catheter to dilate a narrow vessel **10** or by open heart surgery to create a shunt around a blocked vessel. **11**

1. ______________________________

2. ______________________________

3. ______________________________

4. ______________________________

5. ______________________________

6. ______________________________

7. ______________________________

8. ______________________________

9. ______________________________

10. ______________________________

11. ______________________________

Case Study

Below is a case study presentation of a patient with a condition discussed in this chapter. Read the case study and answer the questions below. Some questions will ask for information not included within this chapter. Use your text, a medical dictionary, or any other reference material you choose to answer these questions.

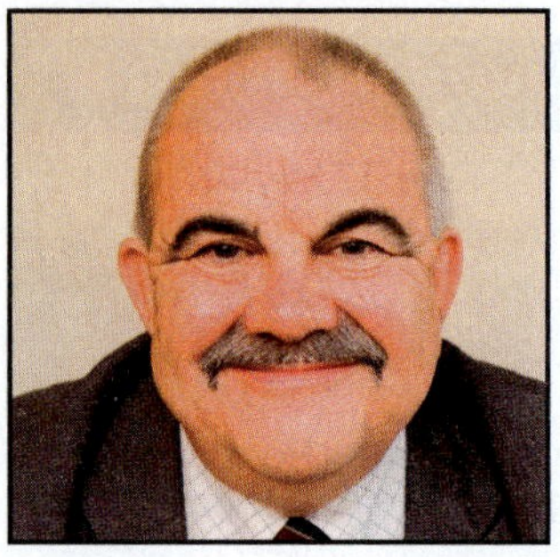
(Christopher Coates/Shutterstock)

Mr. Thomas is a 62-year-old man who has been diagnosed with an acute myocardial infarction with the following symptoms and history. His chief complaint is a persistent, crushing chest pain that radiates to his left arm, jaw, neck, and shoulder blade. He describes the pain, which he has had for the past 12 hours, as a "squeezing" sensation around his heart. He has also suffered nausea, dyspnea, and diaphoresis. He has a low-grade temperature and his blood pressure is within a normal range at 130/82. He states that he smokes two packs of cigarettes a day, is overweight by 50 pounds, and has a family history of hypertension and coronary artery disease. He leads a relatively sedentary lifestyle.

Questions

1. What is the common name for Mr. Thomas's acute condition? Look this condition up in a reference source and include a short description of it.

____

____

2. What do you think the phrase "chief complaint" means?

____

____

3. What is the medical term for this patient's chief complaint? Define this term.

____

____

4. List and define each of the patient's additional symptoms in your own words. (These terms appear in other chapters of this book or use a medical dictionary.)

____

____

5. Using your text as a resource, name and describe three diagnostic tests that may be performed to determine the extent of the patient's heart damage.

____

____

6. What risk factors for developing heart disease does Mr. Thomas have? What changes should he make?

____

____

Practice Exercises

A. Word Building Practice

The combining form **cardi/o** refers to the *heart*. Use it to write a term that means:

1. pertaining to the heart ________________
2. disease of the heart muscle ________________
3. enlargement of the heart ________________
4. fast heart condition ________________
5. slow heart condition ________________
6. record of heart electricity ________________

The combining form **angi/o** refers to the *vessel*. Use it to write a term that means:

7. vessel narrowing ________________
8. vessel inflammation ________________
9. involuntary muscle contraction of a vessel ________________

The combining form **arteri/o** refers to the *artery*. Use it to write a term that means:

10. pertaining to an artery ________________
11. hardening of an artery ________________
12. small artery ________________

Add the appropriate prefix to **carditis** to form the term that matches each definition:

13. inflammation of the inner lining of the heart ________________
14. inflammation of the outer layer of the heart ________________
15. inflammation of the muscle of the heart ________________

B. Anatomical Adjectives

Fill in the blank with the missing noun or adjective.

	Noun	Adjective
1.	aorta	__________
2.	atrium	__________
3.	__________	cardiac
4.	vein	__________
5.	__________	arteriolar
6.	__________	ventricular
7.	valve	__________
8.	heart muscle	__________
9.	venule	__________
10.	__________	coronary
11.	__________	vascular
12.	__________	arterial

C. Complete the Term

For each definition given below, fill in the blank with the word part that completes the term.

Definition	Term
1. record of a vessel	______________gram
2. fast heart condition	tachy ______________
3. heart muscle disease	______________myopathy
4. inflammation of inner lining of heart	______________carditis
5. hardening of an artery	______________sclerosis
6. excessive pressure	hyper ______________
7. fatty substance mass	______________oma
8. vein inflammation	______________itis
9. clot destruction	______________lytic
10. surgical removal of a plug	______________ectomy
11. pertaining to within the heart	______________coronary
12. surgical repair of a valve	______________plasty

D. Complete the Statement

1. The ______________ circulation carries blood between the heart and lungs, while the ______________ circulation carries blood between the heart and the cells and tissues of the body.
2. The ______________ is composed of cardiac muscle.
3. The right and left sides of the heart are divided by the ______________.
4. The atrioventricular valves are the ______________ and ______________. The semilunar valves are the ______________ and ______________.
5. The ______________ is the pacemaker of the heart.
6. The ______________ arteries carry blood to the heart muscle.
7. ______________ is the force exerted by blood against the wall of a blood vessel.
8. A network of tiny blood vessels is referred to as a(n) ______________.

E. Using Abbreviations

Fill in each blank with the appropriate abbreviation.

1. A(n) __________ is an arrhythmia, also called a heart block.
2. In a(n) __________, there is partial or complete occlusion of a coronary artery.
3. A(n) __________ occurs when there is an early contraction of an atrium.
4. A(n) __________ is used to diagnose cardiac arrhythmias.
5. A(n) __________ uses ultrasound to visualize cardiac structures.
6. The coronary artery was dilated during a(n) __________ procedure.
7. During open-heart surgery, __________ is used to oxygenate and circulate blood.
8. Doppler ultrasonography was used to look for a(n) __________.

9. In __________, the myocardium is too weak to efficiently pump blood.

10. __________ means that at birth there is a hole in the septum between two heart chambers.

F. Define the Term

1. catheter ______________________________
2. infarct ______________________________
3. thrombus ______________________________
4. palpitation ______________________________
5. regurgitation ______________________________
6. aneurysm ______________________________
7. cardiac arrest ______________________________
8. fibrillation ______________________________
9. myocardial infarction ______________________________
10. hemorrhoid ______________________________

G. Fill in the Blank

angiography	murmur	varicose veins	echocardiogram
pacemaker	CHF	defibrillation	angina pectoris
Holter monitor	hypertension	MI	CCU

1. Tiffany was born with a congenital condition resulting in an abnormal heart sound called a(n) __________.
2. Joseph suffered an arrhythmia resulting in cardiac arrest. The emergency team used an instrument to give electric shocks to the heart to create a normal heart rhythm. This procedure is called __________.
3. Marguerite has been placed on a low-sodium diet and medication to bring her blood pressure down to a normal range. She suffers from __________.
4. Tony has had an artificial device called a(n) __________ inserted to control the beating of his heart by producing rhythmic electrical impulses.
5. Derrick's physician determined that he had __________ after examining his legs and finding swollen, tortuous veins.
6. Laura has persistent chest pains that require medication. The term for the pain is __________.
7. La Tonya will be admitted to what hospital unit after surgery to correct her heart condition? __________
8. Stephen is going to have a coronary artery bypass graft to correct the blockage in his coronary arteries. He recently suffered a heart attack as a result of this occlusion. His attack is called a(n) __________.
9. Stephen's physician scheduled a(n) __________, an X-ray to determine the extent of his blood vessel damage.
10. Maria is scheduled to have a diagnostic procedure that uses ultrasound to produce an image of the heart valves. She is going to have a(n) __________.
11. Eric must wear a device for 24 hours that will keep track of his heart activity as he performs his normal daily routine. This device is called a(n) __________.
12. Lydia is 82 years old and is suffering from a heart condition that causes weakness, edema, and breathlessness. Her heart failure is the cause of her lung congestion. This condition is called __________.

H. Pharmacology Challenge

Fill in the classification for each drug description, then match the brand name.

Drug Description	Classification	Brand Name
1. ________ prevents arrhythmia	________________	a. tPA
2. ________ reduces cholesterol	________________	b. Coumadin
3. ________ increases force of heart contraction	________________	c. Cardizem
4. ________ increases urine production	________________	d. Nitro-Dur
5. ________ prevents blood clots	________________	e. Tambocor
6. ________ dissolves blood clots	________________	f. Lanoxin
7. ________ relaxes smooth muscle in artery wall	________________	g. Lipitor
8. ________ causes heart to beat less forcefully	________________	h. Lasix

I. Spelling Practice

Some of the following terms are misspelled. Identify the incorrect terms and spell them correctly in the blank provided.

1. cardiomiopathy ________________
2. tackycardia ________________
3. ischemia ________________
4. auscultation ________________
5. arteriosclerosis ________________
6. aneurysm ________________
7. catheterization ________________
8. infraction ________________
9. arhythmia ________________
10. angitis ________________

Labeling Exercises

Image A

Write the labels for this figure on the numbered lines provided.

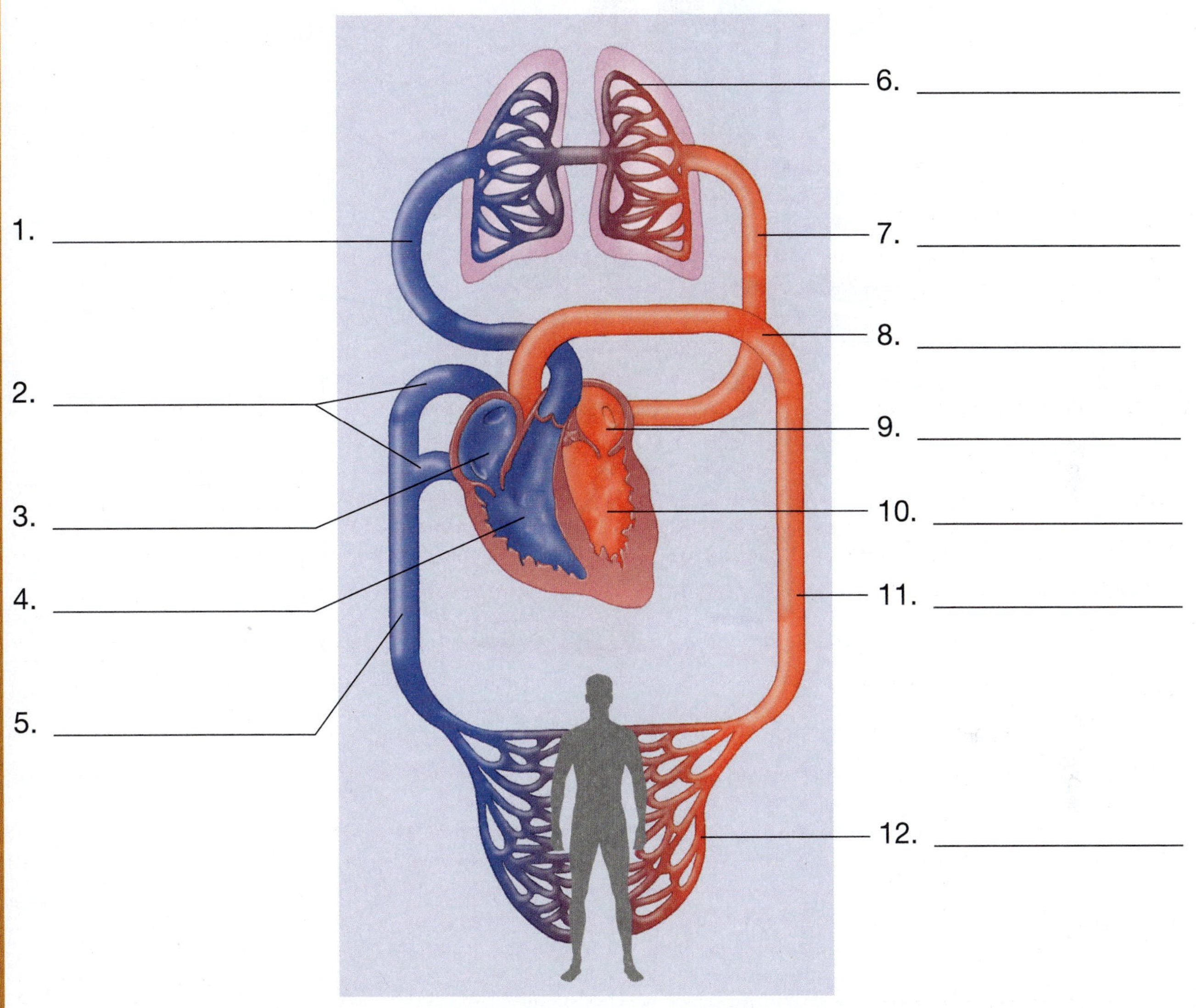

Image B

Write the labels for this figure on the numbered lines provided.

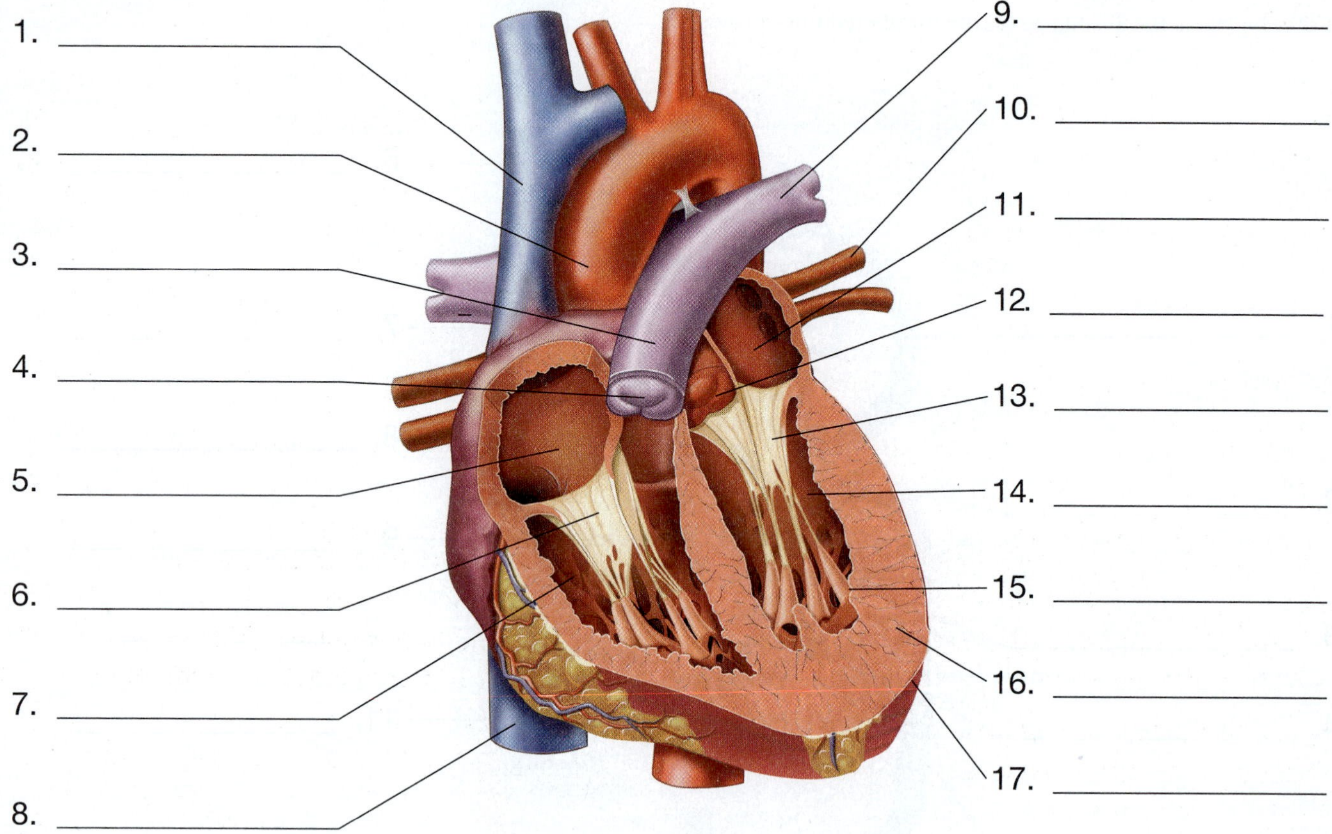

Chapter 6

Blood and the Lymphatic and Immune Systems

Learning Objectives

Upon completion of this chapter, you will be able to

1. Identify and define the combining forms and suffixes introduced in this chapter.
2. Gain the ability to pronounce medical terms and major anatomical structures.
3. List the major components, structures, and organs of the blood and lymphatic and immune systems and their functions.
4. Describe the blood typing systems.
5. Discuss immunity, the immune response, and standard precautions.
6. Identify and define blood and lymphatic and immune system anatomical terms.
7. Identify and define selected blood and lymphatic and immune system pathology terms.
8. Identify and define selected blood and lymphatic and immune system diagnostic procedures.
9. Identify and define selected blood and lymphatic and immune system therapeutic procedures.
10. Identify and define selected medications associated with blood and the lymphatic and immune systems.
11. Define selected abbreviations associated with blood and the lymphatic and immune systems.

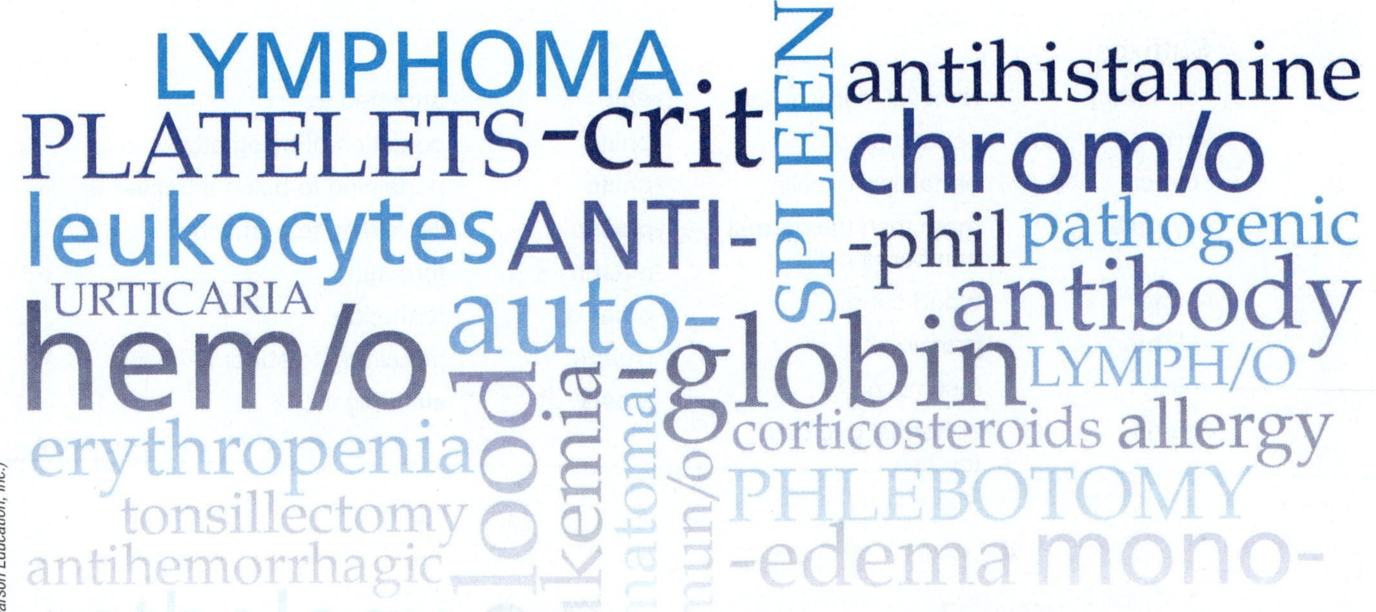

(Pearson Education, Inc.)

AT A GLANCE

Function

Blood transports gases, nutrients, and wastes to all areas of the body either attached to red blood cells or dissolved in the plasma. White blood cells fight infection and disease, and platelets initiate the blood-clotting process.

Organs

The primary components that comprise blood:

formed elements

- **erythrocytes**
- **leukocytes**
- **platelets**

plasma

Word Parts

Presented here are the most common word parts (with their meanings) used to build blood terms. For a more comprehensive list, refer to the Terminology section of this chapter.

Combining Forms

agglutin/o	clumping	**hemat/o**	blood
bas/o	base	**morph/o**	shape
chrom/o	color	**myel/o**	bone marrow, spinal cord
coagul/o	clotting	**neutr/o**	neutral
eosin/o	rosy red	**phag/o**	eat, swallow
fus/o	pouring	**sanguin/o**	blood
granul/o	granules	**septic/o**	infection
hem/o	blood		

Suffixes

-apheresis	removal, carry away	**-phil**	attracted to
-crit	separation of	**-philia**	condition of being attracted to
-cytic	pertaining to cells	**-philic**	pertaining to being attracted to
-cytosis	more than the normal number of cells	**-plastic**	pertaining to formation
		-plastin	formation
-emia	blood condition	**-poiesis**	formation
-globin	protein	**-rrhagic**	pertaining to abnormal flow
-oid	resembling	**-stasis**	standing still
-penia	abnormal decrease, too few		

Blood Illustrated

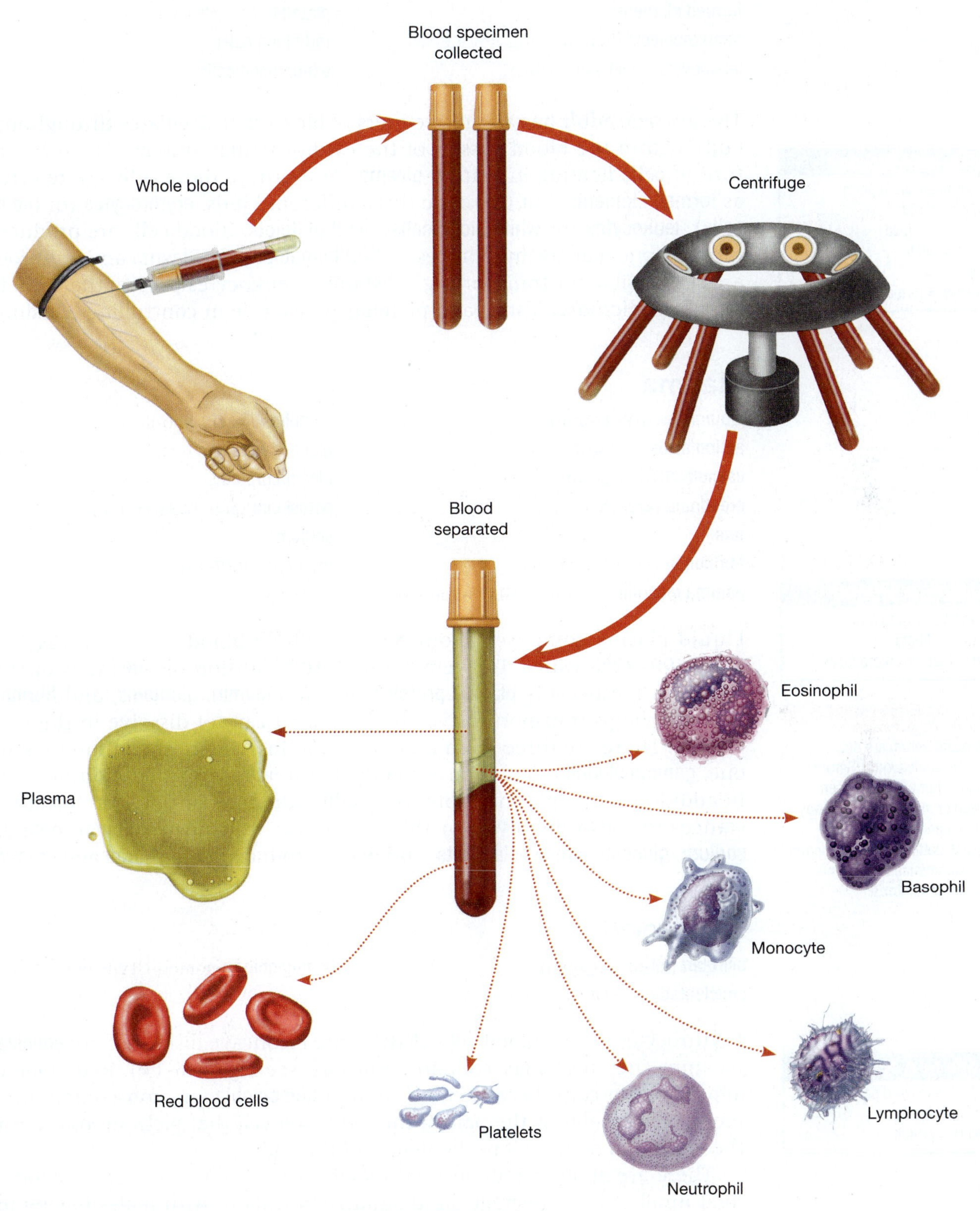

Anatomy and Physiology of Blood

erythrocytes (eh-RITH-roh-sights)
formed elements
hematopoiesis (hee-mah-toh-poy-EE-sis)
leukocytes (LOO-koh-sights)
plasma (PLAZ-mah)
platelets (PLAYT-lets)
red blood cells
white blood cells

What's In A Name?
Look for these word parts:
erythr/o = red
hemat/o = blood
leuk/o = white
-cyte = cell
-poiesis = formation

The average adult has about five liters of blood that circulates throughout the body within the blood vessels of the cardiovascular system. Blood is a mixture of cells floating in watery **plasma**. As a group, these cells are referred to as **formed elements**, but there are three different kinds: **erythrocytes** (or **red blood cells**), **leukocytes** (or **white blood cells**), and **platelets**. Blood cells are produced in the red bone marrow by a process called **hematopoiesis**. Plasma and erythrocytes are responsible for transporting substances, leukocytes protect the body from invading microorganisms, and platelets play a role in controlling bleeding.

Plasma

albumin (al-BYOO-min)
amino acids (ah-MEE-noh)
calcium (KAL-see-um)
creatinine (kree-AT-in-in)
fats
fibrinogen (fye-BRIN-oh-jen)
gamma globulin (GAM-ah / GLOB-yoo-lin)
globulins (GLOB-yoo-lins)
glucose (GLOO-kohs)
plasma proteins
potassium (poh-TASS-ee-um)
sodium
urea (yoo-REE-ah)

What's In A Name?
Look for these word parts:
fibrin/o = fibers
-gen = that which produces

Word Watch
Plasma and *serum* are not interchangeable words. Serum is plasma, but with fibrinogen removed or inactivated. This way it can be handled and tested without it clotting. The term *serum* is also sometimes used to mean antiserum or antitoxin.

Liquid plasma composes about 55% of whole blood in the average adult and is 90–92% water. The remaining 8–10% portion of plasma is dissolved substances, especially **plasma proteins** such as **albumin**, **globulins**, and **fibrinogen**. Albumin helps transport fatty substances that cannot dissolve in the watery plasma. There are three main types of globulins; the most commonly known one, **gamma globulin**, acts as an antibody. Fibrinogen is a blood-clotting protein. In addition to the plasma proteins, smaller amounts of other important substances are also dissolved in the plasma for transport: **calcium**, **potassium**, **sodium**, **glucose**, **amino acids**, **fats**, and waste products such as **urea** and **creatinine**.

Erythrocytes

bilirubin (bil-ih-ROO-bin)
enucleated (ee-NOO-klee-ay-ted)
hemoglobin (hee-moh-GLOH-bin)

What's In A Name?
Look for these word parts:
hem/o = blood
-globin = protein

Erythrocytes, or red blood cells (RBCs), are biconcave disks that are **enucleated**, meaning they no longer contain a nucleus (see Figure 6-1 ■). Red blood cells appear red in color because they contain **hemoglobin**, an iron-containing pigment. Hemoglobin is the part of the red blood cell that picks up oxygen from the lungs and delivers it to the tissues of the body.

There are about 5 million erythrocytes per cubic millimeter of blood. The total number in an average-sized adult is 35 trillion, with males having more red blood cells than females. Erythrocytes have an average lifespan of 120 days, and then the spleen removes the worn-out and damaged ones from circulation. Much of the red blood cell, such as the iron, can be reused, but one portion, **bilirubin**, is a waste product disposed of by the liver.

Erythrocytes

Red blood cells

■ **Figure 6-1** The biconcave disk shape of erythrocytes (red blood cells).

Leukocytes

Basophil

Eosinophil

Monocyte

Neutrophil

Lymphocyte

■ **Figure 6-2** The five different types of leukocytes (white blood cells).

Leukocytes

agranulocytes (ah-GRAN-yoo-loh-sights)
granulocytes (GRAN-yoo-loh-sights)
pathogens (PATH-oh-jenz)

Leukocytes, also referred to as white blood cells (WBCs), provide protection against the invasion of **pathogens** such as bacteria, viruses, and other foreign material. In general, white blood cells have a spherical shape with a large nucleus, and there are about 8,000 per cubic millimeter of blood (see Figure 6-2 ■). There are five different types of white blood cells, each with its own strategy for protecting the body. The five can be subdivided into two categories: **granulocytes** (with granules in the cytoplasm) and **agranulocytes** (without granules in the cytoplasm). The name and function of each type is presented in Table 6-1 ■.

Platelets

agglutinate (ah-GLOO-tih-nayt)
fibrin (FYE-brin)
hemostasis (hee-moh-STAY-sis)
prothrombin (proh-THROM-bin)
thrombin (THROM-bin)
thrombocyte (THROM-boh-sight)
thromboplastin (throm-boh-PLAS-tin)

Platelet, the modern term for **thrombocyte**, refers to the smallest of all the formed blood elements. Platelets are not whole cells, but rather are formed when the

■ **TABLE 6–1** Leukocyte Classification

Leukocyte	Function
Granulocytes	
Basophils (basos) (BAY-soh-fillz)	Release histamine and heparin to damaged tissues
Eosinophils (eosins, eos) (ee-oh-SIN-oh-fillz)	Destroy parasites and increase during allergic reactions
Neutrophils (NOO-troh-fillz)	Engulf foreign and damaged cells (phagocytosis); most numerous of the leukocytes
Agranulocytes	
Monocytes (monos) (MON-oh-sights)	Engulf foreign and damaged cells (phagocytosis)
Lymphocytes (lymphs) (LIM-foh-sights)	Play several different roles in immune response

Med Term Tip

Your body makes about 2 million erythrocytes every second. Of course, it must then destroy 2 million every second to maintain a relatively constant 30 trillion red blood cells.

What's In A Name?

Look for these word parts:
bas/o = base
eosin/o = rosy red
granul/o = granules
lymph/o = lymph
neutr/o = neutral
path/o = disease
-cyte = cell
-gen = that which produces
-phil = attracted to
a- = without
mono- = one

Med Term Tip

A *phagocyte* is a cell that has the ability to ingest (**phag/o** = eat; **-cyte** = cell) and digest bacteria and other foreign particles. This process, *phagocytosis*, is critical for the control of bacteria within the body.

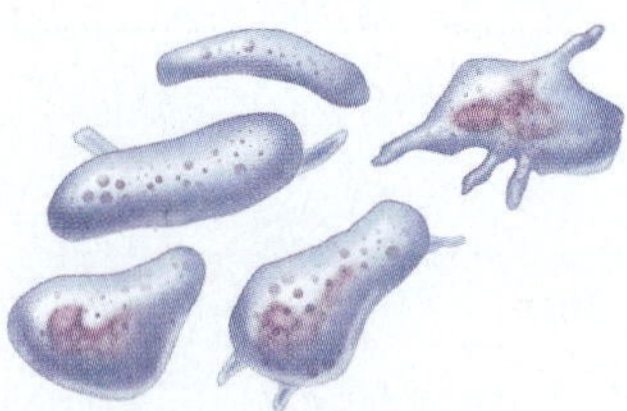

■ **Figure 6-3** Platelet structure.

What's In A Name?

Look for these word parts:
agglutin/o = clumping
hem/o = blood
thromb/o = clot
-cyte = cell
-plastin = formation
-stasis = standing still
pro- = before

cytoplasm of a large precursor cell shatters into small platelike fragments (see Figure 6-3 ■). There are between 200,000 and 300,000 per cubic millimeter in the body.

Platelets play a critical part in the blood-clotting process or **hemostasis**. They **agglutinate** or clump together into small clusters when a blood vessel is cut or damaged. Platelets also release a substance called **thromboplastin**, which, in the presence of calcium, reacts with **prothrombin** (a clotting protein in the blood) to form **thrombin**. Then thrombin, in turn, works to convert fibrinogen to **fibrin**, which eventually becomes the meshlike blood clot.

Blood Typing

ABO system
blood typing
Rh factor

Each person's blood is different due to the presence of antigens or markers on the surface of erythrocytes. Before a person receives a blood transfusion, it is important to do **blood typing**. This laboratory test determines if the donated blood is compatible with the recipient's blood. There are many different subgroups of blood markers, but the two most important ones are the **ABO system** and **Rh factor**.

ABO System

type A
type AB
type B
type O
universal donor
universal recipient

In the ABO blood system, there are two possible red blood cell markers, A and B. A marker is one method by which cells identify themselves. A person with an A marker is said to have **type A** blood. Type A blood produces anti-B antibodies that will attack type B blood. The presence of a B marker indicates **type B** blood and anti-A antibodies (that will attack type A blood). If both markers are present, the blood is **type AB** and does not contain any antibodies. Therefore, type AB blood will not attack any other blood type. The absence of either an A or a B marker results in **type O** blood, which contains both anti-A and anti-B antibodies. Type O blood will attack all other blood types (A, B, and AB). For further information on antibodies, refer to the lymphatic section later in this chapter.

Because type O blood does not have either the A or B marker, its red blood cells will not be attacked by the antibodies in type A, type B, or type AB blood. For this reason, a person with type O blood is referred to as a **universal donor**. In extreme cases, type O blood may be given to a person with any of the other blood types. Similarly, type AB blood is the **universal recipient**. A person with type AB blood has no antibodies against the other blood types and, therefore, in extreme cases, can receive any type of blood.

Rh Factor

Rh-negative
Rh-positive

Rh factor is not as difficult to understand as the ABO system. A person with the Rh factor on his or her red blood cells is said to be **Rh-positive** (Rh+). Since this person has the factor, he or she will not make anti-Rh antibodies. A person without the Rh factor is **Rh-negative** (Rh–) and will produce anti-Rh antibodies. Therefore, an Rh+ person may receive both an Rh+ and an Rh– transfusion, but an Rh– person can receive only Rh– blood.

PRACTICE AS YOU GO

A. Complete the Statement

1. The process whereby cells ingest and destroy bacteria within the body is ________________.
2. The formed elements of blood are the ________________, ________________, and ________________.
3. The fluid portion of blood is called ________________.
4. The medical term for blood clotting is ________________.
5. The two most important subgroups of blood markers are the ________________ and ________________.

Terminology

Word Parts Used to Build Blood Terms

The following lists contain the combining forms, suffixes, and prefixes used to build terms in the remaining sections of this chapter.

Combining Forms

bas/o	base	fus/o	pouring	myel/o	bone marrow
chrom/o	color	hem/o	blood	neutr/o	neutral
coagul/o	clotting	hemat/o	blood	phleb/o	vein
cyt/o	cell	leuk/o	white	sanguin/o	blood
eosin/o	rosy red	lip/o	fat	septic/o	infection
erythr/o	red	lymph/o	lymph	thromb/o	clot
fibrin/o	fibers	morph/o	shape		

Suffixes

-apheresis	removal, carry away	-ic	pertaining to	-philia	condition of being attracted to
-crit	separation of	-ion	action	-philic	pertaining to being attracted to
-cyte	cell	-logy	study of	-plastic	pertaining to formation
-cytic	pertaining to cells	-lytic	destruction	-rrhage	abnormal flow
-cytosis	more than the normal number of cells	-oid	resembling	-rrhagic	pertaining to abnormal flow
-emia	blood condition	-oma	mass	-tic	pertaining to
-globin	protein	-otomy	cutting into		
-ia	condition	-ous	pertaining to		
		-penia	too few		

Prefixes

a-	without	dys-	abnormal	pan-	all
an-	without	homo-	same	poly-	many
anti-	against	hyper-	excessive	trans-	across
auto-	self	hypo-	insufficient		
contra-	against	mono-	one		

Adjective Forms of Anatomical Terms

Term	Word Parts	Definition
basophilic (bay-soh-FILL-ik)	**bas/o** = base **-philic** = pertaining to being attracted to	Pertaining to [a leukocyte] that attracts a basic pH stain
eosinophilic (ee-oh-sin-oh-FILL-ik)	**eosin/o** = rosy red **-philic** = pertaining to being attracted to	Pertaining to [a leukocyte] that attracts a rosy red stain
erythrocytic (eh-rith-roh-SIT-ik)	**erythr/o** = red **-cytic** = pertaining to cells	Pertaining to a red blood cell
fibrinous (FYE-brin-us)	**fibrin/o** = fibers **-ous** = pertaining to	Pertaining to fibers
hematic (hee-MAT-ik)	**hemat/o** = blood **-ic** = pertaining to	Pertaining to blood
leukocytic (loo-koh-SIT-ik)	**leuk/o** = white **-cytic** = pertaining to cells	Pertaining to a white blood cell
lymphocytic (lim-foh-SIT-ik)	**lymph/o** = lymph **-cytic** = pertaining to cells	Pertaining to a [white] cell formed in lymphatic tissue
monocytic (mon-oh-SIT-ik)	**mono-** = one **-cytic** = pertaining to cells	Pertaining to a [white] cell with a single, large nucleus
neutrophilic (noo-troh-FILL-ik)	**neutr/o** = neutral **-philic** = pertaining to being attracted to	Pertaining to [a leukocyte] that attracts a neutral pH stain
sanguineous (sang-GWIN-ee-us)	**sanguin/o** = blood **-ous** = pertaining to **Word Watch** The term *sanguineous* has an unusual spelling; an *e* is added between the word root, **sanguin**, and the suffix, **-ous**.	Pertaining to blood
thrombocytic (throm-boh-SIT-ik)	**thromb/o** = clot **-cytic** = pertaining to cells	Pertaining to a clotting cell; a platelet
thrombotic (throm-BOT-ik)	**thromb/o** = clot **-tic** = pertaining to	Pertaining to a clot

PRACTICE AS YOU GO

B. Give the adjective form for each anatomical structure.

1. Blood ______________________ or ______________________
2. White cell ______________________
3. Clotting cell ______________________
4. Fibers ______________________
5. Red cell ______________________

Pathology

Term	Word Parts	Definition
Medical Specialties		
hematology (hee-mah-TALL-oh-jee)	hemat/o = blood -logy = study of	Branch of medicine specializing in treatment of diseases and conditions of blood; physician is a *hematologist*
Signs and Symptoms		
coagulate (koh-AG-yoo-late)	coagul/o = clotting	To convert from a liquid to a gel or solid, as in blood coagulation
dyscrasia (dis-KRAY-zee-ah)	dys- = abnormal -ia = condition	General term indicating presence of a disease affecting blood
hematoma (hee-mah-TOH-mah)	hemat/o = blood -oma = mass	Collection of blood under skin as result of blood escaping into tissue from damaged blood vessels; commonly referred to as a *bruise*
	Word Watch The term *hematoma* is confusing. Its simple translation is *blood mass.* However, it is used to refer to blood that has leaked out of a blood vessel and has pooled in the tissues causing swelling.	
hemorrhage (HEM-eh-rij)	hem/o = blood -rrhage = abnormal flow	Blood flowing out of blood vessel (i.e., bleeding)
thrombus (THROM-bus)	thromb/o = clot	Hard collection of fibrin, blood cells, and tissue debris that is end result of hemostasis or blood-clotting process; thrombus is helpful to body by stopping bleeding, as in skin laceration; however, it is hurtful to body if it occurs within a blood vessel, as in myocardial infarction; commonly referred to as a *blood clot*
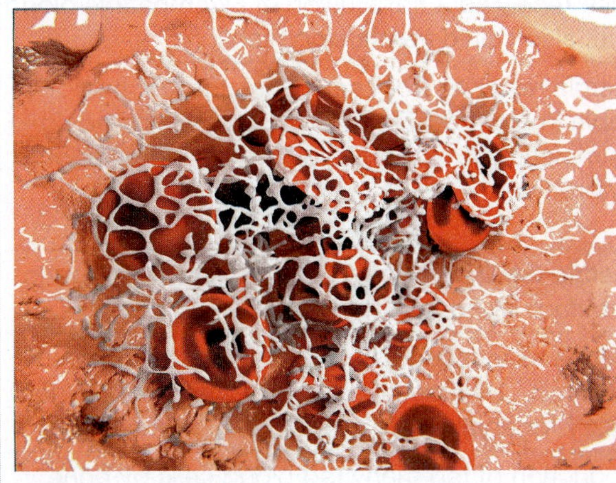		**Figure 6-4** Electronmicrograph showing a thrombus composed of fibrin, red blood cells, and tissue debris. *(Juan Gaertner/Shutterstock)*
Blood		
hemophilia (hee-moh-FILL-ee-ah)	hem/o = blood -philia = condition of being attracted to	Hereditary blood disease in which blood-clotting time is prolonged due to lack of one vital clotting factor; transmitted by sex-linked trait from females to males, appearing almost exclusively in males
hyperlipidemia (high-per-lip-ih-DEE-mee-ah)	hyper- = excessive lip/o = fat -emia = blood condition	Condition of having too high a level of lipids such as cholesterol in bloodstream; risk factor for developing atherosclerosis and coronary artery disease
pancytopenia (pan-sigh-toh-PEE-nee-ah)	pan- = all cyt/o = cell -penia = too few	Having too few of all cells
septicemia (sep-tih-SEE-mee-ah)	septic/o = infection -emia = blood condition	Having bacteria or their toxins in bloodstream; *sepsis* is term that means *putrefaction* or *infection;* commonly referred to as *blood poisoning*

Pathology (continued)

Term	Word Parts	Definition
Erythrocytes		
anemia (ah-NEE-mee-ah)	an- = without -emia = blood condition	Large group of conditions characterized by reduction in number of red blood cells or amount of hemoglobin in blood; results in less oxygen reaching tissues
aplastic anemia (ay-PLAS-tik / ah-NEE-mee-ah)	a- = without -plastic = pertaining to formation an- = without -emia = blood condition	Severe form of anemia that develops as a consequence of loss of functioning red bone marrow; results in decrease in number of all formed elements; treatment may eventually require bone marrow transplant
erythrocytosis (eh-rith-roh-sigh-TOH-sis)	erythr/o = red -cytosis = more than normal number of cells	Condition of having too many red blood cells
erythropenia (eh-rith-roh-PEE-nee-ah)	erythr/o = red -penia = too few	Condition of having too few red blood cells
hemolytic anemia (hee-moh-LIT-ik / ah-NEE-mee-ah)	hem/o = blood -lytic = destruction an- = without -emia = blood condition	Anemia that develops as result of destruction of erythrocytes
hemolytic reaction (hee-moh-LIT-ik)	hem/o = blood -lytic = destruction	Destruction of patient's erythrocytes that occurs when receiving a transfusion of incompatible blood type; also called *transfusion reaction*
hypochromic anemia (high-poh-KROHM-ik / ah-NEE-mee-ah)	hypo- = insufficient chrom/o = color -ic = pertaining to an- = without -emia = blood condition	Anemia resulting from having insufficient hemoglobin in erythrocytes; named because hemoglobin molecule is responsible for dark red color of erythrocytes
iron-deficiency anemia	an- = without -emia = blood condition	Anemia resulting from not having sufficient iron to manufacture hemoglobin
pernicious anemia (PA) (per-NISH-us / ah-NEE-mee-ah)	an- = without -emia = blood condition	Anemia associated with insufficient absorption of vitamin B_{12} by digestive system; vitamin B_{12} is necessary for erythrocyte production
polycythemia vera (pol-ee-sigh-THEE-mee-ah / VAIR-ah)	poly- = many cyt/o = cell hem/o = blood -ia = condition	Production of too many red blood cells by bone marrow; blood becomes too thick to easily flow through blood vessels
sickle cell anemia	an- = without -emia = blood condition	Genetic disorder in which erythrocytes take on abnormal curved or "sickle" shape; cells are fragile and are easily damaged, leading to hemolytic anemia

■ **Figure 6-5** Comparison of normal-shaped erythrocytes and the abnormal sickle shape noted in patients with sickle cell anemia.

Pathology (continued)

Term	Word Parts	Definition
thalassemia (thal-ah-SEE-mee-ah)	-emia = blood condition	Genetic disorder in which body is unable to make functioning hemoglobin, resulting in anemia
Leukocytes		
leukemia (loo-KEE-mee-ah)	leuk/o = white -emia = blood condition	Cancer located in red bone marrow tissue responsible for producing white blood cells; results in large number of abnormal and immature leukocytes circulating in bloodstream
leukocytosis (loo-koh-sigh-TOH-sis)	leuk/o = white -cytosis = more than normal number of cells	Condition of having too many white blood cells
leukopenia (loo-koh-PEE-nee-ah)	leuk/o = white -penia = too few	Condition of having too few white blood cells
lymphocytic leukemia (lim-foh-SIT-ik / loo-KEE-mee-ah)	lymph/o = lymph -cytic = pertaining to cells leuk/o = white -emia = blood condition	Type of leukemia in which abnormal white blood cells are lymphocytes; may be acute (rapid onset and progression) or chronic (slow onset and progression)
myeloid leukemia (MY-eh-loyd / loo-KEE-mee-ah)	myel/o = bone marrow -oid = resembling leuk/o = white -emia = blood condition	Type of leukemia in which abnormal leukocytes are granulocytes (usually neutrophils); may be acute (rapid onset and progression) or chronic (slow onset and progression)
Platelets		
thrombocytopenia (throm-boh-sigh-toh-PEE-nee-ah)	thromb/o = clot cyt/o = cell -penia = too few	Condition of having too few platelets
thrombocytosis (throm-boh-sigh-TOH-sis)	thromb/o = clot -cytosis = more than normal number of cells	Condition of having too many platelets

PRACTICE AS YOU GO

C. Terminology Matching

Match each term to its definition.

1. ________ thalassemia
2. ________ dyscrasia
3. ________ hematoma
4. ________ anemia
5. ________ hemophilia

a. disease in which blood does not clot
b. condition with reduced number of RBCs
c. mass of blood
d. type of anemia
e. general term for blood disorders

Diagnostic Procedures

Term	Word Parts	Definition
Clinical Laboratory Tests		
blood analyzer		Automated machine that analyzes different characteristics of blood specimen, such as complete blood count, erythrocyte sedimentation rate, and blood-clotting tests
blood culture and sensitivity (C&S)		Sample of blood is incubated in laboratory to check for bacterial growth; if bacteria are present, they are identified and tested to determine to which antibiotics they are sensitive
complete blood count (CBC)		Combination of blood tests including red blood cell count (RBC), white blood cell count (WBC), hemoglobin (Hgb), hematocrit (Hct), white blood cell differential, and platelet count
erythrocyte sedimentation rate (ESR, sed rate) (eh-RITH-roh-sight / sed-ih-men-TAY-shun)	**erythr/o** = red **-cyte** = cell	Blood test to determine rate at which mature red blood cells settle out of blood after addition of anticoagulant; indicates presence of inflammatory disease
hematocrit (HCT, Hct, crit) (hee-MAT-oh-krit)	**hemat/o** = blood **-crit** = separation of	Blood test to measure volume of red blood cells (erythrocytes) within total volume of blood
hemoglobin (Hgb, Hb) (hee-moh-GLOH-bin)	**hem/o** = blood **-globin** = protein	Blood test to measure amount of hemoglobin present in given volume of blood
platelet count (PLAYT-let)		Determines number of platelets in given volume of blood
prothrombin time (pro-time, PT) (proh-THROM-bin)	**thromb/o** = clot	Indicates blood's coagulation abilities by measuring how long it takes for a clot to form after prothrombin has been activated
red blood cell count (RBC)		Determines number of erythrocytes in volume of blood; decrease in red blood cells may indicate anemia; increase may indicate polycythemia
red blood cell morphology	**morph/o** = shape **-logy** = study of	Determines diseases such as sickle cell anemia through examination of specimen of blood for abnormalities in shape (morphology) of erythrocytes
white blood cell count (WBC)		Measures number of leukocytes in volume of blood; increase may indicate presence of infection or disease such as leukemia; decrease in white blood cells may be caused by radiation therapy or chemotherapy
white blood cell differential (diff) (diff-er-EN-shal)		Determines number of each variety of leukocytes in volume of blood
Medical Procedures		
bone marrow aspiration (as-pih-RAY-shun)		Removed by aspiration with a needle, a sample of bone marrow is examined for diseases such as leukemia or aplastic anemia
phlebotomy (fleh-BOT-oh-mee)	**phleb/o** = vein **-otomy** = cutting into	Incision into vein in order to remove blood for diagnostic test; also called *venipuncture*

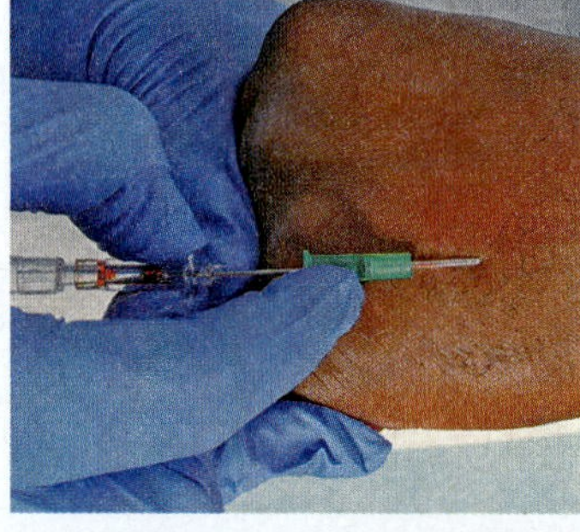

■ **Figure 6-6** Phlebotomist using a needle to withdraw blood. *(Michal Heron/Pearson Education, Inc.)*

Therapeutic Procedures

Term	Word Parts	Definition
Medical Procedures		
autologous transfusion (aw-TALL-oh-gus / trans-FYOO-zhun)	auto- = self	Procedure for collecting and storing patient's own blood several weeks prior to actual need; can then be used to replace blood lost during surgical procedure
blood transfusion (trans-FYOO-zhun)	trans- = across fus/o = pouring -ion = action	Artificial transfer of blood into bloodstream **Med Term Tip** Before a patient receives a blood transfusion, the laboratory performs a **type and cross-match**. This test first double-checks the blood type of both the donor's and recipient's blood. Then a cross-match is performed. This process mixes together small samples of both bloods and observes the mixture for adverse reactions.
bone marrow transplant (BMT)		Patient receives red bone marrow from donor after patient's own bone marrow has been destroyed by radiation or chemotherapy
homologous transfusion (hoh-MALL-oh-gus / trans-FYOO-zhun)	homo- = same	Replacement of blood by transfusion of blood received from another person
packed red cells		Transfusion in which most of plasma, leukocytes, and platelets have been removed, leaving only erythrocytes
plasmapheresis (plaz-mah-fah-REE-sis)	-apheresis = removal, carry away	Method of removing plasma from body without depleting formed elements; whole blood is removed and cells and plasma are separated; cells are returned to patient along with donor plasma transfusion
whole blood		Transfusion of a mixture of both plasma and formed elements

Pharmacology

Vocabulary

Term	Word Parts	Definition
additive		Sum of action of two (or more) drugs given; in this case, total strength of medications is equal to sum of strength of each individual drug
contraindication (kon-trah-in-dih-KAY-shun)	contra- = against	Condition in which particular drug should not be used
drug interaction		Occurs when effect of one drug is altered because it was taken at the same time as another drug
potentiation (poh-ten-shee-AY-shun)		Giving patient a second drug to boost (potentiate) effect of another drug; total strength of drugs is greater than sum of strength of individual drugs

Drugs

Classification	Word Parts	Action	Examples
anticoagulant (an-tye-koh-AG-yoo-lant)	anti- = against coagul/o = clotting	Prevents blood clot formation; commonly referred to as *blood thinner*	heparin, HepLock; warfarin, Coumadin

Pharmacology (continued)

Classification	Word Parts	Action	Examples
antihemorrhagic (an-tye-hem-eh-RAJ-ik)	anti- = against hem/o = blood -rrhagic = pertaining to abnormal flow	Prevents or stops hemorrhaging; *hemostatic agent*	aminocaproic acid, Amicar; vitamin K
antiplatelet agents (an-tee-PLAYT-let)	anti- = against	Interferes with action of platelets; prolongs bleeding time; used to prevent heart attacks and strokes	clopidogrel, Plavix; ticlopidine, Ticlid
fibrinolytic (fye-brin-oh-LIT-ik)	fibrin/o = fibers -lytic = destruction	Able to dissolve existing blood clots	alteplase, Activase; tissue plasminogen activator; Tenecteplase
hematinic (hee-mah-TIN-ik)	hemat/o = blood -ic = pertaining to	Increases number of erythrocytes or amount of hemoglobin in blood	epoetin alfa, Procrit; darbepoetin alfa, Aranesp

PRACTICE AS YOU GO

D. Procedure Matching

Match each procedure term with its definition.

1. ________ phlebotomy
2. ________ ESR
3. ________ plasmapheresis
4. ________ whole blood
5. ________ culture and sensitivity

a. method of removing plasma from the body
b. mixture of plasma and formed elements
c. removal of blood from a vein
d. test for bacterial growth
e. test that indicates presence of inflammatory disease

Abbreviations

ā	before	**CBC**	complete blood count
ac	before meals	**CLL**	chronic lymphocytic leukemia
ALL	acute lymphocytic leukemia	**CML**	chronic myeloid leukemia
AML	acute myeloid leukemia	**diff**	differential
ante	before	**eosins, eos**	eosinophils
basos	basophils	**ESR, sed rate**	erythrocyte sedimentation rate
BMT	bone marrow transplant	**et**	and
c̄	with	**HCT, Hct, crit**	hematocrit

Abbreviations (continued)

Hgb, Hb	hemoglobin	**PMN, polys**	polymorphonuclear neutrophil
lymphs	lymphocytes	**PT, pro-time**	prothrombin time
monos	monocytes	**RBC**	red blood cell
noc	night	**Rh+**	Rh-positive
p̄	after	**Rh–**	Rh-negative
PA	pernicious anemia	**s̄**	without
pc	after meals	**segs**	segmented neutrophils
PCV	packed cell volume	**WBC**	white blood cell

PRACTICE AS YOU GO

E. What's the Abbreviation?

1. acute lymphocytic leukemia ____________________
2. bone marrow transplant ____________________
3. eosinophils ____________________
4. hematocrit ____________________
5. pernicious anemia ____________________
6. complete blood count ____________________
7. differential ____________________
8. white blood cell ____________________
9. night ____________________
10. after meals ____________________

SECTION II: THE LYMPHATIC AND IMMUNE SYSTEMS

AT A GLANCE

Function

The lymphatic system consists of a network of lymph vessels that pick up excess tissue fluid, cleanse it, and return it to the circulatory system. It also picks up fats that have been absorbed by the digestive system. The immune system fights disease and infections.

Organs

The primary structures that comprise the lymphatic and immune systems:

lymph nodes
lymphatic vessels
spleen
thymus gland
tonsils

Word Parts

Presented here are the most common word parts (with their meanings) used to build lymphatic and immune system terms. For a more comprehensive list, refer to the Terminology section of this chapter.

Combining Forms

adenoid/o	adenoids
axill/o	axilla (underarm)
immun/o	protection
inguin/o	groin region
lymph/o	lymph
lymphaden/o	lymph node
lymphangi/o	lymph vessel
nucle/o	nucleus
splen/o	spleen
thym/o	thymus gland
tonsill/o	tonsils

Suffixes

-edema	swelling
-globulin	protein
-phage	to eat
-toxic	pertaining to poison

The Lymphatic and Immune Systems Illustrated

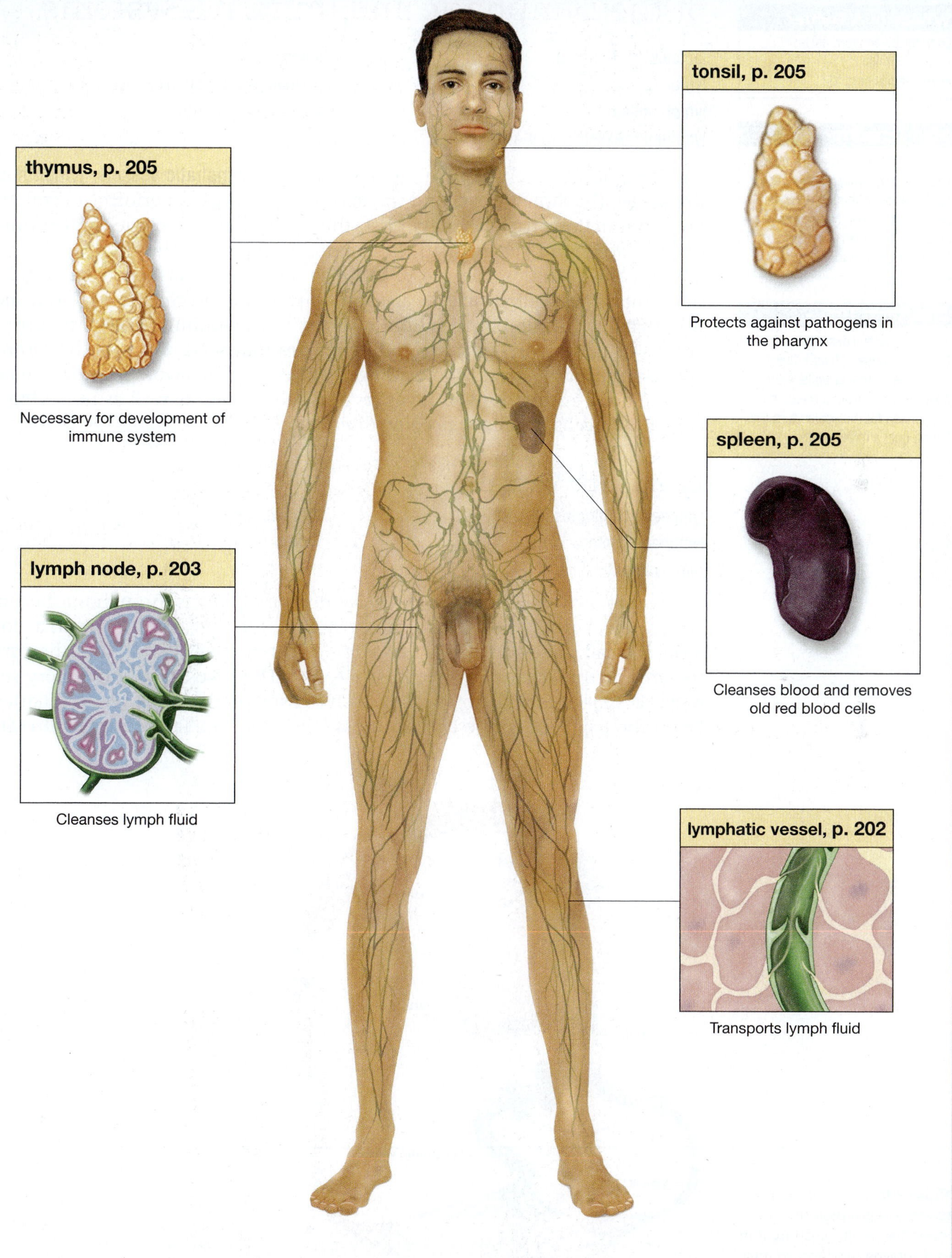

Anatomy and Physiology of the Lymphatic and Immune Systems

What's In A Name?

Look for these word parts:
lact/o = milk
-eal = pertaining to

Med Term Tip

The term *lymph* comes from the Latin word *lympha* meaning *clear spring water.* Although a very pale, clear yellow, lymph appears crystal clear when compared to the other body fluid, blood.

Med Term Tip

The term *lacteal* describes the appearance of lymph fluid inside the lacteal vessels. After absorbing fats from a meal, the suspended fat molecules turn the lymph fluid a milky white.

lacteals (LAK-tee-als)
lymph (LIMF)
lymph nodes
lymphatic vessels (lim-FAT-ik)
spleen
thymus gland (THIGH-mus)
tonsils (TAHN-sulls)

The lymphatic system consists of a network of **lymphatic vessels**, **lymph nodes**, the **spleen**, the **thymus gland**, and the **tonsils**. These organs perform several quite diverse functions for the body. First, they collect excess tissue fluid throughout the body and return it to the circulatory system. The fluid, once inside a lymphatic vessel, is referred to as **lymph**. Lymph vessels located around the small intestines, called **lacteals**, are able to pick up absorbed fats for transport. Additionally, the lymphatic system works with the immune system to form the groups of cells, tissues, organs, and molecules that serve as the body's primary defense against the invasion of pathogens. These systems work together, defending the body against foreign invaders and substances, as well as removing the body's own cells that have become diseased.

Lymphatic Vessels

lymphatic capillaries (KAP-ih-lair-eez)
lymphatic ducts
right lymphatic duct
thoracic duct
valves

The lymphatic vessels form an extensive network of ducts throughout the entire body. However, unlike the circulatory system, these vessels are not in a closed loop. Instead, they serve as one-way pipes conducting lymph from the tissues toward the thoracic cavity (see Figure 6-7 ■). These vessels begin as very small **lymphatic capillaries** in the tissues. Excessive tissue fluid enters these capillaries to begin the trip back to the circulatory system. The capillaries merge into larger

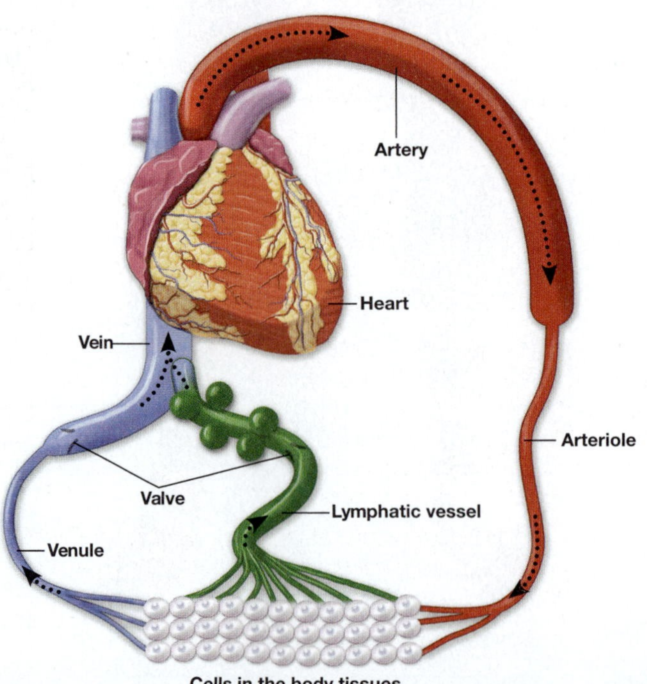

■ **Figure 6-7** Lymphatic vessels (green) pick up excess tissue fluid, purify it in lymph nodes, and return it to the circulatory system.

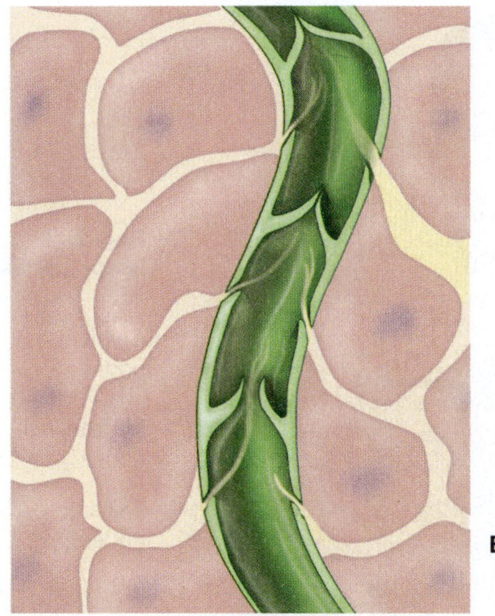

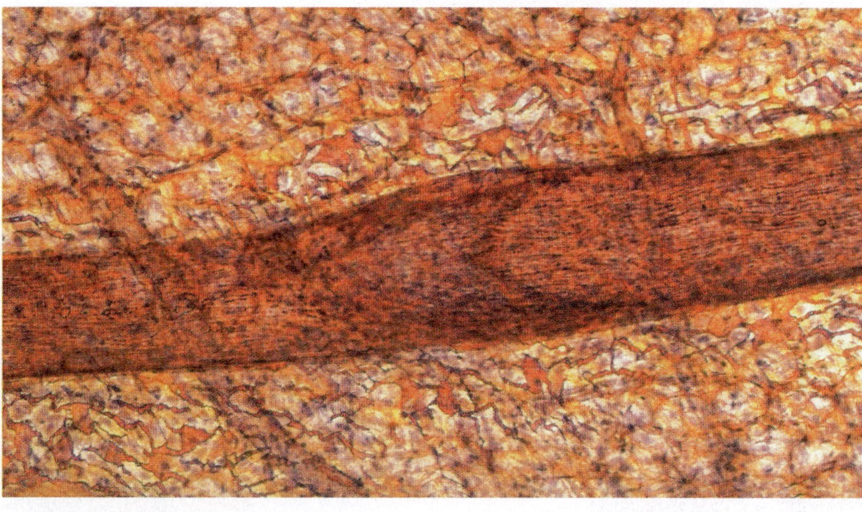

■ **Figure 6-8** A) Lymphatic vessel with valves within tissue cells; B) Photomicrograph of lymphatic vessel with valve clearly visible. *(Michael Abbey/Science Source.)*

lymphatic vessels. This is a very low-pressure system, so these vessels have **valves** along their length to ensure that lymph can only move forward toward the thoracic cavity (see Figure 6-8■). These vessels finally drain into one of two large **lymphatic ducts**, the **right lymphatic duct** or the **thoracic duct**. The smaller right lymphatic duct drains the right arm and the right side of the head, neck, and chest. This duct empties lymph into the right subclavian vein. The larger thoracic duct drains lymph from the rest of the body and empties into the left subclavian vein (see Figure 6-9■).

What's In A Name?

Look for these word parts:
thorac/o = chest
-ic = pertaining to

Med Term Tip

The term *capillary* is also used to describe the minute blood vessels within the circulatory system. This is one of several general medical terms, such as valves, cilia, and hair, that are used across several systems.

Lymph Nodes

lymph glands

Lymph nodes are small organs composed of lymphatic tissue located along the route of the lymphatic vessels. These nodes, also referred to as **lymph glands**, house lymphocytes and antibodies and therefore work to remove pathogens and cell debris as lymph passes through them on its way back to the thoracic cavity (see Figure 6-10■). Lymph nodes also serve to trap and destroy cells from cancerous tumors. Although found throughout the body, lymph nodes are particularly concentrated in several regions. For example, lymph nodes concentrated in the neck region drain lymph from the head. See again Figure 6-9 and Table 6-2■ for a description of some of the most important sites for lymph nodes.

Med Term Tip

In surgical procedures to remove a malignancy from an organ, such as a breast, the adjacent lymph nodes are also tested for cancer. If cancerous cells are found in the tested lymph nodes, the disease is said to have spread or *metastasized.* Tumor cells may then spread to other parts of the body by means of the lymphatic system.

■ **TABLE 6-2** Sites for Lymph Nodes

Name	Location	Function
axillary (AK-sih-lair-ee)	armpits	Drain arms and shoulder region; cancer cells from breasts may be present
cervical (SER-vih-kal)	neck	Drain head and neck; may be enlarged during upper respiratory infections
inguinal (ING-gwih-nal)	groin	Drain legs and lower pelvis
mediastinal (mee-dee-as-TYE-nal)	chest	Drain chest cavity

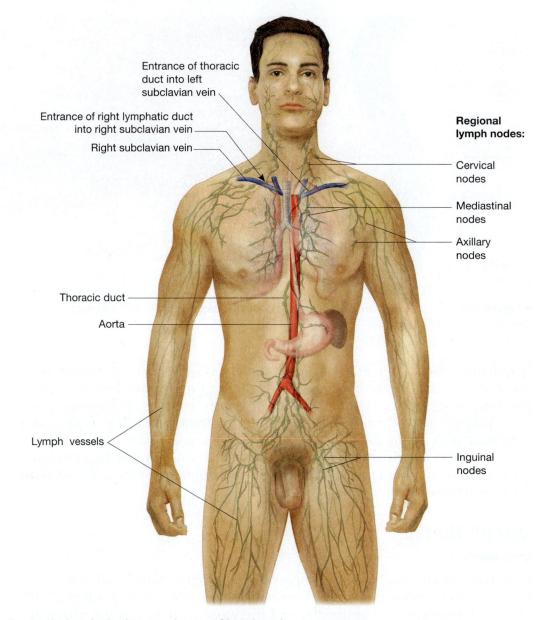

Entrance of thoracic duct into left subclavian vein
Entrance of right lymphatic duct into right subclavian vein
Right subclavian vein
Thoracic duct
Aorta
Lymph vessels
Regional lymph nodes:
Cervical nodes
Mediastinal nodes
Axillary nodes
Inguinal nodes

■ **Figure 6-9** Location of lymph vessels, lymphatic ducts, and areas of lymph node concentrations.

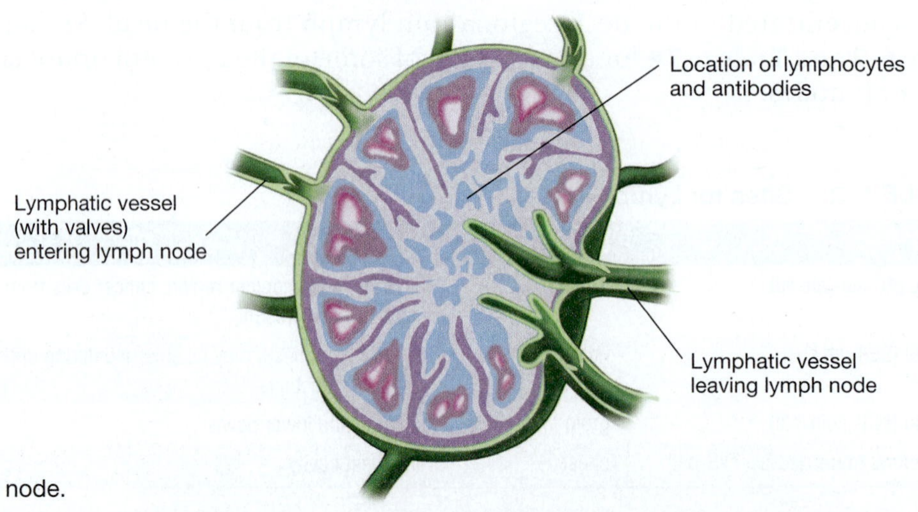

■ **Figure 6-10** Structure of a lymph node.

Tonsils

adenoids (AD-eh-noydz)
lingual tonsils (LING-gwal)
palatine tonsils (PAL-ah-tyne)
pharyngeal tonsils (fair-IN-jee-al)
pharynx (FAIR-inks)

The tonsils are collections of lymphatic tissue located on each side of the throat or **pharynx** (see Figure 6-11 ■). There are three sets of tonsils: **palatine tonsils**, **pharyngeal tonsils** (commonly referred to as the **adenoids**), and **lingual tonsils**. All tonsils contain a large number of leukocytes and act as filters to protect the body from the invasion of pathogens through the digestive or respiratory systems. Tonsils are not vital organs and can safely be removed if they become a continuous site of infection.

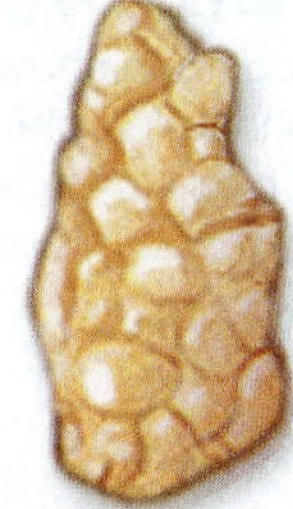

■ **Figure 6-11** The shape of a tonsil.

What's In A Name?
Look for these word parts:
lingu/o = tongue
palat/o = palate
pharyng/o = pharynx
-al = pertaining to
-eal = pertaining to
-ine = pertaining to

Spleen

blood sinuses
macrophages (MAK-roh-fay-jez)

The spleen, located in the upper left quadrant of the abdomen, consists of lymphatic tissue that is highly infiltrated with blood vessels (see Figure 6-12 ■). These vessels spread out into slow-moving **blood sinuses**. The spleen filters out and destroys old red blood cells, recycles the iron, and also stores some of the blood supply for the body. Phagocytic **macrophages** line the blood sinuses in the spleen to engulf and remove pathogens. Because the blood is moving through the organ slowly, the macrophages have time to carefully identify pathogens and worn-out red blood cells. The spleen is also not a vital organ and can be removed due to injury or disease. However, without the spleen, a person's susceptibility to a bloodstream infection may be increased.

What's In A Name?
Look for these word parts:
macro- = large
-phage = to eat

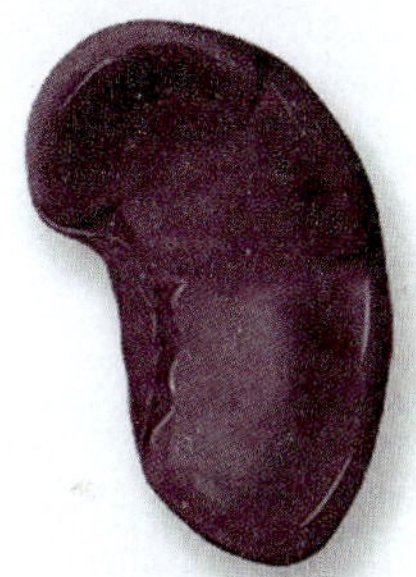

■ **Figure 6-12** The shape of the spleen.

Thymus Gland

T cells
T lymphocytes
thymosin (THIGH-moh-sin)

The thymus gland, located in the upper portion of the mediastinum, is essential for the proper development of the immune system (see Figure 6-13 ■). It assists the body with the immune function and the development of antibodies. This organ's hormone, **thymosin**, changes lymphocytes to **T lymphocytes** (simply called **T cells**), which play an important role in the immune response. The thymus is active in the unborn child and throughout childhood until adolescence, when it begins to shrink in size.

What's In A Name?
Look for these word parts:
lymph/o = lymph
-cyte = cell

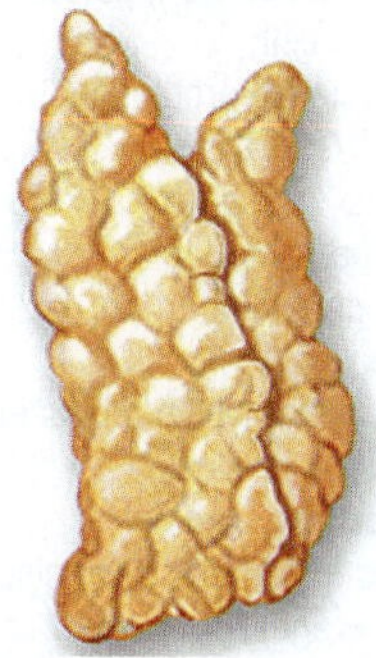

■ **Figure 6-13** The shape of the thymus gland.

Immunity

acquired immunity
active acquired immunity
bacteria (bak-TEE-ree-ah)
cancerous tumors
fungi (FUN-jeye)
immune response
immunity (im-YOO-nih-tee)
immunizations (im-yoo-nih-ZAY-shuns)
natural immunity
passive acquired immunity
protozoans (proh-toh-ZOH-anz)
toxins
vaccinations (vak-sih-NAY-shuns)
viruses

Immunity is the body's ability to defend itself against pathogens, such as **bacteria**, **viruses**, **fungi**, **protozoans**, **toxins**, and **cancerous tumors**. Immunity comes in two forms: **natural immunity** and **acquired immunity**. Natural immunity, also called *innate immunity*, is not specific to a particular disease and does not require prior exposure to the pathogenic agent. A good example of natural immunity is the

What's In A Name?
Look for this word part:
-ous = pertaining to

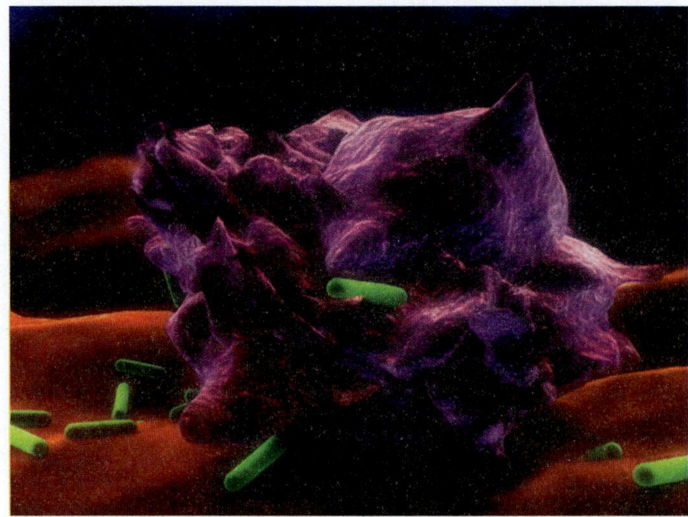

■ **Figure 6-14** Enhanced photomicrograph showing a macrophage (purple) attacking bacillus *Escherichia coli* (green). *(Sebastian Kaulitzki/ Shutterstock)*

macrophage. These leukocytes are present throughout all the tissues of the body, but are concentrated in areas of high exposure to invading bacteria, like the lungs and digestive system. They are very active phagocytic cells, ingesting and digesting any pathogen they encounter (see Figure 6-14■).

Acquired immunity is the body's response to a specific pathogen and may be established either passively or actively. **Passive acquired immunity** results when a person receives protective substances produced by another human or animal. This may take the form of maternal antibodies crossing the placenta to a baby or an antitoxin or gamma globulin injection. **Active acquired immunity** develops following direct exposure to the pathogenic agent. The agent stimulates the body's **immune response**, a series of different mechanisms all geared to neutralize the agent. For example, a person typically can catch chickenpox only once because once the body has successfully fought the virus, it will be able to more quickly recognize and kill it in the future. **Immunizations**, or **vaccinations**, are special types of active acquired immunity. Instead of actually being exposed to the infectious agent and having the disease, a person is exposed to a modified or weakened pathogen that is still capable of stimulating the immune response but not actually causing the disease.

Immune Response

antibody (AN-tih-bod-ee)
antibody-mediated immunity
antigen–antibody complex
antigens (AN-tih-jens)
B cells
B lymphocytes
cell-mediated immunity
cellular immunity
cytotoxic (sigh-toh-TOK-sik)
humoral immunity (HYOO-mor-al)
immunoglobulin (Ig) (im-yoo-noh-GLOB-yoo-lin)
natural killer (NK) cells
pathogenic (path-oh-JEN-ik)

Disease-causing, or **pathogenic**, agents are recognized as being foreign because they display proteins that are different from a person's own natural proteins. Those foreign proteins, called **antigens**, stimulate the immune response. The immune response consists of two distinct and different processes: **humoral immunity** (also called **antibody-mediated immunity**) and **cellular immunity** (also called **cell-mediated immunity**).

Humoral immunity refers to the production of **B lymphocytes**, also called **B cells**, which respond to antigens by producing a protective protein, called an **antibody** (also referred to as an **immunoglobulin**). Antibodies combine with the antigen to form an **antigen–antibody complex**. This complex either targets the foreign

What's In A Name?

Look for these word parts:
cyt/o = cell
immun/o = protection
lymph/o = lymph
path/o = disease
-al = pertaining to
-ar = pertaining to
-cyte = cell
-gen = that which produces
-genic = producing
-globulin = protein
-toxic = pertaining to poison
anti- = against

Med Term Tip

The term *humoral* comes from the Latin word for *liquid*. It is the old-fashioned term to refer to the fluids of the body.

substance for phagocytosis or prevents the infectious agent from damaging healthy cells.

Cellular immunity involves the production of T cells and **natural killer** (NK) **cells**. These defense cells are **cytotoxic**, meaning that they physically attack and destroy pathogenic cells.

Standard Precautions

cross-infection
healthcare-associated infection (HAI)
nosocomial infection (noh-soh-KOH-mee-al)
Occupational Safety and Health Administration (OSHA)
reinfection
self-inoculation

Hospitals and other healthcare settings contain a large number of infective pathogens. Patients and healthcare workers are exposed to each other's pathogens and sometimes become infected. An infection acquired in this manner, as a result of hospital exposure, is referred to as a **nosocomial infection** or a **healthcare-associated infection** (HAI). Nosocomial infections can spread in several ways. **Cross-infection** occurs when a person, either a patient or healthcare worker, acquires a pathogen from another patient or healthcare worker. **Reinfection** takes place when a patient becomes infected again with the same pathogen that originally brought him or her to the hospital. **Self-inoculation** occurs when a person becomes infected in a different part of the body by a pathogen from another part of his or her own body—such as intestinal bacteria spreading to the urethra.

What's In A Name?

Look for these word parts:
-al = pertaining to
re- = again

Med Term Tip

The term *nosocomial* comes from the Greek word *nosokomeion*, meaning hospital.

With the appearance of the hepatitis B virus (HBV) in the mid-1960s and the human immunodeficiency virus (HIV) in the mid-1980s, the fight against spreading infections took on even greater significance. In 1987 the **Occupational Safety and Health Administration** (OSHA) issued mandatory guidelines to ensure that all employees at risk of exposure to body fluids are provided with personal protective equipment. These guidelines state that all human blood, tissue, and body fluids must be treated as if they were infected with HIV, HBV, or other bloodborne pathogens. These guidelines were expanded in 1992, 1996, and 2011 to encourage the fight against not just bloodborne pathogens, but all nosocomial infections spread by contact with blood, mucous membranes, nonintact skin, and all body fluids (including amniotic fluid, vaginal secretions, pleural fluid, cerebrospinal fluid, peritoneal fluid, pericardial fluid, and semen). These guidelines are commonly referred to as the Standard Precautions:

1. Wash or sanitize hands before putting on and after removing gloves, and before and after working with each patient or patient equipment.
2. Wear gloves when in contact with any body fluid, mucous membrane, or nonintact skin, or if you have chapped hands, a rash, or open sores.
3. Wear a nonpermeable gown or apron during procedures that are likely to expose you to any body fluid, mucous membrane, or nonintact skin.
4. Wear a mask and protective equipment or a face shield when in contact with patients who are coughing frequently, or if body fluid droplets or splashes are likely.
5. Wear a facemask and eyewear that seal close to the face during procedures that cause body tissues to be vaporized.
6. Remove for proper cleaning any shared equipment—such as a thermometer, stethoscope, or blood pressure cuff—that has come into contact with body fluids, mucous membrane, or nonintact skin.

Med Term Tip

The simple act of thoroughly washing your hands is the most effective method of preventing the spread of infectious diseases.

PRACTICE AS YOU GO

F. Complete the Statement

1. The organs of the lymphatic system other than lymphatic vessels and lymph nodes are the ______________, ______________, and ______________.
2. The two lymph ducts are the ______________ and ______________.
3. The primary concentrations of lymph nodes are the ______________, ______________, ______________, and ______________ regions.
4. ______________ immunity develops following direct exposure to a pathogen.
5. Humoral immunity is also referred to as ______________ immunity.

Terminology

Word Parts Used to Build Lymphatic and Immune System Terms

The following lists contain the combining forms, suffixes, and prefixes used to build terms in the remaining sections of this chapter.

Combining Forms

adenoid/o	adenoids	lymph/o	lymph	pneumon/o (see Chapter 7)	lung
axill/o	axilla, underarm	lymphaden/o	lymph node	rhin/o	nose
conjunctiv/o (see Chapter 13)	conjunctiva	lymphangi/o	lymph vessel	sarc/o	flesh
cortic/o	outer layer	myel/o	bone marrow	splen/o	spleen
dermat/o	skin	nas/o	nose	thym/o	thymus gland
immun/o	protection	nucle/o	nucleus	tonsill/o	tonsils
inguin/o	groin	path/o	disease		

Suffixes

-al	pertaining to	-graphy	process of recording	-logy	study of
-ar	pertaining to	-ia	condition	-megaly	enlarged
-ary	pertaining to	-iasis	abnormal condition	-oma	tumor
-atic	pertaining to	-ic	pertaining to	-osis	abnormal condition
-ectomy	surgical removal	-itis	inflammation	-pathy	disease
-edema	swelling			-therapy	treatment
-gram	record				

Prefixes

anti-	against	auto-	self	mono-	one

Adjective Form of Anatomical Terms

Term	Word Parts	Definition
axillary (AK-sih-lair-ee)	axill/o = axilla, underarm -ary = pertaining to	Pertaining to underarm region
inguinal (ING-gwih-nal)	inguin/o = groin -al = pertaining to	Pertaining to groin region
lymphangial (lim-FAN-jee-al)	lymphangi/o = lymph vessel -al = pertaining to	Pertaining to lymph vessels
lymphatic (lim-FAT-ik)	lymph/o = lymph -atic = pertaining to	Pertaining to lymph
splenic (SPLEN-ik)	splen/o = spleen -ic = pertaining to	Pertaining to spleen
thymic (THIGH-mik)	thym/o = thymus gland -ic = pertaining to	Pertaining to thymus gland
tonsillar (TAHN-sih-lar)	tonsill/o = tonsils -ar = pertaining to	Pertaining to tonsils

PRACTICE AS YOU GO

G. Give the adjective form for each anatomical structure.

1. Spleen ______________________
2. Lymph ______________________
3. Tonsil ______________________
4. Thymus gland ______________________
5. Lymph vessel ______________________

Pathology

Term	Word Parts	Definition
Medical Specialties		
allergist (AL-er-jist)		Physician who specializes in testing for and treating allergies
immunology (im-yoo-NALL-oh-jee)	immun/o = protection -logy = study of	Branch of medicine concerned with diagnosis and treatment of infectious diseases and other disorders of immune system; physician is an *immunologist*
pathology (pah-THOL-oh-jee)	path/o = disease -logy = study of	Branch of medicine concerned with determining underlying causes and development of diseases; physician is a *pathologist*

Pathology (continued)

Term	Word Parts	Definition
Signs and Symptoms		
hives		Appearance of wheals as part of allergic reaction
inflammation (in-flah-MAY-shun)		Tissues' response to injury from pathogens or physical agents; characterized by redness, pain, swelling, and feeling hot to the touch
lymphedema (limf-eh-DEE-mah)	lymph/o = lymph -edema = swelling	Edema appearing in extremities due to obstruction of lymph flow through lymphatic vessels
splenomegaly (spleh-noh-MEG-ah-lee)	splen/o = spleen -megaly = enlarged	Enlarged spleen
urticaria (er-tih-KAIR-ee-ah)		Severe itching associated with hives, usually linked to food allergy, stress, or drug reactions
Allergic Reactions		
allergic asthma (ah-LER-jik / AZ-mah)	-ic = pertaining to	Inflammation and narrowing of airways triggered by inhaling an allergen; symptoms include wheezing, coughing, and shortness of breath
allergic conjunctivitis (ah-LER-jik / kon-junk-tih-VYE-tis)	-ic = pertaining to conjunctiv/o = conjunctiva -itis = inflammation	Inflammation of the conjunctiva (protective membrane over front of eyeball) caused by allergens in the air
allergic rhinitis (ah-LER-jik / rye-NYE-tis)	-ic = pertaining to rhin/o = nose -itis = inflammation	Allergic reaction caused by inhaling an allergen such as pollen, animal dander, or mold; symptoms may include sneezing, runny nose, congestion, post-nasal drip, cough, and itchy, watery eyes; commonly called *hay fever*
allergy (AL-er-jee)		Hypersensitivity to common substance in environment or to medication; substance causing allergic reaction is called *allergen*
anaphylactic shock (an-ah-fih-LAK-tik)		Life-threatening condition resulting from a severe allergic reaction; examples of instances that may trigger this reaction include bee stings, medications, or ingestion of foods; circulatory and respiratory problems occur, including respiratory distress, hypotension, edema, tachycardia, and convulsions; also called *anaphylaxis*

Figure 6-15 Inflammation as illustrated by cellulitis of the nose. Note that the area is red and swollen. It is also painful and hot to touch. *(ARENA Creative/Shutterstock)*

Word Watch

The terms *inflammation* and *inflammatory* are spelled with two *m*'s, while *inflame* and *inflamed* each have only one *m*. These may be the most commonly misspelled terms by medical terminology students.

Pathology (continued)

Term	Word Parts	Definition
contact dermatitis (der-mah-TYE-tis)	dermat/o = skin -itis = inflammation	Skin irritation caused by skin coming into direct contact with an allergen; symptoms may include redness, itching, rash, and blisters; common allergens are poison ivy, soaps, fragrances, and jewelry
Lymphatic System		
adenoiditis (ad-eh-noyd-EYE-tis)	adenoid/o = adenoids -itis = inflammation	Inflammation of adenoids
autoimmune disease	auto- = self	Disease resulting from body's immune system attacking its own cells as if they were pathogens; examples include systemic lupus erythematosus, rheumatoid arthritis, and multiple sclerosis
elephantiasis (el-eh-fan-TYE-ah-sis)	-iasis = abnormal condition	Inflammation, obstruction, and destruction of lymph vessels resulting in enlarged tissues due to edema
Hodgkin's disease (HD) (HOJ-kins)		Also called *Hodgkin's lymphoma*; cancer of lymphatic cells found in concentration in lymph nodes; named after Thomas Hodgkin, a British physician, who first described it
lymphadenitis (lim-fad-en-EYE-tis)	lymphaden/o = lymph node -itis = inflammation	Inflammation of lymph nodes; referred to as *swollen glands*
lymphadenopathy (lim-fad-eh-NOP-ah-thee)	lymphaden/o = lymph node -pathy = disease	General term for lymph node diseases
lymphangioma (lim-fan-jee-OH-mah)	lymphangi/o = lymph vessel -oma = tumor	Tumor in a lymphatic vessel
lymphoma (lim-FOH-mah)	lymph/o = lymph -oma = tumor	Tumor in lymphatic tissue
mononucleosis (mono) (mon-oh-noo-klee-OH-sis)	mono- = one nucle/o = nucleus -osis = abnormal condition	Acute infectious disease with large number of abnormal mononuclear lymphocytes; caused by Epstein–Barr virus; abnormal liver function may occur; commonly called *kissing disease* since virus can be spread by saliva
non-Hodgkin's lymphoma (NHL)	lymph/o = lymph -oma = tumor	Cancer of lymphatic tissues other than Hodgkin's lymphoma

Med Term Tip

Mononuclear is a term occasionally used to describe any cell that has a large, single, round nucleus, including lymphocytes and monocytes. This is opposed to having a lobed nucleus like the other white blood cells.

Figure 6-16 Photo of the neck of a patient with non-Hodgkin's lymphoma showing swelling associated with enlarged lymph nodes.
(Dr. P. Marazzi/Science Source)

Pathology (continued)

Term	Word Parts	Definition
thymoma (thigh-MOH-mah)	thym/o = thymus gland -oma = tumor	Tumor of thymus gland
tonsillitis (tahn-sill-EYE-tis)	tonsill/o = tonsils -itis = inflammation	Inflammation of tonsils
Immune System		
acquired immunodeficiency syndrome (AIDS) (im-yoo-noh-dih-FIH-shen-see / SIN-drohm)	immun/o = protection	Disease involving defect in cell-mediated immunity system; syndrome of opportunistic infections occurring in final stages of infection with human immunodeficiency virus (HIV); virus attacks T4 lymphocytes and destroys them, reducing person's ability to fight infection
AIDS-related complex (ARC)		Early stage of AIDS; there is a positive test for virus, but only mild symptoms of weight loss, fatigue, skin rash, and anorexia
graft versus host disease (GVHD)		Serious complication of bone marrow transplant (graft); immune cells from donor bone marrow attack recipient's (host's) tissues
human immunodeficiency virus (HIV) (im-yoo-noh-dih-FIH-shen-see)	immun/o = protection	Virus that causes AIDS; also known as a *retrovirus*

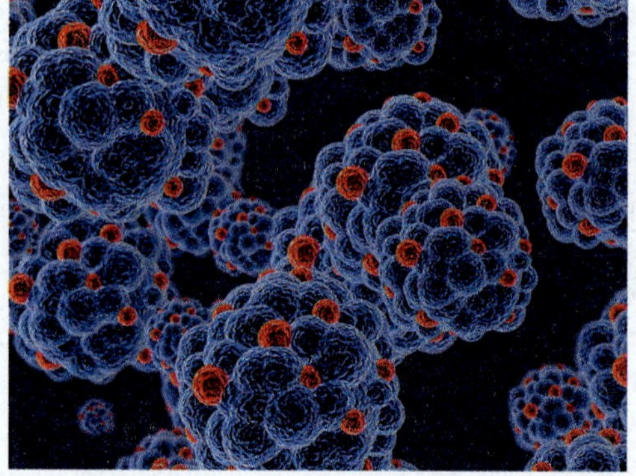

■ **Figure 6-17** Color enhanced scanning electron micrograph of HIV virus (red) infecting T-helper cells (blue). *(Illustration Forest/Shutterstock)*

Term	Word Parts	Definition
immunocompromised (im-yoo-noh-KOM-proh-myzd)	immun/o = protection	Having immune system that is unable to respond properly to pathogens; also called *immunodeficiency disorder*
Kaposi's sarcoma (KS) (KAP-oh-seez / sar-KOH-mah)	sarc/o = flesh -oma = tumor	Form of skin cancer frequently seen in patients with AIDS; consists of brownish-purple papules that spread from skin and metastasize to internal organs; named for dermatologist Moritz Kaposi
multiple myeloma (my-eh-LOH-mah)	myel/o = bone marrow -oma = tumor	Originates in plasma cells (type of lymphocyte responsible for making antibodies); over time, these malignant cells collect in bone marrow, resulting in a bone marrow tumor; may spread to skeleton
opportunistic infections		Infectious diseases associated with patients who have compromised immune systems and therefore lowered resistance to infections and parasites; may be result of HIV infection

Pathology (continued)

Term	Word Parts	Definition
pneumocystis pneumonia (PCP) (noo-moh-SIS-tis / noo-MOH-nee-ah)	pneumon/o = lung -ia = condition	Pneumonia common in patients with weakened immune systems, such as AIDS patients, caused by *Pneumocystis jiroveci* fungus
sarcoidosis (sar-koy-DOH-sis)	-osis = abnormal condition	Autoimmune disease of unknown cause that forms fibrous lesions commonly appearing in lymph nodes, liver, skin, lungs, spleen, eyes, and small bones of hands and feet
severe combined immunodeficiency (SCID)	immun/o = protection	Disease seen in children born with nonfunctioning immune system; often these children are forced to live in sealed sterile rooms
Nosocomial Infections		
carbapenem-resistant Enterobacteriaceae (CRE) **infection** (kar-bah-PEN-em / ree-ZISS-tent / en-ter-oh-bak-teer-ee-AY-see-ee)		Infection by group of bacteria that have resistance to powerful group of antibiotics called *carbapenems;* almost all infections occur in healthcare settings, especially among patients with ventilators, urinary catheters, intravenous catheters, or on long-term antibiotics
Clostridium difficile (C. diff) **infection** (klaw-STRIH-dee-um / dif-ee-SEEL)		Infection with *C. diff* bacteria causes inflammation of colon; symptoms may include diarrhea, nausea, fever, and abdominal pain; most commonly occurs in persons with conditions requiring extended use of antibiotics; infection spread through contact with contaminated feces
methicillin-resistant *Staphylococcus aureus* (MRSA) **infection** (meth-ih-SIL-in / ree-ZISS-tent / staf-ih-loh-KOK-us / OR-ee-iss)		Infecting bacteria are resistant to many common antibiotics, such as methicillin, oxacillin, penicillin, and amoxicillin; spread through contact with contaminated surface, often improperly washed hands

PRACTICE AS YOU GO

H. Terminology Matching

Match each term to its definition.

1. ________ allergy

2. ________ hives

3. ________ Hodgkin's disease

4. ________ sarcoidosis

5. ________ graft vs. host disease

a. seen in an allergic reaction

b. complication of bone marrow transplant

c. a hypersensitivity reaction

d. a type of cancer

e. autoimmune disease

Diagnostic Procedures

Term	Word Parts	Definition
Clinical Laboratory Tests		
antinuclear antibody (ANA) **test** (an-tee-NOO-klee-ar / AN-tee-bod-ee)	anti- = against nucle/o = nucleus -ar = pertaining to	Blood test to assist in diagnosis of autoimmune diseases; antinuclear antibodies are produced by persons with autoimmune disease; presence of these antibodies in blood indicates that person's immune system is attacking body's cells
HIV antigen/antibody immunoassay (im-yoo-noh-ASS-ay)	anti- = against immun/o = protection	Blood test for HIV infection; tests for both HIV antigens and antibodies; foreign viral proteins (HIV antigen) can be detected very shortly after exposure, and antibodies produced by body in response to HIV infection can be detected two to eight weeks after exposure; antibody-only test can also be performed using saliva
Diagnostic Imaging		
lymphangiogram (lim-FAN-jee-oh-gram)	lymphangi/o = lymph vessel -gram = record	X-ray record of lymphatic vessels produced by lymphangiography
lymphangiography (lim-fan-jee-OG-rah-fee)	lymphangi/o = lymph vessel -graphy = process of recording	X-ray taken of lymph vessels after injection of dye into foot; lymph flow through chest is traced
magnetic resonance imaging (MRI) (REZ-oh-nens) ■ **Figure 6-18** Magnetic resonance image (MRI) showing a sagittal view of the brain, oral cavity, nasal cavity, and spinal cord. *(MriMan/Shutterstock)*	-ic = pertaining to	Use of electromagnetic energy to produce image of soft tissues in any plane of body; atoms behave differently when placed in strong magnetic field; when body is exposed to this magnetic field, nuclei of body's atoms emit radio-frequency signals that can be used to create an image
Additional Diagnostic Procedures		
Monospot		Blood test for infectious mononucleosis
skin allergy testing ■ **Figure 6-19** A) Skin allergy testing; patient is exposed to allergens through light scratch in the skin. B) Positive allergy test results. Inflammation indicates person is allergic to that substance. *(Anthony Ricci/Shutterstock)*	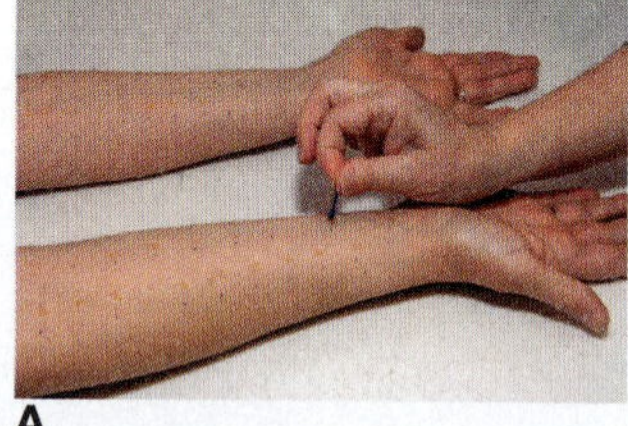 A	Form of allergy testing in which the body is exposed to allergens through light scratch, injection, patch, or prick on skin 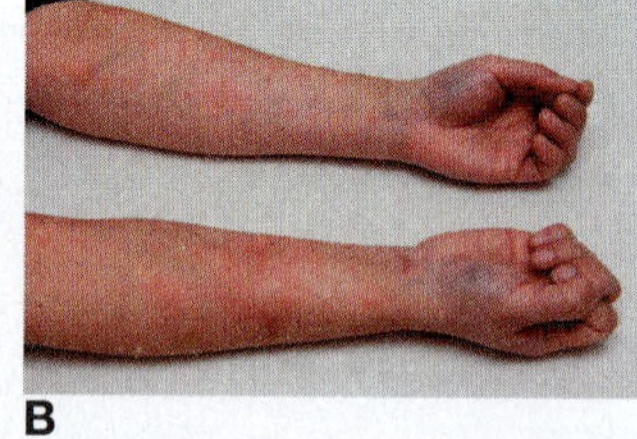 B

Therapeutic Procedures

Term	Word Parts	Definition
Medical Procedures		
allergy shots		Type of immunotherapy; person receives regular injections of tiny amounts of allergen to which he or she is allergic; injection is too small to cause allergic reaction, but large enough to stimulate immune system; over time, person's sensitivity to allergen reduces

Therapeutic Procedures (continued)

Term	Word Parts	Definition
immunotherapy (IM-yoo-noh-thair-ah-pee)	immun/o = protection -therapy = treatment	Giving patient injection of immunoglobulins or antibodies in order to treat disease; antibodies may be produced by another person or animal, for example, antivenom for snake bites; more recent developments include treatments to boost activity of immune system, especially to treat cancer and AIDS
vaccination (vak-sih-NAY-shun)		Exposure to weakened pathogen that stimulates immune response and antibody production in order to confer protection against full-blown disease; also called *immunization*
Surgical Procedures		
adenoidectomy (ad-eh-noyd-EK-toh-mee)	adenoid/o = adenoids -ectomy = surgical removal	Surgical removal of adenoids
lymphadenectomy (lim-fad-eh-NEK-toh-mee)	lymphaden/o = lymph node -ectomy = surgical removal	Surgical removal of lymph node; usually done to test for malignancy
splenectomy (spleh-NEK-toh-mee)	splen/o = spleen -ectomy = surgical removal	Surgical removal of spleen
thymectomy (thigh-MEK-toh-mee)	thym/o = thymus gland -ectomy = surgical removal	Surgical removal of thymus gland
tonsillectomy (tahn-sih-LEK-toh-mee)	tonsill/o = tonsils -ectomy = surgical removal	Surgical removal of tonsils

Pharmacology

Classification	Word Parts	Action	Examples
antihistamine (an-tih-HIST-ah-meen)	anti- = against	Blocks effects of histamine released by body during allergic reaction	cetirizine, Zyrtec; diphenhydramine, Benadryl
corticosteroids (kor-tih-koh-STAIR-oydz)	cortic/o = outer layer	Natural or synthetic adrenal cortex hormone; has very strong anti-inflammatory properties; particularly useful in treating autoimmune diseases	prednisone; methylprednisolone, Solu-Medrol
immunosuppressants (im-yoo-noh-suh-PRESS-antz)	immun/o = protection	Block certain actions of immune system; required to prevent rejection of transplanted organ	mycophenolate mofetil, CellCept; cyclosporine, Neoral
nasal steroids (NAY-zal)	nas/o = nose -al = pertaining to	Nose spray; reduces inflammation and treats symptoms of nasal rhinitis	fluticasone, Flonase; triamcinolone, Nasacort
protease inhibitor drugs (PROH-tee-ays)		Inhibit protease, enzyme that viruses need to reproduce	indinavir, Crixivan; saquinavir, Fortovase
reverse transcriptase inhibitor drugs (trans-KRIP-tays)		Inhibit reverse transcriptase, enzyme needed by viruses to reproduce	lamivudine, Epivir; zidovudine, Retrovir

PRACTICE AS YOU GO

I. Procedure Matching

Match each procedure term with its definition.

1. ________ ANA test
2. ________ vaccination
3. ________ corticosteroid
4. ________ Monospot
5. ________ lymphangiography

a. test for mononucleosis
b. an X-ray
c. immunization
d. has strong anti-inflammatory properties
e. assists in diagnosis of autoimmune disease

Abbreviations

AIDS	acquired immunodeficiency syndrome	**Ig**	immunoglobulins (IgA, IgD, IgE, IgG, IgM)
ANA	antinuclear antibody	**KS**	Kaposi's sarcoma
ARC	AIDS-related complex	**mono**	mononucleosis
C. diff	*Clostridium difficile*	**MRSA**	methicillin-resistant *Staphylococcus aureus*
CRE	carbapenem-resistant *Enterobacteriaceae*	**NHL**	non-Hodgkin's lymphoma
GVHD	graft versus host disease	**NK**	natural killer cells
HAI	healthcare-associated infection	**PCP**	pneumocystis pneumonia
HD	Hodgkin's disease	**SCID**	severe combined immunodeficiency
HIV	human immunodeficiency virus		

PRACTICE AS YOU GO

J. What's the Abbreviation?

1. acquired immunodeficiency syndrome ________
2. AIDS-related complex ________
3. human immunodeficiency virus ________
4. mononucleosis ________
5. Kaposi's sarcoma ________
6. immunoglobulin ________
7. severe combined immunodeficiency syndrome ________
8. pneumocystis pneumonia ________

Chapter Review

Real-World Applications

Medical Record Analysis

This Discharge Summary contains 10 medical terms. Underline each term and write it in the list below the report. Then explain each term as you would to a nonmedical person.

Discharge Summary

Admitting Diagnosis:	Splenomegaly, weight loss, diarrhea, fatigue, chronic cough
Final Diagnosis:	Non-Hodgkin's lymphoma of spleen; splenectomy
History of Present Illness:	Patient is a 36-year-old businessman who was first seen in the office with complaints of feeling generally "run-down," intermittent diarrhea, weight loss, and, more recently, a dry cough. He states he has been aware of these symptoms for approximately six months. Monospot and HIV antigen/antibody immunoassay are both negative. In spite of a 35-pound weight loss, he has abdominal swelling and splenomegaly was detected. He was admitted to the hospital for further evaluation and treatment.
Summary of Hospital Course:	Full-body MRI confirmed splenomegaly and located a 3-cm encapsulated tumor in the spleen. Biopsies taken from the splenic tumor confirmed the diagnosis of non-Hodgkin's lymphoma. The patient underwent splenectomy for removal of the tumor.
Discharge Plans:	Patient was discharged home following recovery from the splenectomy. The abdominal swelling and diarrhea were resolved, but the dry cough persisted. He was referred to a cancer clinic for evaluation for chemotherapy.

	Term	Explanation
1.	______	______
2.	______	______
3.	______	______
4.	______	______
5.	______	______
6.	______	______
7.	______	______
8.	______	______
9.	______	______
10.	______	______

Chart Note Transcription

The chart note below contains 10 phrases that can be reworded with a medical term presented in this chapter. Each phrase is identified with an underline. Determine the medical term and write your answers in the space provided.

Pearson General Hospital Consultation Report

Task Edit View Time Scale Options Help Download Archive Date: 17 May 2017

Current Complaint:	Patient is a 22-year-old female referred to the specialist in treating blood disorders **1** by her internist. Her complaints include fatigue, weight loss, and easy bruising.
Past History:	Patient had normal childhood diseases. She is a college student and was feeling well until symptoms gradually appeared starting approximately three months ago.
Signs and Symptoms:	An immunoassay test for HIV exposure **2** was normal. The measure of the blood's coagulation abilities **3** indicated that the blood took too long to form a clot. A blood test to count all the blood cells **4** reported too few red blood cells **5** and too few clotting cells. **6** There were too many white blood cells, **7** but they were immature and abnormal. A sample of bone marrow obtained for microscopic examination **8** found an excessive number of immature white blood cells.
Diagnosis:	Cancer of the white blood cell–forming bone marrow **9**
Treatment:	Aggressive chemotherapy for the cancer of the white blood cell–forming bone marrow **9** and replacement blood from another person **10** to replace the erythrocytes and platelets.

1. ______
2. ______
3. ______
4. ______
5. ______
6. ______
7. ______
8. ______
9. ______
10. ______

Case Study

Below is a case study presentation of a patient with a condition discussed in this chapter. Read the case study and answer the questions below. Some questions will ask for information not included within this chapter. Use your text, a medical dictionary, or any other reference material you choose to answer these questions.

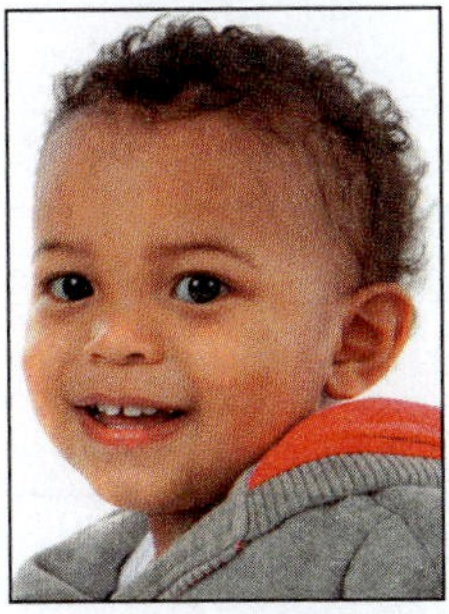

(Flashon Studio/Shutterstock)

A two-year-old boy is being seen by a hematologist. The child's symptoms include the sudden onset of high fevers, thrombopenia, epistaxis, gingival bleeding, petechiae, and ecchymoses after minor traumas. The physician has ordered a bone marrow aspiration to confirm the clinical diagnosis of acute lymphocytic leukemia (ALL). If the diagnosis is positive, the child will be placed immediately on intensive chemotherapy. The physician has informed the parents that treatment produces remission in 90% of children with ALL, especially those between the ages of two and eight.

Questions

1. What pathological condition does the hematologist suspect? Look this condition up in a reference source and include a short description of it.

   ____

   ____

2. List and define each of the patient's presenting symptoms in your own words.

   ____

   ____

3. What diagnostic test did the physician perform? Describe it in your own words.

   ____

   ____

4. Explain the phrase "clinical diagnosis" in your own words.

   ____

   ____

5. If the suspected diagnosis is correct, explain the treatment that will begin.

   ____

   ____

6. What do you think the term *remission* means?

   ____

   ____

Practice Exercises

A. Word Building Practice

The combining form **splen/o** refers to the *spleen.* Use it to write a term that means:

1. enlargement of the spleen ______
2. surgical removal of the spleen ______
3. cutting into the spleen ______

The combining form **lymph/o** refers to the *lymph.* Use it to write a term that means:

4. lymph cells ______
5. tumor of the lymph system ______

The combining form **lymphaden/o** refers to the *lymph nodes.* Use it to write a term that means:

6. disease of a lymph gland ______
7. tumor of a lymph gland ______
8. inflammation of a lymph gland ______

The combining form **immun/o** refers to the *immune system.* Use it to write a term that means:

9. specialist in the study of the immune system ______
10. immune protein ______
11. study of the immune system ______

The combining form **hemat/o** refers to *blood.* Use it to write a term that means:

12. relating to the blood ______
13. blood tumor or mass ______
14. blood formation ______

The combining form **hem/o** refers to *blood.* Use it to write a term that means:

15. blood destruction ______
16. blood protein ______

The suffix **-penia** refers to *too few (cells).* Use it to write a term that means:

17. too few white (cells) ______
18. too few red (cells) ______
19. too few of all cells ______

The suffix **-cytosis** refers to *more than the normal number of cells.* Use it to write a term that means:

20. more than the normal number of white cells ______
21. more than the normal number of red cells ______
22. more than the normal number of clotting cells ______

The suffix **-cyte** refers to *cells.* Use it to write a term that means:

23. red cell ______
24. white cell ______
25. lymph cell ______

B. Using Abbreviations

Fill in each blank with the appropriate abbreviation.

1. The ________________ test showed a low volume of red blood cells.
2. Infection by the ________________ virus may result in ________________, a severe immune system disease.
3. The results of the ________________ indicated the presence of an inflammatory disease.
4. ________________ is a potential complication following a bone marrow transplant.
5. A(n) ________________ was ordered to determine if there was a bacterial infection in the blood.
6. ________________ is a type of pneumonia common in immunocompromised persons.
7. Before surgery, a(n) ________________ was performed to check the blood's coagulation ability.
8. Further tests were needed to determine if the acute leukemia was ________________ or ________________.
9. The formed elements of the blood include ________________, ________________, and platelets.
10. Vitamin B_{12} injections are used to treat ________________.

C. Complete the Term

For each definition given below, fill in the blank with the word part that completes the term.

Definition	Term
1. more than normal number of red cells	erythro ________________
2. blood condition with excessive fat	hyperlipid ________________
3. too few white (cells)	leuko ________________
4. blood protein	hemo ________________
5. cutting into a vein	________________ otomy
6. clot destruction	________________ lytic
7. study of shape	________________ logy
8. separation of blood	hemato ________________
9. study of disease	________________ logy
10. swelling with lymph	lymph ________________
11. lymph vessel tumor	________________ oma
12. protection treatment	________________ therapy
13. surgical removal of tonsils	________________ ectomy
14. bone marrow tumor	________________ oma
15. enlarged spleen	________________ megaly

D. Fill in the Blank

Kaposi's sarcoma	mononucleosis	Hodgkin's disease	aplastic
polycythemia vera	anaphylactic shock	autoimmune diseases	pernicious
pneumocystis	HIV		

1. The condition characterized by the production of too many red blood cells is called ________________.
2. The Epstein–Barr virus is thought to be responsible for ________________ infectious disease.
3. A life-threatening allergic reaction is ________________.
4. The virus responsible for causing AIDS is ________________.
5. A cancer that is seen frequently in AIDS patients is ________________.
6. An ANA test is used to test for ________________.
7. Malignant tumors concentrate in lymph nodes with this disease: ________________.
8. A type of pneumonia seen in AIDS patients is ________________ pneumonia.
9. ________________ anemia is a severe form of anemia caused by nonfunctioning red bone marrow.
10. ________________ anemia is the result of a vitamin B_{12} deficiency.

E. Pharmacology Challenge

Fill in the classification for each drug description, then match the brand name.

	Drug Description	Classification	Brand Name
1.	________ inhibits enzyme needed for viral reproduction	________________	a. HepLock
2.	________ prevents blood clot formation	________________	b. Activase
3.	________ stops bleeding	________________	c. Solu-Medrol
4.	________ blocks effects of histamine	________________	d. Amicar
5.	________ prevents rejection of a transplanted organ	________________	e. Epivir
6.	________ dissolves existing blood clots	________________	f. CellCept
7.	________ increases number of erythrocytes	________________	g. Procrit
8.	________ strong anti-inflammatory properties	________________	h. Zyrtec
9.	________ interferes with action of platelets	________________	i. Plavix

F. Terminology Matching

Match each term to its definition.

1.	________ culture and sensitivity	a. measure of blood's clotting ability
2.	________ hematocrit	b. counts number of each type of blood cell
3.	________ complete blood count	c. examines cells for abnormal shape
4.	________ erythrocyte sedimentation rate	d. checks blood for bacterial growth and best antibiotic to use
5.	________ prothrombin time	e. determines number of each type of white blood cell
6.	________ white cell differential	f. measures percent of whole blood that is red blood cells
7.	________ red cell morphology	g. an indicator of the presence of an inflammatory condition

G. Define the Term

1. immunotherapy __________
2. Monospot __________
3. opportunistic infection __________
4. urticaria __________
5. inflammation __________
6. homologous transfusion __________
7. pernicious anemia __________
8. leukemia __________
9. hemorrhage __________
10. septicemia __________

H. Anatomical Adjectives

Fill in the blank with the missing noun or adjective.

	Noun	Adjective
1.	underarm	__________
2.	blood	__________
3.	__________	lymphangial
4.	__________	fibrinous
5.	__________	splenic
6.	__________	thymic
7.	clotting cell	__________
8.	white cell	__________
9.	red cell	__________
10.	__________	tonsillar

I. Spelling Practice

Some of the following terms are misspelled. Identify the incorrect terms and spell them correctly in the blank provided.

1. tonsilitis __________
2. sanguineous __________
3. immunosuppressants __________
4. sarcoidosis __________
5. inflamation __________
6. phlebotomy __________
7. autolgous __________
8. thrombocytosis __________
9. pancytopeenia __________
10. dyscrasea __________

J. Complete the Statement

1. Erythrocytes contain ______________________, a protein than binds oxygen for transport.
2. The five types of leukocytes are ______________________, ______________________, ______________________, ______________________, and ______________________.
3. ______________________ is the modern term for thrombocyte.
4. Type O blood is the universal ______________________ and Type AB blood is the universal ______________________.
5. Lymphatic vessels located around the intestines are called ______________________.
6. ______________________ are located along lymphatic vessels and work to trap and destroy pathogens.
7. The ______________________ filters out and destroys old erythrocytes.
8. Natural killer cells are part of ______________________ immunity.

MyLab Medical Terminology™

MyLab Medical Terminology is a premium online homework management system that includes a host of features to help you study. Registered users will find:

- A multitude of activities and assignments built within the MyLab platform
- Powerful tools that track and analyze your results—allowing you to create a personalized learning experience
- Videos and audio pronunciations to help enrich your progress
- Streaming lesson presentations (Guided Lectures) and self-paced learning modules
- A space where you and your instructors can check your progress and manage your assignments

Labeling Exercises

Image A

Write the labels for this figure on the numbered lines provided.

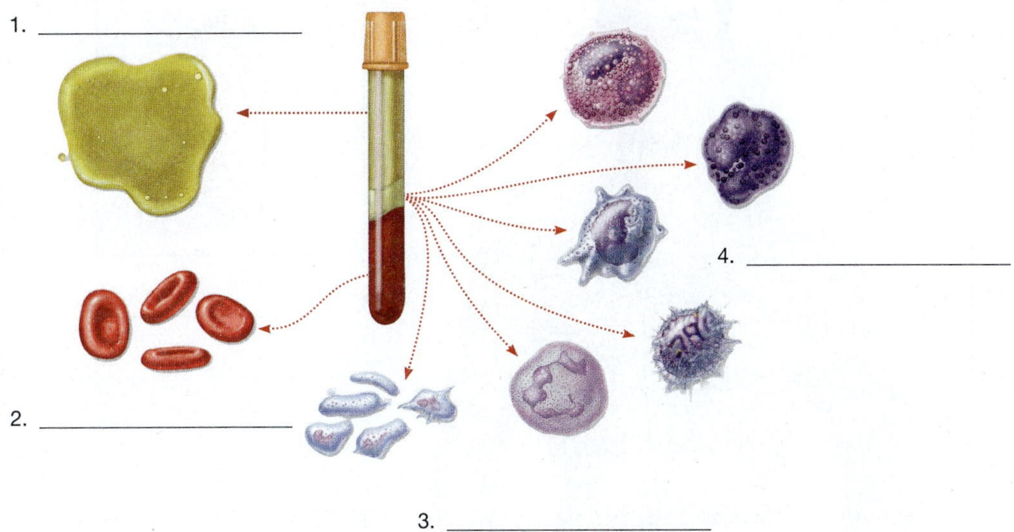

Image B

Write the labels for this figure on the numbered lines provided.

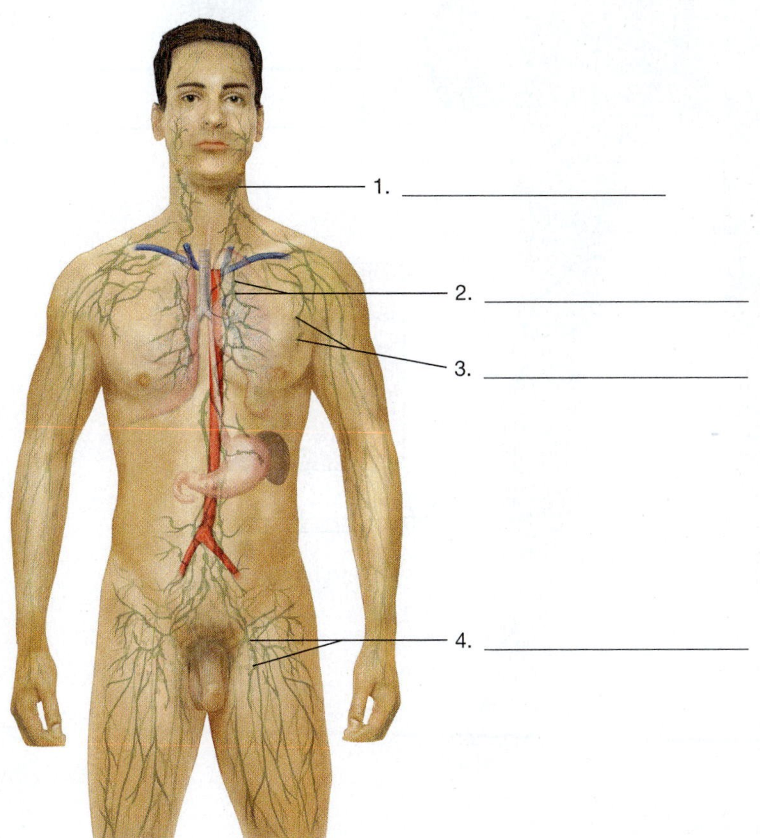

Image C

Write the labels for this figure on the numbered lines provided.

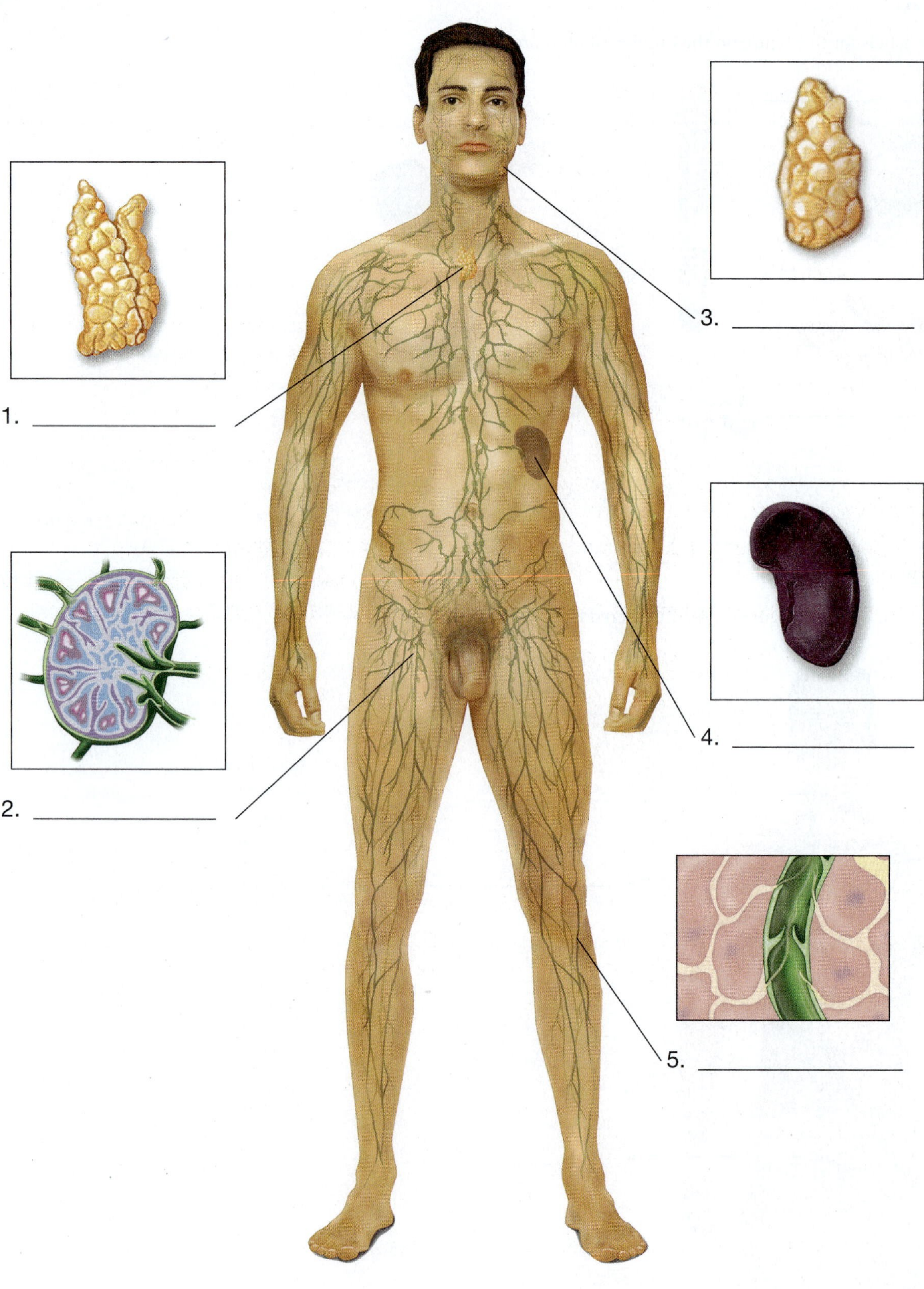

Chapter 7

Respiratory System

Learning Objectives

Upon completion of this chapter, you will be able to

1. Identify and define the combining forms and suffixes introduced in this chapter.
2. Correctly spell and pronounce medical terms and major anatomical structures relating to the respiratory system.
3. Locate and describe the major organs of the respiratory system and their functions.
4. List and describe the lung volumes and capacities.
5. Describe the process of respiration.
6. Identify and define respiratory system anatomical terms.
7. Identify and define selected respiratory system pathology terms.
8. Identify and define selected respiratory system diagnostic procedures.
9. Identify and define selected respiratory system therapeutic procedures.
10. Identify and define selected medications relating to the respiratory system.
11. Define selected abbreviations associated with the respiratory system.

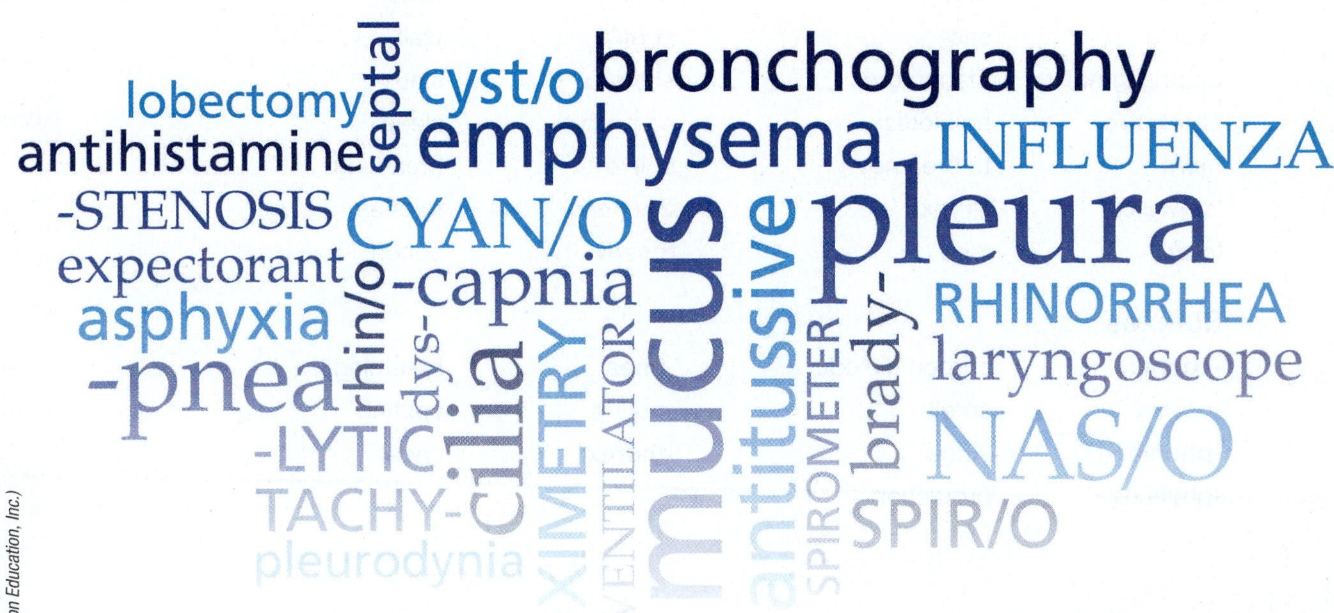

(Pearson Education, Inc.)

RESPIRATORY SYSTEM

AT A GLANCE

Function

The organs of the respiratory system are responsible for bringing fresh air into the lungs, exchanging oxygen for carbon dioxide between the air sacs of the lungs and the bloodstream, and exhaling the stale air.

Organs

The primary structures that comprise the respiratory system:

nasal cavity	**trachea**
pharynx	**bronchial tubes**
larynx	**lungs**

Word Parts

Presented here are the most common word parts (with their meanings) used to build respiratory system terms. For a more comprehensive list, refer to the Terminology section of this chapter.

Combining Forms

aer/o	air	**muc/o**	mucus
alveol/o	alveolus	**nas/o**	nose
anthrac/o	coal	**ox/o, ox/i**	oxygen
atel/o	incomplete	**pharyng/o**	pharynx
bronch/o	bronchus	**pleur/o**	pleura
bronchi/o	bronchus	**pneum/o**	lung, air
bronchiol/o	bronchiole	**pneumon/o**	lung, air
coni/o	dust	**pulmon/o**	lung
cyan/o	blue	**rhin/o**	nose
cyst/o	sac	**sept/o**	wall
diaphragmat/o	diaphragm	**sinus/o**	sinus
epiglott/o	epiglottis	**somn/o**	sleep
hal/o	to breathe	**spir/o**	breathing
laryng/o	larynx	**trache/o**	trachea
lob/o	lobe	**tuss/o**	cough

Suffixes

-capnia	carbon dioxide	**-pnea**	breathing
-osmia	smell	**-ptysis**	spitting
-phonia	voice	**-thorax**	chest
-phylaxis	protection		

Respiratory System Illustrated

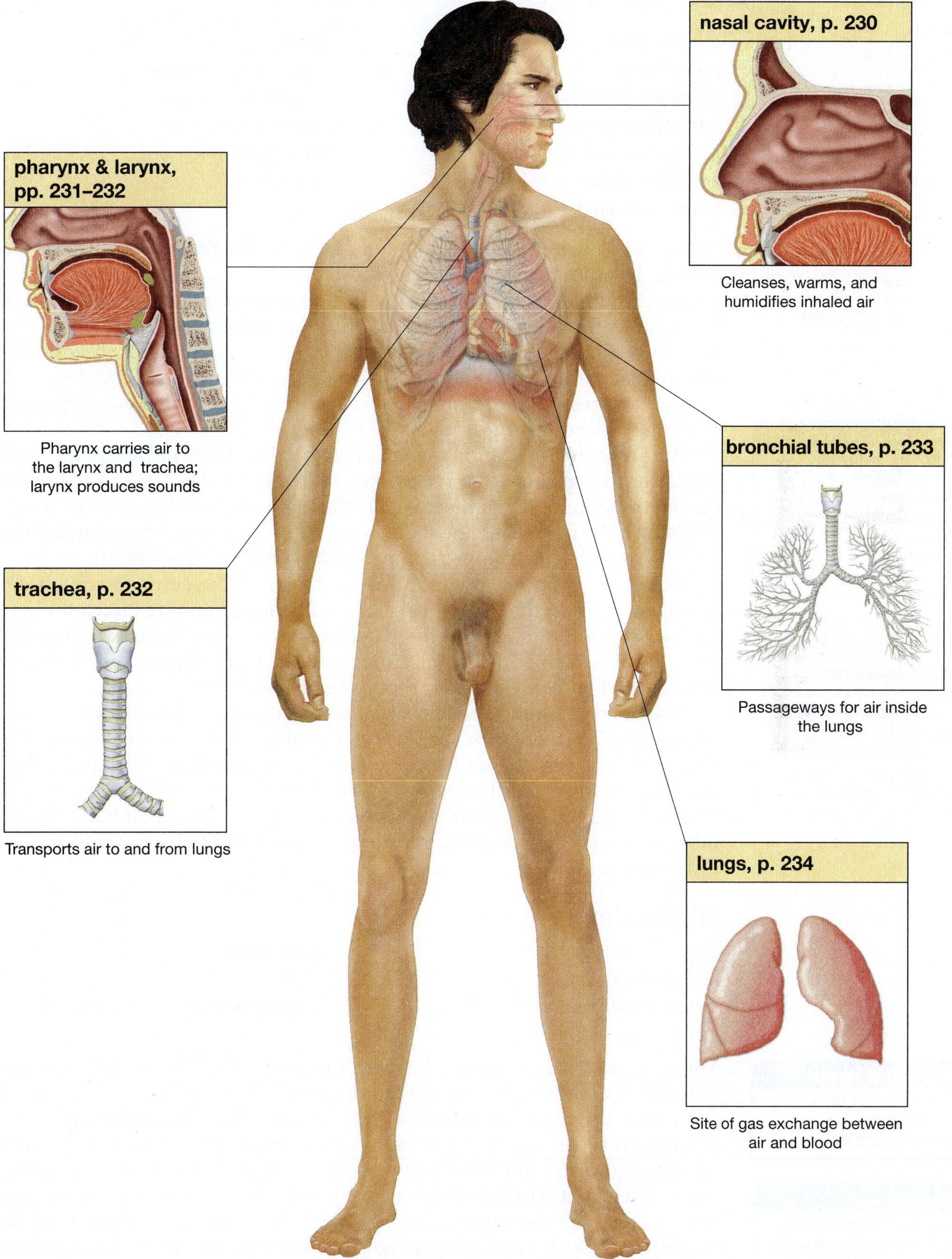

nasal cavity, p. 230
Cleanses, warms, and humidifies inhaled air
pharynx & larynx, pp. 231–232
Pharynx carries air to the larynx and trachea; larynx produces sounds
bronchial tubes, p. 233
Passageways for air inside the lungs
trachea, p. 232
Transports air to and from lungs
lungs, p. 234
Site of gas exchange between air and blood

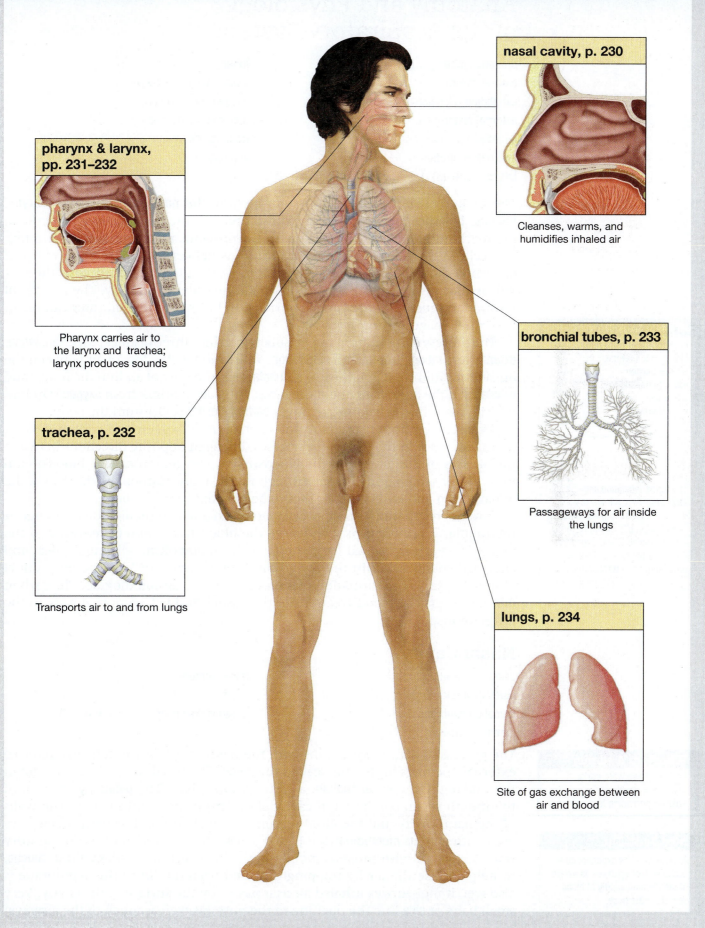

Anatomy and Physiology of the Respiratory System

bronchial tubes (BRONG-kee-al)
carbon dioxide
exhalation (eks-hah-LAY-shun)
external respiration
inhalation (in-hah-LAY-shun)
internal respiration
larynx (LAIR-inks)
lungs
nasal cavity (NAY-zal)
oxygen (OK-sih-jen)
pharynx (FAIR-inks)
trachea (TRAY-kee-ah)
ventilation

The organs of the respiratory system include the **nasal cavity**, **pharynx**, **larynx**, **trachea**, **bronchial tubes**, and **lungs**. These organs function together to perform the mechanical and, for the most part, unconscious mechanism of respiration. The cells of the body require the continuous delivery of oxygen and removal of carbon dioxide. The respiratory system works in conjunction with the cardiovascular system to deliver oxygen to all the cells of the body. The process of respiration must be continuous; interruption for even a few minutes can result in brain damage and/or death.

What's In A Name?

Look for these word parts:
hal/o = to breathe
ox/i = oxygen
-al = pertaining to
di- = two
ex- = outward
in- = inward

The process of respiration can be subdivided into three distinct parts: **ventilation**, **external respiration**, and **internal respiration**. Ventilation is the flow of air between the outside environment and the lungs. **Inhalation** is the flow of air into the lungs, and **exhalation** is the flow of air out of the lungs. Inhalation brings fresh **oxygen** (O_2) into the air sacs, while exhalation removes **carbon dioxide** (CO_2) from the body.

External respiration refers to the exchange of oxygen and carbon dioxide that takes place in the lungs. These gases diffuse in opposite directions between the air sacs of the lungs and the bloodstream. Oxygen enters the bloodstream from the air sacs to be delivered throughout the body. Carbon dioxide leaves the bloodstream and enters the air sacs to be exhaled from the body.

Word Watch

The terms *inhalation* and *inspiration* (**in-** = inward + **spir/o** = breathing) can be used interchangeably. Similarly, the terms *exhalation* and *expiration* (**ex-** = outward + **spir/o** = breathing) are interchangeable.

Internal respiration is the process of oxygen and carbon dioxide exchange at the cellular level when oxygen leaves the bloodstream and is delivered to the tissues. Oxygen is needed for the body cells' metabolism, all the physical and chemical changes within the body that are necessary for life. The by-product of metabolism is the formation of a waste product, carbon dioxide. The carbon dioxide enters the bloodstream from the tissues and is transported back to the lungs for disposal.

Nasal Cavity

cilia (SIL-ee-ah)
mucus (MYOO-kus)
mucous membrane
nares (NAIR-eez)
nasal septum
palate (PAL-et)
paranasal sinuses (pair-ah-NAY-zal)

What's In A Name?

Look for these word parts:
muc/o = mucus
-ous = pertaining to

Med Term Tip

Anyone who has experienced a nosebleed, or *epistaxis*, is aware of the plentiful supply of blood vessels in the nose.

The process of ventilation begins with the nasal cavity. Air enters through two external openings in the nose called the **nares**. The nasal cavity is divided down the middle by the **nasal septum**, a cartilaginous plate. The **palate** in the roof of the mouth separates the nasal cavity above from the mouth below. The walls of the nasal cavity and the nasal septum are made up of flexible cartilage covered with **mucous membrane** (see Figure 7-1 ■). In fact, much of the respiratory tract is covered with mucous membrane, which secretes a sticky fluid, **mucus**, to help cleanse the air by trapping dust and bacteria. Since this membrane is also wet, it moisturizes inhaled air as it passes by the surface of the cavity. Very small hairs or **cilia** line the opening to the nose (as well as much of the airways)

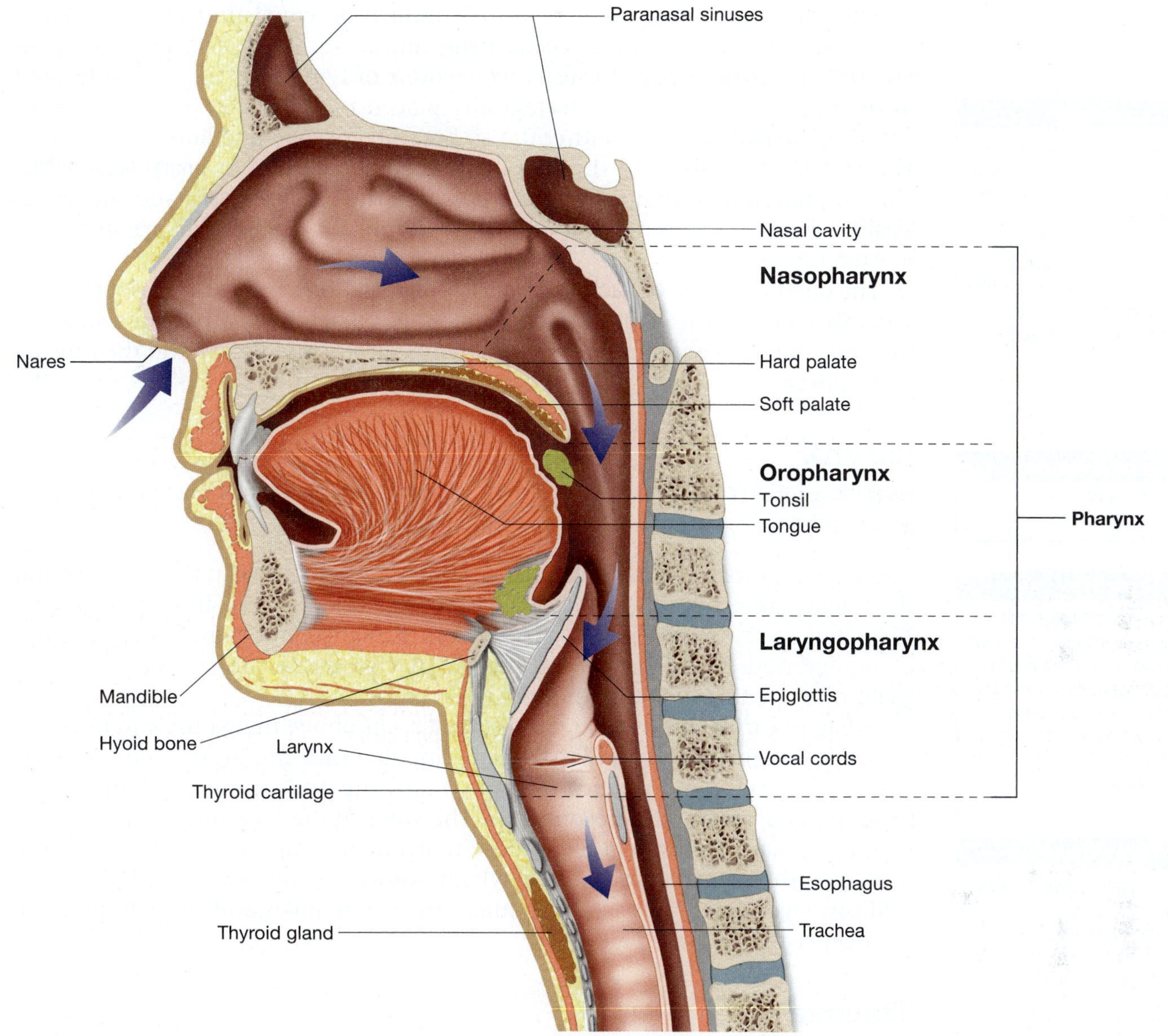

■ **Figure 7-1** Sagittal section of upper respiratory system illustrating the internal anatomy of the nasal cavity, pharynx, larynx, and trachea.

and filter out large dirt particles before they can enter the lungs. Capillaries in the mucous membranes warm inhaled air as it passes through the airways. Additionally, several **paranasal sinuses**, or air-filled cavities, are located within the facial bones. The sinuses act as an echo chamber during sound production and give resonance to the voice.

Word Watch

The term *cilia* means *hair*, and there are other body systems that have cilia or cilialike processes. For example, when discussing the eye, *cilia* means *eyelashes*.

Pharynx

adenoids (AD-eh-noydz)
auditory tube
eustachian tube (yoo-STAY-shee-en)
laryngopharynx (lah-ring-goh-FAIR-inks)
lingual tonsils (LING-gwal)
nasopharynx (nay-zoh-FAIR-inks)
oropharynx (or-oh-FAIR-inks)
palatine tonsils (PAL-ah-tyne)
pharyngeal tonsils (fair-IN-jee-al)

Air next enters the pharynx, also referred to as the *throat*, which is used by both the respiratory and digestive systems. At the end of the pharynx, air enters the trachea while food and liquids are shunted into the esophagus.

What's In A Name?

Look for these word parts:
audit/o = hearing
lingu/o = tongue
-al = pertaining to
-ory = pertaining to

The pharynx is roughly a five-inch-long tube consisting of three parts: the upper **nasopharynx**, middle **oropharynx**, and lower **laryngopharynx** (see again Figure 7-1). Three pairs of tonsils (collections of lymphatic tissue) are located in the pharynx. Tonsils are strategically placed to help keep pathogens from entering the body through either the air breathed or food and liquid swallowed. The nasopharynx, behind the nose, contains the **adenoids** or **pharyngeal tonsils**. The oropharynx, behind the mouth, contains the **palatine tonsils** and the **lingual tonsils**. Tonsils are considered a part of the lymphatic system and are discussed in Chapter 6.

The opening of the **eustachian** or **auditory tube** is also found in the nasopharynx. The other end of this tube is in the middle ear. Each time a person swallows, this tube opens to equalize air pressure between the middle ear and the outside atmosphere.

Med Term Tip

In the early 1970s, it was common practice to remove the tonsils and adenoids in children suffering from repeated infections. However, it is now understood how important these organs are in removing pathogens from the air we breathe and the food we eat. Antibiotic treatment has also reduced the severity of infections.

Larynx

epiglottis (ep-ih-GLOT-iss)
glottis (GLOT-iss)
thyroid cartilage (THIGH-royd / KAR-tih-lij)
vocal cords

The larynx, or *voice box*, is a muscular structure located between the pharynx and the trachea and contains the **vocal cords** (see again Figure 7-1 and Figure 7-2■). The vocal cords are not actually cordlike in structure, but rather they are folds of membranous tissue that produce sound by vibrating as air passes through the **glottis**, the opening between the two vocal cords.

A flap of cartilaginous tissue, the **epiglottis**, sits above the glottis and provides protection against food and liquid being inhaled into the lungs. The epiglottis covers the larynx and trachea during swallowing and shunts food and liquid from the pharynx into the esophagus. The walls of the larynx are composed of several cartilage plates held together with ligaments and muscles. One of these cartilages, the **thyroid cartilage**, forms what is known as the *Adam's apple*. The thyroid cartilage is generally larger in males than in females and helps to produce the deeper male voice.

What's In A Name?

Look for this word part:
epi- = above

Med Term Tip

Stuttering may actually result from faulty neuromuscular control of the larynx. Some stutterers can sing or whisper without difficulty. Both singing and whispering involve movements of the larynx that differ from those required for regular speech.

Med Term Tip

The term *Adam's apple* is thought to come from a fable that when Adam realized he had sinned in the Garden of Eden, he was unable to swallow the apple in his throat.

Trachea

The trachea, also called the *windpipe*, is the passageway for air that extends from the pharynx and larynx down to the main bronchi (see Figure 7-3■). Measuring approximately four inches in length, it is composed of smooth muscle and cartilage rings and is lined by mucous membrane and cilia. Therefore, it also assists in cleansing, warming, and moisturizing air as it travels to the lungs.

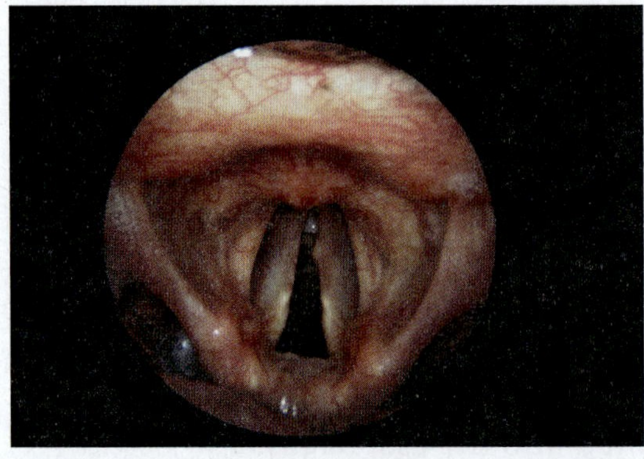

■ **Figure 7-2** The vocal cords within the larynx, superior view from the pharynx. *(CNRI/Science Source)*

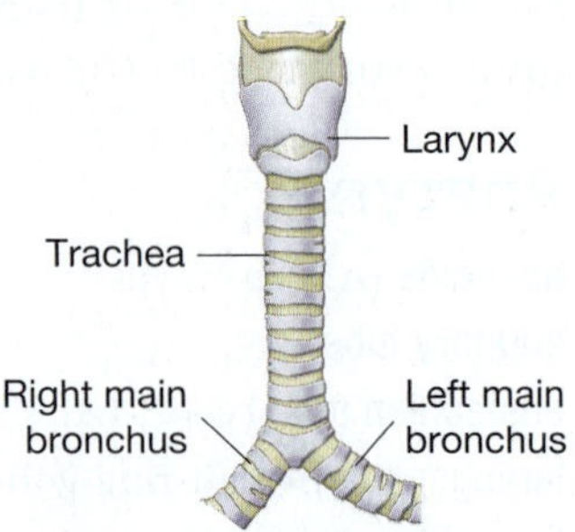

■ **Figure 7-3** Structure of the trachea, which extends from the larynx above to the main bronchi below.

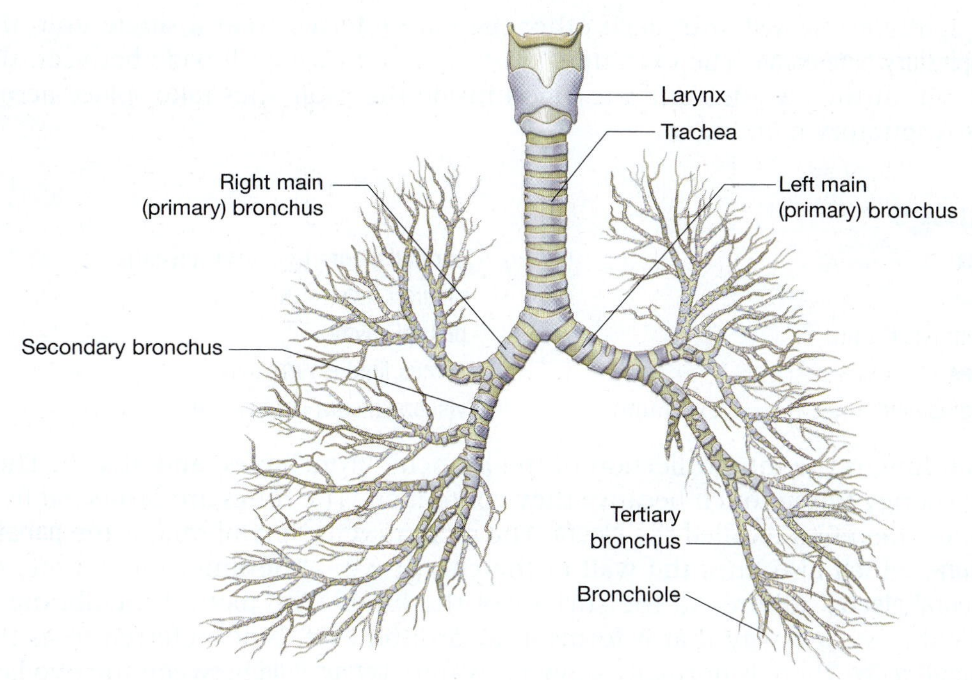

■ **Figure 7-4** The bronchial tree. Note how each main bronchus enters a lung and then branches into smaller and smaller primary bronchi, secondary bronchi, and bronchioles.

Bronchial Tubes

alveoli (al-VEE-oh-lye)
bronchioles (BRONG-kee-ohlz)
bronchus (BRONG-kus)
pulmonary capillaries
respiratory membrane

The distal end of the trachea divides to form the left and right main (primary) bronchi. Each **bronchus** enters one of the lungs and branches repeatedly to form secondary and tertiary bronchi. Each branch becomes narrower until the narrowest branches, the **bronchioles**, are formed (see Figure 7-4 ■). Each bronchiole terminates in a small group of air sacs, called **alveoli**. Each lung has approximately 150 million alveoli. The walls of alveoli are elastic, giving them the ability to expand to hold air and then recoil to their original size. A network of **pulmonary capillaries** from the pulmonary blood vessels tightly encases each alveolus (see Figure 7-5 ■). In fact, the walls of the alveoli and capillaries are

What's In A Name?

Look for these word parts:
bronchi/o = bronchus
-ole = small

Med Term Tip

The respiratory system can be thought of as an upside-down tree and its branches. The trunk of the tree consists of the pharynx, larynx, and trachea. The trachea then divides into two branches, the bronchi. Each bronchus further divides into smaller and smaller branches. In fact, this branching system of tubes is referred to as the *bronchial tree*.

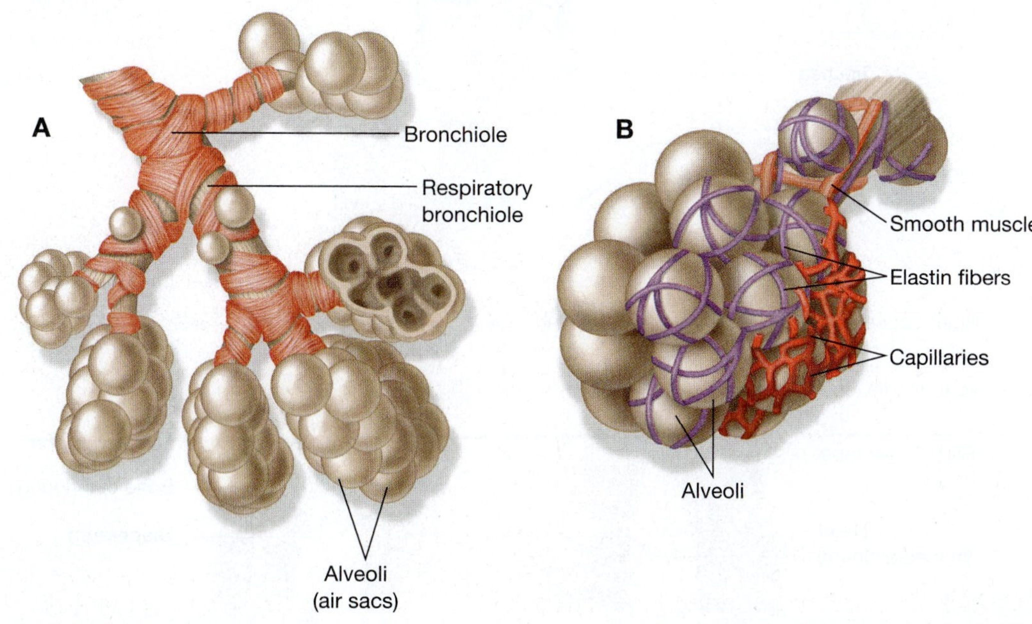

■ **Figure 7-5** A) Each bronchiole terminates in an alveolar sac, a group of alveoli. B) Alveoli encased by network capillaries, forming the respiratory membrane.

so tightly associated with each other they are referred to as a single unit, the **respiratory membrane**. The exchange of oxygen and carbon dioxide between the air within the alveolus and the blood inside the capillaries takes place across the respiratory membrane.

Lungs

apex
base
hilum (HYE-lum)
lobes
mediastinum (mee-dee-as-TYE-num)
parietal pleura (pah-RYE-eh-tal)
pleura (PLOO-rah)
pleural cavity
serous fluid (SEER-us)
visceral pleura (VISS-er-al)

What's In A Name?
Look for these word parts:
pariet/o = cavity wall
viscer/o = internal organs
-al = pertaining to
-ous = pertaining to

Each lung is the total collection of the bronchi, bronchioles, and alveoli. They are spongy to the touch because they contain air. The lungs are protected by a double membrane called the **pleura**. The pleura's outer membrane is the **parietal pleura**, which also lines the wall of the chest cavity. The inner membrane, or **visceral pleura**, adheres to the surface of the lungs. The pleural membrane is folded in such a way that it forms a sac around each lung, referred to as the **pleural cavity**. There is normally slippery, watery **serous fluid** between the two layers of the pleura that reduces friction when the two layers rub together as the lungs repeatedly expand and contract.

The lungs contain divisions or **lobes**. There are three lobes in the larger right lung (right upper, right middle, and right lower lobes) and two in the left lung (left upper and left lower lobes). The pointed superior portion of each lung is the **apex**, while the broader lower area is the **base**. Entry of structures like the bronchi, pulmonary blood vessels, and nerves into each lung occurs along its medial border in an area called the **hilum**. The lungs within the thoracic cavity are protected from puncture and damage by the ribs. The area between the right and left lung is called the **mediastinum** and contains the heart, aorta, esophagus, thymus gland, and trachea. See Figure 7-6 ■ for an illustration of the lungs within the chest cavity.

Med Term Tip
Some of the abnormal lung sounds heard with a stethoscope, such as crackling and rubbing, are made when the parietal and/or visceral pleura become inflamed and rub against one another.

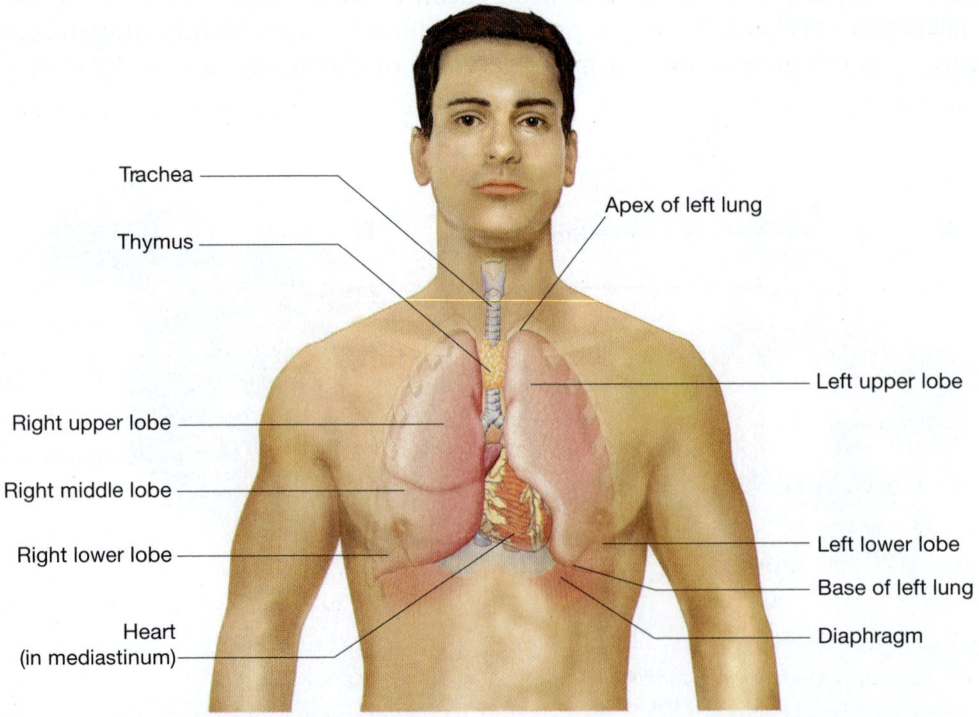

■ **Figure 7-6** Position of the lungs within the thoracic cavity; anterior view illustrating regions of the lungs and their relationship to other thoracic organs.

PRACTICE AS YOU GO

A. Complete the Statement

1. The organs of the respiratory system are ______________, ______________, ______________, ______________, ______________, and ______________.
2. The passageway for food, liquids, and air is the ______________.
3. The ______________ helps to keep food out of the respiratory tract.
4. The right lung has ______________ lobes; the left lung has ______________ lobes.
5. The air sacs at the ends of the bronchial tree are called ______________.
6. The term for the double membrane around the lungs is ______________.
7. The small branches of the bronchi are the ______________ and the air sacs are the ______________.

Lung Volumes and Capacities

pulmonary function test **respiratory therapist**

For some types of medical conditions, like emphysema, it is important to measure the volume of air flowing in and out of the lungs to determine lung capacity. Lung volumes are measured by **respiratory therapists** to aid in determining the functioning level of the respiratory system. Collectively, these measurements are called **pulmonary function tests**. Table 7-1 ■ lists and defines the four lung volumes and four lung capacities.

What's In A Name?
Look for these word parts:
spir/o = breathing
-ory = pertaining to
re- = again

Respiratory Muscles

diaphragm **intercostal muscles** (in-ter-KOS-tal)

Air moves in and out of the lungs due to the difference between the atmospheric pressure and the pressure within the chest cavity. The **diaphragm**, the muscle separating the abdomen from the thoracic cavity, produces this difference

What's In A Name?
Look for these word parts:
cost/o = ribs
-al = pertaining to
inter- = between

■ **TABLE 7-1** Lung Volumes and Capacities

Term	Definition
Tidal volume (TV)	Amount of air that enters lungs in a single inhalation or leaves lungs in a single exhalation of quiet breathing; in an adult this is normally 500 mL*
Inspiratory reserve volume (IRV)	Amount of air that can be forcibly inhaled after normal inspiration; also called *complemental air*, generally measures around 3,000 mL*
Expiratory reserve volume (ERV)	Amount of air that can be forcibly exhaled after normal, quiet exhalation; also called *supplemental air*, approximately 1,000 mL*
Residual volume (RV)	Air remaining in lungs after forced exhalation; about 1,500 mL* in an adult
Inspiratory capacity (IC)	Volume of air inhaled after normal exhale
Functional residual capacity (FRC)	Air that remains in lungs after normal exhalation has taken place
Vital capacity (VC)	Total volume of air that can be exhaled after maximum inhalation; amount will be equal to sum of TV, IRV, and ERV
Total lung capacity (TLC)	Volume of air in lungs after maximal inhalation

*There is a normal range for measurements of volume of air exchanged; numbers given are for average measurement.

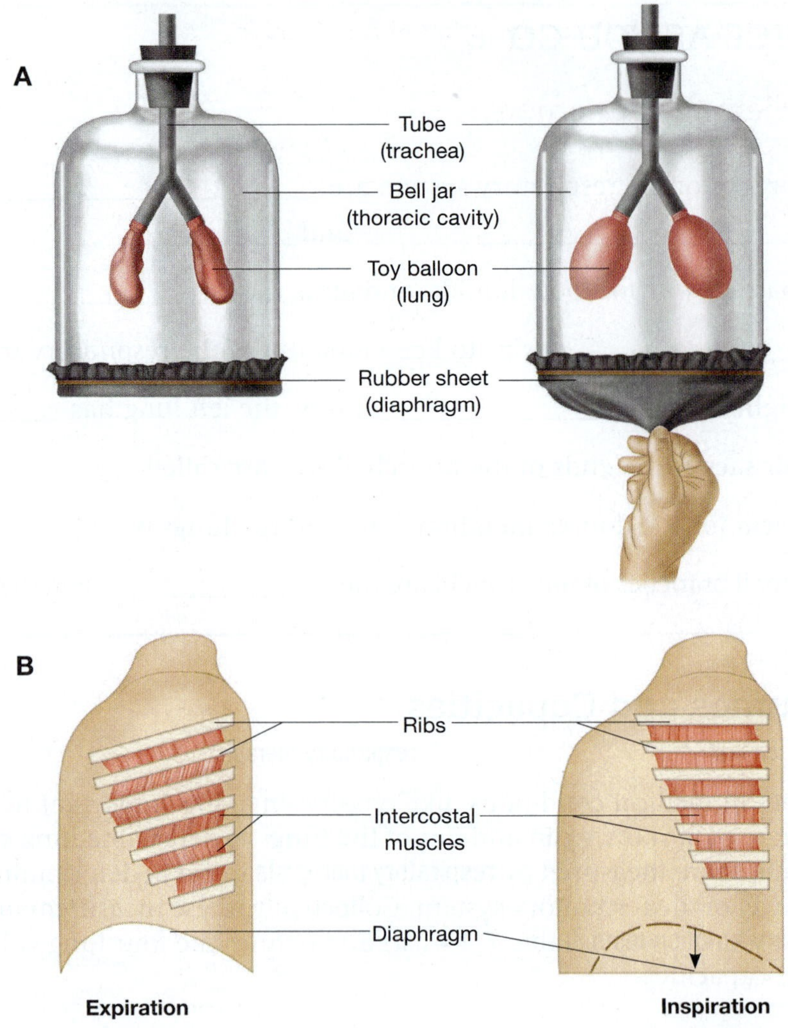

Figure 7-7 A) Bell jar apparatus demonstrating how downward movement of the diaphragm results in air flowing into the lungs. B) Action of the intercostal muscles lifts the ribs to assist the diaphragm in enlarging the volume of the thoracic cavity.

in pressure. To do this, the diaphragm contracts and moves downward. This increase in thoracic cavity volume causes a decrease in pressure, or negative thoracic pressure, within the chest cavity. Air then flows into the lungs (inhalation) to equalize the pressure. The **intercostal muscles** between the ribs assist in inhalation by raising the rib cage to further enlarge the thoracic cavity. See Figure 7-7 ■ for an illustration of the role of the diaphragm in inhalation. Similarly, when the diaphragm and intercostal muscles relax, the thoracic cavity becomes smaller. This produces an increase in pressure within the cavity, or positive thoracic pressure, and air flows out of the lungs, resulting in exhalation. Therefore, a quiet, unforced exhalation is a passive process since it does not require any muscle contraction. When a forceful inhalation or exhalation is required, additional chest and neck muscles become active to create larger changes in thoracic pressure.

Med Term Tip

Diaphragmatic breathing is taught to singers and public speakers. You can practice this type of breathing by allowing your abdomen to expand during inhalation and contract during exhalation while your shoulders remain motionless.

Respiratory Rate

vital signs

Respiratory rate (measured in breaths per minute) is one of the body's **vital signs** (VS), along with heart rate, temperature, and blood pressure. The respiratory rate is normally regulated by the level of CO_2 in the blood. When the CO_2 level is high, breathing is more rapid to expel the excess. Likewise, when CO_2 levels drop, the respiratory rate will also drop.

TABLE 7-2 Respiratory Rates for Different Age Groups

Age	Respirations Per Minute
Newborn	30–60
1-year-old	18–30
16-year-old	16–20
Adult	12–20

When the respiratory rate falls outside the range of normal, it may indicate an illness or medical condition. For example, when a patient is running an elevated temperature and has shortness of breath (SOB) due to pneumonia, the respiratory rate may increase dramatically. Or a brain injury or some medications, such as those for pain, can cause a decrease in the respiratory rate. See Table 7-2 for normal respiratory rate ranges for different age groups.

PRACTICE AS YOU GO

B. Lung Volumes and Capacities Matching

1. ________ tidal volume
2. ________ residual volume
3. ________ vital capacity
4. ________ inspiratory reserve volume
5. ________ total lung capacity
6. ________ expiratory reserve volume
7. ________ inspiratory capacity
8. ________ functional residual capacity

a. air that can be exhaled after a maximum inhalation
b. air forcibly exhaled after normal quiet exhalation
c. air that enters lungs in a single inhalation
d. air still in lungs after normal exhalation
e. air inhaled after normal exhale
f. air in lungs after forced exhalation
g. air in lungs after a maximal inhalation
h. air forcibly inhaled after normal inspiration

Terminology

Word Parts Used to Build Respiratory System Terms

The following lists contain the combining forms, suffixes, and prefixes used to build terms in the remaining sections of this chapter.

Combining Forms

aer/o	air	**atel/o**	incomplete	**carcin/o**	cancer
alveol/o	alveolus	**bi/o**	life	**cardi/o**	heart
angi/o	vessel	**bronch/o**	bronchus	**coni/o**	dust
anthrac/o	coal	**bronchi/o**	bronchus	**cortic/o**	outer layer
arteri/o	artery	**bronchiol/o**	bronchiole	**cyan/o**	blue

Combining Forms (continued)

cyst/o	sac	**myc/o**	fungus	**py/o**	pus
cyt/o	cell	**nas/o**	nose	**rhin/o**	nose
diaphragmat/o	diaphragm	**orth/o**	straight	**sept/o**	wall
embol/o	plug	**ot/o**	ear	**sinus/o**	sinus
epiglott/o	epiglottis	**ox/i**	oxygen	**somn/o**	sleep
fibr/o	fibers	**ox/o**	oxygen	**spir/o**	breathing
hem/o	blood	**pharyng/o**	pharynx	**thorac/o**	chest
hist/o	tissue	**pleur/o**	pleura	**trache/o**	trachea
laryng/o	larynx	**pneum/o**	air	**tuss/o**	cough
lob/o	lobe	**pneumon/o**	lung		
muc/o	mucus	**pulmon/o**	lung		

Suffixes

-al	pertaining to	**-ism**	state of	**-plasm**	formation
-algia	pain	**-itis**	inflammation	**-plasty**	surgical repair
-ar	pertaining to	**-logy**	study of	**-plegia**	paralysis
-ary	pertaining to	**-lytic**	destruction	**-pnea**	breathing
-capnia	carbon dioxide	**-meter**	instrument to measure	**-ptysis**	spitting
-centesis	puncture to withdraw fluid	**-metry**	process of measuring	**-rrhagia**	abnormal flow condition
-dynia	pain	**-oma**	tumor	**-rrhea**	discharge
-eal	pertaining to	**-ory**	pertaining to	**-scope**	instrument for viewing
-ectasis	dilation	**-osis**	abnormal condition	**-scopy**	process of visually examining
-ectomy	surgical removal	**-osmia**	smell	**-spasm**	involuntary muscle contraction
-emia	blood condition	**-ostomy**	surgically create an opening	**-stenosis**	narrowing
-genic	produced by	**-otomy**	cutting into	**-thorax**	chest
-gram	record	**-ous**	pertaining to	**-tic**	pertaining to
-graphy	process of recording	**-phonia**	voice		
-ia	condition	**-phylaxis**	protection		
-ic	pertaining to				

Prefixes

a-	without	**endo-**	within	**poly-**	many
an-	without	**eu-**	normal	**pro-**	before
anti-	against	**hyper-**	excessive	**re-**	again
brady-	slow	**hypo-**	insufficient	**tachy-**	fast
de-	without	**pan-**	all		
dys-	difficult, abnormal	**para-**	beside		

Adjective Forms of Anatomical Terms

Term	Word Parts	Definition
alveolar (al-VEE-oh-lar)	alveol/o = alveolus -ar = pertaining to	Pertaining to alveoli
bronchial (BRONG-kee-al)	bronchi/o = bronchus -al = pertaining to	Pertaining to a bronchus
bronchiolar (brong-KEE-oh-lar)	bronchiol/o = bronchiole -ar = pertaining to	Pertaining to a bronchiole
diaphragmatic (dye-ah-frag-MAT-ik)	diaphragmat/o = diaphragm -ic = pertaining to	Pertaining to diaphragm
epiglottic (ep-ih-GLOT-ik)	epiglott/o = epiglottis -ic = pertaining to	Pertaining to epiglottis
laryngeal (lair-IN-jee-al)	laryng/o = larynx -eal = pertaining to	Pertaining to larynx
lobar (LOH-bar)	lob/o = lobe -ar = pertaining to	Pertaining to a lobe (of the lung)
mucous (MYOO-kus)	muc/o = mucus -ous = pertaining to	Pertaining to mucus
nasal (NAY-zal)	nas/o = nose -al = pertaining to	Pertaining to nose or nasal cavity
nasopharyngeal (nay-zoh-fah-RIN-jee-al)	nas/o = nose pharyng/o = pharynx -eal = pertaining to	Pertaining to nose and pharynx
paranasal (pair-ah-NAY-zal)	para- = beside nas/o = nose -al = pertaining to	Pertaining to beside the nose
pharyngeal (fair-IN-jee-al)	pharyng/o = pharynx -eal = pertaining to	Pertaining to pharynx
pleural (PLOO-ral)	pleur/o = pleura -al = pertaining to	Pertaining to pleura
pulmonary (PULL-mon-air-ee)	pulmon/o = lung -ary = pertaining to	Pertaining to lung
septal (SEP-tal)	sept/o = wall -al = pertaining to	Pertaining to wall (i.e., nasal septum)
thoracic (tho-RASS-ik)	thorac/o = chest -ic = pertaining to	Pertaining to chest
tracheal (TRAY-kee-al)	trache/o = trachea -al = pertaining to	Pertaining to trachea

PRACTICE AS YOU GO

C. Give the adjective form for each anatomical structure.

1. The larynx ____________________
2. The lung ____________________
3. Beside the nose ____________________
4. An alveolus ____________________
5. The nose ____________________
6. The diaphragm ____________________

Pathology

Term	Word Parts	Definition
Medical Specialties		
internal medicine		Branch of medicine involving diagnosis and treatment of diseases and conditions of internal organs such as respiratory system; physician is an *internist*
otorhinolaryngology (ENT) (oh-toh-rye-noh-lair-in-GALL-oh-jee)	ot/o = ear rhin/o = nose laryng/o = larynx -logy = study of	Branch of medicine involving diagnosis and treatment of conditions and diseases of ear, nose, and throat region; physician is *otorhinolaryngologist*; this medical specialty may also be referred to as *otolaryngology*
pulmonology (pull-mon-NALL-oh-jee)	pulmon/o = lung -logy = study of	Branch of medicine involved in diagnosis and treatment of diseases and disorders of respiratory system; physician is *pulmonologist*
respiratory therapy	re- = again spir/o = breathing -ory = pertaining to	Allied health specialty that assists patients with respiratory and cardiopulmonary disorders; duties of *respiratory therapist* include conducting pulmonary function tests, monitoring oxygen and carbon dioxide levels in blood, administering breathing treatments, and ventilator management
thoracic surgery (tho-RASS-ik)	thorac/o = chest -ic = pertaining to	Branch of medicine involving diagnosis and treatment of conditions and diseases of respiratory system by surgical means; physician is *thoracic surgeon*
Signs and Symptoms		
anosmia (an-OZ-mee-ah)	an- = without -osmia = smell	Lack of sense of smell

Pathology (continued)

Term	Word Parts	Definition
anoxia (an-OK-see-ah)	an- = without ox/o = oxygen -ia = condition	Condition of receiving almost no oxygen from inhaled air
aphonia (ah-FOH-nee-ah)	a- = without -phonia = voice	Condition of being unable to produce sounds
apnea (AP-nee-ah)	a- = without -pnea = breathing	Not breathing
asphyxia (as-FIK-see-ah)	a- = without -ia = condition	Lack of oxygen that can lead to unconsciousness and death if not corrected immediately; also called *asphyxiation* or *suffocation*; common causes include drowning, foreign body in respiratory tract, poisoning, and electric shock
aspiration (as-pih-RAY-shun)	spir/o = breathing	Refers to withdrawing fluid from body cavity using suction; for example, using long needle and syringe to withdraw fluid from pleural cavity, or using vacuum pump to remove phlegm from patient's airway; additionally, refers to inhaling food, liquid, or foreign object into airways, which may lead to development of pneumonia
bradypnea (brad-ip-NEE-ah)	brady- = slow -pnea = breathing	Breathing too slowly; low respiratory rate
bronchiectasis (brong-kee-EK-tah-sis)	bronchi/o = bronchus -ectasis = dilation	Dilated bronchus
bronchospasm (BRONG-koh-spazm)	bronch/o = bronchus -spasm = involuntary muscle contraction	Involuntary muscle spasm of smooth muscle in the wall of bronchus
Cheyne–Stokes respiration (CHAIN / STOHKS / res-pir-AY-shun)	re- = again spir/o = breathing	Abnormal breathing pattern in which there are long periods (10–60 seconds) of apnea followed by deeper, more rapid breathing; named for John Cheyne, a Scottish physician, and Sir William Stokes, an Irish surgeon
clubbing		Abnormal widening and thickening of ends of fingers and toes associated with chronic oxygen deficiency; seen in patients with chronic respiratory conditions or circulatory problems
crackles		Abnormal crackling or bubbling sound made during inspiration; usually indicates presence of fluid or mucus in small airways; also called *rales*

Pathology (continued)

Term	Word Parts	Definition
cyanosis (sigh-ah-NOH-sis)	cyan/o = blue -osis = abnormal condition	Refers to bluish tint of skin that is receiving insufficient amount of oxygen or circulation
dysphonia (dis-FOH-nee-ah)	dys- = difficult, abnormal -phonia = voice	Condition of having difficulty producing sounds or producing abnormal sounds
dyspnea (DISP-nee-ah)	dys- = difficult -pnea = breathing	Term describing difficult or labored breathing
epistaxis (ep-ih-STAK-sis)		Nosebleed
eupnea (yoop-NEE-ah)	eu- = normal -pnea = breathing	Normal breathing and respiratory rate
hemoptysis (hee-MOP-tih-sis)	hem/o = blood -ptysis = spitting	To cough up blood or blood-stained sputum
hemothorax (hee-moh-THOH-raks)	hem/o = blood -thorax = chest	Presence of blood in chest cavity
hypercapnia (high-per-KAP-nee-ah)	hyper- = excessive -capnia = carbon dioxide	Condition of having excessive carbon dioxide in body
hyperpnea (high-PERP-nee-ah)	hyper- = excessive -pnea = breathing	Taking deep breaths
hyperventilation (high-per-ven-tih-LAY-shun)	hyper- = excessive	Breathing both too fast (tachypnea) and too deep (hyperpnea)
hypocapnia (high-poh-KAP-nee-ah)	hypo- = insufficient -capnia = carbon dioxide	Insufficient level of carbon dioxide in body; very serious problem because it is presence of carbon dioxide that stimulates respiration, not absence of oxygen; therefore, person with low carbon dioxide levels would respond with increased respiratory rate
hypopnea (high-POP-nee-ah)	hypo- = insufficient -pnea = breathing	Taking shallow breaths

Figure 7-8 A cyanotic infant. Note the bluish tinge to the skin around the lips, chin, and nose.
(St Bartholomew's Hospital, London/Science Source)

Med Term Tip

When divers wish to hold their breath longer, they first hyperventilate (breathe faster and deeper) in order to get rid of as much CO_2 as possible. This will hold off the urge to breathe, allowing a diver to stay submerged longer.

Pathology (continued)

Term	Word Parts	Definition
hypoventilation (high-poh-ven-tih-LAY-shun)	hypo- = insufficient	Breathing both too slow (bradypnea) and too shallow (hypopnea)
hypoxemia (high-pok-SEE-mee-ah)	hypo- = insufficient ox/o = oxygen -emia = blood condition	Condition of having insufficient amount of oxygen in bloodstream
hypoxia (high-POK-see-ah)	hypo- = insufficient ox/o = oxygen -ia = condition	Condition of receiving insufficient amount of oxygen from inhaled air
laryngoplegia (lah-ring-goh-PLEE-jee-ah)	laryng/o = larynx -plegia = paralysis	Paralysis of muscles controlling larynx
orthopnea (or-THOP-nee-ah)	orth/o = straight -pnea = breathing	Term describing dyspnea worsened by lying flat; patient feels able to breathe easier while sitting straight up; common occurrence in those with pulmonary disease
pansinusitis (pan-sigh-nus-EYE-tis)	pan- = all sinus/o = sinus -itis = inflammation	Inflammation of all paranasal sinuses
patent (PAY-tent)		Open or unblocked, such as patent airway
phlegm (FLEM)		Thick mucus secreted by membranes lining respiratory tract; when phlegm is coughed through mouth, is called *sputum*; phlegm is examined for color, odor, and consistency and tested for presence of bacteria, viruses, and fungi
pleural rub (PLOO-ral)	pleur/o = pleura -al = pertaining to	Grating sound made when two layers of pleura rub together during respiration; caused when one surface becomes thicker as a result of inflammation or other disease conditions; rub can be felt through fingertips when placed on chest wall or heard through stethoscope
pleurodynia (ploor-oh-DIN-ee-ah)	pleur/o = pleura -dynia = pain	Pleural pain
pyothorax (pye-oh-THOH-raks)	py/o = pus -thorax = chest	Presence of pus in chest cavity; indicates bacterial infection
rhinitis (rye-NYE-tis)	rhin/o = nose -itis = inflammation	Inflammation of nasal cavity
rhinorrhagia (rye-noh-RAY-jee-ah)	rhin/o = nose -rrhagia = abnormal flow condition	Rapid flow of blood from nose
rhinorrhea (rye-noh-REE-ah)	rhin/o = nose -rrhea = discharge	Discharge from nose; commonly called a *runny nose*
rhonchi (RONG-kigh)		Somewhat musical sound during expiration, often found in asthma or infection; caused by spasms of bronchial tubes; also called *wheezing*

Pathology (continued)

Term	Word Parts	Definition
shortness of breath (SOB)		Term used to indicate patient is having some difficulty breathing; also called *dyspnea*; causes can range from mild SOB after exercise to SOB associated with heart disease
sputum (SPYOO-tum)		Mucus or phlegm coughed up from lining of respiratory tract
stridor (STRY-der)		Harsh, high-pitched, noisy breathing sound made when there is obstruction of bronchus or larynx; found in conditions such as croup in children
tachypnea (tak-ip-NEE-ah)	tachy- = fast -pnea = breathing	Breathing fast; high respiratory rate
thoracalgia (thor-ah-KAL-jee-ah)	thorac/o = chest -algia = pain	Chest pain; does not refer to angina pectoris
tracheostenosis (tray-kee-oh-steh-NOH-sis)	trache/o = trachea -stenosis = narrowing	Narrowing of trachea
Upper Respiratory System		
croup (KROOP)		Acute respiratory condition found in infants and children characterized by barking type of cough or stridor
diphtheria (dif-THEAR-ee-ah)	-ia = condition	Bacterial upper respiratory infection characterized by formation of thick membranous film across throat and high mortality rate; rare now, due to childhood diphtheria, pertussis, and tetanus (DPT) vaccines
laryngitis (lair-in-JYE-tis)	laryng/o = larynx -itis = inflammation	Inflammation of larynx
nasopharyngitis (nay-zoh-fair-in-JYE-tis)	nas/o = nose pharyng/o = pharynx -itis = inflammation	Inflammation of nasal cavity and pharynx; commonly called *common cold*
pertussis (per-TUH-sis)	tuss/o = cough	Infectious bacterial disease of upper respiratory system that children receive immunization against as part of their DPT shots; commonly called *whooping cough*, due to whoop sound made when coughing
pharyngitis (fair-in-JYE-tis)	pharyng/o = pharynx -itis = inflammation	Inflammation of pharynx; commonly called a *sore throat*
rhinomycosis (rye-noh-my-KOH-sis)	rhin/o = nose myc/o = fungus -osis = abnormal condition	Fungal infection of nasal cavity

Med Term Tip

The term *sputum*, from the Latin word meaning *to spit*, now refers to the material coughed up and spit out from the respiratory system.

Pathology (continued)

Term	Word Parts	Definition
Bronchial Tubes		
asthma (AZ-mah)		Disease caused by various conditions, like allergens, and resulting in constriction of bronchial airways, dyspnea, coughing, and wheezing; can cause violent spasms of bronchi (bronchospasms) but generally not life-threatening condition; medication can be very effective
bronchiectasis (brong-kee-EK-tah-sis)	bronchi/o = bronchus -ectasis = dilation	Abnormal enlargement of bronchi; may be result of lung infection; condition can be irreversible and result in destruction of bronchial walls; major symptoms include coughing up large amount of purulent sputum, crackles, and hemoptysis
bronchitis (brong-KIGH-tis)	bronch/o = bronchus -itis = inflammation	Inflammation of a bronchus
bronchogenic carcinoma (brong-koh-JEN-ik / kar-sih-NOH-mah)	bronch/o = bronchus -genic = produced by carcin/o = cancer -oma = tumor	Malignant tumor originating in bronchi; usually associated with history of cigarette smoking
Lungs		
acute respiratory distress syndrome (ARDS)	re- = again spir/o = breathing -ory = pertaining to	Acute respiratory failure in adults characterized by tachypnea, dyspnea, cyanosis, tachycardia, and hypoxemia; may follow trauma, pneumonia, or septic infections; also called *acute respiratory distress syndrome*
anthracosis (an-thrah-KOH-sis)	anthrac/o = coal -osis = abnormal condition	Type of pneumoconiosis that develops from collection of coal dust in lung; also called *black lung* or *miner's lung*
asbestosis (az-bes-TOH-sis)	-osis = abnormal condition	Type of pneumoconiosis that develops from collection of asbestos fibers in lungs; may lead to development of lung cancer
atelectasis (at-eh-LEK-tah-sis)	atel/o = incomplete -ectasis = dilation	Condition in which alveoli in a portion of the lung collapse, preventing respiratory exchange of oxygen and carbon dioxide; can be caused by variety of conditions, including pressure on lung from tumor or other object; term also used to describe failure of newborn's lungs to expand

Med Term Tip

The term *asthma*, from the Greek word meaning *panting*, describes the breathing pattern of a person having an asthma attack.

Lung cancer

Figure 7-9 Color-enhanced X-ray of large malignant tumor in the right lung. *(Wonderisland/Shutterstock)*

Pathology (continued)

Term	Word Parts	Definition
chronic obstructive pulmonary disease (COPD) (PULL-mon-air-ee)	pulmon/o = lung -ary = pertaining to	Progressive, chronic, and usually irreversible group of conditions (often a combination of chronic bronchitis and emphysema) in which lungs have diminished capacity for inhalation and exhalation; person may have dyspnea upon exertion and a cough
cystic fibrosis (CF) (SIS-tik / fye-BROH-sis)	cyst/o = sac -ic = pertaining to fibr/o = fibers -osis = abnormal condition	Hereditary condition causing exocrine glands to malfunction; patient produces very thick mucus that causes severe congestion within lungs, pancreas, and intestine; through more advanced treatment, many children are now living into adulthood with this disease
emphysema (em-fih-SEE-mah)		Pulmonary condition characterized by destruction of walls of alveoli, resulting in fewer, overexpanded air sacs; can occur as a result of long-term heavy smoking; air pollution also worsens disease; patient may not be able to breathe except in sitting or standing position
histoplasmosis (his-toh-plaz-MOH-sis)	hist/o = tissue -plasm = formation -osis = abnormal condition	Pulmonary infection caused by fungus *Histoplasma capsulatum*, found in dust and in droppings of pigeons and chickens
infant respiratory distress syndrome (IRDS)	re- = again spir/o = breathing -ory = pertaining to	Lung condition most commonly found in premature infants characterized by tachypnea and respiratory grunting; condition caused by lack of surfactant necessary to keep lungs inflated; also called *hyaline membrane disease* (HMD) and *respiratory distress syndrome of the newborn*
influenza (flu) (in-floo-EN-zah)		Viral infection of respiratory system characterized by chills, fever, body aches, and fatigue; commonly called the *flu*
Legionnaires' disease (lee-jen-AYRZ)		Severe, often fatal bacterial infection characterized by pneumonia and liver and kidney damage; named after people who came down with it at American Legion convention in 1976
Middle East respiratory syndrome (MERS)		Life-threatening viral respiratory illness first reported in Saudi Arabia in September 2012; symptoms include fever, cough, and shortness of breath
***Mycoplasma* pneumonia** (MY-koh-plaz-mah)	myc/o = fungus -plasm = formation	Less severe but longer-lasting form of pneumonia caused by *Mycoplasma pneumoniae* bacteria; also called *walking pneumonia*

Med Term Tip

Cystic fibrosis received its name from fibrotic cysts that are visible in the pancreas as scarred areas.

Pathology (continued)

Term	Word Parts	Definition
pneumoconiosis (noo-moh-koh-nee-OH-sis)	**pneum/o** = lung **coni/o** = dust **-osis** = abnormal condition	Condition resulting from inhalation of environmental particles that become toxic; can be result of inhaling coal dust (*anthracosis*) or asbestos (*asbestosis*)
pneumonia (noo-MOH-nee-ah)	**pneumon/o** = lung **-ia** = condition	Inflammatory condition of lung that can be caused by bacteria, viruses, fungi, and aspirated substances; results in filling of alveoli and air spaces with fluid
pulmonary edema (PULL-mon-air-ee / eh-DEE-mah)	**pulmon/o** = lung **-ary** = pertaining to	Condition in which lung tissue retains excessive amount of fluid, especially in alveoli; results in dyspnea
pulmonary embolism (PE) (EM-boh-lizm)	**pulmon/o** = lung **-ary** = pertaining to **embol/o** = plug **-ism** = state of	Obstruction of pulmonary artery or one of its branches by embolus (often blood clot broken away from another area of body); may cause infarct in lung tissue
pulmonary fibrosis (fye-BROH-sis)	**pulmon/o** = lung **-ary** = pertaining to **fibr/o** = fibers **-osis** = abnormal condition	Formation of fibrous scar tissue in lungs that leads to decreased ability to expand lungs; may be caused by infections, pneumoconiosis, autoimmune diseases, and toxin exposure
severe acute respiratory syndrome (SARS)	**re-** = again **spir/o** = breathing **-ory** = pertaining to	Acute viral respiratory infection that begins like flu but quickly progresses to severe dyspnea; high fatality rate in persons over age 65; first appeared in China in 2003
silicosis (sil-ih-KOH-sis)	**-osis** = abnormal condition	Type of pneumoconiosis that develops from inhalation of silica (quartz) dust found in quarrying, glasswork, sandblasting, and ceramics
sleep apnea (AP-nee-ah)	**a-** = without **-pnea** = breathing	Condition in which breathing stops repeatedly during sleep long enough to cause drop in oxygen levels in blood
sudden infant death syndrome (SIDS)		Unexpected and unexplained death of apparently well infant under one year of age; child suddenly stops breathing for unknown reasons
tuberculosis (TB) (too-ber-kyoo-LOH-sis)	**-osis** = abnormal condition	Infectious disease caused by bacteria *Mycobacterium tuberculosis*; most commonly affects respiratory system and causes inflammation and calcification in lungs; tuberculosis incidence is on the increase and is seen in many patients with weakened immune systems; multidrug-resistant tuberculosis is a particularly dangerous form of the disease because some bacteria have developed resistance to standard drug therapy
Pleural Cavity		
empyema (em-pye-EE-mah)	**py/o** = pus	Pus within pleural space usually associated with bacterial infection; also called *pyothorax*

Pathology (continued)

Term	Word Parts	Definition
pleural effusion (PLOO-ral / eh-FYOO-zhun)	pleur/o = pleura -al = pertaining to	Abnormal accumulation of fluid in pleural cavity preventing lungs from fully expanding; physicians can detect presence of fluid by tapping chest (percussion) or listening with stethoscope (auscultation)
pleurisy (PLOOR-ih-see)	pleur/o = pleura	Inflammation of pleura characterized by sharp chest pain with each breath; also called *pleuritis*
pneumothorax (noo-moh-THOH-raks)	pneum/o = air -thorax = chest	Collection of air or gas in pleural cavity, possibly resulting in collapse of lung

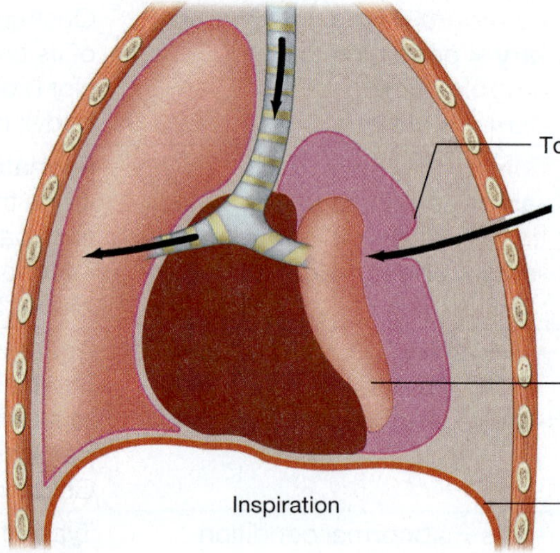

Figure 7-10 Pneumothorax. Figure illustrates how puncture of thoracic wall and tearing of pleural membrane allows air into lung and results in collapsed lung.

PRACTICE AS YOU GO

D. Terminology Matching

Match each term to its definition.

1. ________ inhaling environmental particles
2. ________ whooping cough
3. ________ may result in collapsed lung
4. ________ pus in the pleural space
5. ________ respiratory tract mucus
6. ________ nosebleed
7. ________ cyanosis
8. ________ *Mycoplasma* pneumonia
9. ________ disease with overexpanded air sacs
10. ________ histoplasmosis

a. empyema
b. blue tint to the skin
c. caused by a fungus
d. epistaxis
e. pneumoconiosis
f. emphysema
g. walking pneumonia
h. pneumothorax
i. pertussis
j. phlegm

Diagnostic Procedures

Term	Word Parts	Definition
Clinical Laboratory Tests		
arterial blood gases (ABGs) (ar-TEE-ree-al)	**arteri/o** = artery **-al** = pertaining to	Testing for gases present in blood; generally used to assist in determining levels of oxygen and carbon dioxide in blood
sputum culture and sensitivity (C&S) (SPYOO-tum)		Testing sputum by placing it on culture medium and observing any bacterial growth; specimen is then tested to determine antibiotic effectiveness
sputum cytology (SPYOO-tum / sigh-TALL-oh-jee)	**cyt/o** = cell **-logy** = study of	Examining sputum for malignant cells
Diagnostic Imaging		
bronchogram (BRONG-koh-gram)	**bronch/o** = bronchus **-gram** = record	X-ray record of bronchus produced by bronchography
bronchography (brong-KOG-rah-fee)	**bronch/o** = bronchus **-graphy** = process of recording	X-ray of lung after radiopaque substance inserted into trachea or bronchial tube; resulting X-ray is called *bronchogram*
chest X-ray (CXR)		Taking radiographic picture of lungs and heart from back and sides
pulmonary angiography (PULL-mon-air-ee / an-jee-OG-rah-fee)	**pulmon/o** = lung **-ary** = pertaining to **angi/o** = vessel **-graphy** = process of recording	Injecting dye into blood vessel for purpose of taking X-ray of arteries and veins of lungs
ventilation-perfusion scan (per-FYOO-zhun)		Nuclear medicine diagnostic test especially useful in identifying pulmonary emboli; radioactive air is inhaled for ventilation portion to determine if air is filling entire lung; radioactive intravenous injection shows if blood is flowing to all parts of lung
Endoscopic Procedures		
bronchoscope (BRONG-koh-skohp)	**bronch/o** = bronchus **-scope** = instrument for viewing	Instrument used to view inside bronchus during *bronchoscopy*
bronchoscopy (Bronch) (brong-KOSS-koh-pee)	**bronch/o** = bronchus **-scopy** = process of visually examining	Visual examination of inside of bronchi; uses instrument called *bronchoscope* (see Figure 7-11 ■)
laryngoscope (lah-RING-goh-skohp)	**laryng/o** = larynx **-scope** = instrument for viewing	Instrument used to view inside larynx during *laryngoscopy*
laryngoscopy (lair-in-GOSS-koh-pee)	**laryng/o** = larynx **-scopy** = process of visually examining	Examination of interior of larynx with lighted instrument called *laryngoscope*

Diagnostic Procedures (continued)

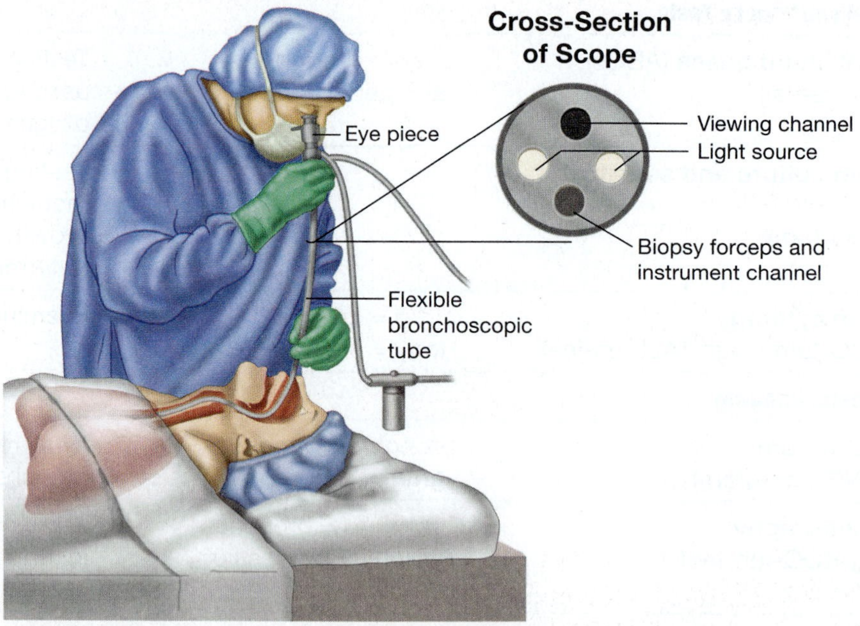

Term	Word Parts	Definition
Figure 7-11 Bronchoscopy. Figure illustrates physician using a bronchoscope to inspect the patient's bronchial tubes. Advances in technology include using a videoscope, which projects the internal view of the bronchus onto a video screen.		
Pulmonary Function Tests		
oximeter (ok-SIM-eh-ter)	**ox/i** = oxygen **-meter** = instrument to measure	Instrument that measures amount of oxygen in bloodstream
oximetry (ok-SIM-eh-tree)	**ox/i** = oxygen **-metry** = process of measuring	Procedure to measure oxygen level in blood using device, an *oximeter*, placed on patient's fingertip or earlobe
pulmonary function test (PFT) (PULL-mon-air-ee)	**pulmon/o** = lung **-ary** = pertaining to	Group of diagnostic tests that give information regarding airflow in and out of lungs, lung volumes, and gas exchange between lungs and bloodstream
spirometer (spy-ROM-eh-ter)	**spir/o** = breathing **-meter** = instrument to measure	Instrument to measure lung capacity used for *spirometry*
spirometry (spy-ROM-eh-tree)	**spir/o** = breathing **-metry** = process of measuring	Procedure to measure lung capacity using *spirometer*
Additional Diagnostic Procedures		
polysomnography (pol-ee-som-NOG-rah-fee)	**poly-** = many **somn/o** = sleep **-graphy** = process of recording	Monitoring patient while sleeping to identify sleep apnea; also called *sleep apnea study*
sweat test		Test for cystic fibrosis; patients with this disease have abnormally large amount of salt in their sweat
tuberculin skin test (TB test) (too-BER-kyoo-lin)		Procedure in which tuberculin purified protein derivative (PPD) is applied under surface of skin to determine if patient has been exposed to tuberculosis; also called a *Mantoux test*

Therapeutic Procedures

Term	Word Parts	Definition
Respiratory Therapy		
aerosol therapy (AIR-oh-sol)	aer/o = air	Medication suspended in mist intended for inhalation; delivered by *nebulizer*, which provides mist for period of time while patient breathes, or *metered-dose inhaler* (MDI), which delivers single puff of mist
continuous positive airway pressure (CPAP)		Machine that supplies constant and steady air pressure through mask; keeps airways continuously open; common treatment for sleep apnea
endotracheal intubation (en-doh-TRAY-kee-al / in-too-BAY-shun)	endo- = within trache/o = trachea -al = pertaining to	Placing of a tube through mouth, through glottis, and into trachea to create patent airway

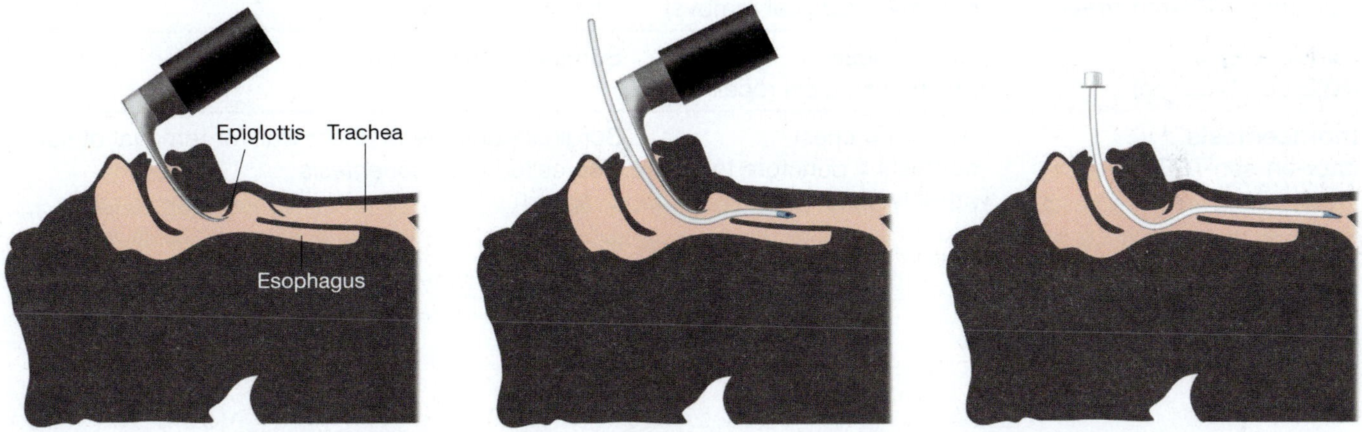

■ Figure 7-12 Endotracheal intubation. First, a lighted scope is used to distinguish the trachea from the esophagus. Next, the tube is placed through the pharynx and into the trachea. Finally, the scope is removed, leaving the tube in place.

Term	Word Parts	Definition
intermittent positive pressure breathing (IPPB)		Method for assisting patients in breathing using mask connected to machine that produces increased positive thoracic pressure
nasal cannula (KAN-yoo-lah)	nas/o = nose -al = pertaining to	Two-pronged plastic device for delivering oxygen into nose; one prong is inserted into each naris
postural drainage	-al = pertaining to	Drainage of secretions from bronchi by placing patient in position that uses gravity to promote drainage; used for treatment of cystic fibrosis and bronchiectasis
supplemental oxygen therapy	-al = pertaining to	Providing patient with additional concentration of oxygen to improve oxygen levels in bloodstream; oxygen may be provided by mask or nasal cannula
ventilator (VEN-tih-lay-ter)		Machine that provides artificial ventilation for patient unable to breathe on his or her own; also called *respirator*
Surgical Procedures		
bronchoplasty (BRONG-koh-plas-tee)	bronch/o = bronchus -plasty = surgical repair	Surgical repair of a bronchus
laryngectomy (lair-in-JEK-toh-mee)	laryng/o = larynx -ectomy = surgical removal	Surgical removal of larynx

Therapeutic Procedures (continued)

Term	Word Parts	Definition
laryngoplasty (lah-RING-goh-plas-tee)	**laryng/o** = larynx **-plasty** = surgical repair	Surgical repair of larynx
lobectomy (loh-BEK-toh-mee)	**lob/o** = lobe **-ectomy** = surgical removal	Surgical removal of a lobe of a lung
pleurectomy (ploor-EK-toh-mee)	**pleur/o** = pleura **-ectomy** = surgical removal	Surgical removal of pleura
pleurocentesis (ploor-oh-sen-TEE-sis)	**pleur/o** = pleura **-centesis** = puncture to withdraw fluid	Procedure involving insertion of needle into pleural space to withdraw fluid; may be treatment for excess fluid accumulating or to obtain fluid for diagnostic examination
pneumonectomy (noo-moh-NEK-toh-mee)	**pneum/o** = lung **-ectomy** = surgical removal	Surgical removal of entire lung
rhinoplasty (RYE-noh-plas-tee)	**rhin/o** = nose **-plasty** = surgical repair	Surgical repair of nose
thoracentesis (thor-ah-sen-TEE-sis)	**thorac/o** = chest **-centesis** = puncture to withdraw fluid	Surgical puncture of chest wall for removal of fluids; also called *thoracocentesis*

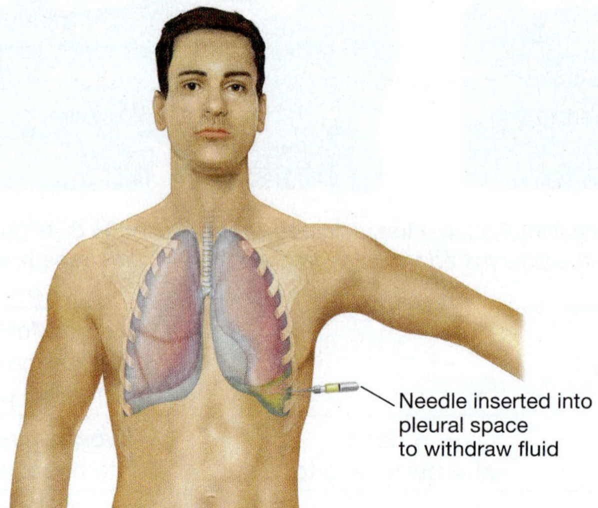

Figure 7-13 Thoracentesis. Insertion of a needle between the ribs to withdraw fluid from the pleural sac at the base of the left lung.

Term	Word Parts	Definition
thoracostomy (thor-ah-KOS-toh-mee)	**thorac/o** = chest **-ostomy** = surgically create an opening	Insertion of tube into chest cavity for purpose of draining off fluid or air; also called *chest tube*
thoracotomy (thor-ah-KOT-oh-mee)	**thorac/o** = chest **-otomy** = cutting into	To cut into chest cavity

Therapeutic Procedures (continued)

Term	Word Parts	Definition
tracheotomy (tray-kee-OT-oh-mee)	**trache/o** = trachea **-otomy** = cutting into	Surgical procedure often performed in emergency that creates opening directly into trachea to allow patient to breathe easier; also called *tracheostomy*

Thyroid cartilage
Trachea
Tracheotomy tube
Epiglottis
Larynx
Esophagus

■ **Figure 7-14** A tracheotomy tube in place, inserted through an opening in the front of the neck and anchored within the trachea.

Term	Word Parts	Definition
Additional Procedures		
cardiopulmonary resuscitation (CPR) (kar-dee-oh-PULL-mon-air-ee / ree-suss-ih-TAY-shun)	**cardi/o** = heart **pulmon/o** = lung **-ary** = pertaining to	Emergency treatment provided by persons trained in CPR and given to patients when their respirations and heart stop; CPR provides oxygen to brain, heart, and other vital organs until medical treatment can restore normal heart and pulmonary function
Heimlich maneuver (HYME-lik)		Technique for removing foreign body from trachea or pharynx by exerting diaphragmatic pressure; named for Henry Heimlich, a U.S. thoracic surgeon
percussion (per-KUH-shun)		Use of fingertips to tap on surface to assess condition beneath; determined in part by feel of surface as it is tapped and sound generated

PRACTICE AS YOU GO

E. Terminology Matching

Match each term to its definition.

1. ________ sweat test	**a.** polysomnography
2. ________ measures oxygen levels in blood	**b.** Mantoux test
3. ________ ventilator	**c.** oximetry
4. ________ test to identify sleep apnea	**d.** puncture chest wall to remove fluid
5. ________ thoracentesis	**e.** respirator
6. ________ tuberculin test	**f.** test for cystic fibrosis

Pharmacology

Vocabulary

Term	Word Parts	Definition
cumulative action		Action that occurs in body when drug is allowed to accumulate or stay in body
prophylaxis (proh-fih-LAK-sis)	**pro-** = before **-phylaxis** = protection	Prevention of disease; for example, antibiotic can be used to prevent occurrence of bacterial infection

Drugs

Classification	Word Parts	Action	Examples
antibiotic (an-tih-bye-AW-tik)	**anti-** = against **bi/o** = life **-tic** = pertaining to	Kills bacteria causing respiratory infections	ampicillin; amoxicillin, Amoxil; ciprofloxacin, Cipro
antihistamine (an-tih-HIST-ah-meen)	**anti-** = against	Blocks effects of histamine released by body during allergy attack	fexofenadine, Allegra; loratadine, Claritin; diphenhydramine, Benadryl
antitussive (an-tih-TUSS-iv)	**anti-** = without **tuss/o** = cough	Relieves urge to cough	hydrocodon, Hycodan; dextromethorphan, Vicks Formula 44
bronchodilator (BRONG-koh-dye-lay-ter)	**bronch/o** = bronchus	Relaxes muscle spasms in bronchial tubes; used to treat asthma	albuterol, Proventil, Ventolin; salmeterol, Serevent
corticosteroids (kor-tih-koh-STAIR-oydz)	**cortic/o** = outer layer, cortex	Reduces inflammation and swelling in respiratory tract	fluticasone, Flonase; mometasone, Nasonex; triamcinolone, Azmacort
decongestant (dee-kon-JES-tant)	**de-** = without	Reduces stuffiness and congestion throughout respiratory system	oxymetazoline, Afrin, Dristan, Sinex; pseudoephedrine, Drixoral, Sudafed
expectorant (ek-SPEK-toh-rent)		Improves ability to cough up mucus from respiratory tract	guaifenesin, Robitussin, Mucinex
mucolytic (myoo-koh-LIT-ik)	**muc/o** = mucus **-lytic** = destruction	Liquefies mucus so it is easier to cough and clear from respiratory tract	N-acetyl-cysteine, Mucomyst

Med Term Tip

There are three accepted pronunciations for the prefix **anti-**, "an-tih," "an-tee," and "an-tye."

Abbreviations

ABGs	arterial blood gases	**MERS**	Middle East respiratory syndrome
ad lib	as desired	**O_2**	oxygen
ARDS	adult (or acute) respiratory distress syndrome	**PE**	pulmonary embolism
Bronch	bronchoscopy	**per**	with
CF	cystic fibrosis	**PFT**	pulmonary function test
CO_2	carbon dioxide	**po**	by mouth
COPD	chronic obstructive pulmonary disease	**PPD**	purified protein derivative
CPAP	continuous positive airway pressure	**prn**	as needed
CPR	cardiopulmonary resuscitation	**R**	respiration
C&S	culture and sensitivity	**RA**	room air
CTA	clear to auscultation	**RDS**	respiratory distress syndrome
CXR	chest X-ray	**RLL**	right lower lobe
d	day	**RML**	right middle lobe
DOE	dyspnea on exertion	**RRT**	registered respiratory therapist
DPT	diphtheria, pertussis, tetanus injection	**RUL**	right upper lobe
ENT	ear, nose, and throat	**RV**	reserve volume
ERV	expiratory reserve volume	**SARS**	severe acute respiratory syndrome
flu	influenza	**SIDS**	sudden infant death syndrome
FRC	functional residual capacity	**SOB**	shortness of breath
HMD	hyaline membrane disease	**TB**	tuberculosis
IC	inspiratory capacity	**TLC**	total lung capacity
IPPB	intermittent positive pressure breathing	**TPR**	temperature, pulse, and respiration
IRDS	infant respiratory distress syndrome	**TV**	tidal volume
IRV	inspiratory reserve volume	**URI**	upper respiratory infection
LLL	left lower lobe	**VC**	vital capacity
LUL	left upper lobe	**VS**	vital signs
MDI	metered-dose inhaler		

PRACTICE AS YOU GO

F. What's the Abbreviation?

1. upper respiratory infection __________
2. pulmonary function test __________
3. oxygen __________
4. carbon dioxide __________
5. chronic obstructive pulmonary disease __________
6. bronchoscopy __________
7. tuberculosis __________
8. infant respiratory distress syndrome __________

Chapter Review

Real-World Applications

Medical Record Analysis

This Pulmonology Consultation Report contains 12 medical terms. Underline each term and write it in the list below the report. Then explain each term as you would to a nonmedical person.

Pulmonology Consultation Report

Reason for Consultation:	Evaluation of increasingly severe asthma
History of Present Illness:	Patient is a 10-year-old male who first presented to the Emergency Room with dyspnea, coughing, and wheezing at seven years of age. Attacks are increasing in frequency, and there do not appear to be any precipitating factors such as exercise. No other family members are asthmatics.
Results of Physical Examination:	Patient is currently in the ER with marked dyspnea, cyanosis around the lips, prolonged expiration, and a hacking cough producing thick phlegm. Auscultation revealed rhonchi throughout lungs. ABGs indicate hypoxemia. Spirometry reveals moderately severe airway obstruction during expiration. This patient responded to Proventil and he is beginning to cough less and breathe with less effort.
Assessment:	Acute asthma attack with severe airway obstruction. There is no evidence of infection. In view of increasing severity and frequency of attacks, all his medications should be reevaluated for effectiveness and all attempts to identify precipitating factors should be made.
Recommendations:	Patient is to continue to use Proventil for relief of bronchospasms. Instructions for taking medications and controlling severity of asthma attacks were carefully reviewed with the patient and his family.

	Term	Explanation
1.	______________	______________
2.	______________	______________
3.	______________	______________
4.	______________	______________
5.	______________	______________
6.	______________	______________
7.	______________	______________
8.	______________	______________
9.	______________	______________
10.	______________	______________
11.	______________	______________
12.	______________	______________

Chart Note Transcription

The chart note below contains 11 phrases that can be reworded with a medical term presented in this chapter. Each phrase is identified with an underline. Determine the medical term and write your answers in the space provided.

Pearson General Hospital Emergency Room Record

Task Edit View Time Scale Options Help Download Archive Date: 17 May 2017

Current Complaint:	A 43-year-old female was brought to the Emergency Room by her family. She complained of painful and labored breathing, **1** rapid breathing, **2** and fever. Symptoms began three days ago, but have become much worse during the past 12 hours.
Past History:	Patient is a mother of three and a business executive. She has had no surgeries or previous serious illnesses.
Signs and Symptoms:	Temperature is 103°F, respiratory rate is 20 breaths/minute, blood pressure is 165/98, and heart rate is 90 bpm. A blood test to measure the levels of oxygen in the blood **3** indicates a marked low level of oxygen in the blood. **4** The process of listening to body sounds **5** of the lungs revealed abnormal crackling sounds **6** over the left lower chest. She is producing large amounts of pus-filled **7** mucus coughed up from the respiratory tract **8** and a chest X-ray **9** shows a large cloudy patch in the lower lobe of the left lung.
Diagnosis:	Left lower lobe inflammatory condition of the lungs caused by bacterial infection **10**
Treatment:	Patient was started on intravenous antibiotics. She also required a tube placed through the mouth to create an airway **11** for three days.

1. ______________________________

2. ______________________________

3. ______________________________

4. ______________________________

5. ______________________________

6. ______________________________

7. ______________________________

8. ______________________________

9. ______________________________

10. ______________________________

11. ______________________________

Case Study

Below is a case study presentation of a patient with a condition discussed in this chapter. Read the case study and answer the questions below. Some questions will ask for information not included within this chapter. Use your text, a medical dictionary, or any other reference material you choose to answer these questions.

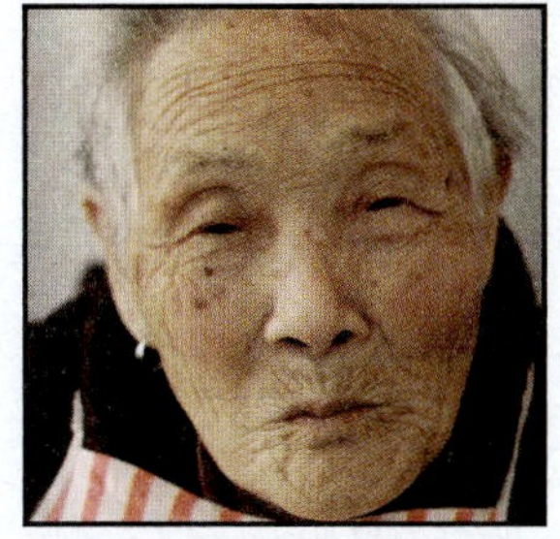

(Real444/E+/Getty Images)

An 88-year-old female was seen in the physician's office complaining of dyspnea, dizziness, orthopnea, elevated temperature, and a cough. Lung auscultation revealed crackles over the right bronchus. CXR revealed fluid in the RUL. The patient was sent to the hospital with an admitting diagnosis of pneumonia. Vital signs upon admission were temperature 102°F, pulse 100 BPM and rapid, respirations 24 breaths/min and labored, blood pressure 180/110. She was treated with IV antibiotics and IPPB. She responded well to treatment and was released home to her family with oral antibiotics on the third day.

Questions

1. What was this patient's admitting diagnosis? Look up this condition in a reference source and include a short description of it.

____

____

2. List and define each of the patient's presenting symptoms in your own words.

____

____

3. Define auscultation and CXR. Describe what each revealed in your own words.

____

____

4. What does the term *vital signs* mean? Describe this patient's vital signs.

____

____

5. Describe the treatments this patient received while in the hospital in your own words.

____

____

6. Explain the change in the patient's medication when she was discharged home.

____

____

Practice Exercises

A. Complete the Statement

1. The primary function of the respiratory system is ______________________.
2. The movement of air in and out of the lungs is called ______________________.
3. *External respiration* is defined as ______________________.
4. *Internal respiration* is defined as ______________________.
5. The muscle that divides the thoracic cavity from the abdominal cavity is the ______________________.
6. Total lung capacity means ______________________.
7. Tidal volume means ______________________.
8. Residual volume means ______________________.
9. The organs of the respiratory system are ______________________.
10. The four vital signs are ____________, ____________, ____________, and ____________.

B. Word Building Practice

The combining form **rhin/o** refers to the *nose*. Use it to write a term that means:

1. inflammation of the nose ______________________
2. discharge from the nose ______________________
3. surgical repair of the nose ______________________

The combining form **laryng/o** refers to the *larynx* or *voice box*. Use it to write a term that means:

4. inflammation of the larynx ______________________
5. spasm of the larynx ______________________
6. visual examination of the larynx ______________________
7. pertaining to the larynx ______________________
8. removal of the larynx ______________________
9. surgical repair of the larynx ______________________
10. paralysis of the larynx ______________________

The combining form **bronch/o** refers to the *bronchus*. Use it to write a term that means:

11. pertaining to bronchus ______________________
12. inflammation of the bronchus ______________________
13. visually examine the interior of the bronchus ______________________
14. produced by bronchus ______________________
15. spasm of the bronchus ______________________

The combining form **thorac/o** refers to the *chest*. Use it to write a term that means:

16. cutting into the chest ______________________
17. chest pain ______________________
18. pertaining to chest ______________________

The combining form **trache/o** refers to the *trachea*. Use it to write a term that means:

19. cutting into the trachea ____________________
20. narrowing of the trachea ____________________
21. pertaining to inside the trachea ____________________

The suffix **-pnea** means *breathing*. Use this suffix to write a medical term that means:

22. difficult or labored breathing ____________________
23. rapid breathing ____________________
24. can breathe only in an upright position ____________________
25. lack of breathing ____________________

C. Complete the Term

For each definition given below, fill in the blank with the word part that completes the term.

	Definition	Term
1.	lack of sense of smell	an ____________
2.	breathing too slowly	brady ____________
3.	paralysis of the larynx	____________plegia
4.	to cough up and spit out blood	hemo ____________
5.	abnormal flow of blood from the nose	rhino ____________
6.	abnormal voice	dys____________
7.	commonly called a *sore throat*	____________itis
8.	dilation of bronchi	____________ectasis
9.	commonly called *black lung*	____________osis
10.	air in the chest	____________thorax
11.	instrument to measure oxygen	____________meter
12.	process of visually examining the voice box	____________scopy
13.	process to withdraw fluid from the pleura	pleuro____________
14.	pertaining to heart and lung	____________ary
15.	narrowing of the windpipe	____________stenosis

D. Name that Term

1. the process of breathing in ______________________
2. spitting up of blood ______________________
3. blood clot in the pulmonary artery ______________________
4. inflammation of a sinus ______________________
5. sore throat ______________________
6. air in the pleural cavity ______________________
7. whooping cough ______________________
8. cutting into the pleura ______________________
9. pain in the pleural region ______________________
10. common cold ______________________

E. Using Abbreviations

Fill in each blank with the appropriate abbreviation.

1. He went to see a(n) ______________________ for his recurring throat and sinus infections.
2. ______________________ is a chronic condition with reduced capacity for inhaling and exhaling.
3. It was discovered at birth that the child had ______________________, a malfunction of the exocrine glands.
4. ______________________ is also called HMD.
5. A(n) ______________________ obstructs a pulmonary artery.
6. ______________________ is the unexpected and unexplained death of a newborn.
7. A(n) ______________________ tests the amount of oxygen and carbon dioxide in the blood.
8. The area of pneumonia could be seen on the ______________________.
9. Due to her difficulty breathing, the doctor ordered a(n) ______________________, a group of diagnostic tests.
10. A(n) ______________________ machine is a common treatment for sleep apnea.

F. Fill in the Blank

anthracosis	sputum cytology	cardiopulmonary resuscitation	patent
thoracentesis	respirator	ventilation-perfusion scan	rhonchi
supplemental oxygen	hyperventilation		

1. When the patient's breathing and heart stopped, the paramedics began ______________________.
2. The physician performed a ______________________ to remove fluid from the chest.
3. A ______________________ is also called a ventilator.
4. The patient received ______________________ through a nasal cannula.
5. An endotracheal intubation was performed to establish a ______________________ airway.
6. A ______________________ is a particularly useful test to identify a pulmonary embolus.

7. The result of the ____________________ was negative for cancer.

8. ____________________ involves tachypnea and hyperpnea.

9. ____________________ are wheezing lung sounds.

10. Miners are at risk of developing ____________________.

G. Pharmacology Challenge

Fill in the classification for each drug description, then match the brand name.

	Drug Description	Classification	Brand Name
1.	__________ Reduces stuffiness and congestion	____________________	a. Hycodan
2.	__________ Relieves the urge to cough	____________________	b. Flonase
3.	__________ Kills bacteria	____________________	c. Cipro
4.	__________ Improves ability to cough up mucus	____________________	d. Ventolin
5.	__________ Liquefies mucus	____________________	e. Allegra
6.	__________ Relaxes bronchial muscle spasms	____________________	f. Afrin
7.	__________ Blocks allergy attack	____________________	g. Robitussin
8.	__________ Reduces inflammation and swelling	____________________	h. Mucomyst

H. Anatomical Adjectives

Fill in the blank with the missing noun or adjective.

Noun	Adjective
1. air sacs	____________________
2. ____________________	pulmonary
3. chest	____________________
4. ____________________	bronchial
5. windpipe	____________________
6. ____________________	epiglottic
7. mucus	____________________
8. throat	____________________
9. ____________________	bronchiolar
10. ____________________	septal

I. Spelling Practice

Some of the following terms are misspelled. Identify the incorrect terms and spell them correctly in the blank provided.

1. nasopharyngial ______
2. asphyxia ______
3. canula ______
4. hemoptosis ______
5. bronchodilater ______
6. rhinorrhagia ______
7. polysomnography ______
8. bronchiectasis ______
9. tuberculosis ______
10. pneumoconosis ______

Labeling Exercises

Image A

Write the labels for this figure on the numbered lines provided.

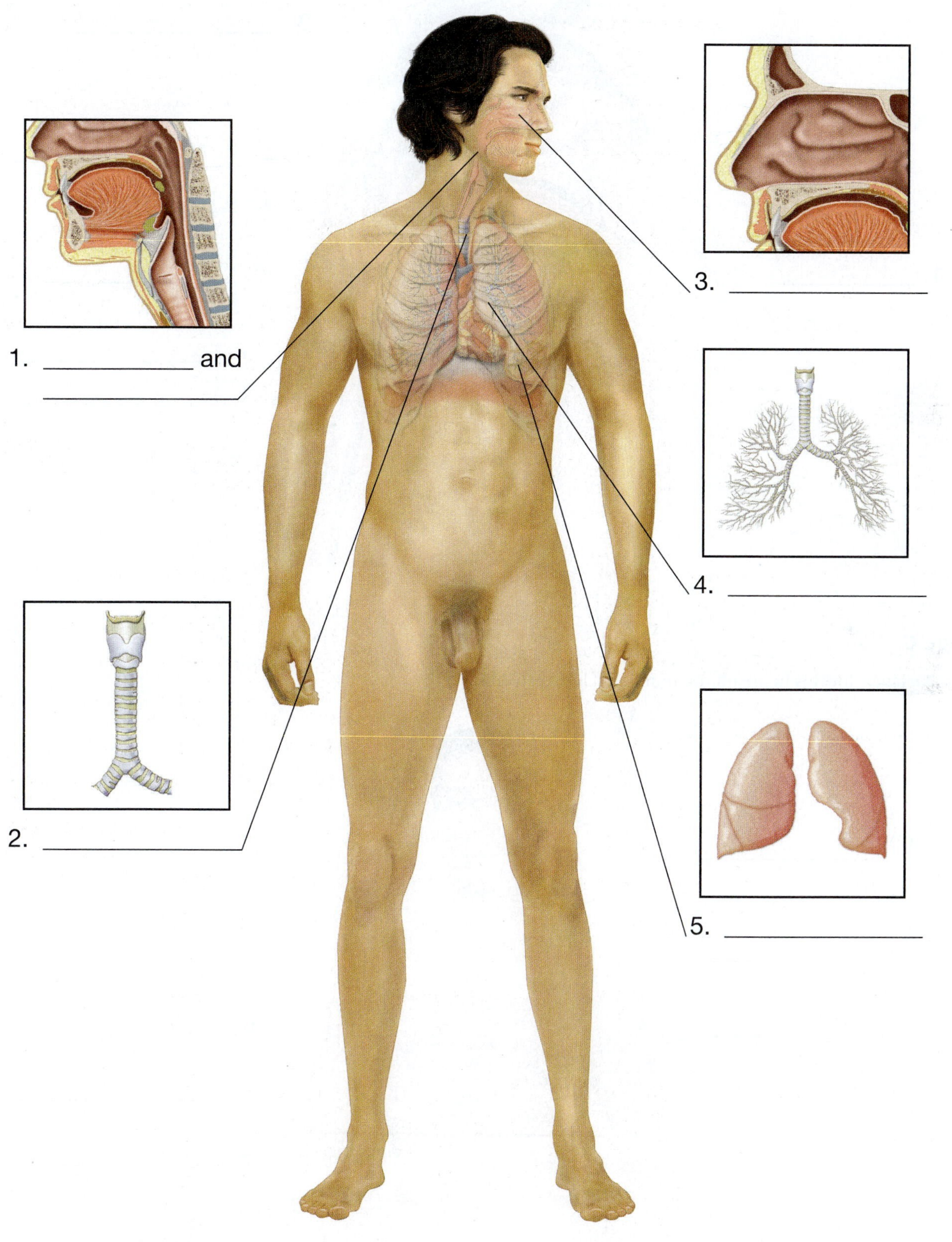

Image B

Write the labels for this figure on the numbered lines provided.

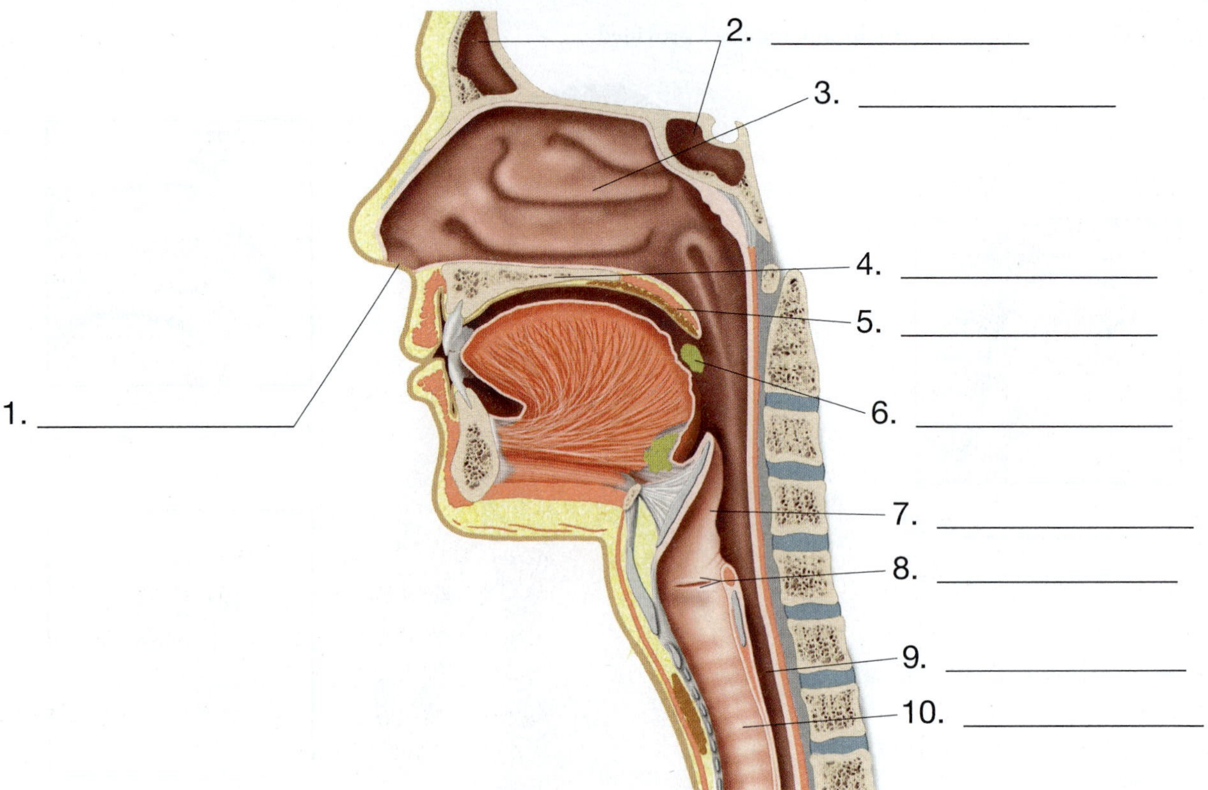

Image C

Write the labels for this figure on the numbered lines provided.

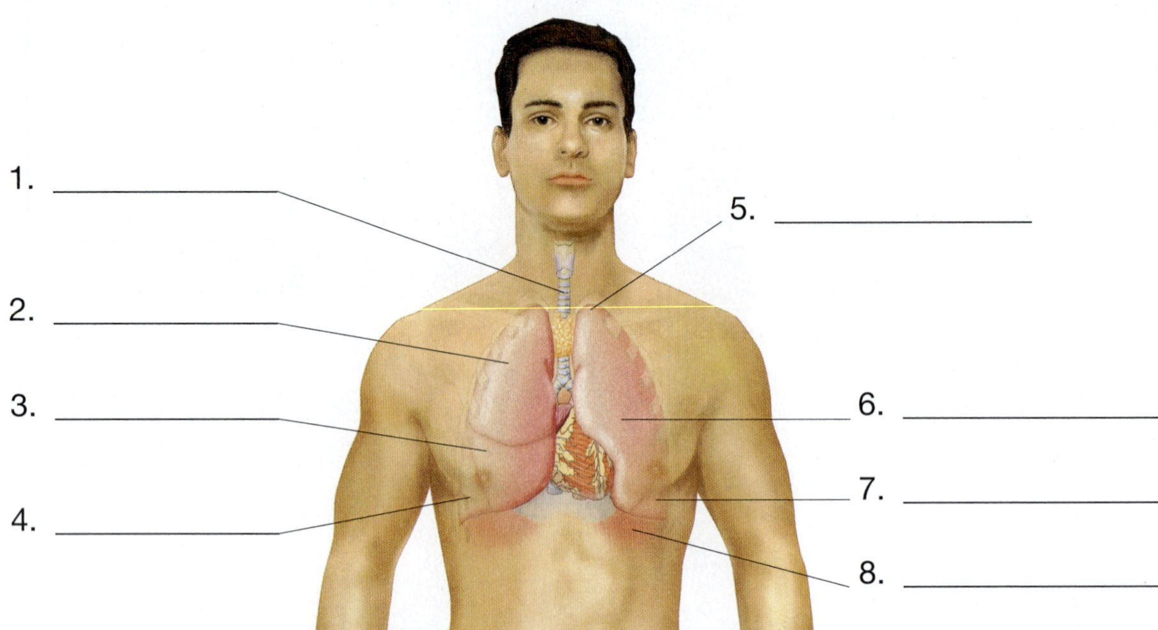

Chapter 8

Digestive System

Learning Objectives

Upon completion of this chapter, you will be able to

1. Identify and define the combining forms and suffixes introduced in this chapter.
2. Correctly spell and pronounce medical terms and major anatomical structures relating to the digestive system.
3. Locate and describe the major organs of the digestive system and their functions.
4. Identify the shape and function of each type of tooth.
5. Describe the function of the accessory organs of the digestive system.
6. Identify and define digestive system anatomical terms.
7. Identify and define selected digestive system pathology terms.
8. Identify and define selected digestive system diagnostic procedures.
9. Identify and define selected digestive system therapeutic procedures.
10. Identify and define selected medications relating to the digestive system.
11. Define selected abbreviations associated with the digestive system.

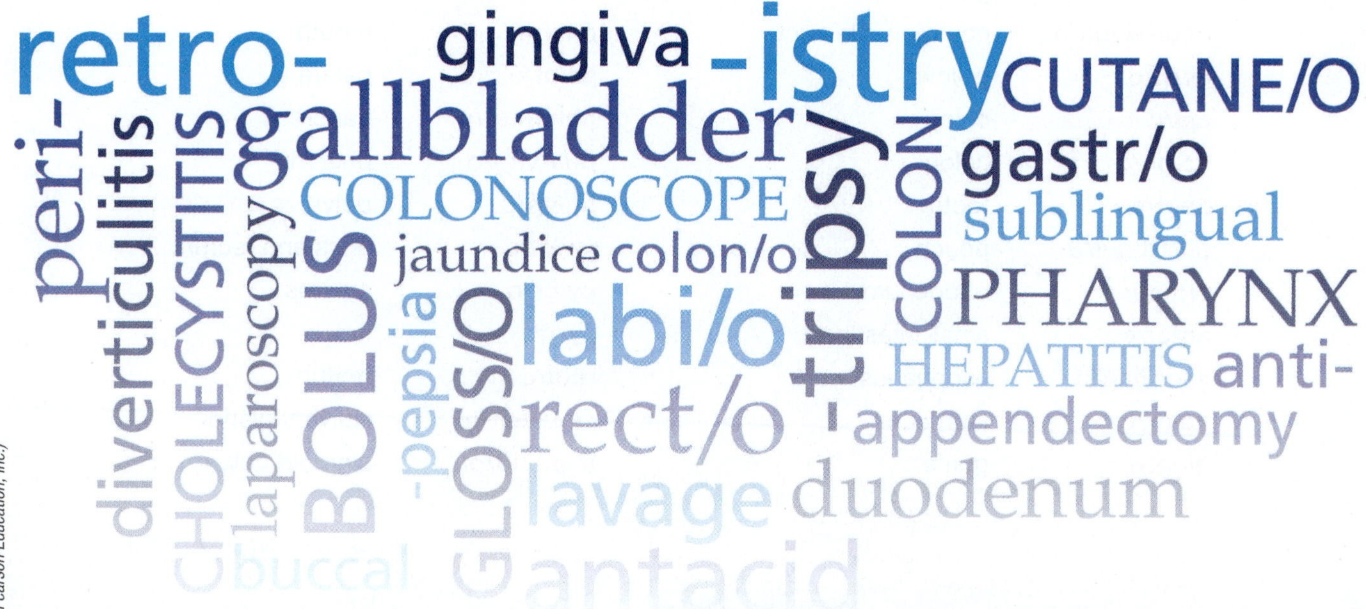

(Pearson Education, Inc.)

DIGESTIVE SYSTEM

AT A GLANCE

Function

The digestive system begins breaking down food through mechanical and chemical digestion. After being digested, nutrient molecules are absorbed into the body and enter the bloodstream; any food not digested or absorbed is eliminated as solid waste.

Organs

The primary structures that comprise the digestive system:

anus
esophagus
gallbladder (GB)
large intestine
liver
mouth
oral cavity
pancreas
pharynx
salivary glands
small intestine
stomach

Word Parts

Presented here are the most common word parts (with their meanings) used to build digestive system terms. For a more comprehensive list, refer to the Terminology section of this chapter.

Combining Forms

an/o	anus
append/o	appendix
appendic/o	appendix
bar/o	weight
bucc/o	cheek
cec/o	cecum
cholangi/o	bile duct
chol/e	bile, gall
cholecyst/o	gallbladder
choledoch/o	common bile duct
cirrh/o	yellow
col/o	colon
colon/o	colon
dent/o	tooth
diverticul/o	pouch
duoden/o	duodenum
enter/o	small intestine
esophag/o	esophagus
gastr/o	stomach
gingiv/o	gums
gloss/o	tongue
hepat/o	liver
ile/o	ileum
jejun/o	jejunum
labi/o	lip
lapar/o	abdomen
lingu/o	tongue
lith/o	stone
odont/o	tooth
or/o	mouth
palat/o	palate
pancreat/o	pancreas
pharyng/o	pharynx
polyp/o	polyp
proct/o	anus and rectum
pylor/o	pylorus
pyr/o	fire
rect/o	rectum
sialaden/o	salivary gland
sigmoid/o	sigmoid colon

(continued on page 270)

Digestive System Illustrated

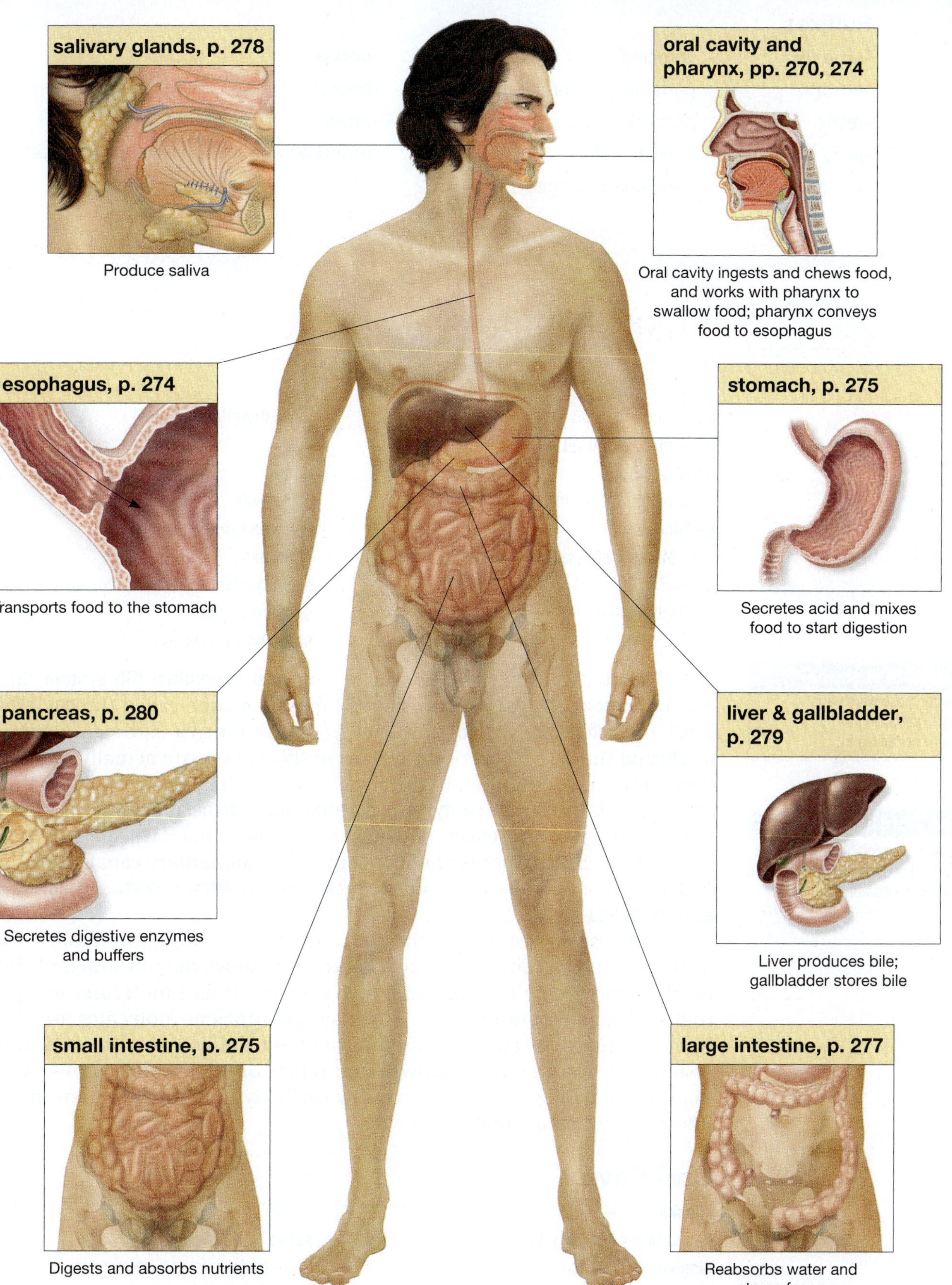

salivary glands, p. 278
Produce saliva
oral cavity and pharynx, pp. 270, 274
Oral cavity ingests and chews food, and works with pharynx to swallow food; pharynx conveys food to esophagus
esophagus, p. 274
Transports food to the stomach
stomach, p. 275
Secretes acid and mixes food to start digestion
pancreas, p. 280
Secretes digestive enzymes and buffers
liver & gallbladder, p. 279
Liver produces bile; gallbladder stores bile
small intestine, p. 275
Digests and absorbs nutrients
large intestine, p. 277
Reabsorbs water and stores feces

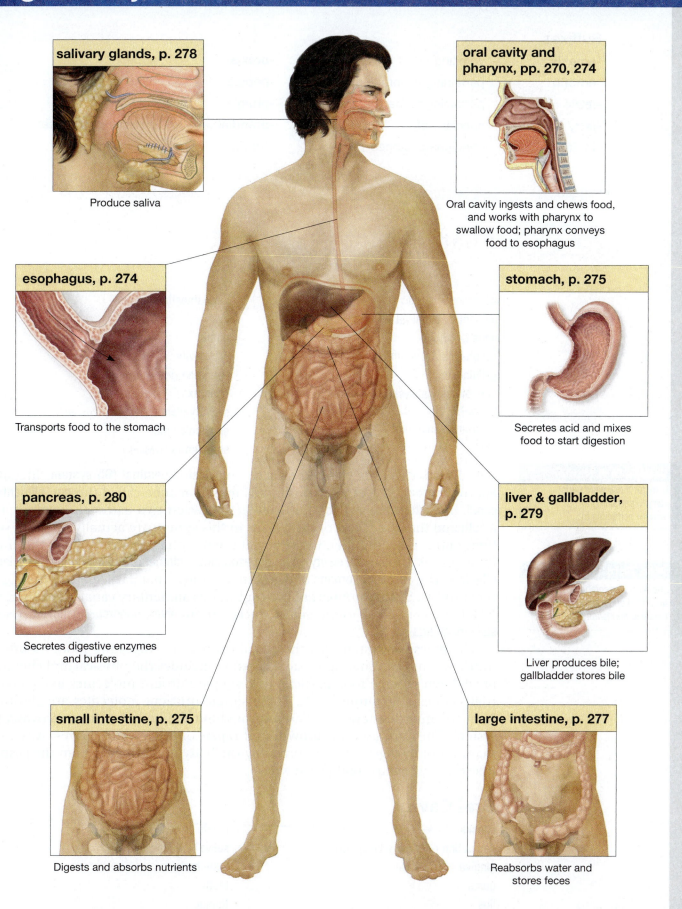

(continued from page 268)

Suffixes

-emesis	vomiting	**-orexia**	appetite
-emetic	pertaining to vomiting	**-pepsia**	digestion
-iatric	pertaining to medical treatment	**-phagia**	eat, swallow
-istry	specialty of	**-prandial**	pertaining to a meal
-lithiasis	condition of stones	**-tripsy**	surgical crushing

Anatomy and Physiology of the Digestive System

accessory organs
alimentary canal (al-ih-MEN-tah-ree)
anus (AY-nus)
esophagus (eh-SOFF-ah-gus)
gallbladder
gastrointestinal system (gas-troh-in-TESS-tih-nal)
gastrointestinal tract
gut
large intestine
liver
mouth
oral cavity
pancreas (PAN-kree-as)
pharynx (FAIR-inks)
salivary glands (SAL-ih-vair-ee)
small intestine
stomach (STUM-ak)

What's In A Name?

Look for these word parts:
-ary = pertaining to
-ory = pertaining to

Med Term Tip

The term *alimentary* comes from the Latin term *alimentum* meaning *nourishment.*

The digestive system, also known as the **gastrointestinal (GI) system**, includes approximately 30 feet of a continuous muscular tube called the **gut**, **alimentary canal**, or **gastrointestinal tract** that stretches between two external openings, the **mouth** and the **anus**. Most of the organs in this system are actually different sections of this tube. In order, beginning at the mouth and continuing to the anus, these organs are the **oral cavity**, **pharynx**, **esophagus**, **stomach**, **small intestine**, and **large intestine.** The **accessory organs** of digestion are those that participate in the digestion process, but are not part of the continuous alimentary canal. These organs, which are connected to the gut by ducts, are the **liver**, **pancreas**, **gallbladder**, and **salivary glands.**

The digestive system has three main functions: digesting food, absorbing nutrients, and eliminating waste. Digestion includes the physical and chemical breakdown of large food particles into simple nutrient molecules like glucose, triglycerides, and amino acids. These simple nutrient molecules are absorbed from the intestines and circulated throughout the body by the cardiovascular system. They are used for growth and repair of organs and tissues. Any food that cannot be digested or absorbed by the body is eliminated from the gastrointestinal system as solid waste.

Oral Cavity

cheeks
deglutition (dee-gloo-TISH-un)
gingiva (JIN-jih-vah)
gums
lips
mastication (mass-tih-KAY-shun)
palate (PAL-et)
saliva (suh-LYE-vah)
taste buds
teeth
tongue
uvula (YOO-vyoo-lah)

Digestion begins when food enters the mouth and is mechanically broken up by **mastication,** the chewing movements of the **teeth**. The muscular **tongue** moves the food within the mouth and mixes it with **saliva** (see Figure 8-1 ■). Saliva contains digestive enzymes to break down carbohydrates, and slippery lubricants to make food easier for **deglutition** (swallowing). **Taste buds**, found on the surface of the tongue, can distinguish the bitter, sweet, sour, salty, and umami (savory) flavors in food. The roof of the oral cavity is known as the **palate** and is subdivided into the hard palate (the bony anterior portion) and the soft palate (the flexible posterior portion). Hanging down from the posterior edge of the soft palate is the **uvula**. The uvula serves two important functions. First, it has a role in speech production and, second, it is the location of the gag reflex. This reflex is stimulated when food enters the throat without swallowing (e.g., laughing with food in the mouth). It is important because swallowing also results in the epiglottis covering the larynx to prevent food from entering the lungs (see Figure 8-2 ■). The **cheeks** form the lateral walls of this cavity and the **lips** are the anterior opening. The entire oral cavity is lined with mucous membrane, a portion of which forms the **gums**, or **gingiva**, that combine with connective tissue to cover the jawbone and seal off the teeth in their bony sockets.

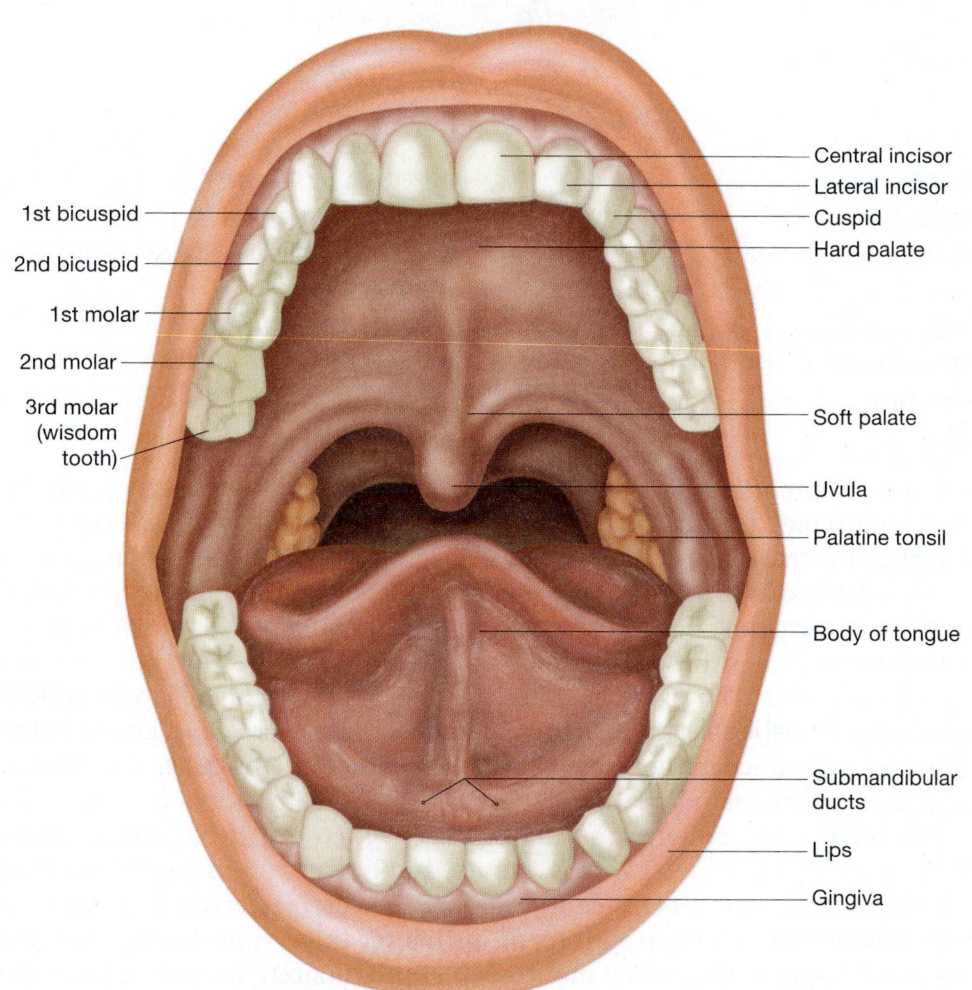

■ **Figure 8-1** Anatomy of structures of the oral cavity.

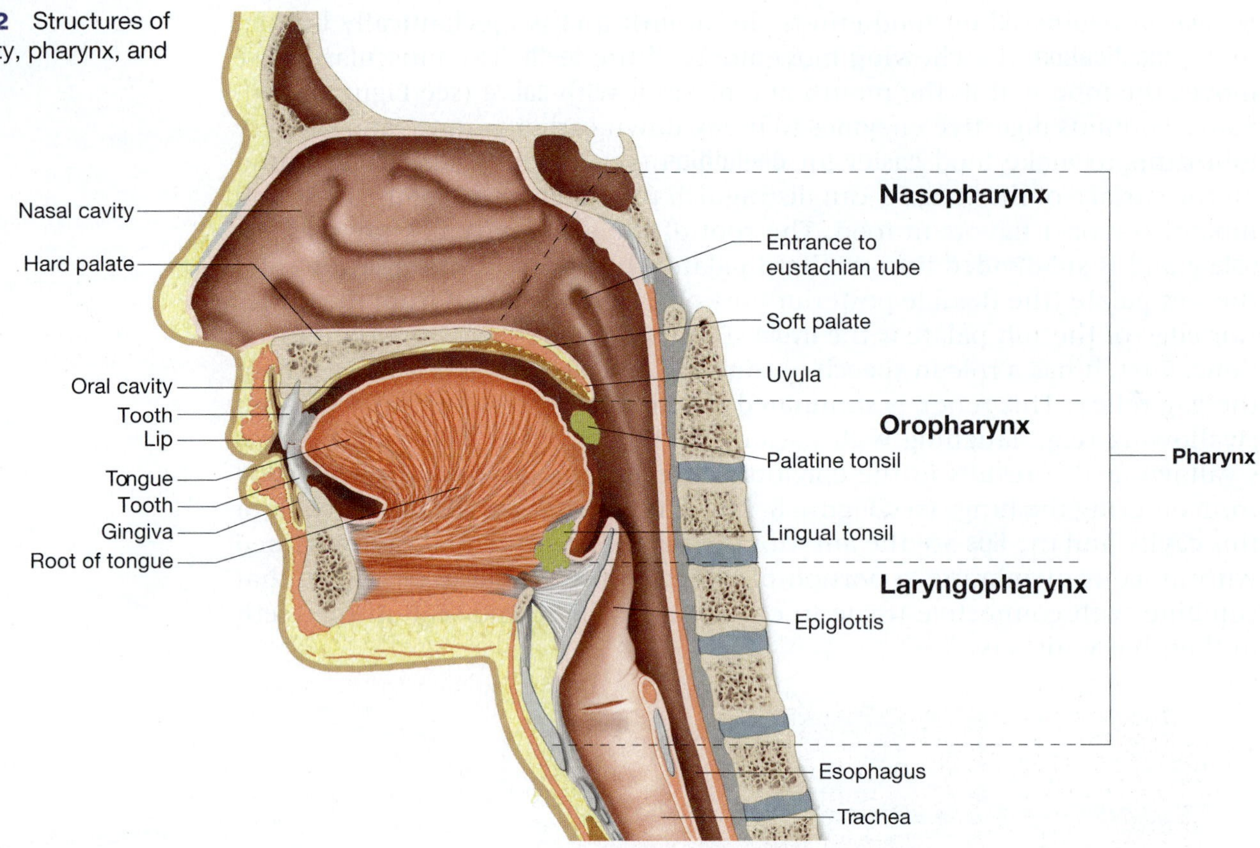

■ **Figure 8-2** Structures of the oral cavity, pharynx, and esophagus.

What's In A Name?

Look for these word parts:
cis/o = to cut
bi- = two
in- = inward
pre- = before

Med Term Tip

There are three different molars, simply referred to as the first, second, and third molars. However, the third molar has a more common name, the wisdom tooth. Not every person forms all four wisdom teeth. Unfortunately, most people do not have enough room in their jaws for the third molars to properly erupt through the gum, a condition requiring surgical removal of the third molar, referred to as an *impacted wisdom tooth*.

Med Term Tip

The combining form **dent/o** means *teeth*. Hence we have terms such as *dentist* and *dentistry*. The combining form **odont/o** also means *teeth* and, when combined with **orth/o**, which means *straight*, we have the specialty of *orthodontics*, or straightening teeth.

Teeth

bicuspids (bye-KUSS-pids)
canines (KAY-nines)
cementum (seh-MEN-tum)
crown
cuspids (KUSS-pids)
deciduous teeth (dih-SID-joo-us)
dentin (DEN-tin)
enamel
incisors (in-SIGH-zers)
molars (MOH-lars)
periodontal ligaments (pair-ee-oh-DON-tal)
permanent teeth
premolars (pree-MOH-lars)
pulp cavity
root
root canal

Teeth are an important part of the first stage of digestion. The teeth in the front of the mouth bite, tear, or cut food into small pieces. These cutting teeth include the **cuspids** (or **canines**) and the **incisors** (see Figure 8-3 ■). The remaining posterior teeth grind and crush food into even finer pieces. These grinding teeth include the **bicuspids** (or **premolars**) and the **molars**. A tooth can be subdivided into the **crown** and the **root**. The crown is that part of the tooth visible above the gum line; the root is below the gum line. The root is anchored in the bony socket of the jaw by **cementum** and tiny **periodontal ligaments**. The crown of the tooth is covered by a layer of **enamel**, the hardest substance in the body. Under the enamel layer is **dentin**, the substance that makes up the main bulk of the tooth. The hollow interior of a tooth is called the **pulp cavity** in the crown and the **root canal** in the root. These cavities contain soft tissue made up of blood vessels, nerves, and lymph vessels (see Figure 8-4 ■).

Humans have two sets of teeth. The first set, often referred to as *baby teeth*, are **deciduous teeth**. There are 20 teeth in this set that erupt through the gums between the ages of six and 28 months. At approximately six years of age, these teeth begin to fall out and are replaced by the 32 **permanent teeth**. This replacement process continues until about 18–20 years of age.

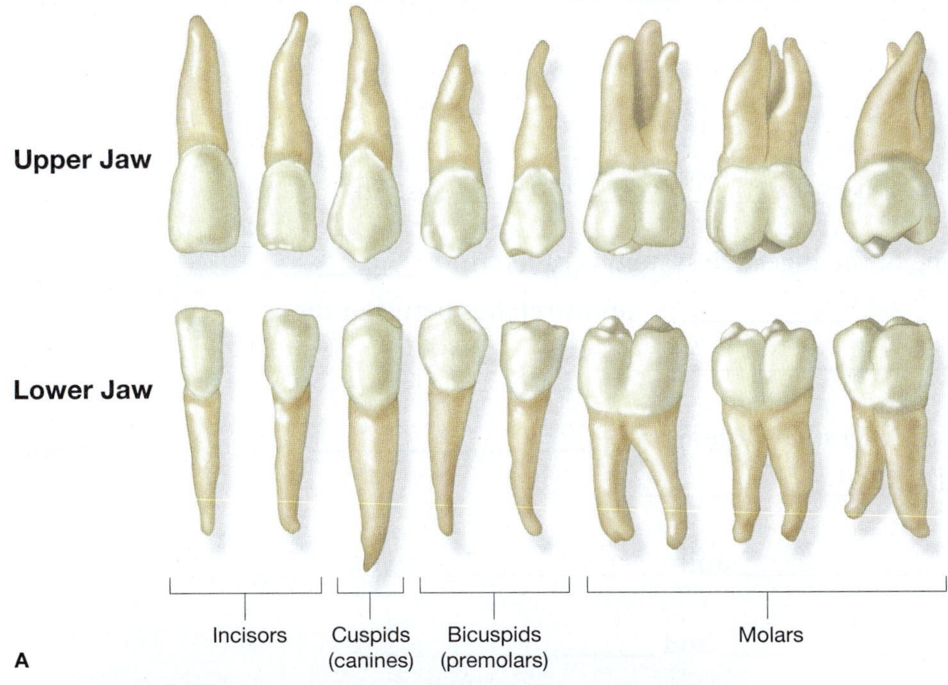

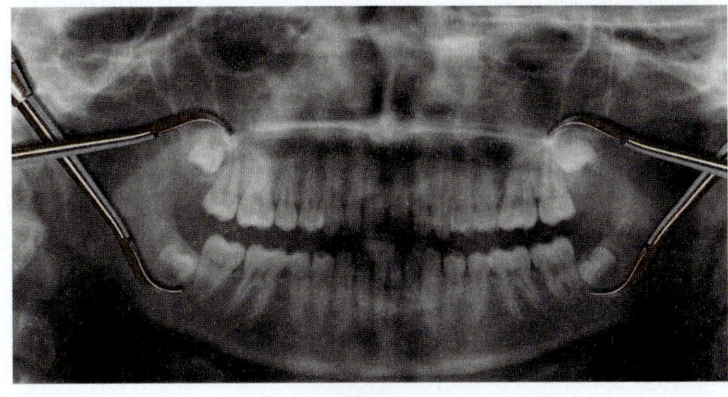

■ **Figure 8-3** A) The name and shape of the adult teeth. These teeth represent those found in the right side of the mouth. Those of the left side would be a mirror image. The incisors and cuspids are cutting teeth. The bicuspids and molars are grinding teeth. B) X-ray scan of all teeth. Note the four wisdom teeth (third molars) that have not erupted. *(Mkarco/Shutterstock)*

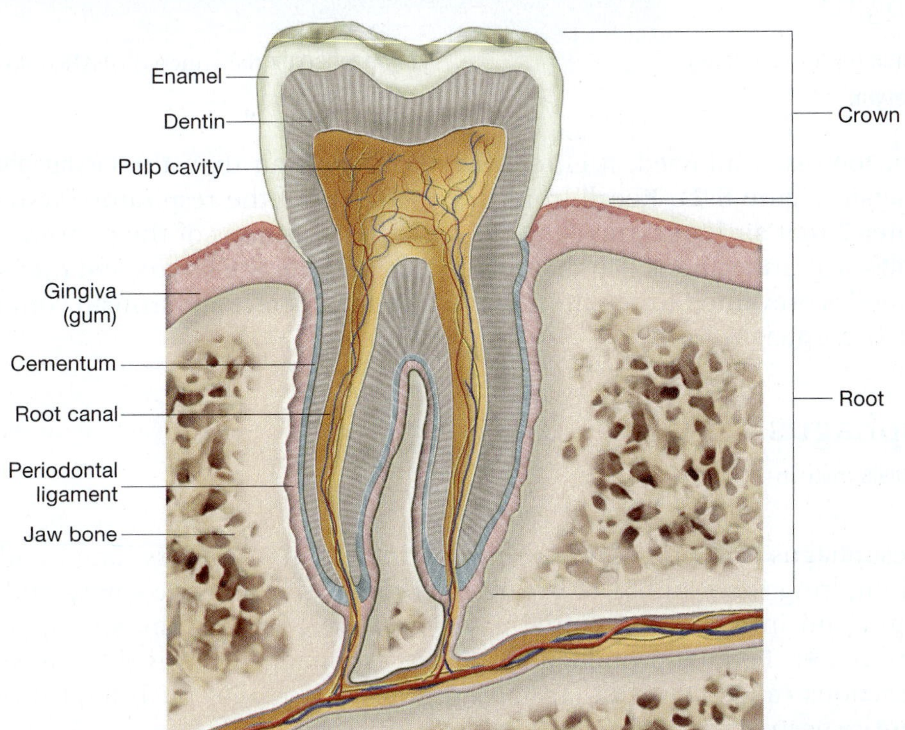

■ **Figure 8-4** An adult tooth, longitudinal view showing internal structures of the crown and root.

PRACTICE AS YOU GO

A. Complete the Statement

1. The digestive system is also known as the ____________________ system.
2. The continuous muscular tube of the digestive system is called the ____________________, ____________________, or ____________________ and stretches between the ____________________ and ____________________.
3. The three main functions of the digestive system are ____________________, ____________________, and ____________________.
4. The cutting teeth are ____________________ and ____________________.
5. The grinding teeth are ____________________ and ____________________.
6. The ____________________ of a tooth is above the gum line and the ____________________ is below the gum line.
7. The hardest substance in the body is ____________________.
8. There are 20 ____________________ teeth and 32 ____________________ teeth.

Pharynx

epiglottis (ep-ih-GLOT-iss)
oropharynx
laryngopharynx (lah-ring-goh-FAIR-inks)

What's In A Name?
Look for these word parts:
laryng/o = larynx
or/o = mouth
epi- = above

When food is swallowed, it enters the **oropharynx** and then the **laryngopharynx** (see again Figure 8-2). Recall from the discussion of the respiratory system in Chapter 7 that air is also traveling through these portions of the pharynx. The **epiglottis** is a cartilaginous flap that folds down to cover the larynx and trachea so that food is prevented from entering the respiratory tract and instead continues into the esophagus.

Esophagus

peristalsis (pair-ih-STALL-sis)

Med Term Tip
It takes about seven seconds for swallowed food to reach the stomach.

The esophagus is a muscular tube measuring about 10 inches long in adults. Food entering the esophagus is carried through the thoracic cavity and diaphragm and into the abdominal cavity, where it enters the stomach (see Figure 8-5 ■). Food is propelled along the esophagus by wavelike muscular contractions called **peristalsis**. In fact, peristalsis works to push food through the entire gastrointestinal tract.

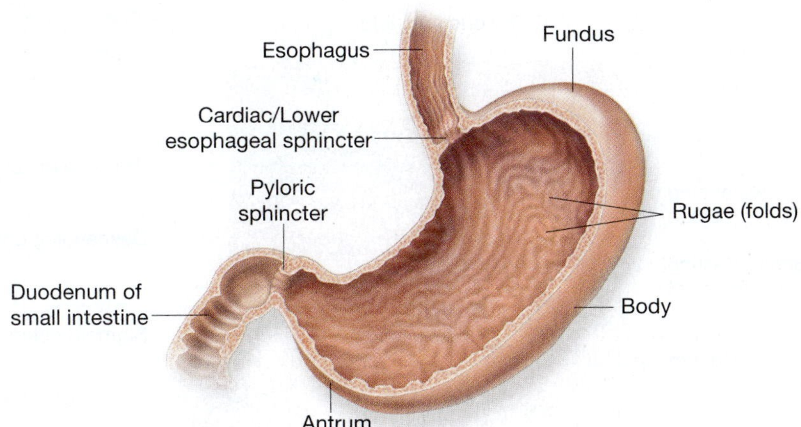

■ **Figure 8-5** The stomach, longitudinal view, showing regions and internal structures.

Stomach

antrum (AN-trum)
body
cardiac sphincter (KAR-dee-ak / SFINGK-ter)
chyme (KIME)
fundus (FUN-dus)
gastroesophageal sphincter (gas-troh-eh-soff-ah-JEE-al / SFINGK-ter)
hydrochloric acid
lower esophageal sphincter (eh-soff-ah-JEE-al / SFINGK-ter)
pyloric sphincter (pye-LOR-ik / SFINGK-ter)
rugae (ROO-jee)
sphincters (SFINGK-ters)

The stomach, a J-shaped muscular organ that acts as a bag or sac to collect and churn food with digestive juices, is composed of three parts: the **fundus** or upper region, the **body** or main portion, and the **antrum** or lower region (see again Figure 8-5). The folds in the lining of the stomach are called **rugae**. When the stomach fills with food, the rugae stretch out and disappear. **Hydrochloric acid** (HCl) is secreted by glands in the mucous membrane lining of the stomach. Food mixes with hydrochloric acid and other gastric juices to form a liquid mixture called **chyme**, which then passes through the remaining portion of the digestive system.

Entry into and exit from the stomach is controlled by muscular valves called **sphincters**. These valves open and close to ensure that food can only move forward down the gut tube. The **cardiac sphincter**, named for its proximity to the heart, is located between the esophagus and the fundus; also called the **lower esophageal sphincter** (LES) or **gastroesophageal sphincter**, it keeps food from flowing backward into the esophagus. During the processes of regurgitation and vomiting (they are not quite the same), the brain causes both of these sphincters to relax, thereby allowing stomach contents to flow backward.

The antrum tapers off into the **pyloric sphincter**, which regulates the passage of food into the small intestine. Only a small amount of the chyme is allowed to enter the small intestine with each opening of the sphincter for two important reasons. First, the small intestine is much narrower than the stomach and cannot hold as much as can the stomach. Second, the chyme is highly acidic and must be thoroughly neutralized as it leaves the stomach.

What's In A Name?

Look for these word parts:
cardi/o = heart
hydr/o = water
-ac = pertaining to
-ic = pertaining to

Med Term Tip

It is easier to remember the function of the pyloric sphincter when you note that **pylor/o** means *gatekeeper*. This gatekeeper controls the forward movement of food. Sphincters are rings of muscle that can be opened and closed to control entry and exit from hollow organs like the stomach, colon, and bladder.

Small Intestine

duodenum (doo-oh-DEE-num/doo-OD-eh-num)
ileocecal valve (il-ee-oh-SEE-kal)
ileum (IL-ee-um)
jejunum (jeh-JOO-num)
microvilli (my-kroh-VILL-eye)
villi (VILL-eye)

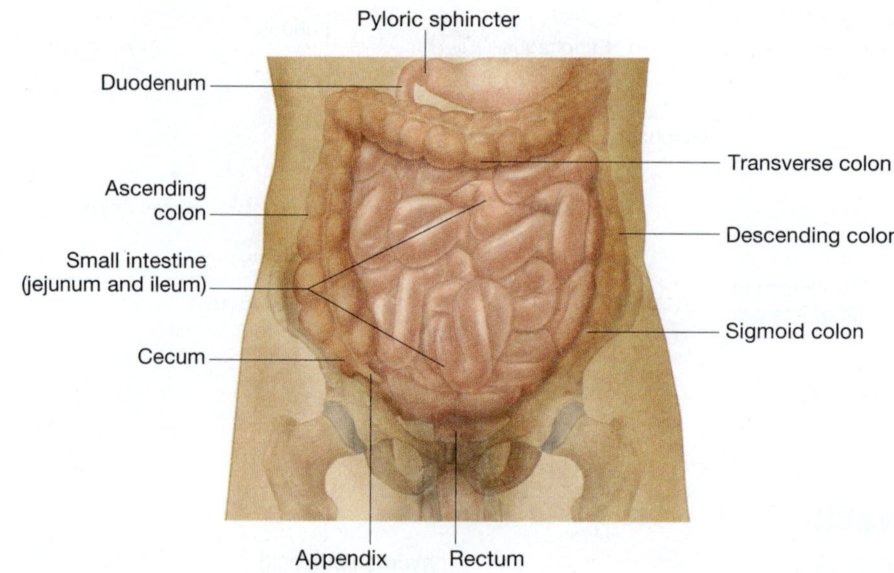

Figure 8-6 The small intestine. Anterior view of the abdominopelvic cavity illustrating how the three sections of small intestine—duodenum, jejunum, ileum—begin at the pyloric sphincter and end at the colon, but are not arranged in an orderly fashion.

Word Watch

Be careful not to confuse the word root **ile/o** meaning *ileum*, a portion of the small intestine, and **ili/o** meaning *ilium*, a pelvic bone.

The small intestine, or small bowel, is the major site of digestion and absorption of nutrients from food. It is located between the pyloric sphincter and the colon (see Figure 8-6 ■). The small intestine is very efficient at absorbing nutrients due to its structure. First, the lining is highly folded into finger-like projections called **villi** (see Figure 8-7 ■). Then each surface cell of a villus is covered in more projections called **microvilli**. Together, these projections give the small intestine a surface area roughly the size of a tennis court! Because the small intestine is concerned with absorption of food products, an abnormality in this organ may result in malnutrition. The small intestine, with an average length of 20 feet, is the longest portion of the alimentary canal and has three sections: the **duodenum**, the **jejunum**, and the **ileum**.

- The duodenum extends from the pyloric sphincter to the jejunum, and is about 10–12 inches long. Digestion is completed in the duodenum after the liquid chyme from the stomach is mixed with digestive juices from the pancreas and gallbladder.
- The jejunum, or middle portion, extends from the duodenum to the ileum and is about eight feet long.

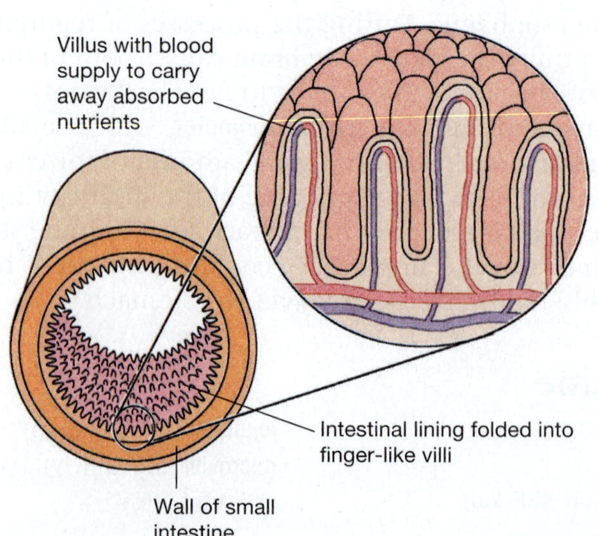

Figure 8-7 Section of small intestine wall illustrating arrangement of villi.
(Mohammed Ali. Pearson India Education Services Pvt. Ltd)

- The ileum is the last portion of the small intestine and extends from the jejunum to the colon. At 12 feet in length, it is the longest portion of the small intestine. The ileum connects to the colon with a sphincter called the **ileocecal valve.**

Large Intestine

anal canal (AY-nal)
anal sphincter (AY-nal / SFINGK-ter)
ascending colon
cecum (SEE-kum)
colon (KOH-lon)
defecation
descending colon
feces (FEE-seez)
rectum (REK-tum)
sigmoid colon (SIG-moyd)
transverse colon
vermiform appendix (VER-mih-form / ah-PEN-diks)

Fluid that remains after the complete digestion and absorption of nutrients in the small intestine enters the large intestine (see Figure 8-8 ■). Most of this fluid is water that is reabsorbed into the body. The material that remains after absorption is solid waste called **feces** (or stool). This is the product evacuated in a bowel movement (BM).

The large intestine is approximately 5 feet long and extends from the ileocecal valve to the anus; this includes the **cecum**, **colon**, **rectum**, and **anal canal**. The cecum is a pouch or saclike area in the first 2–3 inches at the beginning of the colon. The **vermiform appendix** is a small worm-shaped outgrowth at the end of the cecum. The colon consists of the **ascending colon**, **transverse colon**, **descending colon**, and **sigmoid colon**. The ascending colon on the right side extends from the cecum to the lower border of the liver. The transverse colon moves horizontally across the upper abdomen toward the spleen. The descending colon then travels down the left side of the body to where the sigmoid colon begins. The sigmoid colon curves in an S-shape back to the midline of the body and ends at the rectum. The rectum, where feces are stored, leads into the anal canal, which contains the **anal sphincter**. This sphincter consists of rings of voluntary and involuntary muscles to control the evacuation of feces or **defecation**.

Med Term Tip

We can survive without a portion of the small intestine. For example, in cases of cancer, much of the small intestine and/or colon may have to be removed. The surgeon then creates an opening between the remaining intestine and the abdominal wall. The combining form for the section of intestine connected to the abdominal wall and the suffix **-ostomy** are used to describe this procedure. For example, if a person has a *jejunostomy*, the jejunum is connected to the abdominal wall and the ileum (and remainder of the gut tube) has been removed.

Word Watch

The term *colon* refers to only a portion of the large intestine. However, you should be aware that many people use it incorrectly as a general term referring to the entire intestinal system, both small and large intestines.

Med Term Tip

It was long thought that the appendix was a vestigial organ (meaning that it had lost its original function). However, recent research indicates that the appendix serves as a reservoir for beneficial intestinal bacteria. Because of its shape and location, the bacteria in it are protected from being flushed out of the gut during episodes of diarrhea.

Med Term Tip

The term *defecation* comes from the Latin word meaning *to remove the dregs*.

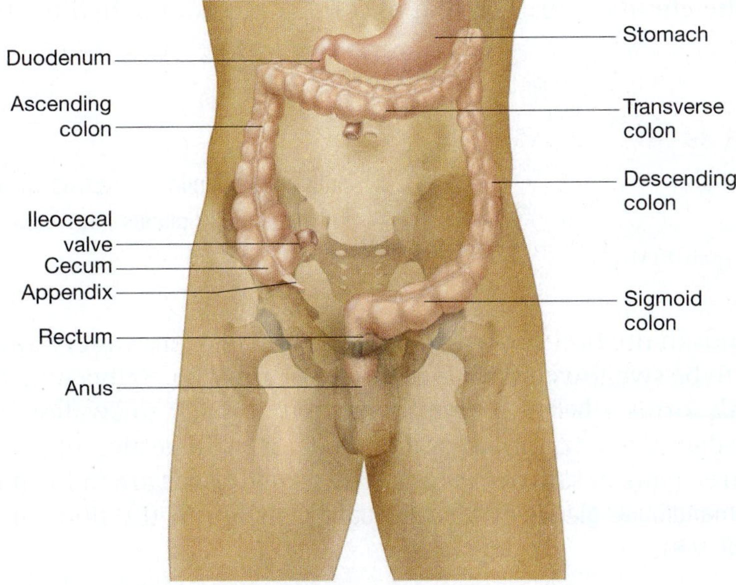

■ **Figure 8-8** The regions of the colon beginning with the cecum and ending at the anus.

PRACTICE AS YOU GO

B. Complete the Statement

1. When food is swallowed, it enters the ____________________.
2. Food is propelled through the gut by wavelike muscular contractions called ____________________.
3. Food in the stomach is mixed with ____________________ and other gastric juices to form a watery mixture called ____________________.
4. The three sections of small intestine, in order, are the ____________________, ____________________, and ____________________.
5. Structures called ____________________ greatly increase the surface area of the small intestine.
6. The large intestine extends from the ____________________ to the ____________________, and includes the ____________________, ____________________, and ____________________.
7. The S-shaped section of colon that curves back toward the rectum is called the ____________________ colon.
8. The evacuation of feces is called ____________________.

Med Term Tip

In anatomy, the term *accessory* generally means that the structure is auxiliary to a more important structure. This is not true for these organs. Digestion would not be possible without the digestive juices produced by these organs.

Accessory Organs of the Digestive System

As described earlier, the accessory organs of the digestive system are the salivary glands, the liver, the pancreas, and the gallbladder. In general, these organs function by producing much of the digestive fluids and enzymes necessary for the chemical breakdown of food. Each is attached to the gut tube by a duct.

Salivary Glands

amylase (AM-il-ace)
bolus
parotid glands (pah-ROT-id)
sublingual glands (sub-LING-gwal)
submandibular glands (sub-man-DIB-yoo-lar)

Salivary glands in the oral cavity produce saliva. This very watery and slick fluid allows food to be swallowed with less danger of choking. Saliva mixed with food in the mouth forms a **bolus**, chewed food that is ready to swallow. Saliva also contains the digestive enzyme **amylase** that begins the digestion of carbohydrates. There are three pairs of salivary glands. The **parotid glands** are in front of the ears, and the **submandibular glands** and **sublingual glands** are in the floor of the mouth (see Figure 8-9 ■).

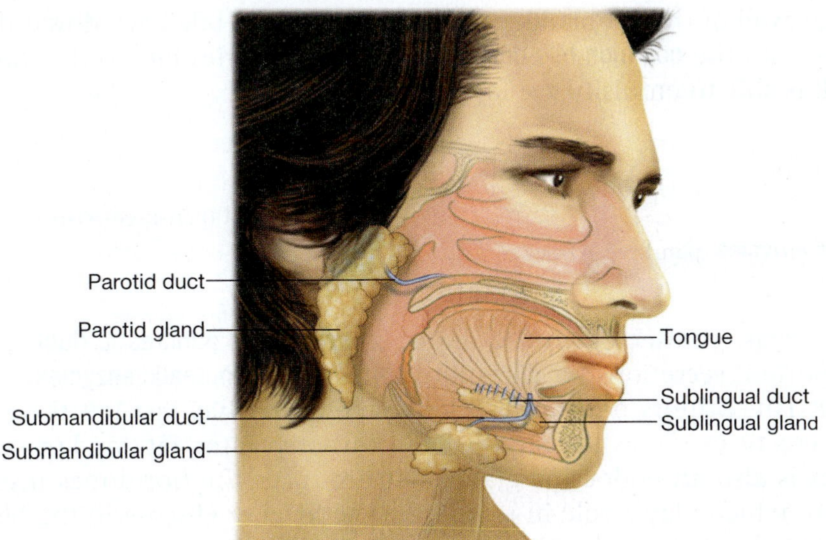

■ **Figure 8-9** The salivary glands: parotid, sublingual, and submandibular. This image shows the position of each gland and its duct emptying into the oral cavity.

Liver

bile (BYE-al) **emulsification** (ee-mull-sih-fih-KAY-shun)

The liver, a large organ located in the right upper quadrant of the abdomen, has several functions including processing the nutrients absorbed by the intestines, detoxifying harmful substances in the body, and producing **bile** (see Figure 8-10 ■). Bile is important for the digestion of fats and lipids because it breaks up large fat globules into much smaller droplets, making them easier to digest in the watery environment inside the intestines. This process is called **emulsification**.

Med Term Tip

The liver weighs about four pounds and has so many important functions that people cannot live without it. It has become a major transplant organ. The liver is also able to regenerate itself. You can lose more than half of your liver, and it will regrow.

Gallbladder

common bile duct **cystic duct** (SIS-tik)
hepatic duct (heh-PAT-ik)

Bile produced by the liver is stored in the gallbladder (GB). As the liver produces bile, it travels down the **hepatic duct** and up the **cystic duct** into the gallbladder (see again Figure 8-10). In response to the presence of fat in the chyme, the

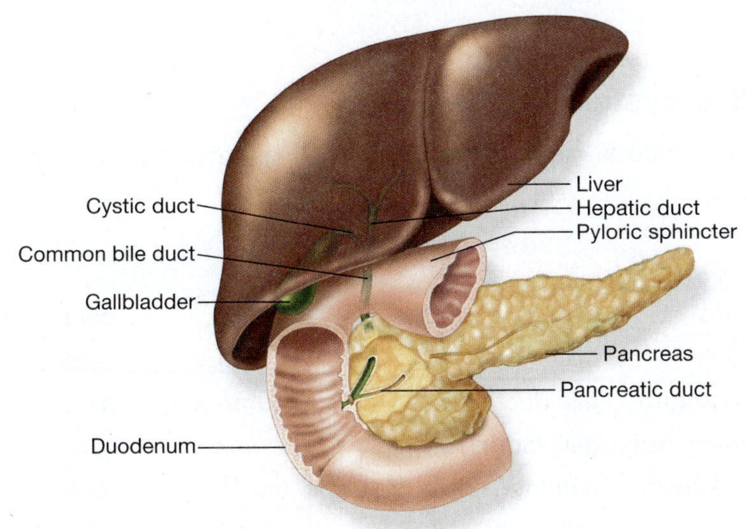

■ **Figure 8-10** The liver, gallbladder, and pancreas. Image shows the relationship of these three organs and their ducts to the duodenum.

muscular wall of the gallbladder contracts and sends bile back down the cystic duct and into the **common bile duct** (CBD), which carries bile to the duodenum where it is able to emulsify the fat in chyme.

Pancreas

buffers

pancreatic enzymes (pan-kree-AT-ik / EN-zimes)

pancreatic duct (pan-kree-AT-ik)

The pancreas, connected to the duodenum by the **pancreatic duct**, produces two important secretions for digestion: **buffers** and **pancreatic enzymes** (see again Figure 8-10). Buffers neutralize acidic chyme that has just left the stomach, and pancreatic enzymes chemically digest carbohydrates, fats, and proteins. The pancreas is also an endocrine gland that produces the hormones insulin and glucagon, which play a role in regulating the level of glucose in the blood and are discussed in further detail in Chapter 11.

PRACTICE AS YOU GO

C. Complete the Statement

1. The accessory organs of the digestive system are the ____________________, ____________________, ____________________, and ____________________.
2. Saliva contains the digestive enzyme ____________________, which begins the digestion of ____________________.
3. ____________________ produced by the liver is responsible for the ____________________ of fats and is stored in the ____________________.
4. The pancreas is connected to the ____________________ and secretes ____________________ and ____________________ for digestion.

Terminology

Word Parts Used to Build Digestive System Terms

The following lists contain the combining forms, suffixes, and prefixes used to build terms in the remaining sections of this chapter.

Combining Forms

an/o	anus	**cec/o**	cecum	**col/o**	colon
append/o	appendix	**chol/e**	bile	**colon/o**	colon
appendic/o	appendix	**cholangi/o**	bile duct	**cutane/o**	skin
bar/o	weight	**cholecyst/o**	gallbladder	**cyst/o**	sac
bucc/o	cheek	**choledoch/o**	common bile duct	**dent/o**	tooth
carcin/o	cancer	**cirrh/o**	yellow	**diverticul/o**	pouch

Combining Forms (continued)

duoden/o	duodenum
enter/o	small intestine
esophag/o	esophagus
gastr/o	stomach
gingiv/o	gums
gloss/o	tongue
hem/o	blood
hemat/o	blood
hepat/o	liver
ile/o	ileum
inguin/o	groin
jejun/o	jejunum
labi/o	lip
lapar/o	abdomen
lingu/o	tongue
lith/o	stone
mandibul/o	mandible
nas/o	nose
odont/o	tooth
or/o	mouth
orth/o	straight
palat/o	palate
pancreat/o	pancreas
pharyng/o	pharynx
polyp/o	polyp
proct/o	anus and rectum
pylor/o	pylorus
pyr/o	fire
rect/o	rectum
sialaden/o	salivary gland
sigmoid/o	sigmoid colon
ven/o	vein

Suffixes

-ac	pertaining to
-al	pertaining to
-algia	pain
-ar	pertaining to
-centesis	process of removing fluid
-eal	pertaining to
-ectomy	surgical removal
-emesis	vomiting
-emetic	pertaining to vomiting
-gram	record
-graphy	process of recording
-iatric	pertaining to medical treatment
-ic	pertaining to
-istry	specialty of
-itis	inflammation
-lithiasis	condition of stones
-logy	study of
-oma	tumor
-orexia	appetite
-osis	abnormal condition
-ostomy	surgically create an opening
-otomy	cutting into
-ous	pertaining to
-pepsia	digestion
-pexy	surgical fixation
-phagia	eat, swallow
-plasty	surgical repair
-plegia	paralysis
-prandial	pertaining to a meal
-ptosis	drooping
-scope	instrument to view
-scopic	pertaining to visually examining
-scopy	process of viewing
-tripsy	surgical crushing

Prefixes

a-	without
an-	without
anti-	against
brady-	slow
dys-	abnormal, painful, difficult
endo-	within
ex-	outward
hyper-	excessive
hypo-	below
in-	inward
intra-	within
per-	through
peri-	around
poly-	many
post-	after
re-	again
retro-	backward
sub-	under
trans-	across

Adjective Forms of Anatomical Terms

Term	Word Parts	Definition
anal	an/o = anus -al = pertaining to **Word Watch** Be careful when using the combining form **an/o** meaning *anus* and the prefix **an-** meaning *without.*	Pertaining to anus
buccal (BUK-al)	bucc/o = cheek -al = pertaining to	Pertaining to cheeks
buccolabial (buk-oh-LAY-bee-al)	bucc/o = cheek labi/o = lip -al = pertaining to	Pertaining to cheeks and lips
cecal (SEE-kal)	cec/o = cecum -al = pertaining to	Pertaining to cecum
cholecystic (koh-lee-SIS-tik)	cholecyst/o = gallbladder -ic = pertaining to	Pertaining to gallbladder
colonic (koh-LON-ik)	colon/o = colon -ic = pertaining to	Pertaining to colon
colorectal (kohl-oh-REK-tal)	col/o = colon rect/o = rectum -al = pertaining to	Pertaining to colon and rectum
cystic (SIS-tik)	cyst/o = sac -ic = pertaining to	Pertaining to gallbladder **Med Term Tip** The combining form **cyst/o** refers to the sac-like shape of the gallbladder.
dental (DEN-tal)	dent/o = tooth -al = pertaining to	Pertaining to teeth
duodenal (doo-oh-DEE-nal / doo-OD-eh-nal)	duoden/o = duodenum -al = pertaining to	Pertaining to duodenum
enteric (en-TAIR-ik)	enter/o = small intestine -ic = pertaining to	Pertaining to small intestine
esophageal (eh-soff-ah-JEE-al)	esophag/o = esophagus -eal = pertaining to	Pertaining to esophagus
gastric (GAS-trik)	gastr/o = stomach -ic = pertaining to	Pertaining to stomach
gastrointestinal (GI) (gas-troh-in-TESS-tih-nal)	gastr/o = stomach -al = pertaining to	Pertaining to stomach and intestines
gingival (JIN-jih-vul)	gingiv/o = gums -al = pertaining to	Pertaining to gums
glossal (GLOSS-al)	gloss/o = tongue -al = pertaining to	Pertaining to tongue
hepatic (heh-PAT-ik)	hepat/o = liver -ic = pertaining to	Pertaining to liver
hypoglossal (high-poh-GLOSS-al)	hypo- = under gloss/o = tongue -al = pertaining to	Pertaining to under tongue
ileal (IL-ee-al)	ile/o = ileum -al = pertaining to	Pertaining to ileum
ileocecal (il-ee-oh-SEE-kal)	ile/o = ileum cec/o = cecum -al = pertaining to	Pertaining to ileum and cecum

Adjective Forms of Anatomical Terms (continued)

Term	Word Parts	Definition
jejunal (jeh-JOO-nal)	jejun/o = jejunum -al = pertaining to	Pertaining to jejunum
labial (LAY-bee-al)	labi/o = lips -al = pertaining to	Pertaining to lips
lingual (LING-gwal)	lingu/o = tongue -al = pertaining to	Pertaining to tongue
nasogastric (nay-zoh-GAS-trik)	nas/o = nose gastr/o = stomach -ic = pertaining to	Pertaining to nose and stomach
oral (OR-al)	or/o = mouth -al = pertaining to	Pertaining to mouth
pancreatic (pan-kree-AT-ik)	pancreat/o = pancreas -ic = pertaining to	Pertaining to pancreas
periodontal (pair-ee-oh-DON-tal)	peri- = around odont/o = tooth -al = pertaining to	Pertaining to around teeth
pharyngeal (fair-IN-jee-al)	pharyng/o = pharynx -eal = pertaining to	Pertaining to pharynx
pyloric (pye-LOR-ik)	pylor/o = pylorus -ic = pertaining to	Pertaining to pylorus
rectal (REK-tal)	rect/o = rectum -al = pertaining to	Pertaining to rectum
sigmoidal (sig-MOYD-al)	sigmoid/o = sigmoid colon -al = pertaining to	Pertaining to sigmoid colon
sublingual (sub-LING-gwal)	sub- = under lingu/o = tongue -al = pertaining to	Pertaining to under tongue
submandibular (sub-man-DIB-yoo-lar)	sub- = under mandibul/o = mandible -ar = pertaining to	Pertaining to under mandible

PRACTICE AS YOU GO

D. Give the adjective form for each anatomical structure.

1. The duodenum ______
2. Nose and stomach ______
3. The liver ______
4. The pancreas ______
5. The gallbladder ______
   or ______
6. Under the tongue ______
7. The esophagus ______
8. The sigmoid colon ______

Pathology

Term	Word Parts	Definition
Medical Specialties		
dentistry	dent/o = tooth -istry = specialty of	Branch of healthcare involved with prevention, diagnosis, and treatment of conditions involving teeth, jaw, and mouth; practitioner is a *dentist*
gastroenterology (gas-troh-en-ter-ALL-oh-jee)	gastr/o = stomach enter/o = small intestine -logy = study of	Branch of medicine involved in diagnosis and treatment of diseases and disorders of digestive system; physician is a *gastroenterologist*
oral surgery	or/o = mouth -al = pertaining to	Branch of dentistry that uses surgical means to treat dental conditions; specialist is an *oral surgeon*
orthodontics (or-thoh-DON-tiks)	orth/o = straight odont/o = tooth -ic = pertaining to	Branch of dentistry concerned with correction of problems with tooth alignment; specialist is an *orthodontist*
periodontics (pair-ee-oh-DON-tiks)	peri- = around odont/o = tooth -ic = pertaining to	Branch of dentistry concerned with treating conditions involving gums and tissues surrounding the teeth; specialist is a *periodontist*
proctology (prok-TALL-oh-jee)	proct/o = anus and rectum -logy = study of	Branch of medicine involved in diagnosis and treatment of diseases and disorders of anus and rectum; physician is a *proctologist*
Signs and Symptoms		
anorexia (an-oh-REK-see-ah)	an- = without -orexia = appetite	General term meaning loss of appetite that may accompany other conditions; also used to refer to *anorexia nervosa*, which is characterized by severe weight loss from excessive dieting
aphagia (ah-FAY-jee-ah)	a- = without -phagia = eat, swallow	Being unable to swallow or eat
ascites (ah-SIGH-teez)		Collection or accumulation of fluid in the peritoneal cavity
bradypepsia (brad-ee-PEP-see-ah)	brady- = slow -pepsia = digestion	Having a slow digestive system
cachexia (kuh-KEK-see-ah)		Loss of weight and generalized wasting that occurs during a chronic disease
cholecystalgia (koh-lee-sis-TAL-jee-ah)	cholecyst/o = gallbladder -algia = pain	Having gallbladder pain
constipation (kon-stih-PAY-shun)		Experiencing difficulty in defecation or infrequent defecation
dentalgia (den-TAL-jee-ah)	dent/o = tooth -algia = pain	Tooth pain
diarrhea (dye-ah-REE-ah)		Passing of frequent, watery, or bloody bowel movements; usually accompanies gastrointestinal (GI) disorders
dysorexia (dis-oh-REK-see-ah)	dys- = abnormal -orexia = appetite	Abnormal appetite; usually a diminished appetite

Pathology (continued)

Term	Word Parts	Definition
dyspepsia (dis-PEP-see-ah)	dys- = painful -pepsia = digestion	Indigestion; commonly called an *upset stomach*
dysphagia (dis-FAY-jee-ah)	dys- = difficult -phagia = eat, swallow	Having difficulty swallowing or eating
emesis (EM-eh-sis)	*Emesis* is the Latin term meaning *to vomit*	Vomiting; the expulsion of stomach contents through the mouth
eructation (ee-ruk-TAY-shun)		Burping of gas or stomach acid into the mouth; belching
flatulence (FLAT-choo-lents)	**Med Term Tip** The term *flatulence* comes from the Latin word *flatus*, meaning *to blow.*	Presence of excess gas in stomach or intestines; may be passed through the anus
gastralgia (gas-TRAL-jee-ah)	gastr/o = stomach -algia = pain	Stomach pain
hematemesis (hee-mah-TEM-eh-sis)	hemat/o = blood -emesis = vomiting	Vomiting blood
hematochezia (hee-mat-oh-KEE-zee-ah)	hemat/o = blood	Passing bright red blood in the stool
hyperemesis (high-per-EM-eh-sis)	hyper- = excessive -emesis = vomiting	Excessive vomiting
jaundice (JAWN-dis)		Yellow cast to the skin, mucous membranes, and whites of the eyes caused by deposit of bile pigment from too much bilirubin in the blood; bilirubin is a waste product produced when worn-out red blood cells are broken down; may be symptom of a disorder such as gallstones blocking the common bile duct or carcinoma of the liver; also called *icterus*
melena (meh-LEE-nah)		Passage of dark tarry stool; color is result of digestive enzymes working on blood in the gastrointestinal tract
nausea (NAW-zee-ah)	**Med Term Tip** The term *nausea* comes from the Greek word for *seasickness.*	Urge to vomit
obesity		Having too much body fat leading to a body weight that is above a healthy level; person whose weight interferes with normal activity and body function has *morbid obesity*
polyphagia (pol-ee-FAY-jee-ah)	poly- = many -phagia = eat, swallow	Excessive eating; eating too much
postprandial (pp) (post-PRAN-dee-al)	post- = after -prandial = pertaining to a meal	After a meal

Pathology (continued)

Term	Word Parts	Definition
pyrosis (pye-ROH-sis)	**pyr/o** = fire **-osis** = abnormal condition	Pain and burning sensation usually caused by stomach acid splashing up into the esophagus; commonly called *heartburn*
regurgitation (ree-ger-jih-TAY-shun)	**re-** = again	Return of fluids and solids from the stomach into the mouth
Oral Cavity		
aphthous ulcers (AF-thus)		Painful ulcers in the mouth of unknown cause; commonly called *canker sores*
cleft lip (KLEFT)		Congenital anomaly in which upper lip and jawbone fail to fuse in the midline, leaving an open gap; often seen along with cleft palate; corrected with surgery
cleft palate (KLEFT / PAL-et)		Congenital anomaly in which roof of the mouth has a split or fissure; corrected with surgery
dental caries (KAIR-eez)	**dent/o** = tooth **-al** = pertaining to	Gradual decay and disintegration of teeth caused by bacteria; may lead to abscessed teeth; commonly called a *tooth cavity*
gingivitis (jin-jih-VIGH-tis)	**gingiv/o** = gums **-itis** = inflammation	Inflammation of the gums
herpes labialis (HER-peez / lay-bee-AL-iss)	**labi/o** = lip	Infection of the lip by herpes simplex virus type 1 (HSV-1); also called *fever blisters* or *cold sores*
periodontal disease (pair-ee-oh-DON-tal)	**peri-** = around **odont/o** = tooth **-al** = pertaining to	Disease of supporting structures of the teeth, including gums and bones; most common cause of tooth loss
sialadenitis (sigh-al-ad-eh-NIGH-tis)	**sialaden/o** = salivary gland **-itis** = inflammation	Inflammation of a salivary gland
Pharynx and Esophagus		
esophageal varices (eh-soff-ah-JEE-al / VAIR-ih-seez)	**esophag/o** = esophagus **-eal** = pertaining to	Enlarged and swollen varicose veins in lower end of the esophagus; if these rupture, serious hemorrhage results; often related to liver disease
gastroesophageal reflux disease (GERD) (gas-troh-eh-soff-ah-JEE-al / REE-fluks)	**gastr/o** = stomach **esophag/o** = esophagus **-eal** = pertaining to	Acid from the stomach flows backward up into the esophagus, causing inflammation and pain
pharyngoplegia (fah-ring-oh-PLEE-jee-ah)	**pharyng/o** = pharynx **-plegia** = paralysis	Paralysis of throat muscles
Stomach		
gastric carcinoma (GAS-trik / kar-sih-NOH-mah)	**gastr/o** = stomach **-ic** = pertaining to	Cancerous tumor in the stomach
gastritis (gas-TRYE-tis)	**gastr/o** = stomach **-itis** = inflammation	Stomach inflammation
gastroenteritis (gas-troh-en-ter-EYE-tis)	**gastr/o** = stomach **enter/o** = small intestine **-itis** = inflammation	Inflammation of stomach and small intestine

Pathology (continued)

Term	Word Parts	Definition
hiatal hernia (high-AY-tal / HER-nee-ah)	**-al** = pertaining to	Protrusion of the stomach through the diaphragm (also called a *diaphragmatocele*) and extending into the thoracic cavity; gastroesophageal reflux disease is a common symptom

■ **Figure 8-11** A hiatal hernia or diaphragmatocele. A portion of the stomach protrudes through the diaphragm into the thoracic cavity.

Term	Word Parts	Definition
peptic ulcer disease (PUD) (PEP-tik / UL-ser)	**-ic** = pertaining to	Ulcer occurring in lower portion of esophagus, stomach, and/or duodenum; thought to be caused by acid of gastric juices; initial damage to protective lining of the stomach may be caused by *Helicobacter pylori* (*H. pylori*) bacterial infection; if ulcer extends all the way through the wall of the stomach, it is called a *perforated ulcer*, which requires immediate surgery to repair

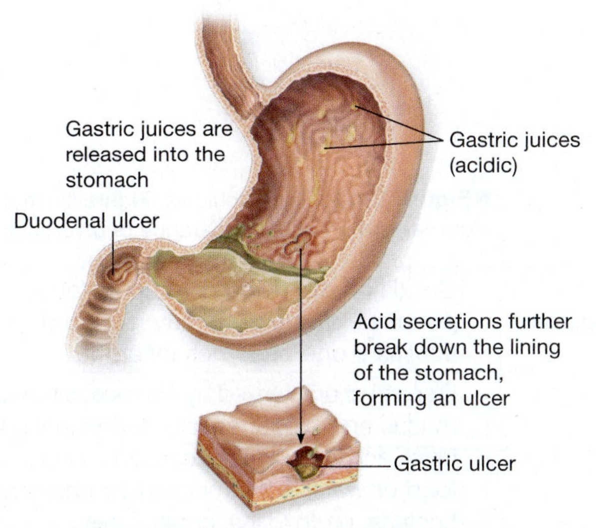
Gastric juices are released into the stomach
Gastric juices (acidic)
Duodenal ulcer
Acid secretions further break down the lining of the stomach, forming an ulcer
Gastric ulcer
A

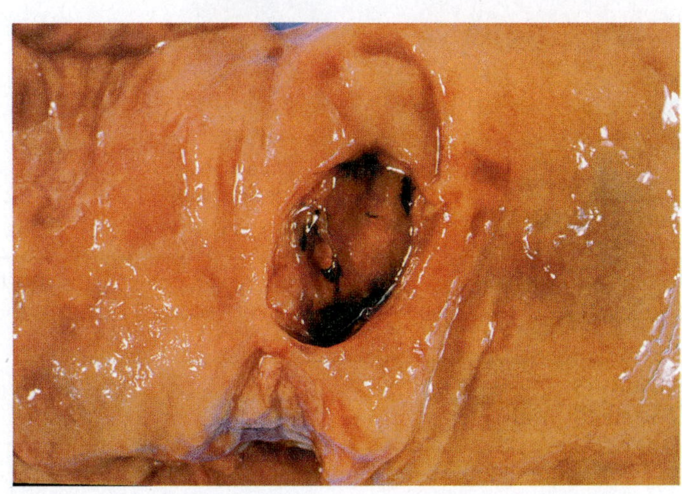
B

■ **Figure 8-12** A) Figure illustrating the location and appearance of a peptic ulcer in both the stomach and the duodenum. B) Photomicrograph illustrating a gastric ulcer. *(Dr. E. Walker/Science Source)*

Pathology (continued)

Term	Word Parts	Definition
Small Intestine and Large Intestine		
anal fistula (FIS-tyoo-lah)	**an/o** = anus **-al** = pertaining to	Abnormal tube-like passage from surface around anal opening directly into the rectum
appendicitis (ah-pen-dih-SIGH-tis)	**appendic/o** = appendix **-itis** = inflammation	Inflammation of the appendix; may require an *appendectomy*
bowel incontinence (in-KON-tih-nens)		Inability to control defecation
celiac disease (SEE-lee-ak)	**-ac** = pertaining to	Autoimmune condition affecting the small intestine; caused by reaction to eating gluten (protein found in wheat, rye, and barley); symptoms may include abdominal bloating and pain, diarrhea, and nutritional deficiencies
colorectal carcinoma (kohl-oh-REK-tal / kar-sih-NOH-mah)	**col/o** = colon **rect/o** = rectum **-al** = pertaining to **carcin/o** = cancer **-oma** = tumor	Cancerous tumor originating in colon or rectum
Crohn's disease (KROHNZ)		Form of chronic inflammatory bowel disease affecting primarily ileum and/or colon; also called *regional ileitis*; autoimmune condition affects all layers of bowel wall and results in scarring and thickening of the gut wall
diverticulitis (dye-ver-tik-yoo-LYE-tis)	**diverticul/o** = pouch **-itis** = inflammation	Inflammation of a *diverticulum* (outpouching off the gut), especially in the colon; inflammation often results when food becomes trapped within the pouch
		■ Figure 8-13 Diverticulosis. Figure illustrates external and internal appearance of diverticula.
diverticulosis (dye-ver-tik-yoo-LOH-sis)	**diverticul/o** = pouch **-osis** = abnormal condition	Condition of having diverticula (outpouches off the gut); may lead to *diverticulitis* if one becomes inflamed
dysentery (DIS-en-tair-ee)		Disease characterized by diarrhea, often with mucus and blood, severe abdominal pain, fever, and dehydration; caused by ingesting food or water contaminated by chemicals, bacteria, protozoans, or parasites
enteritis (en-ter-EYE-tis)	**enter/o** = small intestine **-itis** = inflammation	Inflammation of the small intestine

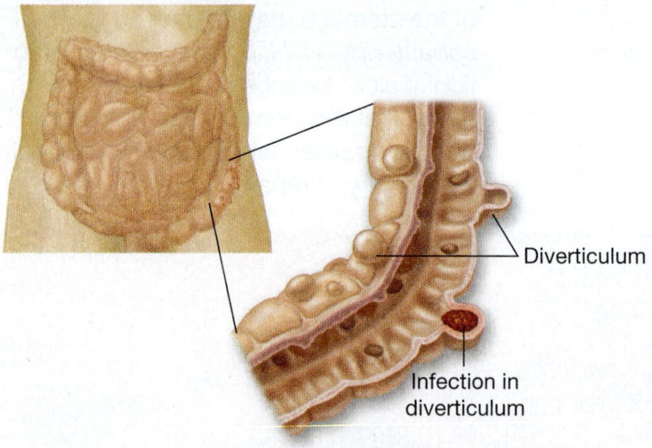

Pathology (continued)

Term	Word Parts	Definition
hemorrhoids (HEM-oh-roydz)	**hem/o** = blood	Varicose veins in rectum and anus
ileus (IL-ee-us)		Severe abdominal pain, inability to pass stool, vomiting, and abdominal distension as a result of intestinal blockage; blockage can be a physical block such as a tumor or failure of bowel contents to move forward due to loss of peristalsis (nonmechanical blockage); may require surgery to reverse blockage
inguinal hernia (ING-gwih-nal / HER-nee-ah) **Figure 8-14** An inguinal hernia. A portion of the small intestine is protruding through the abdominal muscles into the groin region.	**inguin/o** = groin **-al** = pertaining to Loop of intestine protruding through opening in abdominal muscles	Hernia or protrusion of a loop of small intestine into inguinal (groin) region through a weak spot in abdominal muscle wall that develops into a hole; may become *incarcerated* or *strangulated* if muscle tightens down around loop of intestine and cuts off its blood flow
intussusception (in-tuh-suh-SEP-shun) **Figure 8-15** Intussusception. A short length of small intestine has telescoped into itself.	**in-** = inward 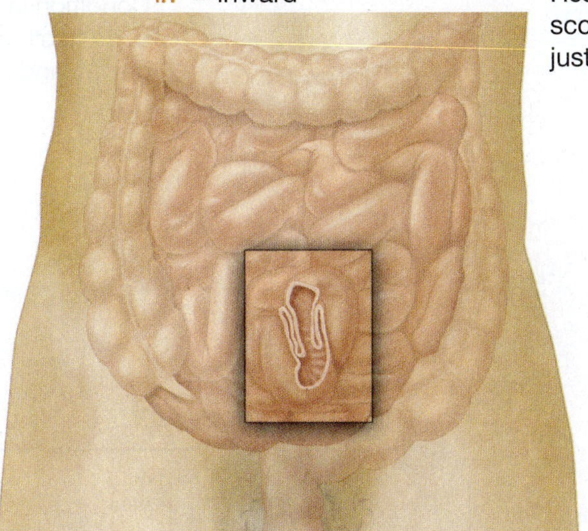	Result of the intestine slipping or telescoping into another section of intestine just below it; more common in children
irritable bowel syndrome (IBS)		Disturbance in functions of the intestine from unknown causes; symptoms generally include abdominal discomfort and alteration in bowel activity; also called *spastic colon* or *functional bowel disorder*

Pathology (continued)

Term	Word Parts	Definition
polyposis (pol-ee-POH-sis)	polyp/o = polyp -osis = abnormal condition	Presence of small tumors, called **polyps**, containing a pedicle or stemlike attachment in mucous membranes of the large intestine (colon); may be precancerous

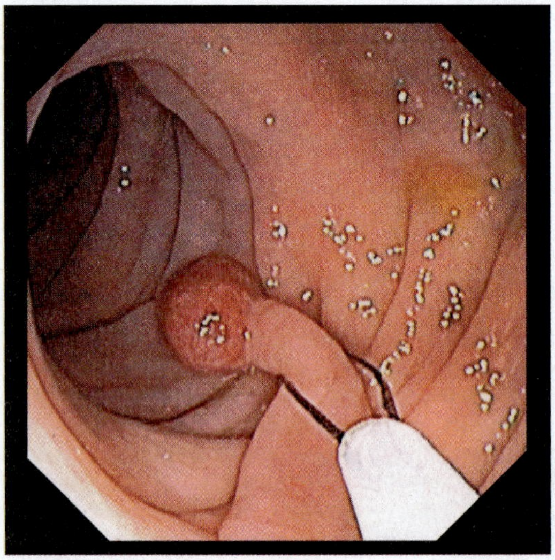

■ **Figure 8-16** Endoscopic view of a polyp in the colon. Note the mushroom-like shape, an enlarged top growing at the end of a stem. It is being removed by means of a wire loop slipped over the polyp and then tightened to cut it off. *(David M. Martin, M.D./ Science Source)*

Term	Word Parts	Definition
proctoptosis (prok-top-TOH-sis)	proct/o = rectum and anus -ptosis = drooping	Prolapsed or drooping rectum and anus
ulcerative colitis (UL-ser-ah-tiv / koh-LYE-tis)	col/o = colon -itis = inflammation	Chronic inflammatory condition resulting in numerous ulcers formed on mucous membrane lining of the colon; cause is unknown; also known as *inflammatory bowel disease* (IBD)
volvulus (VOL-vyoo-lus)		Condition in which the bowel twists upon itself, causing an obstruction; painful and requires immediate surgery

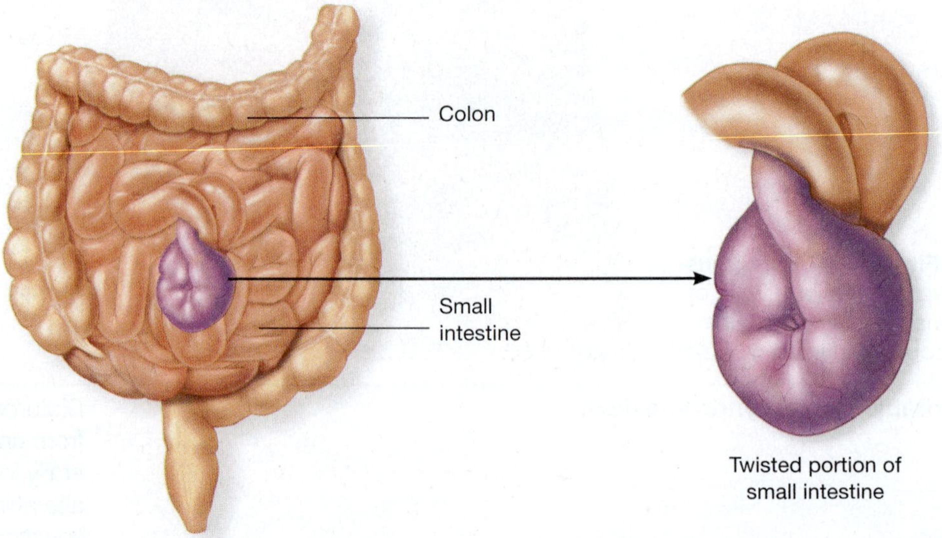

■ **Figure 8-17** Volvulus. A length of small intestine has twisted around itself, cutting off blood circulation to the twisted loop.

Pathology (continued)

Term	Word Parts	Definition
Accessory Organs		
cholecystitis (koh-lee-sis-TYE-tis)	cholecyst/o = gallbladder -itis = inflammation	Inflammation of the gallbladder; most commonly caused by gallstones in gallbladder or common bile duct that block flow of bile
cholelithiasis (koh-lee-lih-THIGH-ah-sis)	chol/e = bile -lithiasis = condition of stones	Presence of gallstones; may or may not cause symptoms such as *cholecystalgia*

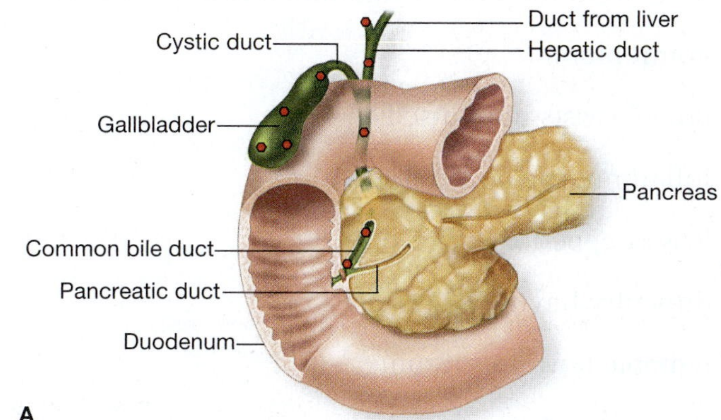

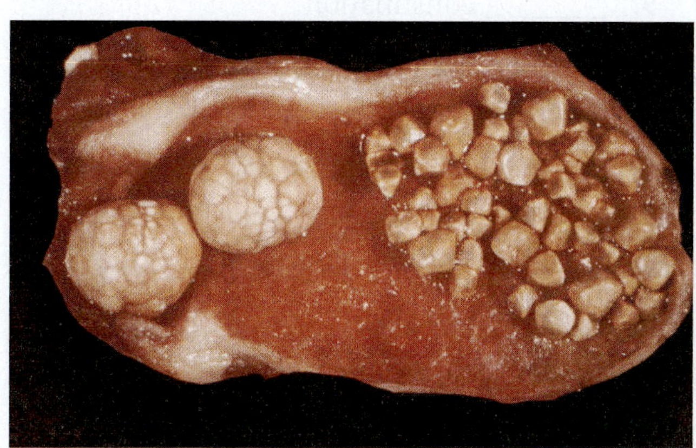

Figure 8-18 A) Common sites for cholelithiasis. B) A gallbladder specimen with multiple gallstones., *(Clinical Photography, Central Manchester University Hospitals NHS Foundation Trust, UK/Science Source)*

Term	Word Parts	Definition
cirrhosis (sih-ROH-sis)	cirrh/o = yellow -osis = abnormal condition	Chronic disease of the liver associated with failure of the liver to function properly
hepatitis (hep-ah-TYE-tis)	hepat/o = liver -itis = inflammation	Inflammation of the liver, usually due to viral infection; different viruses are transmitted by different routes, such as sexual contact or from exposure to blood or fecally contaminated water or food
hepatoma (hep-ah-TOH-mah)	hepat/o = liver -oma = tumor	Liver tumor
pancreatitis (pan-kree-ah-TYE-tis)	pancreat/o = pancreas -itis = inflammation	Inflammation of the pancreas

PRACTICE AS YOU GO

E. Terminology Matching

Match each term to its definition.

1. ________ anorexia
2. ________ hematemesis
3. ________ pyrosis
4. ________ obesity
5. ________ constipation
6. ________ melena
7. ________ ascites
8. ________ cirrhosis
9. ________ spastic colon
10. ________ polyposis
11. ________ volvulus
12. ________ hiatal hernia
13. ________ ulcerative colitis
14. ________ dysentery
15. ________ jaundice

a. excess body weight
b. chronic liver disease
c. heartburn
d. small colon tumors
e. fluid accumulation in abdominal cavity
f. vomit blood
g. bowel twists upon itself
h. inflammatory bowel disease
i. loss of appetite
j. difficulty having BM
k. irritable bowel syndrome
l. dark tarry stool
m. yellow skin color
n. bloody diarrhea
o. diaphragmatocele

Diagnostic Procedures

Term	Word Parts	Definition
Clinical Laboratory Tests		
alanine transaminase (ALT) (AL-ah-neen / trans-AM-ih-nase)		Enzyme normally present in the blood; blood levels are increased in persons with liver disease
aspartate transaminase (AST) (as-PAR-tate / trans-AM-ih-nase)		Enzyme normally present in the blood; blood levels are increased in persons with liver disease
fecal occult blood test (FOBT) (uh-CULT)	-al = pertaining to	Laboratory test on feces to determine if microscopic amounts of blood are present; also called *hemoccult* or *stool guaiac*
***H. pylori* antibody test** (pye-LOR-ee)	anti- = against	Laboratory test used to diagnose *H. pylori* infection that may be associated with peptic ulcer disease; may be performed on stool, breath, or tissue sample

Diagnostic Procedures (continued)

Term	Word Parts	Definition
ova and parasites (O&P) (OH-vah / PAIR-ah-sights)		Laboratory examination of feces with a microscope for presence of parasites or their eggs
serum bilirubin (SEER-um / bil-ih-ROO-bin)		Blood test to determine amount of waste product bilirubin in bloodstream; elevated levels indicate liver disease
stool culture		Laboratory test of feces to determine if any pathogenic bacteria are present
tissue transglutaminase (tTG) **antibody test** (trans-GLOO-tah-mih-nays)		Laboratory blood test for celiac disease; tests for presence of antibodies formed in autoimmune response to gluten
Diagnostic Imaging		
bitewing X-ray		X-ray taken with a part of film holder held between the teeth and parallel to the teeth
cholecystogram (koh-lee-SIS-toh-gram)	cholecyst/o = gallbladder -gram = record	X-ray image of the gallbladder
intravenous cholecystography (in-trah-VEE-nus / koh-lee-sis-TOG-rah-fee)	intra- = within ven/o = vein -ous = pertaining to cholecyst/o = gallbladder -graphy = process of recording	Dye is administered intravenously to patient allowing for X-ray visualization of gallbladder and bile ducts
lower gastrointestinal series (lower GI series)	gastr/o = stomach -al = pertaining to ■ **Figure 8-19** X-ray of the colon taken during a barium enema. *(Kaling2100/Shutterstock)*	X-ray image of colon and rectum is taken after administration of barium (Ba), a radiopaque dye, by enema; also called a *barium enema* (BE, BaE)
percutaneous transhepatic cholangiography (PTC) (per-kyoo-TAY-nee-us / trans-heh-PAT-ik / koh-lan-jee-OG-rah-fee)	per- = through cutane/o = skin -ous = pertaining to trans- = across hepat/o = liver -ic = pertaining to cholangi/o = bile duct -graphy = process of recording	Procedure in which contrast medium is injected directly into the liver to visualize the bile ducts; used to detect obstructions such as gallstones in the common bile duct

Diagnostic Procedures (continued)

Term	Word Parts	Definition
upper gastrointestinal (UGI) **series**	gastr/o = stomach -al = pertaining to	Patient is administered a barium (Ba) contrast material orally and then X-rays are taken to visualize esophagus, stomach, and duodenum; also called a *barium swallow*
Endoscopic Procedures		
colonoscope (koh-LON-oh-skohp)	colon/o = colon -scope = instrument to view	Instrument used to view the colon
colonoscopy (koh-lon-OSS-koh-pee)	colon/o = colon -scopy = process of viewing	Flexible fiberscope called a *colonoscope* is passed through anus, rectum, and colon; used to examine upper portion of the colon; polyps and small growths can be removed during this procedure (see again Figure 8-16)
endoscopic retrograde cholangiopancreatography (ERCP) (en-doh-SKOP-ik / RET-roh-grayd / koh-lan-jee-oh-pan-kree-ah-TOG-rah-fee)	endo- = within -scopic = pertaining to visually examining retro- = backward cholangi/o = bile duct pancreat/o = pancreas -graphy = process of recording	Procedure using an endoscope to visually examine hepatic duct, common bile duct, and pancreatic duct; first an endoscope is passed through patient's mouth, esophagus, and stomach until it reaches the duodenum, where the pancreatic and common bile ducts empty; then a thin catheter is passed through the endoscope and into ducts (in retrograde direction); contrast dye is then used to visualize these ducts on an X-ray
esophagogastroduodenoscopy (EGD) (eh-soff-ah-goh-gas-troh-doo-od-eh-NOSS-koh-pee)	esophag/o = esophagus gastr/o = stomach duoden/o = duodenum -scopy = process of viewing	Use of flexible fiberoptic endoscope to visually examine esophagus, stomach, and beginning of the duodenum
gastroscope (GAS-troh-skohp)	gastr/o = stomach -scope = instrument to view	Instrument used to view inside the stomach
gastroscopy (gas-TROSS-koh-pee)	gastr/o = stomach -scopy = process of viewing	Procedure in which flexible *gastroscope* is passed through the mouth and down the esophagus in order to visualize inside the stomach; used to diagnose peptic ulcers and gastric carcinoma
laparoscope (LAP-ah-roh-skohp)	lapar/o = abdomen -scope = instrument to view	Instrument used to view inside the abdomen
laparoscopy (lap-ar-OSS-koh-pee)	lapar/o = abdomen -scopy = process of viewing	*Laparoscope* is passed into abdominal wall through a small incision; abdominal cavity is then visually examined for tumors and other conditions with this lighted instrument; also called *peritoneoscopy*
sigmoidoscope (sig-MOYD-oh-skohp)	sigmoid/o = sigmoid colon -scope = instrument to view	Instrument used to view inside the sigmoid colon

Diagnostic Procedures (continued)

Term	Word Parts	Definition
sigmoidoscopy (sig-moy-DOSS-koh-pee)	**sigmoid/o** = sigmoid colon **-scopy** = process of viewing	Procedure using flexible *sigmoido-scope* to visually examine the sigmoid colon; commonly done to diagnose cancer and polyps
Additional Diagnostic Procedures		
body mass index (BMI)		Method of determining if person's weight is healthy (neither under, nor overweight); calculated by dividing person's weight in kilograms by his or her height in square meters; there are many online calculators; a BMI below 18.5 is underweight, 18.5–24.9 is healthy, 25.0–29.9 is overweight, 30.0–39.9 is obese, and over 40 is morbid obesity
paracentesis (pair-ah-sen-TEE-sis)	**-centesis** = process of removing fluid	Insertion of a needle into abdominal cavity to withdraw fluid; tests to diagnose diseases may be conducted on the fluid

Therapeutic Procedures

Term	Word Parts	Definition
Dental Procedures		
bridge		Dental appliance to replace missing teeth; attached to adjacent teeth for support
crown		Artificial covering for a tooth that is created to replace original enamel covering of the tooth
denture (DEN-chur)	**dent/o** = tooth	Partial or complete set of artificial teeth that are set in plastic materials; acts as substitute for natural teeth and related structures
extraction	**ex-** = outward	Removing or "pulling" of teeth
gingivectomy (jin-jih-VEK-toh-mee)	**gingiv/o** = gums **-ectomy** = surgical removal	Surgical removal of gum tissue that has pulled away from the teeth and may lead to periodontal disease
implant (IM-plant)		Prosthetic device placed in the jaw to which a tooth or denture may be anchored
root canal	**-al** = pertaining to	Dental treatment involving pulp cavity of the root of a tooth; procedure is used to save a tooth that is badly infected or abscessed
Medical Procedures		
enema (EN-eh-mah)		Injection of fluid through the rectum and into the large intestine for purpose of cleansing bowel for testing, treating constipation, or administering drugs
gavage (guh-VAHZH)		Use of nasogastric (NG) tube to place liquid nourishment directly into the stomach

Therapeutic Procedures (continued)

Term	Word Parts	Definition
lavage (lah-VAHZH)		Use of nasogastric (NG) tube to wash out the stomach, for example, after ingestion of dangerous substances
nasogastric intubation (NG tube) (nay-zoh-GAS-trik / in-too-BAY-shun)	nas/o = nose gastr/o = stomach -ic = pertaining to in- = inward	Procedure in which a flexible catheter is inserted into the nose and down the esophagus to the stomach; may be used for feeding or to suction out stomach fluids
total parenteral nutrition (TPN) (pah-REN-ter-al)	-al = pertaining to	Providing 100% of patient's nutrition intravenously; used when patient is unable to eat
Surgical Procedures		
anastomosis (ah-nas-toh-MOH-sis)		To surgically create a connection between two organs or vessels; for example, joining together two cut ends of the intestines after a section is removed
appendectomy (ap-en-DEK-toh-mee)	append/o = appendix -ectomy = surgical removal	Surgical removal of the appendix
bariatric surgery (bare-ee-AT-rik)	bar/o = weight -iatric = pertaining to medical treatment	Group of surgical procedures designed to treat morbid (extreme) obesity by reducing size of the stomach or diverting food from passing through a portion of the alimentary canal
cholecystectomy (koh-lee-sis-TEK-toh-mee)	cholecyst/o = gallbladder -ectomy = surgical removal	Surgical removal of the gallbladder
choledocholithotripsy (koh-led-oh-koh-LITH-oh-trip-see)	choledoch/o = common bile duct lith/o = stone -tripsy = surgical crushing	Crushing of a gallstone in the common bile duct
colectomy (koh-LEK-toh-mee)	col/o = colon -ectomy = surgical removal	Surgical removal of the colon
colostomy (koh-LOSS-toh-mee)	col/o = colon -ostomy = surgically create an opening	Surgical creation of an opening of some portion of the colon through the abdominal wall to the outside surface; fecal material (stool) drains into a bag worn on the abdomen

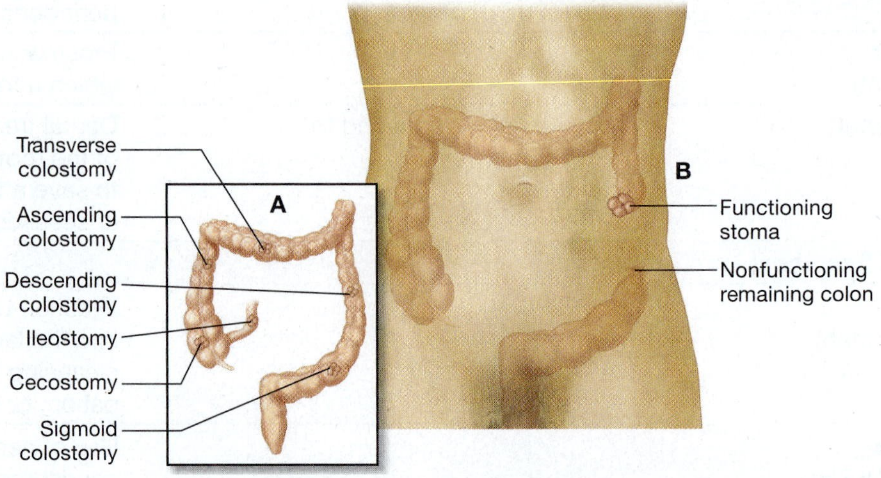

Figure 8-20 A) The colon illustrating various ostomy sites. B) Colostomy in the descending colon, illustrating functioning stoma and nonfunctioning distal sigmoid colon and rectum.

Therapeutic Procedures (continued)

Term	Word Parts	Definition
diverticulectomy (dye-ver-tik-yoo-LEK-toh-mee)	**diverticul/o** = pouch **-ectomy** = surgical removal	Surgical removal of a diverticulum
exploratory laparotomy (ek-SPLOR-ah-tor-ee / lap-ah-ROT-oh-mee)	**lapar/o** = abdomen **-otomy** = cutting into	Abdominal operation for purpose of examining abdominal organs and tissues for signs of disease or other abnormalities
fistulectomy (fis-tyoo-LEK-toh-mee)	**-ectomy** = surgical removal	Removal of an anal fistula
gastric banding	**gastr/o** = stomach **-ic** = pertaining to	Laparoscopic bariatric surgical procedure that places a restrictive band (commonly called a *lap-band*) around top portion of the stomach; leads to eating smaller meals and less food by reducing ability of the stomach to expand and hold food
gastric bypass	**gastr/o** = stomach **-ic** = pertaining to	Bariatric surgical procedure that divides the stomach into small upper portion and larger lower portion; small intestine is then connected to small upper portion; food bypasses most of the stomach and duodenum; small stomach seriously limits amount of food eaten and bypassing the duodenum reduces fat absorption
gastrectomy (gas-TREK-toh-mee)	**gastr/o** = stomach **-ectomy** = surgical removal	Surgical removal of the stomach
gastric stapling	**gastr/o** = stomach **-ic** = pertaining to	Procedure that closes off a large section of the stomach with rows of staples; results in much smaller stomach to assist very obese patients to lose weight
gastrostomy (gas-TROSS-toh-mee)	**gastr/o** = stomach **-ostomy** = surgically create an opening	Surgical procedure to create opening in the stomach
hemorrhoidectomy (hem-oh-royd-EK-toh-mee)	**-ectomy** = surgical removal	Surgical removal of hemorrhoids from anorectal area
hernioplasty (her-nee-oh-PLAS-tee)	**-plasty** = surgical repair	Surgical repair of a hernia; also called *herniorrhaphy*
ileostomy (il-ee-OSS-toh-mee)	**ile/o** = ileum **-ostomy** = surgically create an opening	Surgical creation of an opening in the ileum
laparoscopic cholecystectomy (lap-ar-oh-SKOP-ik / koh-lee-sis-TEK-toh-mee)	**lapar/o** = abdomen **-scopic** = pertaining to visually examining **cholecyst/o** = gallbladder **-ectomy** = surgical removal	Surgical removal of the gallbladder through a very small abdominal incision with assistance of a laparoscope
laparotomy (lap-ah-ROT-oh-mee)	**lapar/o** = abdomen **-otomy** = cutting into	Surgical incision into the abdomen
liver transplant		Transplant of a liver from a donor
palatoplasty (PAL-ah-toh-plas-tee)	**palat/o** = palate **-plasty** = surgical repair	Surgical repair of the palate

Therapeutic Procedures (continued)

Term	Word Parts	Definition
pharyngoplasty (fah-RING-oh-plas-tee)	pharyng/o = pharynx -plasty = surgical repair	Surgical repair of the throat
proctopexy (PROK-toh-pek-see)	proct/o = rectum and anus -pexy = surgical fixation	Surgical fixation of the rectum and anus

PRACTICE AS YOU GO

F. Procedure Matching

Match each procedure term with its definition.

1. ________ serum bilirubin
2. ________ lavage
3. ________ bariatric surgery
4. ________ proctopexy
5. ________ lower GI series
6. ________ paracentesis
7. ________ fecal occult blood test
8. ________ laparoscopy

a. withdraws fluid from abdominal cavity
b. barium enema
c. visually examines abdominal cavity
d. stool guaiac
e. treatment for obesity
f. elevated levels indicate liver disease
g. to wash out the stomach
h. surgical fixation of rectum and anus

Pharmacology

Classification	Word Parts	Action	Examples
anorexiant (an-oh-REKS-ee-ant)	an- = without -orexia = appetite	Treats obesity by suppressing appetite	phendimetrazine, Adipost, Obezine; phentermine, Zantryl, Adipex
antacid	anti- = against	Used to neutralize stomach acids	calcium carbonate, Tums; aluminum hydroxide and magnesium hydroxide, Maalox, Mylanta
antidiarrheal (an-tee-dye-ah-REE-al)	anti- = against -al = pertaining to	Used to control diarrhea	loperamide, Imodium; diphenoxylate and atropine, Lomotil; kaolin/pectin, Kaopectate
antiemetic (an-tye-ee-MEH-tik)	anti- = against -emetic = pertaining to vomiting	Treats nausea and vomiting and motion sickness	prochlorperazine, Compazine; promethazine, Phenergan
herpes antivirals	anti- = against	Treat herpes simplex infection	valacyclovir, Valtrex; famcyclovir, Famvir; acyclovir, Zovirax

Pharmacology (continued)

Classification	Word Parts	Action	Examples
H_2-receptor antagonist	anti- = against	Used to treat peptic ulcers and gastroesophageal reflux disease; when stimulated, H_2-receptors increase production of stomach acid; using an antagonist to block these receptors results in low acid level in the stomach	ranitidine, Zantac; cimetidine, Tagamet; famotidine, Pepcid
laxative **Med Term Tip** The term *laxative* comes from the Latin term meaning *to relax*.		Treats constipation by stimulating a bowel movement	senosides, Senokot; psyllium, Metamucil
proton pump inhibitors		Used to treat peptic ulcers and gastroesophageal reflux disease; blocks the stomach's ability to secrete acid	esomeprazole, Nexium; omeprazole, Prilosec

Abbreviations

ac	before meals	**HDV**	hepatitis D virus
ALT	alanine transaminase	**HEV**	hepatitis E virus
AST	aspartate transaminase	**HSV-1**	herpes simplex virus type 1
Ba	barium	**IBD**	inflammatory bowel disease
BaE	barium enema	**IBS**	irritable bowel syndrome
BE	barium enema	**IVC**	intravenous cholangiography
BM	bowel movement	**N&V**	nausea and vomiting
BMI	body mass index	**NG**	nasogastric (tube)
BS	bowel sounds	**NPO**	nothing by mouth
CBD	common bile duct	**O&P**	ova and parasites
EGD	esophagogastroduodenoscopy	**pc**	after meals
ERCP	endoscopic retrograde cholangiopancreatography	**PO**	by mouth
FOBT	fecal occult blood test	**pp**	postprandial
GB	gallbladder	**PTC**	percutaneous transhepatic cholangiography
GERD	gastroesophageal reflux disease	**PUD**	peptic ulcer disease
GI	gastrointestinal	**q**	every
H. pylori	*Helicobacter pylori*	**qam**	every morning
HAV	hepatitis A virus	**qh**	every hour
HBV	hepatitis B virus	**TPN**	total parenteral nutrition
HCl	hydrochloric acid	**tTG**	tissue transglutaminase
HCV	hepatitis C virus	**UGI**	upper gastrointestinal series

PRACTICE AS YOU GO

G. What's the Abbreviation?

1. nasogastric ____________________
2. gastrointestinal ____________________
3. hepatitis B virus ____________________
4. fecal occult blood test ____________________
5. inflammatory bowel disease ____________________
6. herpes simplex virus type 1 ____________________
7. aspartate transaminase ____________________
8. after meals ____________________
9. peptic ulcer disease ____________________
10. gastroesophageal reflux disease ____________________

Chapter Review

Real-World Applications

Medical Record Analysis

This Gastroenterology Consultation Report contains 12 medical terms. Underline each term and write it in the list below the report. Then explain each term as you would to a nonmedical person.

Gastroenterology Consultation Report

Reason for Consultation:	Evaluation of recurrent epigastric pain with anemia and melena.
History of Present Illness:	Patient is a 56-year-old male. He reports a long history of mild dyspepsia characterized by burning epigastric pain, especially when his stomach is empty. This pain has been temporarily relieved by over-the-counter antacids. Approximately two weeks ago, the pain became significantly worse and he noted that his stool was dark and tarry.
Results of Physical Examination:	CBC indicates anemia, and a fecal occult blood test is positive for blood. A blood test for *Helicobacter pylori* is positive. Gastroscopy located an ulcer in the lining of the stomach. This ulcer is 1.5 cm in diameter and deep. There is evidence of active bleeding from the ulcer.
Assessment:	Peptic ulcer disease
Recommendations:	A gastrectomy to remove the ulcerated portion of the stomach is indicated because the ulcer is already bleeding.

	Term	Explanation
1.	______________	______________________________
2.	______________	______________________________
3.	______________	______________________________
4.	______________	______________________________
5.	______________	______________________________
6.	______________	______________________________
7.	______________	______________________________
8.	______________	______________________________
9.	______________	______________________________
10.	______________	______________________________
11.	______________	______________________________
12.	______________	______________________________

Chart Note Transcription

The chart note below contains 12 phrases that can be reworded with a medical term presented in this chapter. Each phrase is identified with an underline. Determine the medical term and write your answers in the space provided.

Pearson General Hospital Consultation Report

Task Edit View Time Scale Options Help Download Archive Date: 17 May 2017

Current Complaint:	Patient is a 74-year-old female seen by a <u>physician who specializes in the treatment of the gastrointestinal tract</u> **1** with complaints of severe lower abdominal pain and extreme <u>difficulty with having a bowel movement</u>. **2**
Past History:	Patient has a history of the <u>presence of gallstones</u> **3** requiring <u>surgical removal of the gallbladder</u> **4** 10 years ago and chronic <u>acid backing up from the stomach into the esophagus</u>. **5**
Signs and Symptoms:	The patient's abdomen is distended with <u>fluid collecting in the abdominal cavity</u>. **6** <u>X-ray of the colon after inserting barium dye with an enema</u> **7** revealed <u>the presence of multiple small tumors growing on a stalk</u> **8** throughout the colon. <u>Visual examination of the colon by a scope inserted through the rectum</u> **9** was performed, and biopsies taken for microscopic examination located a tumor.
Diagnosis:	Carcinoma of the <u>section of colon between the descending colon and the rectum</u> **10**
Treatment:	<u>Surgical removal of the colon</u> **11** between the descending colon and the rectum with <u>the surgical creation of an opening of the colon through the abdominal wall</u>. **12**

1. ______________________

2. ______________________

3. ______________________

4. ______________________

5. ______________________

6. ______________________

7. ______________________

8. ______________________

9. ______________________

10. ______________________

11. ______________________

12. ______________________

Case Study

Below is a case study presentation of a patient with a condition discussed in this chapter. Read the case study and answer the questions below. Some questions will ask for information not included within this chapter. Use your text, a medical dictionary, or any other reference material you choose to answer these questions.

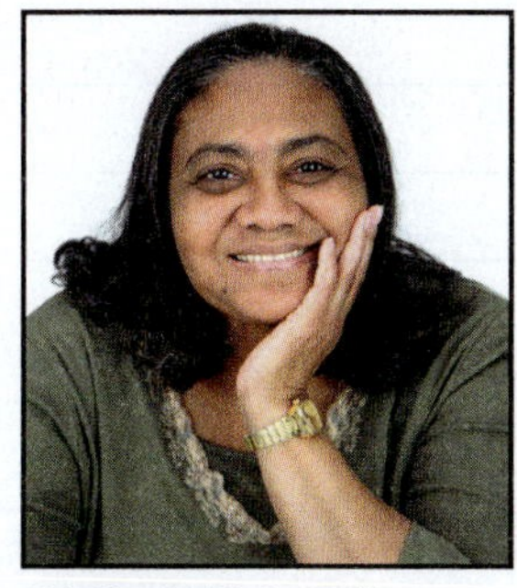

(Rob Marmion/Shutterstock)

A 60-year-old obese female has come into the ER due to severe RUQ pain for the past two hours. Patient also reports increasing nausea but denies emesis. Patient states she has been told she has cholelithiasis by her family physician following a milder episode of this pain two years ago. In addition to severe pain, patient displays a moderate degree of scleral jaundice. Abdominal ultrasound identified acute cholecystitis and a large number of gallstones. Because of the jaundice, a PTC was performed and confirmed choledocholithiasis. Patient was sent to surgery for laparoscopic cholecystectomy to remove the gallbladder and all gallstones. She recovered without incident.

Questions

1. Define each of the patient's symptoms.

____

____

2. The patient has severe RUQ pain. What organs are located in the RUQ?

____

____

3. After reading the definition of jaundice, what is most likely causing this patient to have it?

____

____

4. Describe the diagnostic imaging procedures this patient received.

____

____

5. What is the difference between *cholelithiasis* and *cholecystitis?*

____

____

6. The patient's gallbladder was removed laparoscopically. What does that mean?

____

____

Practice Exercises

A. Word Building Practice

The combining form **gastr/o** refers to the *stomach*. Use it to write a term that means:

1. inflammation of the stomach ______
2. study of the stomach and small intestine ______
3. removal of the stomach ______
4. visual exam of the stomach ______
5. stomach pain ______
6. enlargement of the stomach ______
7. cutting into the stomach ______

The combining form **esophag/o** refers to the *esophagus*. Use it to write a term that means:

8. inflammation of the esophagus ______
9. visual examination of the esophagus ______
10. surgical repair of the esophagus ______
11. pertaining to the esophagus ______
12. surgical removal (of part) of esophagus ______

The combining form **proct/o** refers to the *rectum* and *anus*. Use it to write a term that means:

13. surgical fixation of the rectum and anus ______
14. drooping of the rectum and anus ______
15. inflammation of the rectum and anus ______
16. specialist in the study of the rectum and anus ______

The combining form **cholecyst/o** refers to the *gallbladder*. Use it to write a term that means:

17. removal of the gallbladder ______
18. condition of having gallbladder stones ______
19. gallbladder stone surgical crushing ______
20. gallbladder inflammation ______

The combining form **lapar/o** refers to the *abdomen*. Use it to write a term that means:

21. instrument to view inside the abdomen ______
22. cutting into the abdomen ______
23. visual examination of the abdomen ______

The combining form **hepat/o** refers to the *liver*. Use it to write a term that means:

24. liver tumor ______
25. enlargement of the liver ______
26. pertaining to the liver ______
27. inflammation of the liver ______

The combining form **pancreat/o** refers to the *pancreas*. Use it to write a term that means:

28. inflammation of the pancreas ____________________
29. pertaining to the pancreas ____________________

The combining form **col/o** refers to the *colon*. Use it to write a term that means:

30. surgically create an opening in the colon ____________________
31. inflammation of the colon ____________________

B. Complete the Term

For each definition given below, fill in the blank with the word part that completes the term.

Definition	Term
1. surgical repair of the throat	____________plasty
2. liver tumor	____________oma
3. surgical removal of the stomach	____________ectomy
4. abnormal condition of polyps	____________osis
5. instrument to view inside sigmoid colon	____________scope
6. after a meal	post ____________
7. record of the gallbladder	____________gram
8. inflammation of the pancreas	____________itis
9. salivary gland inflammation	____________itis
10. without appetite	____________
11. vomiting blood	hemat____________
12. slow digestion	brady____________
13. study of stomach and small intestine	____________logy
14. difficult eating/swallowing	dys____________
15. pertaining to around the tooth	peri____________al

C. Using Abbreviations

Fill in each blank with the appropriate abbreviation.

1. As the colon was no longer functioning, __________ was given via a(n) __________ tube.
2. Peter had to drink barium to have a(n) __________ series.
3. The physician thought the patient may have intestinal parasites, so a(n) __________ was ordered.
4. __________ is commonly called *spastic colon*.
5. The diagnosis of __________ was confirmed after the ulcer was observed during a gastroscopy.
6. Stomach acid splashing up into the esophagus resulted in the development of __________.
7. The child complained of severe __________ because of having the stomach flu.
8. Persons with liver disease may have increased levels of __________ and __________ in the blood.
9. The __________ is also called a *hemoccult*.
10. After colon surgery, the nurses watched for the first __________ to know that the colon was functioning properly.

D. Define the Term

1. colonoscopy ______________________
2. bitewing X-ray ______________________
3. hematochezia ______________________
4. serum bilirubin ______________________
5. cachexia ______________________
6. lavage ______________________
7. hernioplasty ______________________
8. extraction ______________________
9. choledocholithotripsy ______________________
10. anastomosis ______________________

E. Fill in the Blank

colonoscopy	barium swallow	lower GI series
gastric stapling	colostomy	colectomy
total parenteral nutrition	choledocholithotripsy	liver biopsy
ileostomy	fecal occult blood test	intravenous cholecystography

1. Excising a small piece of hepatic tissue for microscopic examination is called a(n) ________________.
2. When a surgeon performs a total or partial colectomy for cancer, she may have to create an opening on the surface of the skin for fecal matter to leave the body. This procedure is called a(n) ________________.
3. Another name for an upper GI series is a(n) ________________.
4. Mr. White has had a radiopaque material placed into his colon by means of an enema for the purpose of viewing his colon. This procedure is called a(n) ________________.
5. A(n) ________________ is the surgical removal of the colon.
6. Jessica has been on a red meat–free diet in preparation for a test of her feces for the presence of hidden blood. This test is called a(n) ________________.
7. Dr. Mendez uses equipment to crush gallstones in the common bile duct. This procedure is called a(n) ________________.
8. Mrs. Alcazar required ________________ because she could not eat following her intestinal surgery.
9. Mr. Bright had ________________ to treat his morbid obesity.
10. Visualizing the gallbladder and bile ducts by injecting a dye into the patient's arm is called a(n) ________________.
11. Passing an instrument into the anus and rectum in order to see the colon is called a(n) ________________.
12. Ms. Fayne suffers from Crohn's disease, which has necessitated the removal of much of her small intestine. She has had a surgical passage created for the external disposal of waste material from the ileum. This is called a(n) ________________.

F. Terminology Matching

Match each term to its definition.

1. ________ denture	a. tooth decay
2. ________ cementum	b. prosthetic device used to anchor a tooth
3. ________ root canal	c. inflammation of the gums
4. ________ crown	d. full set of artificial teeth
5. ________ bridge	e. portion of the tooth covered by enamel
6. ________ implant	f. replacement for missing teeth
7. ________ gingivitis	g. anchors root in bony socket of jaw
8. ________ dental caries	h. surgery on the tooth pulp

G. Pharmacology Challenge

Fill in the classification for each drug description, then match the brand name.

Drug Description	Classification	Brand Name
1. ________ Controls diarrhea	________________	a. Pepcid
2. ________ Blocks stomach's ability to secrete acid	________________	b. Obezine
3. ________ Treats motion sickness	________________	c. Metamucil
4. ________ Blocks acid-producing receptors	________________	d. Compazine
5. ________ Suppresses appetite	________________	e. Maalox
6. ________ Stimulates a bowel movement	________________	f. Imodium
7. ________ Neutralizes stomach acid	________________	g. Valtrex
8. ________ Treats herpes simplex infection	________________	h. Nexium

H. Spelling Practice

Some of the following terms are misspelled. Identify the incorrect terms and spell them correctly in the blank provided.

1. gastrointestinal ________________
2. salivery ________________
3. ileocecal ________________
4. submandibuler ________________
5. cachexia ________________
6. cholecystalgia ________________
7. diverticulosis ________________
8. proctoptisis ________________
9. laparoscopy ________________
10. antidiarheal ________________

I. Anatomical Adjectives

Fill in the blank with the missing noun or adjective.

	Noun	Adjective
1.	cheek	__________
2.	gallbladder	__________
3.	__________	jejunal
4.	__________	colorectal
5.	under the tongue	__________
6.	__________	enteric
7.	__________	pancreatic
8.	tooth	__________
9.	__________	labial
10.	__________	sigmoidal
11.	throat	__________
12.	stomach	__________
13.	__________	duodenal
14.	liver	__________
15.	mouth	__________

J. Complete the Statement

1. The pancreas secretes __________ and __________ to aid in digestion.
2. The gallbladder stores __________ produced by the __________.
3. Saliva contains the digestive enzyme __________.
4. The colon extends from the __________ to the __________.
5. The major site for digestion and absorption of nutrients is the __________.
6. The __________ regulates the passage of food into the small intestine.
7. __________ is the wavelike muscular contractions that move food through the esophagus.
8. The __________ prevents food from entering the respiratory tract.
9. The biting teeth are the __________ and __________. The grinding teeth are the __________ and __________.
10. Another term for the gums is __________.

Labeling Exercises

Image A

Write the labels for this figure on the numbered lines provided.

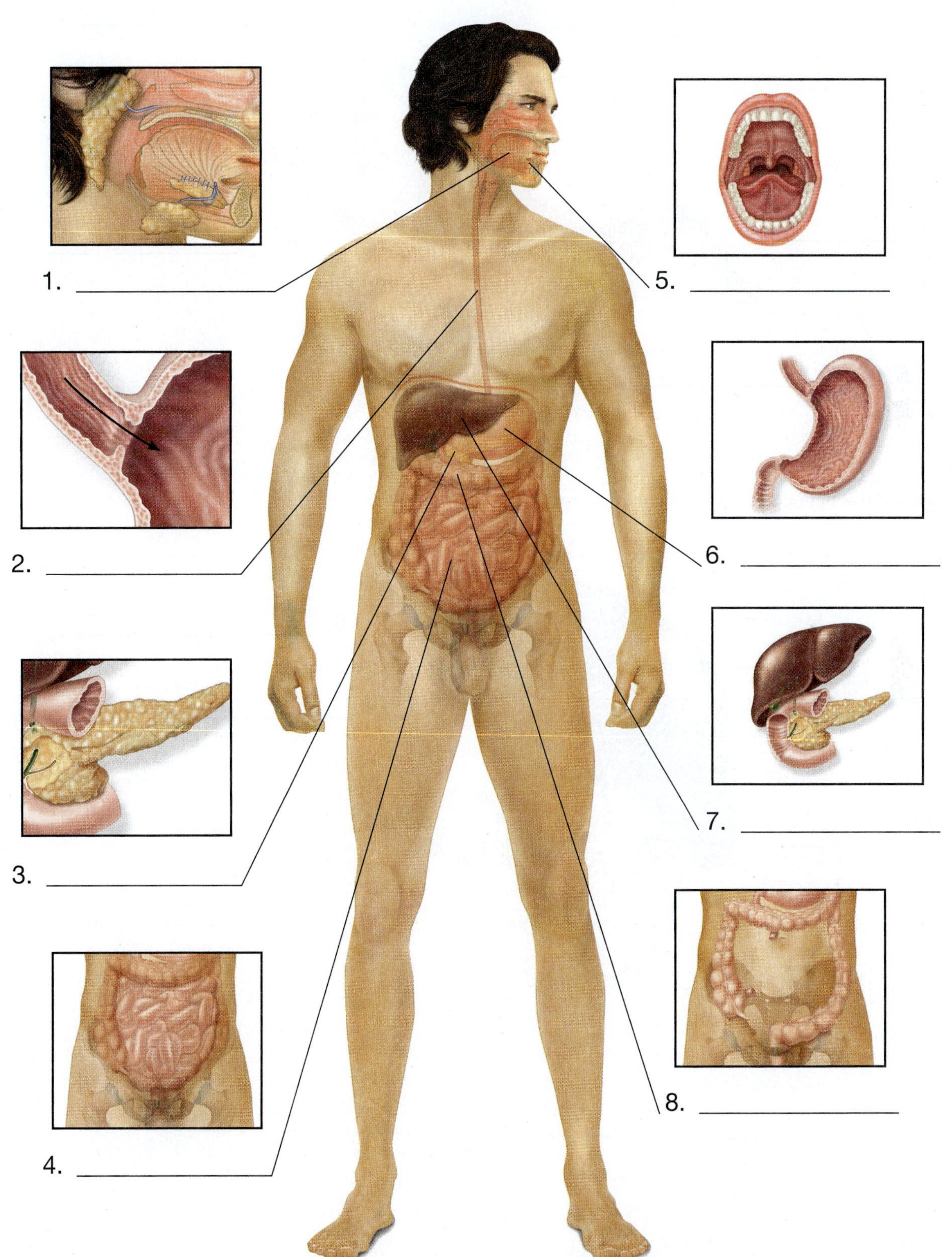

Image B

Write the labels for this figure on the numbered lines provided.

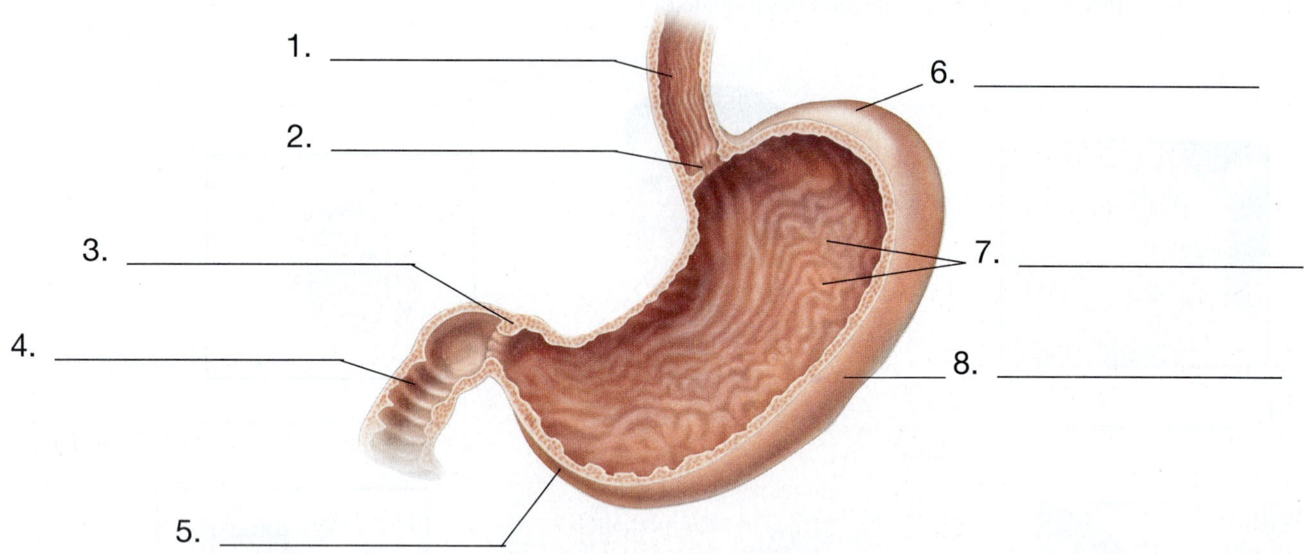

Image C

Write the labels for this figure on the numbered lines provided.

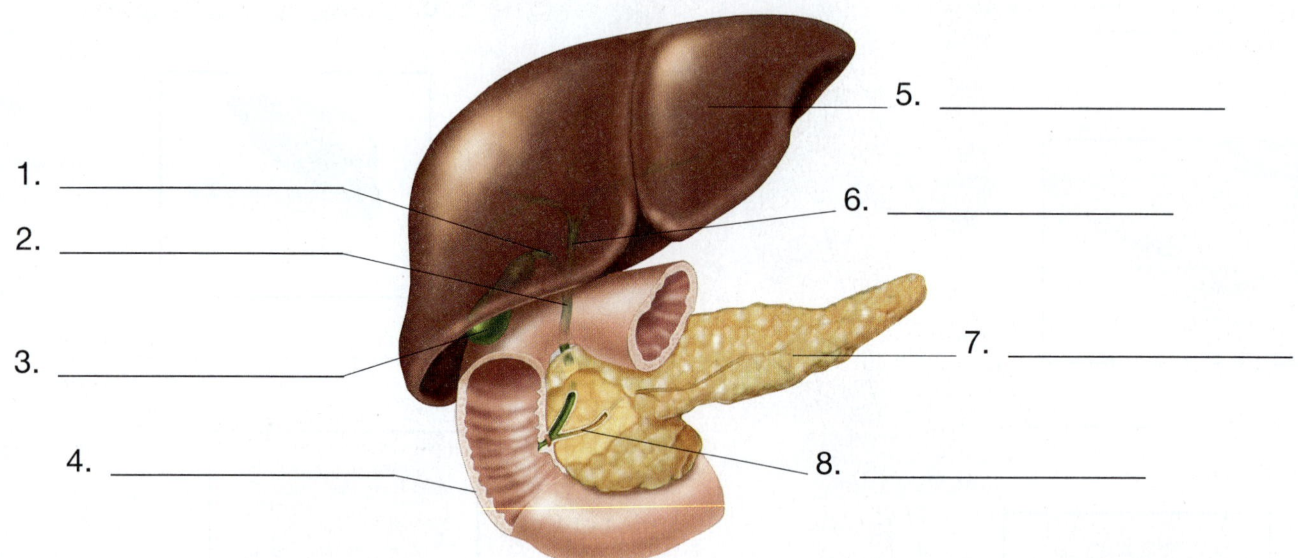

Chapter 9

Urinary System

Learning Objectives

Upon completion of this chapter, you will be able to

1. Identify and define the combining forms and suffixes introduced in this chapter.
2. Correctly spell and pronounce medical terms and major anatomical structures relating to the urinary system.
3. Locate and describe the major organs of the urinary system and their functions.
4. Describe the nephron and the mechanisms of urine production.
5. Identify the characteristics of urine and a urinalysis.
6. Identify and define urinary system anatomical terms.
7. Identify and define selected urinary system pathology terms.
8. Identify and define selected urinary system diagnostic procedures.
9. Identify and define selected urinary system therapeutic procedures.
10. Identify and define selected medications relating to the urinary system.
11. Define selected abbreviations associated with the urinary system.

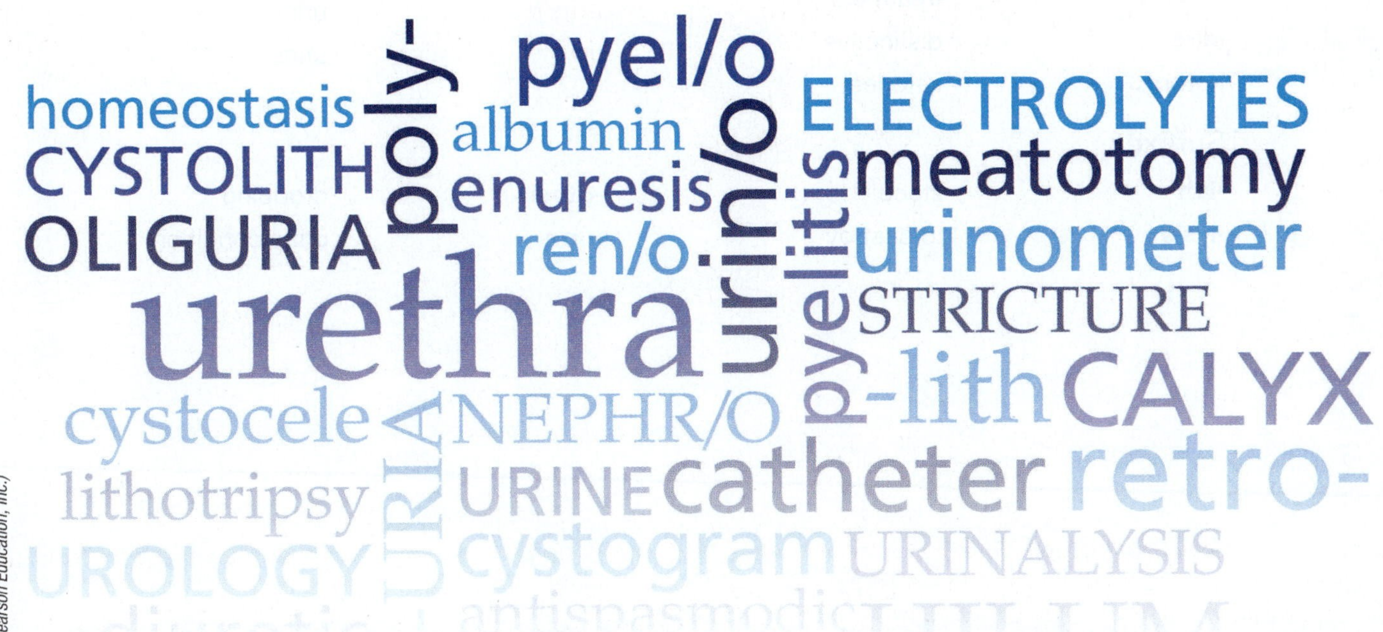

(Pearson Education, Inc.)

URINARY SYSTEM

AT A GLANCE

Function

The urinary system is responsible for maintaining a stable internal environment for the body. In order to achieve this state, the urinary system removes waste products, adjusts water and electrolyte levels, and maintains the correct pH.

Organs

The primary structures that comprise the urinary system:

kidneys

ureters

urethra

urinary bladder

Word Parts

Presented here are the most common word parts (with their meanings) used to build urinary system terms. For a more comprehensive list, refer to the Terminology section of this chapter.

Combining Forms

azot/o	nitrogenous waste
bacteri/o	bacteria
corpor/o	body
cyst/o	urinary bladder
genit/o	genitals
glomerul/o	glomerulus
glycos/o	sugar, glucose
home/o	sameness
hydr/o	water
iatr/o	physician, medicine, treatment
idi/o	distinctive
keton/o	ketones
meat/o	meatus
nephr/o	kidney
noct/i	night
olig/o	scanty
protein/o	protein
pyel/o	renal pelvis
ren/o	kidney
tox/o	poison
ureter/o	ureter
urethr/o	urethra
urin/o	urine
ur/o	urine

Suffixes

-lith	stone
-lysis	to destroy
-ptosis	drooping
-uria	urine condition

Urinary System Illustrated

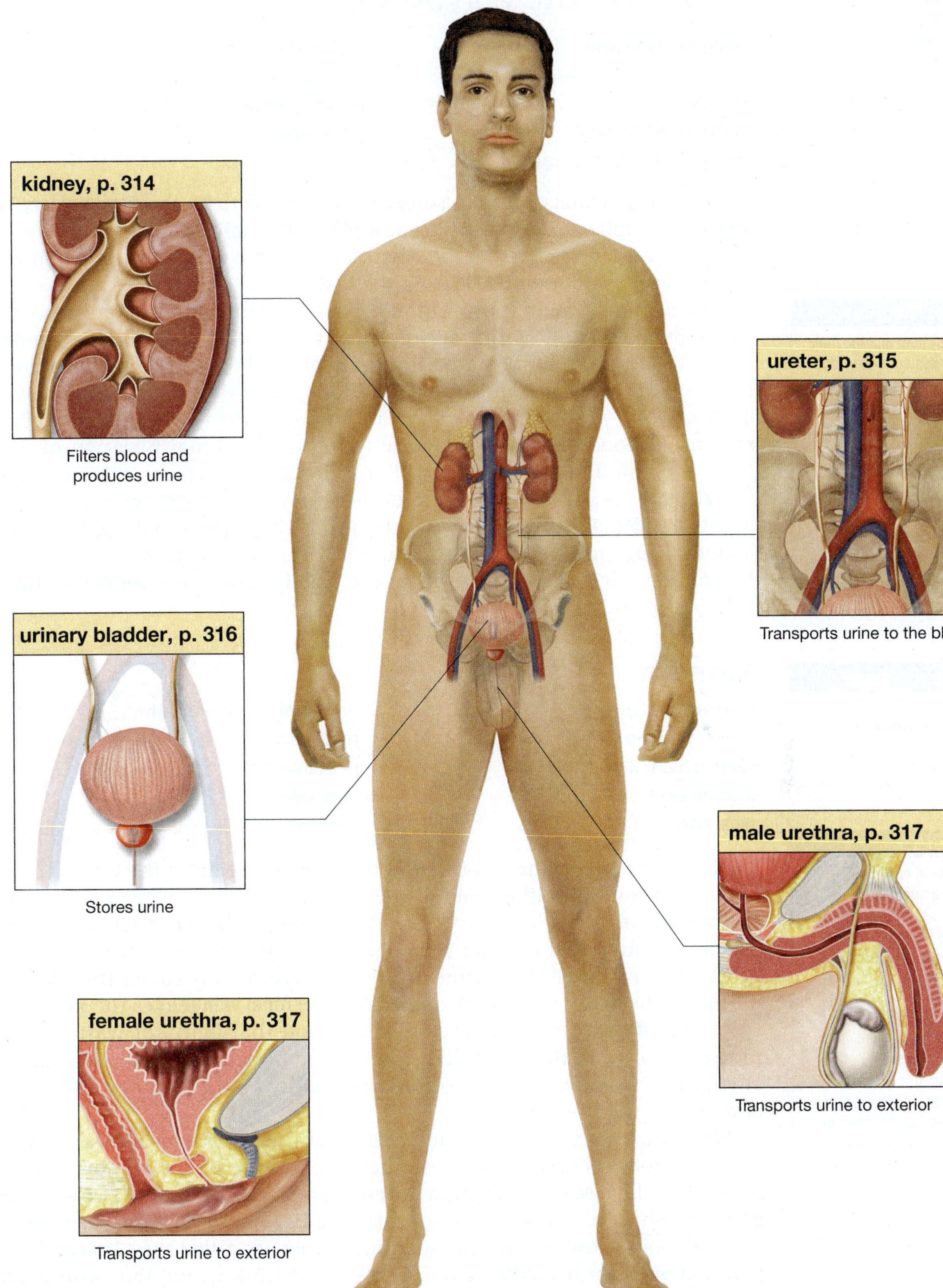

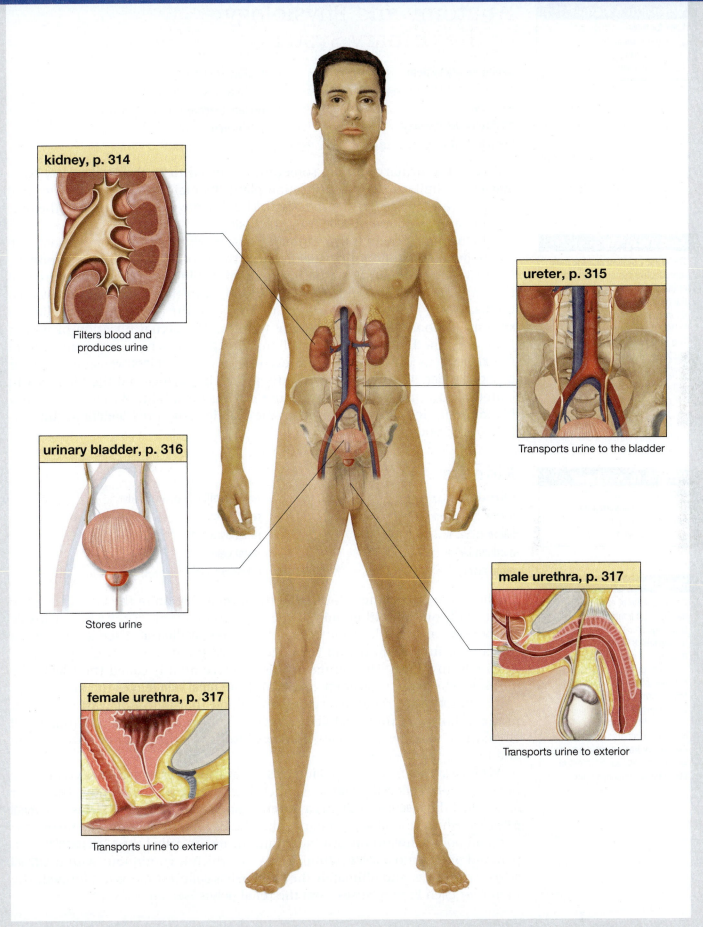

What's In A Name?

Look for these word parts:
genit/o = genitals
urin/o = urine
-ary = pertaining to

Anatomy and Physiology of the Urinary System

genitourinary system (jen-ih-toh-YOO-rih-nair-ee)
kidneys
nephrons (NEF-ronz)
uremia (yoo-REE-mee-ah)
ureters (YOO-reh-ters)
urethra (yoo-REE-thrah)
urinary bladder (YOO-rih-nair-ee)
urine (YOO-rin)

Think of the urinary system, sometimes referred to as the **genitourinary** (GU) **system**, as similar to a water filtration plant. Its main function is to filter and remove waste products from the blood. These waste materials result in the production and excretion of **urine** from the body.

The urinary system is one of the hardest working systems of the body. All the body's metabolic processes result in the production of waste products. These waste products are a natural part of life but quickly become toxic if they are allowed to build up in the blood, resulting in a condition called **uremia**. Waste products in the body are removed through a very complicated system of blood vessels and kidney tubules. The actual filtration of wastes from the blood takes place in millions of **nephrons**, which make up each of the **kidneys**. As urine drains from each kidney, the **ureters** transport it to the **urinary bladder**. The body is constantly producing urine, and the bladder can collect up to one quart of this liquid during the night. When the urinary bladder empties, urine moves from the bladder down the **urethra** to the outside of the body.

Med Term Tip

The urinary system and the male reproductive system share some of the same organs, particularly the urethra. Hence, the term *genitourinary* (GU) is sometimes used to describe the urinary system. The reproductive system is discussed in Chapter 10.

Kidneys

calyx (KAY-liks)
cortex (KOR-teks)
hilum (HYE-lum)
medulla (meh-DULL-ah)
renal artery
renal papilla (pah-PILL-ah)
renal pelvis
renal pyramids
renal vein
retroperitoneal (ret-roh-pair-ih-toh-NEE-al)

What's In A Name?

Look for these word parts:
peritone/o = peritoneum
-al = pertaining to
retro- = behind

The body has two kidneys located in the lumbar region of the back above the waist, with one on either side of the vertebral column. They are not inside the peritoneal sac, a location referred to as **retroperitoneal**. Each kidney has a concave or indented area on the edge toward the center that gives the kidney its bean shape. The center of this concave area is called the **hilum**. The hilum is where the **renal artery** enters and the **renal vein** leaves the kidney (see Figure 9-1 ■). The renal artery delivers blood that is full of waste products to the kidney and the renal vein returns the now cleansed blood to general circulation. Narrow tubes called *ureters* also leave the kidneys at the hilum and lead to the bladder.

When a surgeon cuts into a kidney, several structures or areas are visible. The outer portion, called the **cortex**, is much like a shell for the kidney. The inner area called the **medulla**, contains a dozen or so triangular-shaped areas, the **renal pyramids**, which resemble their namesake, the Egyptian pyramids. The tip of each pyramid points inward toward the hilum. At its tip, called the **renal papilla**, each pyramid opens into a **calyx** (plural is *calyces*), which is continuous with the **renal pelvis**. The calyces and ultimately the renal pelvis collect urine as it is formed. The ureter for each kidney arises from the renal pelvis (see Figure 9-2 ■).

Med Term Tip

From the time of early man, there has been an interest in urine. Drawings on cave walls and hieroglyphics in Egyptian pyramids reveal interest in urine as a means of determining the physical state of the body. Some of the first doctors, called *pisse prophets*, believed that examining the urine would help treat a patient. Now urologists treat disorders of the urinary tract in both men and women, as well as disorders of the male reproductive tract.

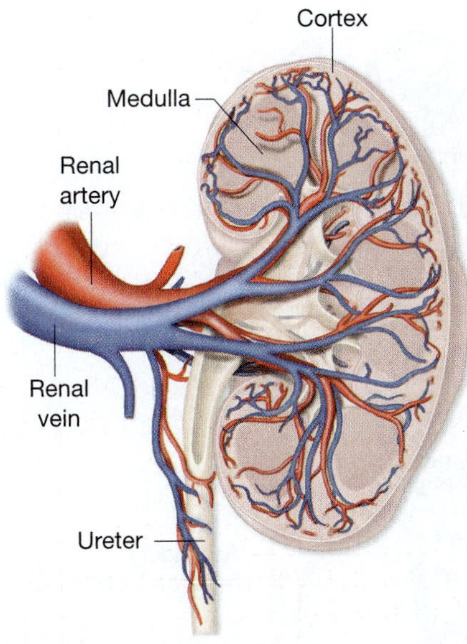

■ **Figure 9-1** Kidney structure. Longitudinal section showing the renal artery entering and the renal vein and ureter exiting at the hilum of the kidney.

■ **Figure 9-2** Longitudinal section of a kidney illustrating the internal structures.

Nephrons

afferent arteriole (AF-er-ent)
Bowman's capsule
collecting tubule
distal convoluted tubule (DIS-tal / kon-voh-LOOT-ed)
efferent arteriole (EF-er-ent)
glomerular capsule (gloh-MAIR-yoo-ler)
glomerulus (gloh-MAIR-yoo-lus)
loop of Henle
nephron loop
proximal convoluted tubule (PROK-sim-al / kon-voh-LOOT-ed)
renal corpuscle (KOR-pus-el)
renal tubule

The functional or working unit of the kidney is the nephron. There are more than one million of these microscopic structures in each human kidney. Each nephron consists of the **renal corpuscle** and the **renal tubule** (see Figure 9-3 ■). The renal corpuscle is the blood-filtering portion of the nephron. It has a double-walled cuplike structure called the **glomerular capsule** (also known as **Bowman's capsule**) that encases a ball of capillaries called the **glomerulus**. An **afferent arteriole** carries blood to the glomerulus, and an **efferent arteriole** carries blood away from the glomerulus.

Water and substances that were removed from the bloodstream in the renal corpuscle flow into the renal tubules to finish the urine production process. This continuous tubule is divided into four sections: the **proximal convoluted tubule**, followed by the narrow **nephron loop** (also known as the **loop of Henle**), then the **distal convoluted tubule**, and finally the **collecting tubule**.

Ureters

As urine drains out of the renal pelvis it enters the ureter, which carries it down to the urinary bladder (see Figure 9-4 ■). Ureters are very narrow tubes measuring less than ¼-inch wide and 10–12 inches long that extend from the renal pelvis to the urinary bladder. Mucous membrane lines the ureters just as it lines most passages that open to the external environment.

Med Term Tip

The kidney bean is so named because it resembles a kidney in shape. Each organ weighs four to six ounces, is two to three inches wide, and approximately one inch thick, and is about the size of your fist. In most people, the left kidney is slightly higher and larger than the right kidney. Functioning kidneys are necessary for life, but it is possible to live with only one working kidney.

What's In A Name?

Look for these word parts:
dist/o = away from
proxim/o = near to
-al = pertaining to

Med Term Tip

Afferent, meaning *moving toward*, and *efferent*, meaning *moving away from*, are terms used when discussing moving either toward or away from the central point in many systems. For example, there are afferent and efferent nerves in the nervous system.

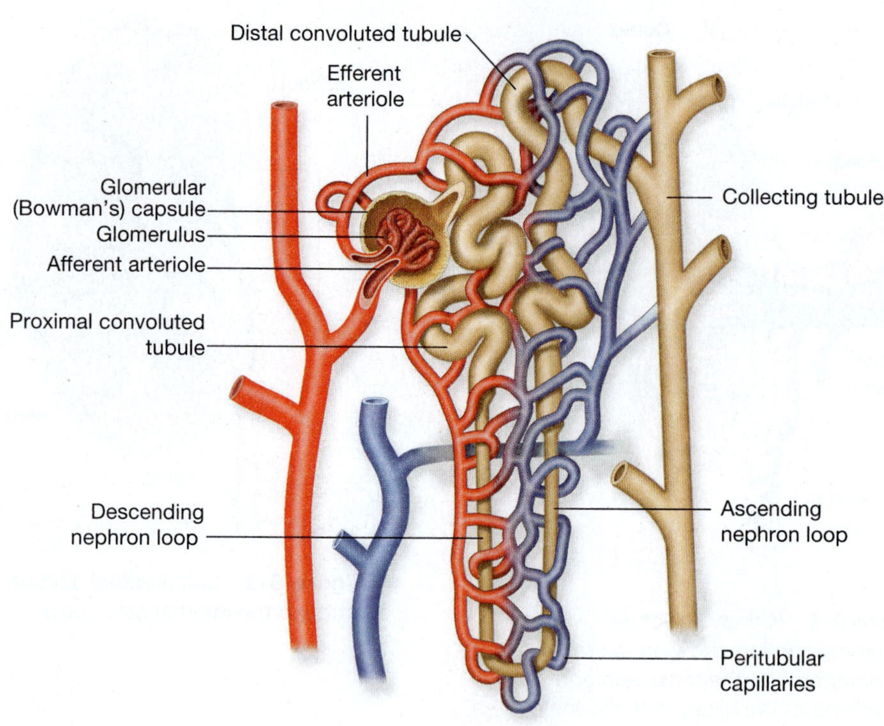

■ **Figure 9-3** The structure of a nephron, illustrating the nephron structure in relation to the circulatory system.

What's In A Name?

Look for these word parts:
ex- = outward
in- = inward
-al = pertaining to

Word Watch

The terms *ureter* and *urethra* are frequently confused. Remember that there are two ureters carrying urine from the kidneys into the bladder. There is only one urethra, and it carries urine from the bladder to the outside of the body.

Med Term Tip

Terms such as *micturition*, *voiding*, and *urination* all mean basically the same thing—the process of releasing urine from the body.

Urinary Bladder

external sphincter (SFINGK-ter)
internal sphincter
rugae (ROO-jee)
urination

The urinary bladder is an elastic muscular sac that lies in the base of the pelvis just behind the pubic symphysis (see Figure 9-5 ■). It is composed of three layers of smooth muscle tissue lined with mucous membrane containing **rugae**, or folds, that allow it to stretch. The bladder receives the urine directly from the ureters, stores it, and excretes it by **urination** through the urethra.

Generally, an adult bladder signals the urge to void (or empty the bladder) when it contains 300–400 mL of urine. Involuntary muscle action causes the bladder to contract and the **internal sphincter** to relax. The internal sphincter prevents the bladder from emptying at the wrong time. Voluntary action controls

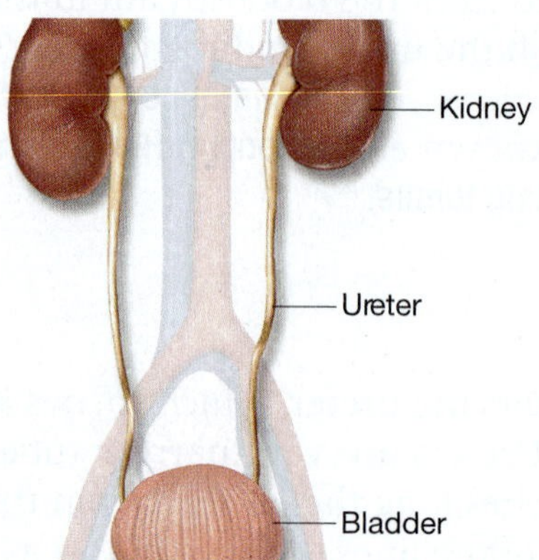

■ **Figure 9-4** The ureters extend from the kidneys to the urinary bladder.

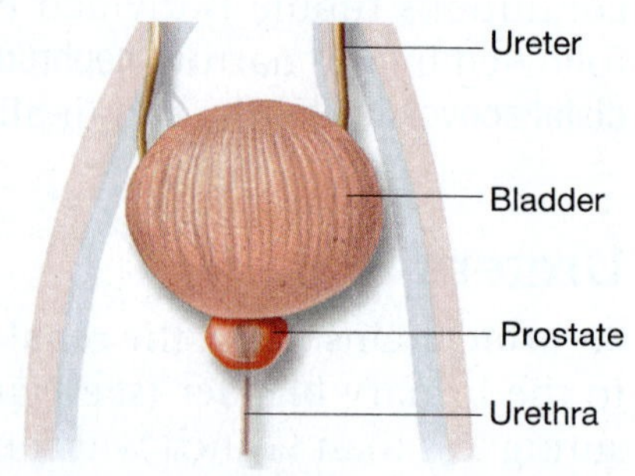

■ **Figure 9-5** The structure of the urinary bladder. (Note the prostate gland.)

the **external sphincter**, which opens on demand to allow the intentional emptying of the bladder. The act of controlling the emptying of urine is developed sometime after a child is two years of age.

Urethra

urinary meatus (mee-AY-tus)

The urethra is a tubular canal that carries the flow of urine from the bladder to the outside of the body (see Figure 9-6 ■). The external opening through which urine passes out of the body is called the **urinary meatus**. Mucous membrane also lines the urethra as it does other structures of the urinary system. This is one of the reasons that bladder infections may spread up the urinary tract. The urethra is one to two inches long in the female and eight inches long in the male. In a woman it functions only as the outlet for urine and is located in front of the vagina. In the male, however, it has two functions: an outlet for urine and the passageway for semen to leave the body.

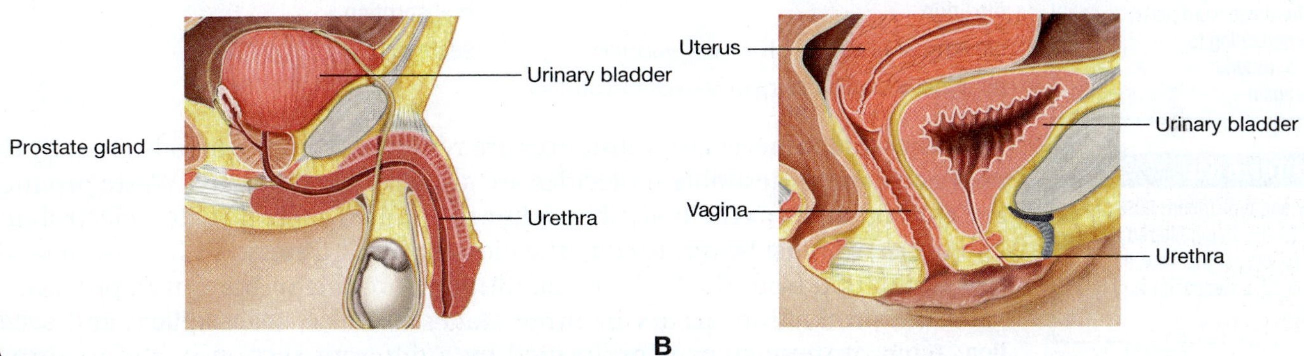

■ **Figure 9-6** A) The male urethra extends from the urinary bladder in the floor of the pelvis through the penis to the urinary meatus. B) The much shorter female urethra extends from the urinary bladder to the floor of the pelvis and exits just in front of the vaginal opening.

PRACTICE AS YOU GO

A. Complete the Statement

1. The functional or working units of the kidneys are the ______________________.
2. The glomerular capsule is also called ______________________ and the nephron loop is also called the ______________________.
3. The urinary bladder is composed of three layers of ______________________ tissue.
4. The term that describes the location of the kidneys is ______________________.
5. The glomerular capsule surrounds the ______________________.
6. The tip of each renal pyramid opens into a(n) ______________________.
7. There are ______________________ ureters and ______________________ urethra.
8. Urination can also be referred to as ______________________ or ______________________.

Role of Kidneys in Homeostasis

electrolytes (ee-LEK-troh-lites)
homeostasis (hoh-mee-oh-STAY-sis)

> **What's In A Name?**
> Look for these word parts:
> **home/o** = sameness
> **-stasis** = standing still

> **Med Term Tip**
> Mucous membranes will carry infections up the urinary tract from the urinary meatus and urethra into the bladder and eventually up the ureters and to the kidneys if not stopped. It is never wise to ignore a simple bladder infection or what is called *cystitis.*

The kidneys are responsible for **homeostasis** or balance in the body. They continually adjust the chemical conditions in the body, allowing humans to survive. Because of its interaction with the bloodstream and its ability to excrete substances from the body, the urinary system maintains the body's proper balance of water (H_2O) and chemicals. If the body is low on water, the kidneys conserve it, or in the opposite case, if there is excess water in the body, the kidneys excrete the excess. In addition to water, the kidneys regulate the level of **electrolytes**—small biologically important molecules such as sodium (Na^+), potassium (K^+), chloride (Cl^-), and bicarbonate (HCO_3^-). Finally, the kidneys play an important role in maintaining the correct pH range within the body, making sure it does not become too acidic or too alkaline. The kidneys accomplish these important tasks through the production of urine.

Stages of Urine Production

filtration
glomerular filtrate (gloh-MAIR-yoo-ler)
peritubular capillaries (pair-ih-TOO-byoo-lar)
reabsorption
secretion

> **What's In A Name?**
> Look for these word parts:
> **-ar** = pertaining to
> **peri-** = around
> **re-** = again

> **Med Term Tip**
> At any one time, about 20% of your blood is being filtered by your kidneys. In this way, all your blood is cleansed every few minutes.

> **Med Term Tip**
> The amount of water and other fluids processed by the kidneys each day is astonishing. Approximately 190 quarts of fluid are filtered out of the glomerular blood every day. Most of this fluid returns to the body through the reabsorption process. About 99% of the water that leaves the blood each day through the filtration process returns to the blood by proximal tubule reabsorption.

As wastes and unnecessary substances are removed from the bloodstream by the nephrons, many desirable molecules are also removed initially. Waste products are eliminated from the body, but other substances such as water, electrolytes, and nutrients must be returned to the bloodstream. Urine, in its final form ready for elimination from the body, is the ultimate product of this entire process.

Urine production occurs in three stages: **filtration**, **reabsorption**, and **secretion**. Each of these steps is performed by a different section of the nephrons (see Figure 9-7 ■).

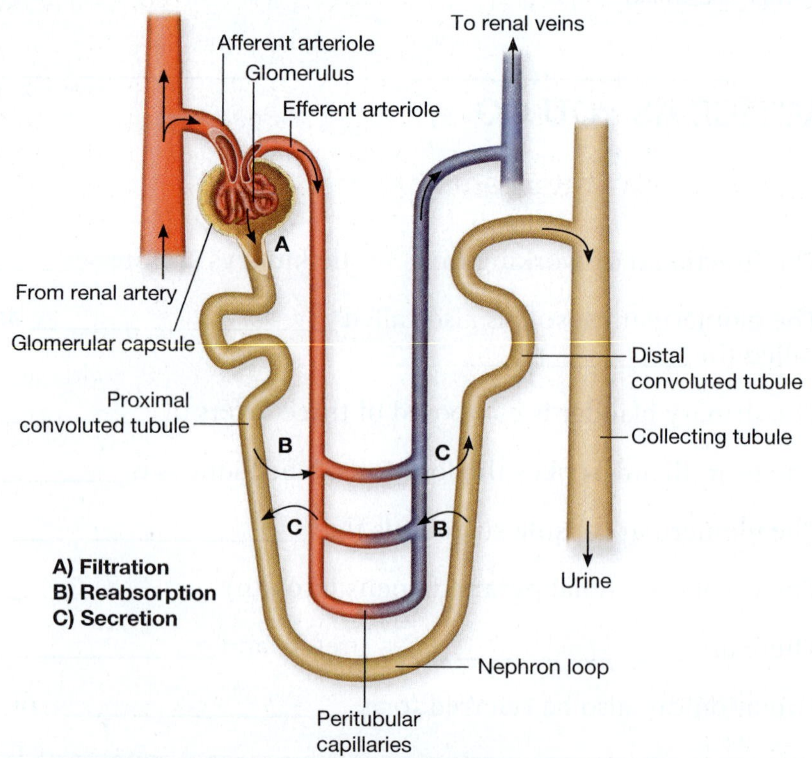

■ **Figure 9-7** The three stages of urine production: filtration, reabsorption, and secretion.

1. **Filtration.** The first stage is the filtering of particles, which occurs in the renal corpuscle. The pressure of blood flowing through the glomerulus forces material out of the bloodstream, through the wall of the glomerular capsule, and into the renal tubules. This fluid in the tubules is called the **glomerular filtrate** and consists of water, electrolytes, nutrients such as glucose and amino acids, wastes, and toxins.
2. **Reabsorption.** After filtration, the filtrate passes through the four sections of the tubule. As the filtrate moves along its twisted journey, most of the water and much of the electrolytes and nutrients are reabsorbed into the **peritubular capillaries**, a capillary bed that surrounds the renal tubules. They can then reenter the circulating blood.
3. **Secretion.** The final stage of urine production occurs when the special cells of the renal tubules secrete ammonia, uric acid, and other waste substances directly into the renal tubule. Urine formation is now finished; it passes into the collecting tubules, renal papilla, calyx, renal pelvis, and ultimately into the ureter.

Urine

albumin (al-BYOO-min)
nitrogenous wastes (nigh-TROJ-eh-nus)
specific gravity
urinalysis (yoo-rih-NAL-ih-sis)

Normal urine color may vary from almost clear, pale yellow, to deep gold, depending on how dilute it is. As it is being produced and collecting in the bladder, it is sterile. However, as it passes through the urethra to the outside, it may become contaminated by bacteria. Although it is 95% water, it also contains many dissolved substances, such as electrolytes, toxins, and **nitrogenous wastes**, the by-products of muscle metabolism. At times the urine also contains substances that should not be there, such as glucose, blood, or **albumin**, a protein that should remain in the blood. This is the reason for performing a **urinalysis**, a physical and chemical analysis of urine, which gives medical personnel important information regarding disease processes occurring in a patient. Normally, during a 24-hour period the output of urine will be 1,000–2,000 mL, depending on the amount of fluid consumed and the general health of the person. Normal urine is acidic because this is one way the body disposes of excess acids. **Specific gravity** indicates the amount of dissolved substances in urine. The specific gravity of pure water is 1.000. The specific gravity of urine varies from 1.001 to 1.030. Highly concentrated urine has a higher specific gravity, while the specific gravity of very dilute urine is close to that of water. See Table 9-1 ■ for the normal values for urine testing and Table 9-2 ■ for abnormal findings.

What's In A Name?

Look for these word parts:
urin/o = urine
-lysis = to destroy
-ous = pertaining to

Med Term Tip

The color, odor, volume, and sugar content of urine have been examined for centuries. Color charts for urine were developed by 1140, and "taste testing" was common in the late 17th century. By the 19th century, urinalysis was a routine part of a physical examination.

■ TABLE 9-1 Normal Values for Urinalysis Testing

Element	Normal Findings
Color	Straw-colored, pale yellow to deep gold
Odor	Aromatic
Appearance	Clear
Specific gravity	1.001–1.030
pH	5.0–8.0
Protein	Negative to trace
Glucose	None
Ketones	None
Blood	Negative

TABLE 9-2 Abnormal Urinalysis Findings

Element	Implications
Color	Color varies depending on patient's fluid intake and output or medication; brown or black urine color indicates a serious disease process
Odor	Fetid or foul odor may indicate infection, while fruity odor may be found in diabetes mellitus, dehydration, or starvation; other odors may be due to medication or foods
Appearance	Cloudiness may mean that infection is present
Specific gravity	Concentrated urine has a higher specific gravity; dilute urine, such as can be found with diabetes insipidus, acute tubular necrosis, or salt-restricted diets, has a lower specific gravity
pH	pH value below 7.0 (acidic) is common in urinary tract infections, metabolic or respiratory acidosis, diets high in fruits or vegetables, or administration of some drugs; pH higher than 7.0 (basic or alkaline) is common in metabolic or respiratory alkalosis, fever, high-protein diets, and taking ascorbic acid
Protein	Protein may indicate glomerulonephritis or preeclampsia in a pregnant woman
Glucose	Small amounts of glucose may be present as result of eating a high-carbohydrate meal, stress, pregnancy, and taking some medications, such as aspirin or corticosteroids; higher levels may indicate poorly controlled diabetes, Cushing's syndrome, or infection
Ketones	Presence of ketones may indicate poorly controlled diabetes, dehydration, starvation, or ingestion of large amounts of aspirin
Blood	Blood may indicate glomerulonephritis, cancer of urinary tract, some types of anemia, taking of some medications (such as blood thinners), arsenic poisoning, reactions to transfusion, trauma, burns, and convulsions

PRACTICE AS YOU GO

B. Complete the Statement

1. The kidneys are responsible for ____________________ or the balance in the body.
2. The three stages of urine production are ____________________, ____________________, and ____________________.
3. Na^+, K^+, and Cl^- are collectively known as ____________________.
4. The capillary bed surrounding the renal tubules is called the ____________________ capillaries.
5. ____________________ indicates the amount of dissolved substances in urine.
6. Nitrogenous wastes are the by-products of ____________________ metabolism.

Terminology

Word Parts Used to Build Urinary System Terms

The following lists contain the combining forms, suffixes, and prefixes used to build terms in the remaining sections of this chapter.

Combining Forms

azot/o	nitrogenous waste	**corpor/o**	body	**hem/o**	blood
bacteri/o	bacteria	**cyst/o**	bladder, pouch	**hemat/o**	blood
bi/o	life	**glomerul/o**	glomerulus	**hydr/o**	water
carcin/o	cancer	**glycos/o**	sugar	**iatr/o**	medicine

Combining Forms (continued)

idi/o	distinctive	**noct/i**	night	**tox/o**	poison
keton/o	ketones	**olig/o**	scanty	**ur/o**	urine
lith/o	stone	**peritone/o**	peritoneum	**ureter/o**	ureter
meat/o	meatus	**protein/o**	protein	**urethr/o**	urethra
necr/o	death	**py/o**	pus	**urin/o**	urine
nephr/o	kidney	**pyel/o**	renal pelvis	**ven/o**	vein
neur/o	nerve	**ren/o**	kidney		

Suffixes

-al	pertaining to	**-lith**	stone	**-pathy**	disease
-algia	pain	**-lithiasis**	condition of stones	**-pexy**	surgical fixation
-ar	pertaining to	**-logy**	study of	**-plasty**	surgical repair
-ary	pertaining to	**-lysis**	to destroy (to break down)	**-ptosis**	drooping
-cele	protrusion	**-malacia**	abnormal softening	**-rrhagia**	abnormal flow condition
-eal	pertaining to	**-megaly**	enlarged	**-sclerosis**	hardening
-ectasis	dilated	**-meter**	instrument to measure	**-scope**	instrument to visually examine
-ectomy	surgical removal	**-oma**	tumor	**-scopy**	process of visually examining
-emia	blood condition	**-ory**	pertaining to	**-stenosis**	narrowing
-genic	producing	**-osis**	abnormal condition	**-tic**	pertaining to
-gram	record	**-ostomy**	surgically create an opening	**-tripsy**	surgical crushing
-graphy	process of recording	**-otomy**	cutting into	**-uria**	urine condition
-ic	pertaining to	**-ous**	pertaining to		
-itis	inflammation				

Prefixes

an-	without	**extra-**	outside of	**poly-**	many
anti-	against	**intra-**	within	**retro-**	backward
dys-	painful, difficult				

Adjective Forms of Anatomical Terms

Term	Word Parts	Definition
cystic (SIS-tik)	cyst/o = bladder -ic = pertaining to **Word Watch** The adjective *cystic* may be used to refer to the urinary bladder, the gallbladder, or a cyst.	Pertaining to bladder
glomerular (gloh-MAIR-yoo-ler)	glomerul/o = glomerulus -ar = pertaining to	Pertaining to a glomerulus
meatal (mee-AY-tal)	meat/o = meatus -al = pertaining to	Pertaining to meatus
pyelitic (pye-eh-LIT-ik)	pyel/o = renal pelvis -tic = pertaining to	Pertaining to renal pelvis
renal (REE-nal)	ren/o = kidney -al = pertaining to	Pertaining to kidney
ureteral (yoo-REE-ter-al)	ureter/o = ureter -al = pertaining to **Word Watch** Be particularly careful when using the three very similar combining forms: **uter/o** meaning *uterus*, **ureter/o** meaning *ureter*, and **urethr/o** meaning *urethra*.	Pertaining to ureter
urethral (yoo-REE-thral)	urethr/o = urethra -al = pertaining to	Pertaining to urethra
urinary (YOO-rih-nair-ee)	urin/o = urine -ary = pertaining to	Pertaining to urine

PRACTICE AS YOU GO

C. Give the adjective form for each term.

1. The ureter ____________________
2. The kidney ____________________
3. A glomerulus ____________________
4. Urine ____________________
5. The urethra ____________________

Pathology

Term	Word Parts	Definition
Medical Specialties		
nephrology (neh-FROL-oh-jee)	nephr/o = kidney -logy = study of	Branch of medicine involved in diagnosis and treatment of diseases and disorders of the kidney; physician is a *nephrologist*
urology (yoo-RALL-oh-jee)	ur/o = urine -logy = study of	Branch of medicine involved in diagnosis and treatment of diseases and disorders of the urinary system (and male reproductive system); physician is a *urologist*
Signs and Symptoms		
anuria (an-YOO-ree-ah)	an- = without -uria = urine condition	Complete suppression of urine formed by the kidneys and a complete lack of urine excretion
azotemia (az-oh-TEE-mee-ah)	azot/o = nitrogenous waste -emia = blood condition	Accumulation of nitrogenous waste in bloodstream; occurs when the kidney fails to filter these wastes from the blood
bacteriuria (bak-teer-ee-YOO-ree-ah)	bacteri/o = bacteria -uria = urine condition	Presence of bacteria in the urine
calculus (KAL-kyoo-lus)		Stone formed within an organ by accumulation of mineral salts; found in kidney, renal pelvis, ureters, bladder, or urethra; plural is *calculi*
cystalgia (sis-TAL-jee-ah)	cyst/o = bladder -algia = pain	Urinary bladder pain
cystolith (SIS-toh-lith)	cyst/o = bladder -lith = stone	Bladder stone
cystorrhagia (sis-toh-RAY-jee-ah)	cyst/o = bladder -rrhagia = abnormal flow condition	Abnormal bleeding from the urinary bladder
diuresis (dye-yoo-REE-sis)		Increased formation and excretion of urine
dysuria (dis-YOOR-ee-ah)	dys- = painful, difficult -uria = urine condition	Difficult or painful urination

■ **Figure 9-8** Photograph of sectioned kidney specimen illustrating extensive renal calculi. *(Dr. E. Walker/Science Source)*

Word Watch

Be careful using the combining forms **cyst/o** meaning *bladder* and **cyt/o** meaning *cell.*

Pathology (continued)

Term	Word Parts	Definition
enuresis (en-yoo-REE-sis)		Involuntary discharge of urine after age by which bladder control should have been established; usually occurs by age five; *nocturnal enuresis* refers to bed-wetting at night
frequency		Greater-than-normal occurrence in urge to urinate, without increase in total daily volume of urine; frequency is indication of inflammation of bladder or urethra
glycosuria (gly-koh-SOO-ree-ah)	glycos/o = sugar -uria = urine condition	Presence of sugar in the urine
hematuria (hee-mah-TOO-ree-ah)	hemat/o = blood -uria = urine condition	Presence of blood in the urine
hesitancy		Decrease in force of urine stream, often with difficulty initiating flow; often a symptom of blockage along the urethra, such as enlarged prostate gland
ketonuria (kee-toh-NYOOR-ee-ah)	keton/o = ketones -uria = urine condition	Presence of ketones in urine; occurs when body burns fat instead of glucose for energy, such as in uncontrolled diabetes mellitus
nephrolith (NEF-roh-lith)	nephr/o = kidney -lith = stone	Kidney stone
nephromalacia (nef-roh-mah-LAY-shee-ah)	nephr/o = kidney -malacia = abnormal softening	Kidney is abnormally soft
nephromegaly (nef-roh-MEG-ah-lee)	nephr/o = kidney -megaly = enlarged	Kidney is enlarged
nephrosclerosis (nef-roh-skleh-ROH-sis)	nephr/o = kidney -sclerosis = hardening	Kidney tissue has become hardened
nocturia (nok-TOO-ree-ah)	noct/i = night -uria = urine condition	Having to urinate frequently during the night
oliguria (ol-ig-YOO-ree-ah)	olig/o = scanty -uria = urine condition	Producing too little urine
polyuria (pol-ee-YOO-ree-ah)	poly- = many -uria = urine condition	Producing unusually large volume of urine
proteinuria (proh-teen-YOO-ree-ah)	protein/o = protein -uria = urine condition	Presence of protein in urine
pyuria (pye-YOO-ree-ah)	py/o = pus -uria = urine condition	Presence of pus in urine
renal colic (KOL-ik)	ren/o = kidney -al = pertaining to -ic = pertaining to	Pain caused by kidney stone; can be excruciating pain and generally requires medical treatment
stricture (STRIK-chur)		Narrowing of passageway in the urinary system
uremia (yoo-REE-mee-ah)	ur/o = urine -emia = blood condition	Accumulation of waste products (especially nitrogenous wastes) in bloodstream; associated with renal failure

Pathology (continued)

Term	Word Parts	Definition
ureterectasis (yoo-ree-ter-EK-tah-sis)	ureter/o = ureter -ectasis = dilated	Ureter is stretched out or dilated
ureterolith (yoo-REE-teh-roh-lith)	ureter/o = ureter -lith = stone	Stone in the ureter
ureterostenosis (yoo-ree-ter-oh-steh-NOH-sis)	ureter/o = ureter -stenosis = narrowing	Ureter has become narrow
urethralgia (yoo-ree-THRAL-jee-ah)	urethr/o = urethra -algia = pain	Urethral pain
urethrorrhagia (yoo-ree-throh-RAY-jee-ah)	urethr/o = urethra -rrhagia = abnormal flow condition	Abnormal bleeding from the urethra
urethrostenosis (yoo-ree-throh-steh-NOH-sis)	urethr/o = urethra -stenosis = narrowing	Urethra has become narrow
urgency (ER-jen-see)		Feeling need to urinate immediately
urinary incontinence (in-KON-tih-nens)	urin/o = urine -ary = pertaining to	Involuntary release of urine; in some patients, indwelling catheter is inserted into the bladder for continuous urine drainage

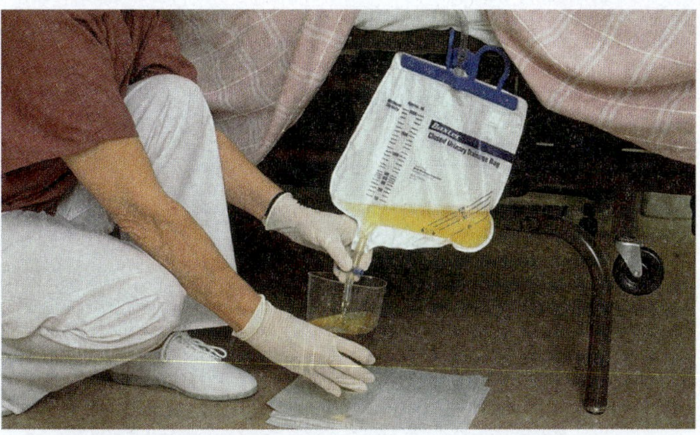

■ **Figure 9-9** Healthcare worker draining urine from a bladder catheter bag. *(Michal Heron/Pearson Education, Inc.)*

Term	Word Parts	Definition
urinary retention	urin/o = urine -ary = pertaining to	Inability to fully empty the bladder; often indicates blockage in the urethra
Kidney		
acute tubular necrosis (ATN) (neh-KROH-sis)	-ar = pertaining to necr/o = death -osis = abnormal condition	Damage to and potential death of the renal tubules due to presence of toxins in urine or to ischemia; results in oliguria
diabetic nephropathy (neh-FROP-ah-thee)	-ic = pertaining to nephr/o = kidney -pathy = disease	Accumulation of damage to the glomerulus capillaries due to chronic high blood sugars of diabetes mellitus
glomerulonephritis (gloh-mair-yoo-loh-neh-FRYE-tis)	glomerul/o = glomerulus nephr/o = kidney -itis = inflammation	Inflammation of the kidney (primarily of the glomerulus); since the glomerular membrane is inflamed, it becomes more permeable and will allow protein and blood cells to enter the filtrate; results in protein in urine (proteinuria) and hematuria

Pathology (continued)

Term	Word Parts	Definition
hydronephrosis (high-droh-neh-FROH-sis)	hydr/o = water nephr/o = kidney -osis = abnormal condition	Distention of the renal pelvis due to urine collecting in the kidney; often result of obstruction of a ureter
nephritis (neh-FRYE-tis)	nephr/o = kidney -itis = inflammation	Kidney inflammation
nephrolithiasis (nef-roh-lith-EYE-ah-sis)	nephr/o = kidney -lithiasis = condition of stones	Presence of calculi in the kidney; usually begins with solidification of salts present in urine
nephroma (neh-FROH-mah)	nephr/o = kidney -oma = tumor	Kidney tumor
nephropathy (neh-FROP-ah-thee)	nephr/o = kidney -pathy = disease	General term describing presence of kidney disease
nephroptosis (nef-rop-TOH-sis)	nephr/o = kidney -ptosis = drooping	Downward displacement of the kidney out of its normal location; commonly called a *floating kidney*
nephrotic syndrome (NS)	nephr/o = kidney -tic = pertaining to	Damage to the glomerulus resulting in protein appearing in urine, proteinuria, and corresponding decrease in protein in bloodstream; also called *nephrosis*
polycystic kidneys (pol-ee-SIS-tik)	poly- = many cyst/o = pouch -ic = pertaining to	Formation of multiple cysts (pouches) within kidney tissue; results in destruction of normal kidney tissue and uremia
■ **Figure 9-10** Photograph of a polycystic kidney on the left compared to a normal kidney on the right. *(Arthur Glauberman/ Science Source)*	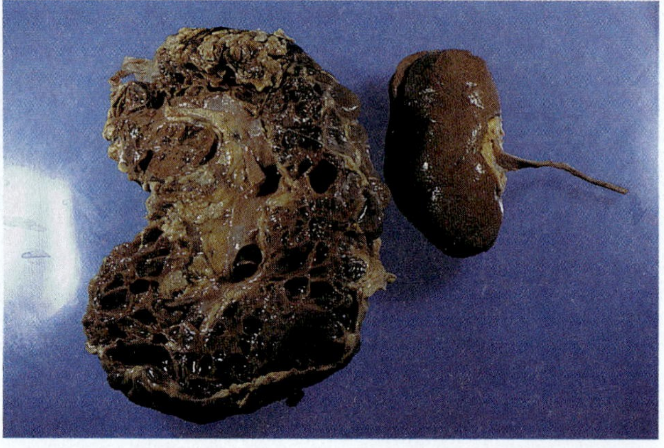	
pyelitis (pye-eh-LYE-tis)	pyel/o = renal pelvis -itis = inflammation	Renal pelvis inflammation
pyelonephritis (pye-eh-loh-neh-FRYE-tis)	pyel/o = renal pelvis nephr/o = kidney -itis = inflammation	Inflammation of the renal pelvis and the kidney; one of most common types of kidney disease; may be result of lower urinary tract infection that moved up to the kidney by way of the ureter; large quantities of white blood cells and bacteria in urine are possible; blood (hematuria) may even be present in urine in this condition; can occur with any untreated or persistent case of cystitis
renal cell carcinoma	ren/o = kidney -al = pertaining to carcin/o = cancer -oma = tumor	Cancerous tumor that arises from kidney tubule cells

Pathology (continued)

Term	Word Parts	Definition
renal failure	ren/o = kidney -al = pertaining to	Inability of the kidneys to filter wastes from the blood, resulting in uremia; may be acute or chronic; major reason for patient being placed on dialysis
Wilms' tumor (VILMZ)		Malignant kidney tumor found most often in children; also called *nephroblastoma*
Urinary Bladder		
bladder cancer		Cancerous tumor that arises from cells lining the bladder; major sign is hematuria
bladder neck obstruction (BNO)		Blockage of the bladder outlet; often caused by enlarged prostate gland in males
cystitis (sis-TYE-tis)	cyst/o = bladder -itis = inflammation	Urinary bladder inflammation
cystocele (SIS-toh-seel)	cyst/o = bladder -cele = protrusion	Protrusion (or herniation) of the urinary bladder into wall of the vagina
interstitial cystitis (in-ter-STISH-al / sis-TYE-tis)	-al = pertaining to cyst/o = bladder -itis = inflammation	Disease of unknown cause in which there is inflammation and irritation of the bladder; most commonly seen in middle-aged women
neurogenic bladder (noo-roh-JEN-ik)	neur/o = nerve -genic = producing	Loss of nervous control that leads to retention; may be caused by spinal cord injury or multiple sclerosis
urinary tract infection (UTI)	urin/o = urine -ary = pertaining to	Infection, usually from bacteria, of any organ of the urinary system; most often begins with cystitis and may ascend into ureters and kidneys; most common in women because of shorter urethra

PRACTICE AS YOU GO

D. Terminology Matching

Match each term to its definition.

1. __________ Wilms' tumor
2. __________ azotemia
3. __________ urinary retention
4. __________ nephroptosis
5. __________ nocturia
6. __________ incontinence
7. __________ hydronephrosis
8. __________ urgency
9. __________ nephrolithiasis
10. __________ polycystic kidney disease

a. kidney stones
b. feeling need to urinate immediately
c. childhood malignant kidney tumor
d. swelling of kidney due to urine collecting in renal pelvis
e. involuntary release of urine
f. frequent urination at night
g. excess nitrogenous waste in bloodstream
h. inability to fully empty bladder
i. a floating kidney
j. multiple cysts in the kidneys

Diagnostic Procedures

Term	Word Parts	Definition
Clinical Laboratory Tests		
albumin/creatinine ratio (ACR)		Screening test for persons at risk (e.g., diabetics) for developing kidney disease; measures amount of albumin and creatinine in urine; there is a high level of albumin in the blood, but almost none is excreted in urine; creatinine, a waste product of muscle metabolism, is excreted into urine at a relatively constant rate; if ratio of these two substances increases, it is an early warning sign of kidney disease
blood urea nitrogen (BUN) (yoo-REE-ah / NIGH-troh-jen)		Blood test to measure kidney function by level of nitrogenous waste (urea) in the blood
clean catch specimen (CC) **Word Watch** Note that the abbreviation for clean catch uses capital letters. Lower case, cc, is the abbreviation for chief complaint.		Urine sample obtained after cleaning off urinary opening and catching or collecting a urine sample in midstream (halfway through urination process) to minimize contamination from genitalia
creatinine clearance (kree-AT-in-in)		Test of kidney function; creatinine is a waste product cleared from bloodstream by the kidneys; for this test, urine is collected for 24 hours, and amount of creatinine in urine is compared to amount of creatinine that remains in bloodstream
estimated glomerular filtration rate (eGFR) (gloh-MAIR-yoo-ler)	glomerul/o = glomerulus -ar = pertaining to	Test to measure kidney function; measures level of creatinine, a waste product of muscle metabolism, in urine and uses this in a formula that estimates how well glomeruli are filtering water out of bloodstream
urinalysis (U/A, UA) (yoo-rih-NAL-ih-sis)	urin/o = urine -lysis = to destroy (to break down)	Laboratory test consisting of physical, chemical, and microscopic examination of urine
urine culture and sensitivity (C&S)		Laboratory test of urine for bacterial infection; attempt to grow bacteria on culture medium in order to identify it and determine to which antibiotics it is sensitive
urinometer (yoor-ih-NOM-eh-ter)	urin/o = urine -meter = instrument to measure	Instrument to measure specific gravity of urine; part of urinalysis
Diagnostic Imaging		
cystogram (SIS-toh-gram)	cyst/o = bladder -gram = record	X-ray record of the urinary bladder
cystography (sis-TOG-rah-fee)	cyst/o = bladder -graphy = process of recording	Process of instilling contrast material or dye into the bladder by catheter to visualize the urinary bladder on X-ray

Diagnostic Procedures (continued)

Term	Word Parts	Definition
excretory urography (EU) (EKS-kreh-tor-ee / yoo-ROG-rah-fee)	-ory = pertaining to ur/o = urine -graphy = process of recording	Injecting dye into bloodstream and then taking X-ray to trace action of the kidney as it excretes dye in the urine
intravenous pyelography (IVP) (in-trah-VEE-nus / pye-eh-LOG-rah-fee)	intra- = within ven/o = vein -ous = pertaining to pyel/o = renal pelvis -graphy = process of recording	Diagnostic X-ray procedure in which dye is injected into a vein and then X-rays are taken to visualize the renal pelvis as dye is removed by the kidney
kidneys, ureters, bladder (KUB)		X-ray taken of the abdomen demonstrating kidneys, ureters, and bladder without using any contrast dye; also called *flat-plate abdomen*
nephrogram (NEF-roh-gram)	nephr/o = kidney -gram = record	X-ray record of the kidney
pyelogram (PYE-eh-loh-gram)	pyel/o = renal pelvis -gram = record	X-ray record of the renal pelvis
retrograde pyelography (RP) (RET-roh-grayd / pye-eh-LOG-rah-fee)	retro- = backward pyel/o = renal pelvis -graphy = process of recording	Diagnostic X-ray procedure in which dye is inserted through the urethra to outline bladder, ureters, and renal pelvis
Figure 9-11 Retrograde pyelogram X-ray. Radiopaque dye outlines urinary bladder, ureters, and renal pelvis. Bladder, right kidney, and both ureters appear normal. Left kidney appears abnormal. *(Jarva Jar/ Shutterstock)*	R	
voiding cystourethrography (VCUG) (sis-toh-yoo-ree-THROG-rah-fee)	cyst/o = bladder urethr/o = urethra -graphy = process of recording	X-ray taken to visualize the urethra while patient is voiding after contrast dye is placed in the bladder
Endoscopic Procedure		
cystoscope (SIS-toh-skohp)	cyst/o = bladder -scope = instrument to visually examine	Instrument used to visually examine inside of the urinary bladder
cystoscopy (cysto) (sis-TOSS-koh-pee)	cyst/o = bladder -scopy = process of visually examining	Visual examination of the urinary bladder using instrument called *cystoscope*
urethroscope (yoo-REE-throh-skohp)	urethr/o = urethra -scope = instrument to visually examine	Instrument to visually examine inside of the urethra

Therapeutic Procedures

Term	Word Parts	Definition
Medical Treatments		
catheter (KATH-eh-ter)		Flexible tube inserted into body for purpose of moving fluids into or out of body; most commonly refers to tube threaded through the urethra into the bladder to withdraw urine (see again Figure 9-9)
catheterization (cath) (kath-eh-ter-ih-ZAY-shun)		Insertion of tube through the urethra and into the urinary bladder for purpose of withdrawing urine or inserting dye
extracorporeal shockwave lithotripsy (ESWL) (eks-trah-kor-POR-ee-al / shockwave / LITH-oh-trip-see)	extra- = outside of corpor/o = body -eal = pertaining to lith/o = stone -tripsy = surgical crushing	Use of ultrasound waves from outside the body to break up stones; process does not require invasive surgery
hemodialysis (HD) (hee-moh-dye-AL-ih-sis)	hem/o = blood	Use of artificial kidney machine that filters the blood of a person to remove waste products; use of this technique in patients who have defective kidneys is lifesaving

■ **Figure 9-12** Extracorporeal shockwave lithotripsy, a noninvasive procedure using high-frequency sound waves to shatter kidney stones.

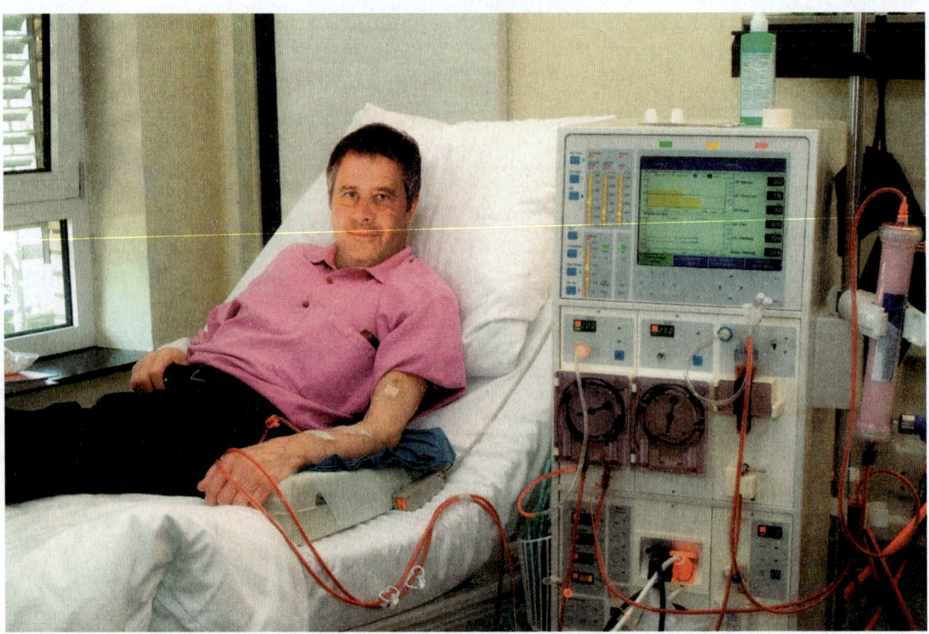

■ **Figure 9-13** Patient undergoing hemodialysis. Patient's blood passes through hemodialysis machine for cleansing and is then returned to the body. *(Gopixa/Shutterstock)*

Therapeutic Procedures (continued)

Term	Word Parts	Definition
peritoneal dialysis (pair-ih-toh-NEE-al / dye-AL-ih-sis)	**peritone/o** = peritoneum **-al** = pertaining to	Removal of toxic waste substances from body by placing warm, chemically balanced solutions into peritoneal cavity; wastes are filtered out of blood across peritoneum; used in treating renal failure and certain poisonings

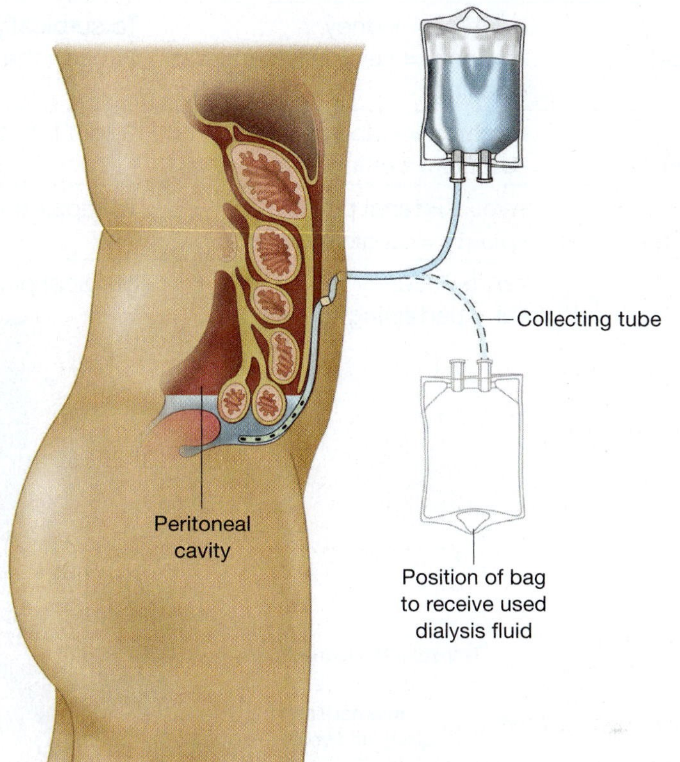

Figure 9-14 Peritoneal dialysis. Chemically balanced solution is placed into the abdominal cavity to draw impurities out of the bloodstream. It is removed after several hours.

Surgical Treatments

Term	Word Parts	Definition
cystectomy (sis-TEK-toh-mee)	**cyst/o** = bladder **-ectomy** = surgical removal	Surgical removal of the urinary bladder
cystopexy (SIS-toh-pek-see)	**cyst/o** = bladder **-pexy** = surgical fixation	Surgical fixation of the urinary bladder; performed to correct cystocele
cystoplasty (SIS-toh-plas-tee)	**cyst/o** = bladder **-plasty** = surgical repair	To repair a defect in the urinary bladder by surgical means
cystostomy (sis-TOSS-toh-mee)	**cyst/o** = bladder **-ostomy** = surgically create an opening	To surgically create opening into the urinary bladder through the abdominal wall
cystotomy (sis-TOT-oh-mee)	**cyst/o** = bladder **-otomy** = cutting into	To cut into the urinary bladder
lithotomy (lith-OT-oh-mee)	**lith/o** = stone **-otomy** = cutting into	To cut into an organ for purpose of removing a stone
lithotripsy (LITH-oh-trip-see)	**lith/o** = stone **-tripsy** = surgical crushing	Physical destruction of a stone in urinary system by crushing or sound waves
meatotomy (mee-ah-TOT-oh-mee)	**meat/o** = meatus **-otomy** = cutting into	To cut into the meatus in order to enlarge opening of the urethra
nephrectomy (neh-FREK-toh-mee)	**nephr/o** = kidney **-ectomy** = surgical removal	Surgical removal of a kidney

Therapeutic Procedures (continued)

Term	Word Parts	Definition
nephrolithotomy (nef-roh-lith-OT-oh-mee)	nephr/o = kidney lith/o = stone -otomy = cutting into	To cut into the kidney in order to remove stones
nephropexy (NEF-roh-pek-see)	nephr/o = kidney -pexy = surgical fixation	Surgical fixation of a kidney to anchor it in its normal anatomical position
nephrostomy (neh-FROS-toh-mee)	nephr/o = kidney -ostomy = surgically create an opening	To surgically create an opening into the kidney through the abdominal wall
nephrotomy (neh-FROT-oh-mee)	nephr/o = kidney -otomy = cutting into	To cut into the kidney
pyeloplasty (PYE-eh-loh-plas-tee)	pyel/o = renal pelvis -plasty = surgical repair	To repair the renal pelvis by surgical means
renal transplant	ren/o = kidney -al = pertaining to	Surgical placement of a donor kidney

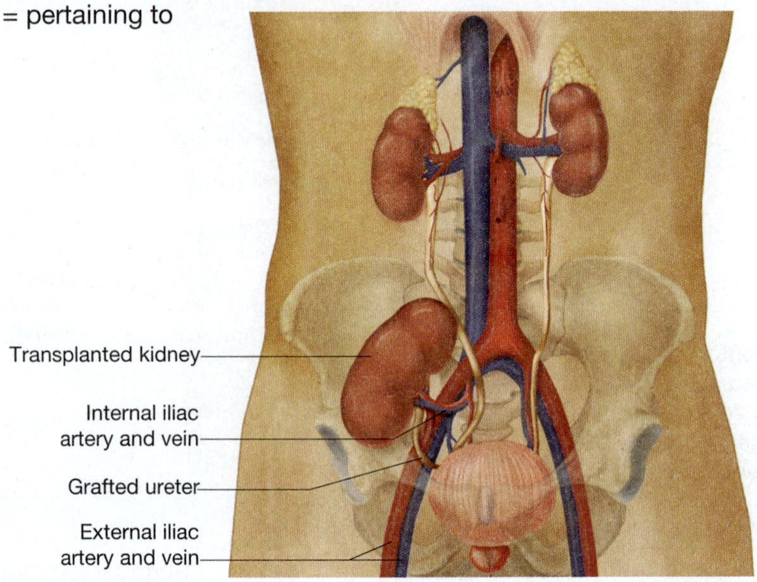

■ **Figure 9-15** Figure illustrates location utilized for implantation of donor kidney.

PRACTICE AS YOU GO

E. Procedure Matching

Match each procedure term with its definition.

1. ____________ clean catch specimen
2. ____________ hemodialysis
3. ____________ pyeloplasty
4. ____________ urinometer
5. ____________ lithotripsy
6. ____________ cystoscopy
7. ____________ catheter
8. ____________ kidneys, ureters, bladder

a. measures specific gravity
b. abdominal X-ray
c. visual examination of the bladder
d. a flexible tube inserted into the body
e. removes waste products from blood
f. method of obtaining urine sample
g. crushing of a stone
h. surgical repair of the renal pelvis

Pharmacology

Vocabulary

Term	Word Parts	Definition
antidote (AN-tih-doht)	**anti-** = against	Substance that will neutralize poisons or their side effects
iatrogenic (eye-ah-troh-JEN-ik)	**iatr/o** = physician, medicine, treatment **-genic** = producing	Usually unfavorable response resulting from physician's actions, taking of medication, or a treatment
idiosyncrasy (id-ee-oh-SIN-krah-see)	**idi/o** = distinctive	Unusual or abnormal response to drug or food
side effect		Response to drug other than effect desired; also called *adverse reaction*
toxicity (tok-SISS-ih-tee)	**tox/o** = poison	Extent or degree to which a substance is poisonous

Drugs

Classification	Word Parts	Action	Examples
antibiotic	**anti-** = against **bi/o** = life **-tic** = pertaining to	Used to treat bacterial infections of the urinary tract	ciprofloxacin, Cipro; nitrofurantoin, Macrobid
antispasmodic (an-tye-spaz-MOD-ik)	**anti-** = against **-ic** = pertaining to	Used to prevent or reduce bladder muscle spasms	oxybutynin, Ditropan; neostigmine, Prostigmine
diuretic (dye-yoo-REH-tik)	**-tic** = pertaining to	Increases volume of urine produced by the kidneys; useful in treatment of edema, kidney failure, heart failure, and hypertension	furosemide, Lasix; spironolactone, Aldactone

Abbreviations

ACR	albumin/creatinine ratio	**C&S**	culture and sensitivity
AGN	acute glomerulonephritis	**cysto**	cystoscopy
AKI	acute kidney injury	**eGFR**	estimated glomerular filtration rate
ARF	acute renal failure	**ESRD**	end-stage renal disease
ATN	acute tubular necrosis	**ESWL**	extracorporeal shockwave lithotripsy
BNO	bladder neck obstruction	**EU**	excretory urography
BUN	blood urea nitrogen	**GU**	genitourinary
CAPD	continuous ambulatory peritoneal dialysis	HCO_3^-	bicarbonate
cath	catheterization	**HD**	hemodialysis
CC	clean catch urine specimen	H_2O	water
Cl^-	chloride	**I&O**	intake and output
CRF	chronic renal failure	**IPD**	intermittent peritoneal dialysis

Abbreviations (continued)

IVP	intravenous pyelogram	**NS**	nephrotic syndrome
K^+	potassium	**pH**	acidity or alkalinity of urine
KUB	kidneys, ureters, bladder	**RP**	retrograde pyelogram
mcg	microgram	**SG, sp. gr.**	specific gravity
mEq	milliequivalent	**U/A, UA**	urinalysis
mg	milligram	**UC**	urine culture
mL	milliliter	**UTI**	urinary tract infection
Na^+	sodium	**VCUG**	voiding cystourethrography

PRACTICE AS YOU GO

F. What Does it Stand For?

1. KUB ____________
2. cath ____________
3. cysto ____________
4. GU ____________
5. ESWL ____________
6. UTI ____________
7. UC ____________
8. RP ____________
9. ARF ____________
10. BUN ____________
11. CRF ____________
12. H_2O ____________

Chapter Review

Real-World Applications

Medical Record Analysis

This Discharge Summary contains 13 medical terms. Underline each term and write it in the list below the report. Then explain each term as you would to a nonmedical person.

Discharge Summary

Admitting Diagnosis:	Severe right side pain and hematuria
Final Diagnosis:	Pyelonephritis right kidney, complicated by chronic cystitis
History of Present Illness:	Patient has long history of frequent bladder infections, but denies any recent lower pelvic pain or dysuria. Earlier today he had rapid onset of severe right side pain and is unable to stand fully erect. His temperature was 101°F, and his skin was sweaty and flushed. He was admitted from the ER for further testing and diagnosis.
Summary of Hospital Course:	Clean catch urinalysis revealed gross hematuria and pyuria, but no albuminuria. A culture and sensitivity was ordered to identify the pathogen and an antibiotic was started. Cystoscopy showed evidence of chronic cystitis, bladder irritation, and a bladder neck obstruction. The obstruction appears to be congenital and the probable cause of the chronic cystitis. The patient was catheterized to ensure complete emptying of the bladder, and fluids were encouraged. Patient responded well to the antibiotic therapy and fluids, and his symptoms improved.
Discharge Plans:	Patient was discharged home after three days in the hospital. He was switched to an oral antibiotic for the pyelonephritis and chronic cystitis. A repeat urinalysis is scheduled for next week. After all inflammation is corrected, will repeat cystoscopy to reevaluate bladder neck obstruction.

	Term	Explanation
1.	______	______
2.	______	______
3.	______	______
4.	______	______
5.	______	______
6.	______	______
7.	______	______
8.	______	______
9.	______	______
10.	______	______
11.	______	______
12.	______	______
13.	______	______

Chart Note Transcription

The chart note below contains 11 phrases that can be reworded with a medical term presented in this chapter. Each phrase is identified with an underline. Determine the medical term and write your answers in the space provided.

Pearson General Hospital Consultation Report

Task Edit View Time Scale Options Help Download Archive Date: 17 May 2017

Current Complaint:	A 36-year-old male was seen by the specialist in the treatment of diseases of the urinary system **1** because of right flank pain and blood in the urine. **2**
Past History:	Patient has a history of bladder infection; **3** denies experiencing any symptoms for two years.
Signs and Symptoms:	A technique used to obtain an uncontaminated urine sample **4** obtained for laboratory analysis of the urine **5** revealed blood in the urine, but no pus in the urine. **6** A kidney X-ray made after inserting dye into the bladder **7** was normal on the left, but dye was seen filling the right tube between the kidney and bladder **8** only halfway to the kidney.
Diagnosis:	Stone in the tube between the kidney and the bladder **9** on the right
Treatment:	Patient underwent the use of ultrasound waves to break up stones. **10** Pieces of dissolved kidney stones **11** were flushed out, after which symptoms resolved.

1. ______________________________

2. ______________________________

3. ______________________________

4. ______________________________

5. ______________________________

6. ______________________________

7. ______________________________

8. ______________________________

9. ______________________________

10. ______________________________

11. ______________________________

Case Study

Below is a case study presentation of a patient with a condition discussed in this chapter. Read the case study and answer the questions below. Some questions will ask for information not included within this chapter. Use your text, a medical dictionary, or any other reference material you choose to answer these questions.

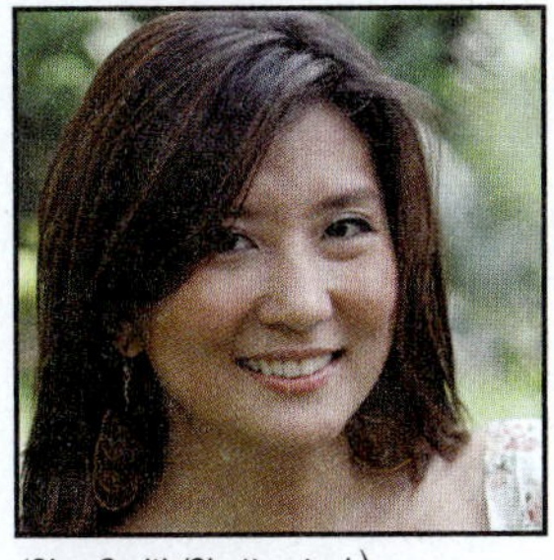

(Gina Smith/Shutterstock)

A 32-year-old female is seen in the urologist's office because of a fever, chills, and generalized fatigue. She also reported urgency, frequency, dysuria, and hematuria. In addition, she noticed that her urine was cloudy with a fishy odor. The physician ordered the following tests: a clean catch specimen for a U/A, a urine C&S, and a KUB. The U/A revealed pyuria, bacteriuria, and a slightly acidic pH. A common type of bacteria was grown in the culture. X-rays reveal acute pyelonephritis resulting from cystitis, which has spread up to the kidney from the bladder. The patient was placed on an antibiotic and encouraged to "push fluids" by drinking two liters of water a day.

Questions

1. This patient has two urinary system infections in different locations; name them. Which one caused the other and how?

   ____

   ____

2. List and define each of the patient's presenting symptoms in your own words.

   ____

   ____

3. What diagnostic tests did the urologist order? Describe them in your own words.

   ____

   ____

4. Explain the results of each diagnostic test in your own words.

   ____

   ____

5. What were the physician's treatment instructions for this patient? Explain the purpose of each treatment.

   ____

   ____

6. Describe the normal appearance of urine.

   ____

   ____

Practice Exercises

A. Word Building Practice

The combining form **nephr/o** refers to *kidney*. Use it to write a term that means:

1. surgical fixation of the kidney ____________
2. X-ray record of the kidney ____________
3. condition of kidney stones ____________
4. removal of a kidney ____________
5. inflammation of the kidney ____________
6. kidney disease ____________
7. hardening of the kidney ____________

The combining form **cyst/o** refers to the *urinary bladder*. Use it to write a term that means:

8. inflammation of the bladder ____________
9. abnormal flow condition from the bladder ____________
10. surgical repair of the bladder ____________
11. instrument to view inside the bladder ____________
12. bladder pain ____________

The combining form **pyel/o** refers to the *renal pelvis*. Use it to write a term that means:

13. surgical repair of the renal pelvis ____________
14. inflammation of the renal pelvis ____________
15. X-ray record of the renal pelvis ____________

The combining form **ureter/o** refers to one or both of the *ureters*. Use it to write a term that means:

16. a ureteral stone ____________
17. ureter dilation ____________
18. ureter narrowing ____________

The combining form **urethr/o** refers to the *urethra*. Use it to write a term that means:

19. urethra inflammation ____________
20. instrument to view inside the urethra ____________

The suffix **-uria** refers to a *urine condition*. Use it to write a term that means:

21. condition of scanty urine ____________
22. condition of blood in the urine ____________
23. condition of protein in the urine ____________
24. condition of sugar in the urine ____________
25. condition of pus in the urine ____________

B. Complete the Term

For each definition given below, fill in the blank with the word part that completes the term.

	Definition	Term
1.	surgical fixation of the bladder	____________pexy
2.	surgical crushing of a stone	____________tripsy
3.	surgical repair of renal pelvis	____________plasty
4.	to destroy (break down) urine	____________lysis
5.	drooping kidney	nephro____________
6.	pus urine condition	py____________
7.	dilated ureter	____________ectasis
8.	inflammation of kidney glomerulus	____________nephritis
9.	cutting into the meatus	____________otomy
10.	pain in the urethra	____________algia

C. Pharmacology Challenge

Fill in the classification for each drug description, then match the brand name.

	Drug Description	Classification	Brand Name
1.	________ Reduces bladder muscle spasms	____________	a. Lasix
2.	________ Treats bacterial infections	____________	b. Ditropan
3.	________ Increases volume of urine produced	____________	c. Cipro

D. Define the Term

1. micturition ____________
2. diuretic ____________
3. renal colic ____________
4. catheterization ____________
5. pyelitis ____________
6. glomerulonephritis ____________
7. lithotomy ____________
8. enuresis ____________
9. meatotomy ____________
10. diabetic nephropathy ____________
11. urinalysis ____________
12. hesitancy ____________

E. Name that Term

1. absence of urine ______________________
2. blood in the urine ______________________
3. kidney stone ______________________
4. crushing a stone ______________________
5. inflammation of the urethra ______________________
6. pus in the urine ______________________
7. bacteria in the urine ______________________
8. painful urination ______________________
9. ketones in the urine ______________________
10. protein in the urine ______________________
11. (too) much urine ______________________

F. Using Abbreviations

Fill in each blank with the appropriate abbreviation.

1. During __________ an artificial kidney machine filters waste from the blood.
2. __________ breaks up kidney stones without surgery.
3. A(n) __________ was performed to look for the source of bladder bleeding.
4. Manuel was concerned about having a(n) __________ because he is allergic to the dye injected into a vein.
5. A(n) __________ is an X-ray also called a flat-plate abdomen.
6. The __________ showed no bacteria growing in the urine.
7. The __________ was caused by an enlarged prostate gland.
8. Her __________ began as simple cystitis, but ascended the ureters and infected her kidneys.

G. Fill in the Blank

renal transplant	ureterectomy	intravenous pyelogram (IVP)
cystostomy	pyelolithectomy	nephropexy
renal biopsy	cystoscopy	urinary tract infection

1. Juan suffered from chronic renal failure. His sister, Maria, donated one of her normal kidneys to him, and he had a(n) ____________________.
2. Anesha's floating kidney needed surgical fixation. Her physician performed a surgical procedure known as ____________________.

3. Kenya's physician stated that she had a general infection that he referred to as a UTI. The full name for this infection is ____________________.
4. Surgeons operated on Robert to remove calculi from his renal pelvis. The name of this surgery is ____________________.
5. Charles had to have a small piece of his kidney tissue removed so that the physician could perform a microscopic evaluation. This procedure is called a(n) ____________________.
6. Naomi had to have one of her ureters removed due to a stricture. This procedure is called ____________________.
7. The physician had to create a temporary opening between Eric's bladder and his abdominal wall. This procedure is called ____________________.
8. Sally's bladder was visually examined using a special instrument. This procedure is called a(n) ____________________.
9. The doctors believe that Jacob has a tumor of the right kidney. They are going to do a test called a(n) ____________________ that requires them to inject a radiopaque contrast medium intravenously so that they can see the kidney on X-ray.

H. Anatomical Adjectives

Fill in the blank with the missing noun or adjective.

Noun	Adjective
1. ____________________	cystic
2. ureter	____________________
3. ____________________	urinary
4. kidney	____________________
5. ____________________	glomerular
6. ____________________	pyelitic
7. meatus	____________________
8. urethra	____________________

I. Spelling Practice

Some of the following terms are misspelled. Identify the incorrect terms and spell them correctly in the blank provided.

1. glycosuria ____________________
2. nephrosklerosis ____________________
3. cystorrhagia ____________________
4. ureterectasis ____________________
5. incontinance ____________________

6. hydronephrosis ______________________________
7. cystoseal ______________________________
8. cathaterization ______________________________
9. hemodialysis ______________________________
10. lithotripsey ______________________________

J. Complete the Statement

1. The by-products of muscle metabolism, ______________, are removed from the body in urine.
2. The filtration stage of urine production takes place in the ______________.
3. The kidneys regulate the levels of ______________, such as sodium and potassium.
4. The folds in the lining of the bladder are called ______________.
5. The nephron loop is also known as the ______________.
6. There is one __________ leading away from the urinary bladder and two __________ leading into it.
7. In the kidney, the renal artery enters and the renal vein and ureter exit at the ______________.
8. The outer portion of the kidney is the ______________ and the inner area is the ______________.

MyLab Medical Terminology™

MyLab Medical Terminology is a premium online homework management system that includes a host of features to help you study. Registered users will find:

- A multitude of activities and assignments built within the MyLab platform
- Powerful tools that track and analyze your results—allowing you to create a personalized learning experience
- Videos and audio pronunciations to help enrich your progress
- Streaming lesson presentations (Guided Lectures) and self-paced learning modules
- A space where you and your instructors can check your progress and manage your assignments

Labeling Exercises

Image A

Write the labels for this figure on the numbered lines provided.

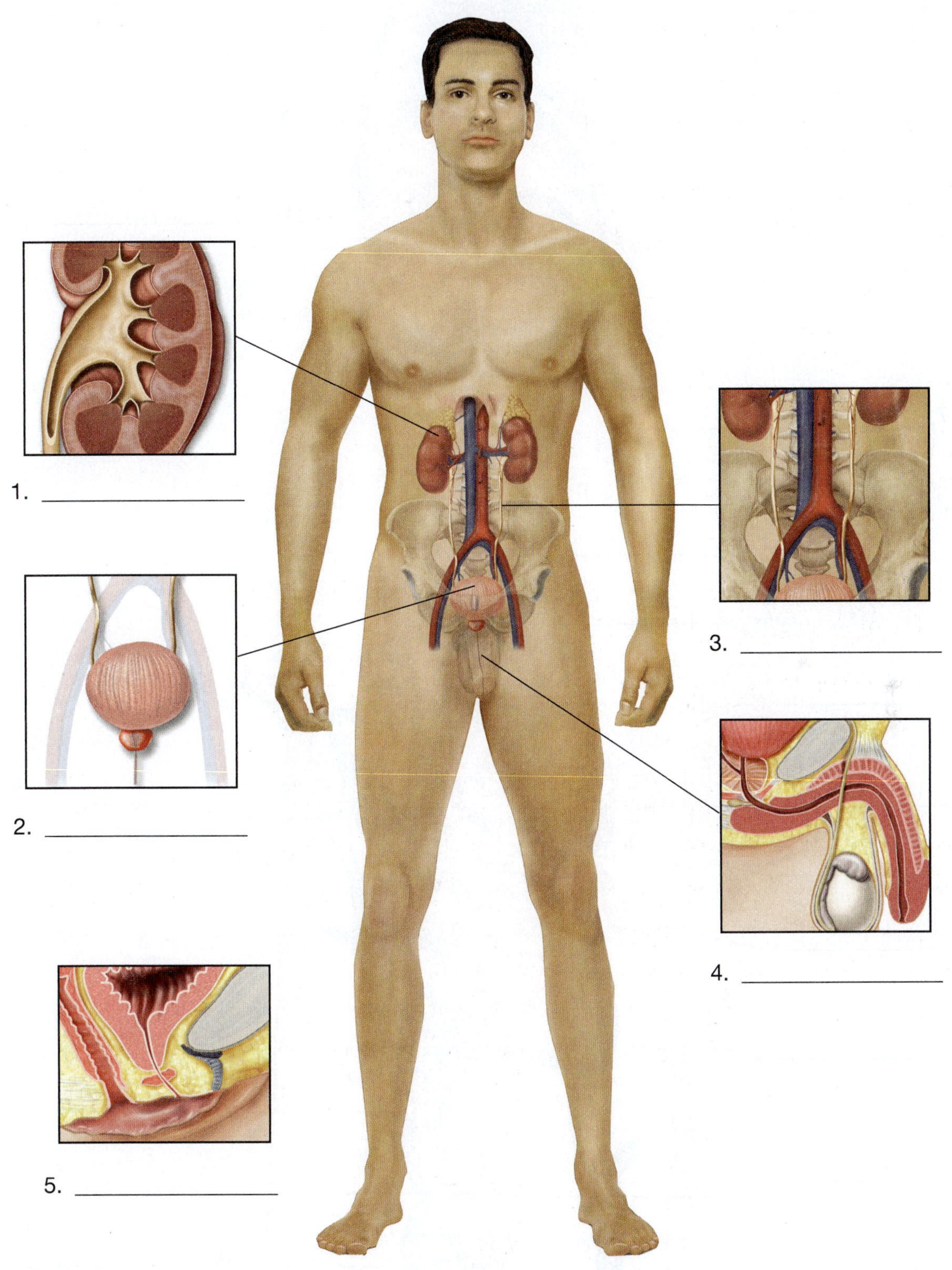

Image B

Write the labels for this figure on the numbered lines provided.

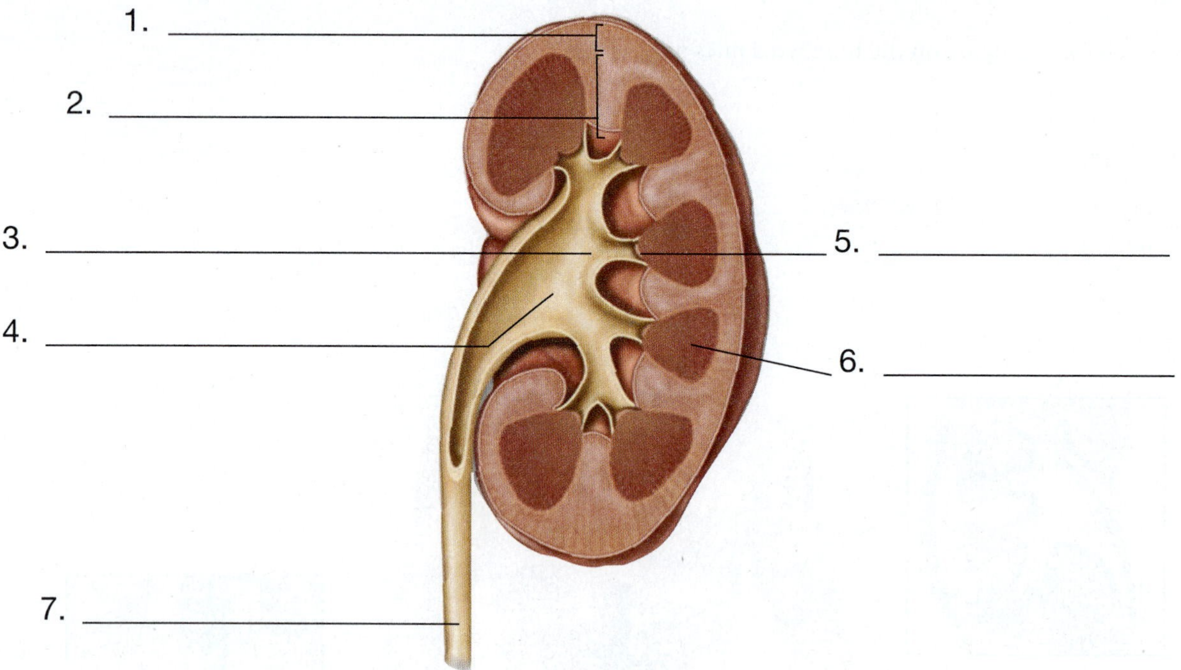

Image C

Write the labels for this figure on the numbered lines provided.

1. ______
2. ______
3. ______
4. ______
5. ______
6. ______
7. ______
8. ______
9. ______
10. ______

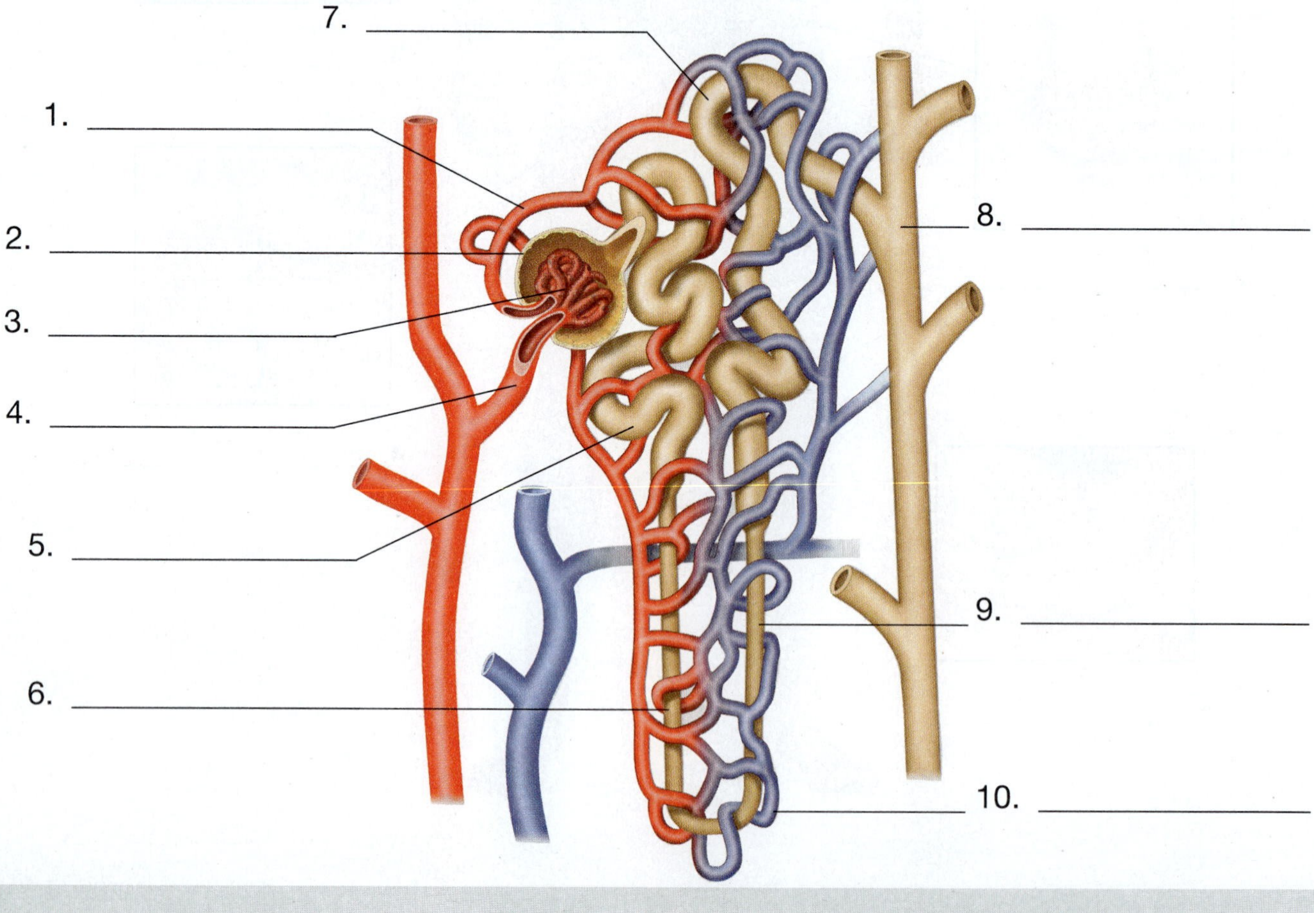

Chapter 10

Reproductive System

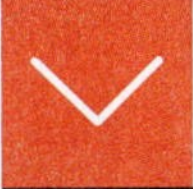

Learning Objectives

Upon completion of this chapter, you will be able to

1. Identify and define the combining forms, suffixes, and prefixes introduced in this chapter.
2. Correctly spell and pronounce medical terms and major anatomical structures relating to the reproductive systems.
3. Locate and describe the major organs of the reproductive systems and their functions.
4. Use medical terms to describe circumstances relating to pregnancy.
5. Identify and define reproductive system anatomical terms.
6. Identify and define selected reproductive system pathology terms.
7. Identify the symptoms and origin of sexually transmitted diseases.
8. Identify and define selected reproductive system diagnostic procedures.
9. Identify and define selected reproductive system therapeutic procedures.
10. Identify and define selected medications relating to the reproductive systems.
11. Define selected abbreviations associated with the reproductive systems.

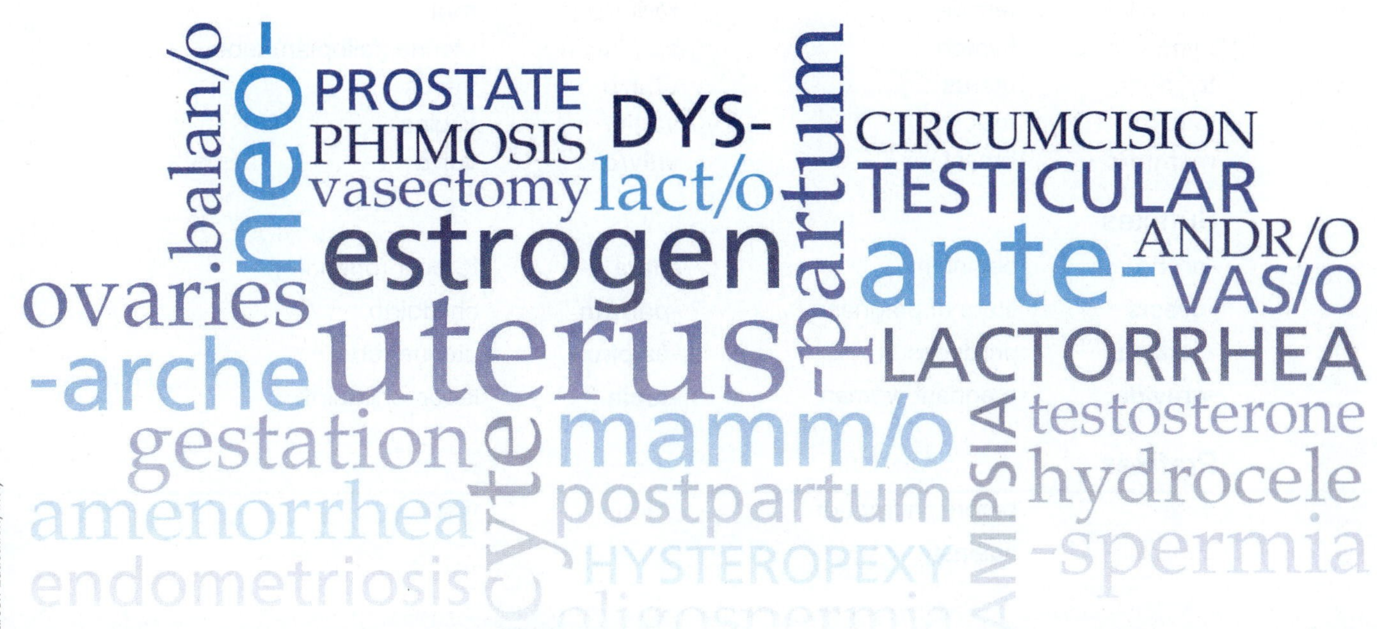

(Pearson Education, Inc.)

SECTION I: FEMALE REPRODUCTIVE SYSTEM

AT A GLANCE

Function

The female reproductive system produces ova (the female reproductive cells), provides a location for fertilization and growth of a baby, and secretes female sex hormones. In addition, the breasts produce milk to nourish the newborn.

Organs

The primary structures that comprise the female reproductive system:

ovaries	**vagina**
uterine tubes	**vulva**
uterus	**breasts**

Word Parts

Presented here are the most common word parts (with their meanings) used to build female reproductive system terms. For a more comprehensive list, refer to the Terminology section of this chapter.

Combining Forms

amni/o	amnion	**mast/o**	breast
cervic/o	neck, cervix	**men/o**	menses, menstruation
chori/o	chorion	**metr/o**	uterus
colp/o	vagina	**nat/o**	birth
culd/o	cul-de-sac	**o/o**	ovum
dilat/o	to widen	**oophor/o**	ovary
embry/o	embryo	**ov/o, ov/i**	ovum
episi/o	vulva	**ovari/o**	ovary
estr/o	female	**pareun/o**	sexual intercourse
fet/o	fetus	**perine/o**	perineum
gynec/o	female	**radic/o**	root
hymen/o	hymen	**salping/o**	uterine (fallopian) tubes
hyster/o	uterus	**uter/o**	uterus
lact/o	milk	**vagin/o**	vagina
mamm/o	breast	**vulv/o**	vulva

Suffixes

-arche	beginning	**-para**	to bear (offspring)
-cyesis	state of pregnancy	**-partum**	childbirth
-genesis	produces	**-salpinx**	uterine tube
-gravida	pregnant woman	**-tocia**	labor, childbirth

Prefixes

ante-	before, in front of	**primi-**	first
contra-	against		

Female Reproductive System Illustrated

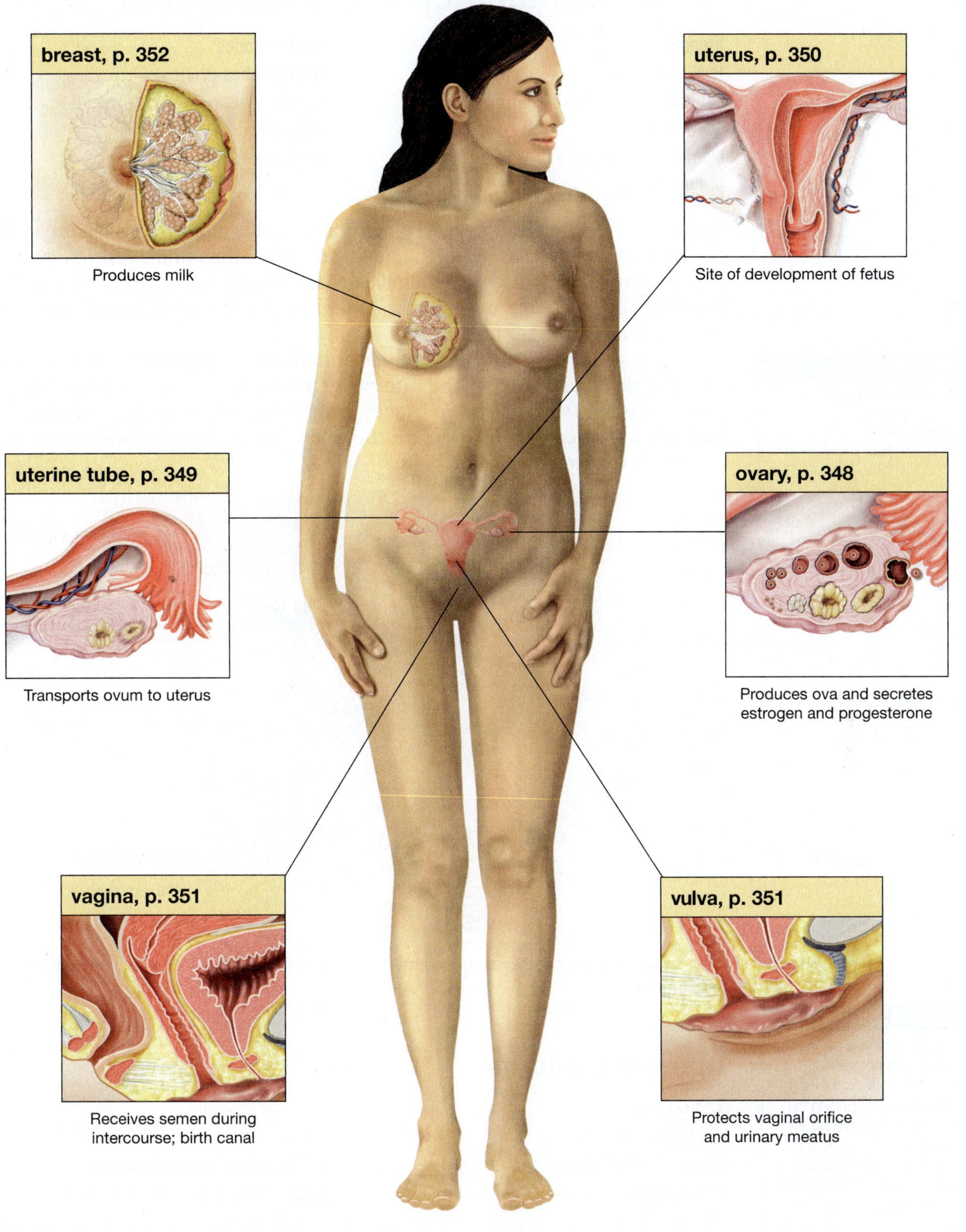

Anatomy and Physiology of the Female Reproductive System

breasts
fertilization
genitalia (jen-ih-TAY-lee-ah)
ova (OH-vah)
ovaries (OH-vah-reez)
pregnancy
sex hormones
uterine tubes (YOO-ter-in)
uterus (YOO-ter-us)
vagina (vah-JIGH-nah)
vulva (VUL-vah)

The female reproductive system plays many vital functions that ensure the continuation of the human race. First, it produces **ova**, the female reproductive cells. It then provides a place for **fertilization** to occur and for a baby to grow during **pregnancy**. The **breasts** provide nourishment for the newborn. Finally, this system secretes the female **sex hormones**.

What's In A Name?
Look for these word parts:
genit/o = genitals
-al = pertaining to

This system consists of both internal and external **genitalia**, or reproductive organs (see Figure 10-1 ■). The internal genitalia are located in the pelvic cavity and consist of the **uterus**, two **ovaries**, two **uterine tubes**, and the **vagina**, which extends to the external surface of the body. The external genitalia are collectively referred to as the **vulva**.

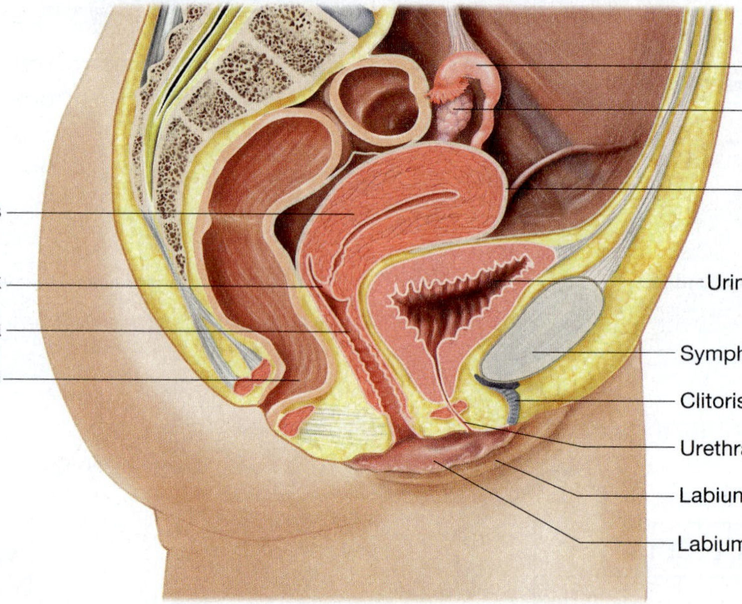

■ **Figure 10-1** The female reproductive system, sagittal view showing organs of the system in relation to the urinary bladder and rectum.

Med Term Tip
The singular for egg is *ovum.* The plural term for many eggs is *ova.* The term *ova* is not used exclusively when discussing the human reproductive system. For instance, testing the stool for ova and parasites is used to detect the presence of parasites or their ova in the digestive tract, a common cause for severe diarrhea. Ova are produced in the ovary by a process called *oogenesis* (**o/o** = ovum and **-genesis** = produces).

Internal Genitalia

Ovaries

estrogen (ESS-troh-jen)
follicle-stimulating hormone (FALL-ih-kl)
luteinizing hormone (LOO-teh-nigh-zing)
oocyte (OH-oh-sight)
ovulation (ov-yoo-LAY-shun)
progesterone (proh-JES-ter-ohn)

There are two ovaries, one located on each side of the uterus within the pelvic cavity (see again Figure 10-1). These are small almond-shaped glands that produce ova (singular is *ovum*) and the female sex hormones (see Figure 10-2 ■). In humans approximately every 28 days hormones from the anterior pituitary,

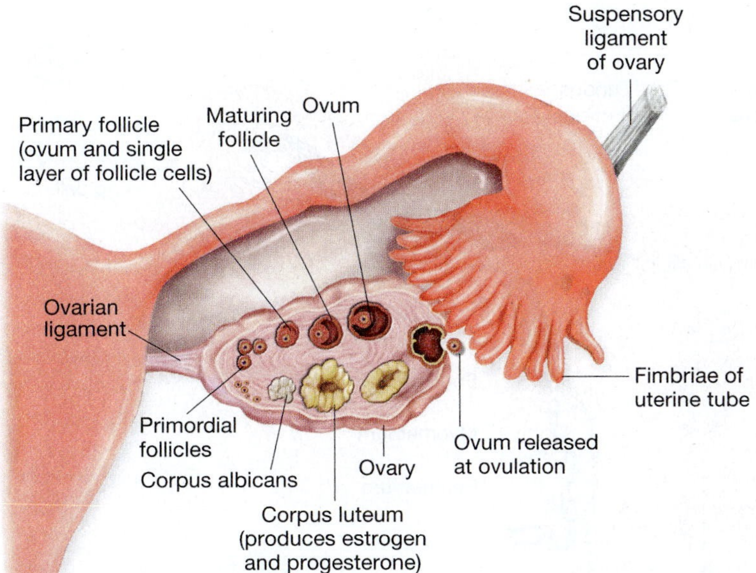

■ **Figure 10-2** Structure of the ovary and uterine (fallopian) tube. Figure illustrates stages of ovum development and the relationship of the ovary to the uterine tube.

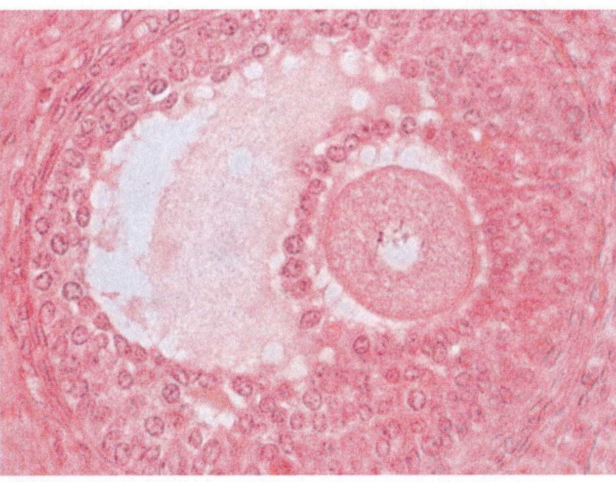

■ **Figure 10-3** Photomicrograph of human ovary showing ovum in its follicle prior to ovulation. *(Anna Jurkovska/Shutterstock)*

follicle-stimulating hormone (FSH) and **luteinizing hormone** (LH), stimulate maturation of an ovum and trigger **ovulation**, the process by which one ovary releases an ovum (or **oocyte**) (see Figure 10-3 ■). The principal female sex hormones produced by the ovaries, **estrogen** and **progesterone**, stimulate the lining of the uterus to be prepared to receive a fertilized ovum. These hormones are also responsible for the female secondary sexual characteristics.

What's In A Name?

Look for these word parts:
estr/o = female
o/o = ovum
ov/o = ovum
-cyte = cell
-gen = that which produces
pro- = before

Uterine Tubes

conception (kon-SEP-shun)
fallopian tubes (fah-LOH-pee-an)
fimbriae (FIM-bree-ee)
oviducts (OH-vih-dukts)

The uterine tubes, also called the **fallopian tubes** or **oviducts**, are approximately 4 inches (10 cm) long and run from the area around each ovary to either side of the upper portion of the uterus (see Figure 10-4 ■ and Figure 10-5 ■). As they near the ovaries, the unattached ends of these two tubes expand into finger-like projections called **fimbriae**. The fimbriae catch an ovum after ovulation and direct it into

What's In A Name?

Look for this word part:
ov/i = ovum

Med Term Tip

When the fertilized egg adheres or implants to the uterine tube instead of moving into the uterus, a condition called *tubal pregnancy* exists. There is not enough room in the uterine tube for the fetus to grow normally. Implantation of the fertilized egg in any location other than the uterus is called an *ectopic pregnancy. Ectopic* is a general term meaning *in the wrong place.*

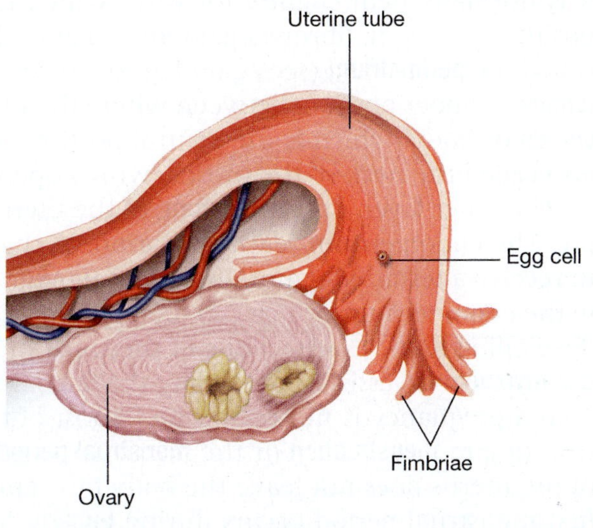

■ **Figure 10-4** Uterine (fallopian) tube, showing released ovum within the uterine tube.

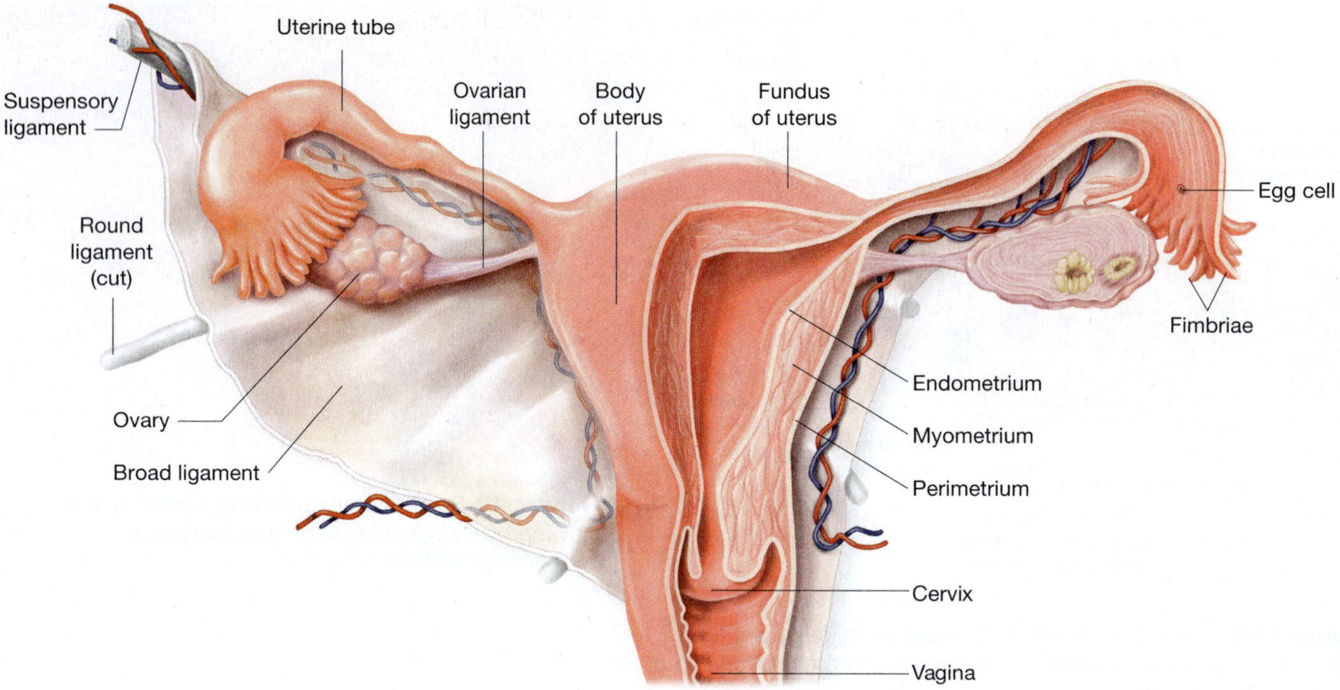

Figure 10-5 The uterus. Cutaway view shows regions of the uterus and cervix and its relationship to the uterine (fallopian) tubes and vagina.

the uterine tube. The uterine tube can then propel the ovum from the ovary to the uterus so that it can implant. The meeting of the egg and sperm, called fertilization or **conception**, normally takes place within the upper one-half of the uterine tubes.

Uterus

anteflexion (an-tee-FLEK-shun)
cervix (SER-viks)
corpus (KOR-pus)
endometrium (en-doh-MEE-tree-um)
fundus (FUN-dus)
menarche (men-AR-kee)
menopause (MEN-oh-pawz)
menstrual period (MEN-stroo-al)
menstruation (men-stroo-AY-shun)
myometrium (my-oh-MEE-tree-um)
perimetrium (pair-ih-MEE-tree-um)
puberty (PYOO-ber-tee)

> **What's In A Name?**
> Look for these word parts:
> **flex/o** = to bend
> **men/o** = menses
> **metr/o** = uterus
> **my/o** = muscle
> **-al** = pertaining to
> **-arche** = beginning
> **-ion** = action
> **ante-** = in front of
> **endo-** = inner
> **peri-** = around

The uterus is a hollow, pear-shaped organ that contains a thick muscular wall, a mucous membrane lining, and a rich supply of blood (see again Figure 10-5). Located in the center of the pelvic cavity between the bladder and the rectum, it is normally bent slightly forward, which is called **anteflexion**, and is held in position by strong fibrous ligaments anchored in the outer layer of the uterus, called the **perimetrium** (see again Figure 10-5). The uterus has three sections: the **fundus** or upper portion, between where the uterine tubes connect to the uterus; **corpus** or body, which is the central portion; and **cervix** (Cx), or lower portion, also called the neck of the uterus, which opens into the vagina.

The inner layer, or **endometrium**, of the uterine wall contains a rich blood supply. The endometrium reacts to hormonal changes every month that prepare it to receive a fertilized ovum. In a normal pregnancy the fertilized ovum implants in the endometrium, which can then provide nourishment and protection for the developing fetus. Contractions of the thick muscular walls of the uterus, called the **myometrium**, assist in propelling the fetus through the birth canal at delivery.

> **Med Term Tip**
> During pregnancy, the height of the fundus is an important measurement for estimating the stage of pregnancy and the size of the fetus. Following birth, massaging the fundus with pressure applied in a circular pattern stimulates the uterine muscle to contract to help stop bleeding. Patients may be more familiar with a common term for uterus, *womb.* However, the correct medical term is *uterus.*

If a pregnancy is not established, most of the endometrium is sloughed off, resulting in **menstruation** or the **menstrual period**. During a pregnancy, the lining of the uterus does not leave the body but remains to nourish the fetus. A girl's first menstrual period occurs during **puberty** (the sequence of events by which a child becomes a young adult capable of reproduction) and is called **menarche**. In the United States, the average age for menarche is 12½ years. The ending of menstrual activity and childbearing years is called **menopause**. This generally occurs between the ages of 40 and 55.

Word Watch

Be careful using the combining forms **uter/o** meaning *uterus* and **ureter/o** meaning *ureter*.

Vagina

Bartholin's glands (BAR-toh-linz)
hymen (HIGH-men)
vaginal orifice (VAJ-in-al / OR-ih-fis)

The vagina is a muscular tube lined with mucous membrane that extends from the cervix of the uterus to the outside of the body (see Figure 10-6 ■). The vagina allows for the passage of the menstrual flow. In addition, during intercourse, it receives the male's penis and semen, which is the fluid containing sperm. The vagina also serves as the birth canal through which the baby passes during a normal vaginal birth.

The **hymen** is a thin membranous tissue that partially covers the external vaginal opening or **vaginal orifice**. This membrane may be broken by the use of tampons, during physical activity, or during sexual intercourse. A pair of glands (called **Bartholin's glands**) are located on either side of the vaginal orifice and secrete mucus for lubrication during intercourse.

Vulva

clitoris (KLIT-oh-ris)
erectile tissue (ee-REK-tile)
labia majora (LAY-bee-ah / mah-JOR-ah)
labia minora (LAY-bee-ah / mih-NOR-ah)
perineum (pair-ih-NEE-um)
urinary meatus (YOO-rih-nair-ee / mee-AY-tus)

Word Watch

Be careful using the combining forms **colp/o** meaning *vagina* and **culd/o** meaning *cul-de-sac* (rectouterine pouch).

The vulva is a general term that refers to the group of structures that make up the female external genitalia. The **labia majora** and **labia minora** are paired folds of skin (each side of the pair would use the singular labium majora or labium minora) that serve as protection for the genitalia, the vaginal orifice, and the **urinary meatus** (see Figure 10-7 ■). Since the urinary tract and the reproductive organs are located in proximity to one another and each contains mucous membranes that can transport infection, there is a danger of infection entering the urinary tract. The **clitoris** is a small organ containing sensitive **erectile tissue** that is aroused during sexual stimulation and corresponds to the glans penis in the male. The region between the vaginal orifice and the anus is referred to as the **perineum**.

What's In A Name?

Look for these word parts:
labi/o = lip
urin/o = urine
-ary = pertaining to

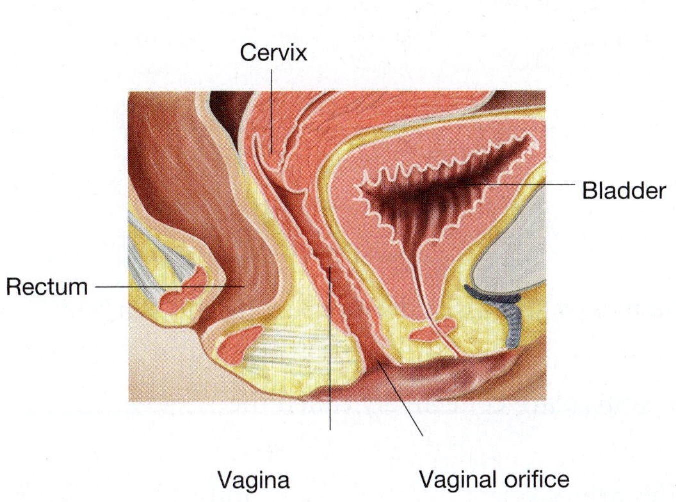

■ **Figure 10-6** The vagina, sagittal section showing the location of the vagina and its relationship to the cervix, uterus, rectum, and bladder.

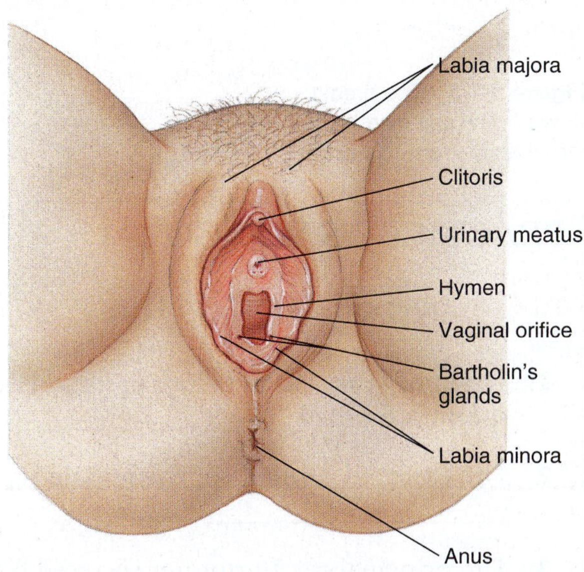

■ **Figure 10-7** The vulva, illustrating how the labia majora and labia minora cover and protect the vaginal orifice, clitoris, and urinary meatus.

Breast

areola (ah-REE-oh-lah)
lactation (lak-TAY-shun)
lactiferous ducts (lak-TIF-er-us)
lactiferous glands (lak-TIF-er-us)
mammary glands (MAM-ah-ree)
nipple
nurse

What's In A Name?

Look for these word parts:
lact/o = milk
mamm/o = breast
-ous = pertaining to
-ary = pertaining to

The breasts, or **mammary glands**, play a vital role in the reproductive process because they produce milk, a process called **lactation**, to nourish the newborn. The size of the breasts, which varies greatly from woman to woman, has no bearing on the ability to **nurse** or feed a baby. Milk is produced by the **lactiferous glands** and is carried to the **nipple** by the **lactiferous ducts** (see Figure 10-8 ■). The **areola** is the pigmented area around the nipple. As long as the breast is stimulated by the nursing infant, the breast will continue to secrete milk.

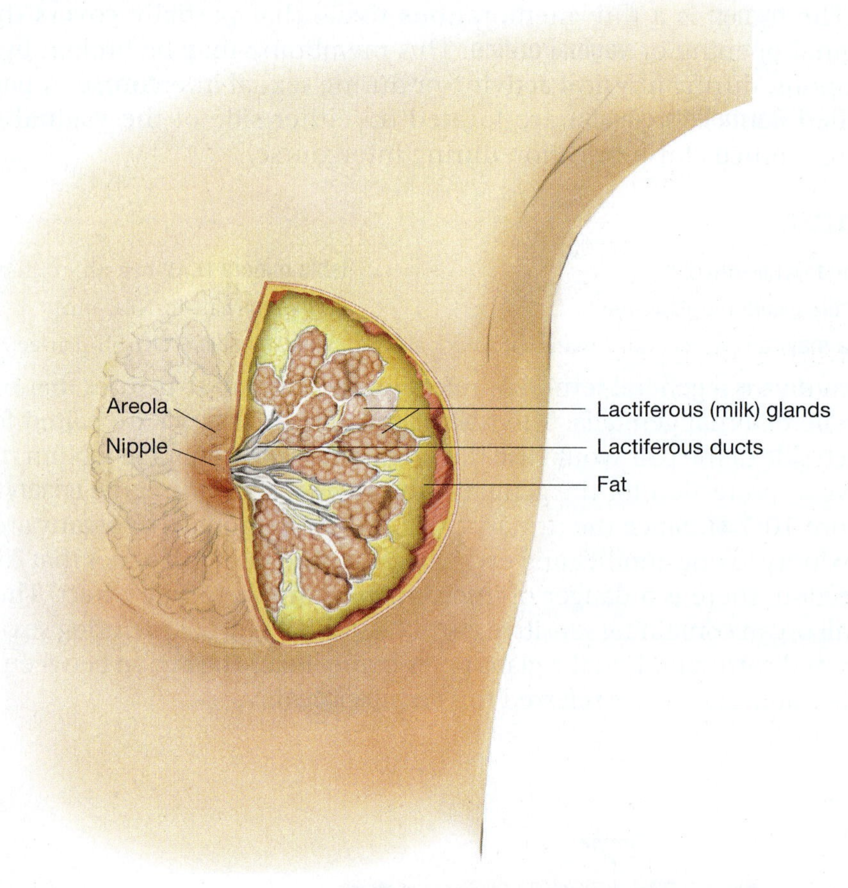

■ **Figure 10-8** The breast, cutaway view showing both internal and external features.

PRACTICE AS YOU GO

A. Complete the Statement

1. The tubes that extend from the outer edges of the uterus and assist in transporting the ova and sperm are called ____________________.
2. The external genitalia of the female reproductive system are collectively called the ____________________.
3. The principal sex hormones secreted by the ovaries are ____________________ and ____________________.

4. The cessation of menstruation is called ____________________.

5. The female sex cell is a(n) ____________________.

6. The inner lining of the uterus is called the ____________________.

7. The ____________________ is a membrane that may be broken by the use of tampons.

8. The process of ____________________ produces milk to nourish the infant.

Pregnancy

amnion (AM-nee-on)
amniotic fluid (am-nee-OT-ik)
chorion (KOH-ree-on)
embryo (EM-bree-oh)
fetus (FEE-tus)
gestation (jess-TAY-shun)
placenta (plah-SEN-tah)
premature
umbilical cord (um-BIL-ih-kal)

Pregnancy refers to the period of time during which a fetus grows and develops in its mother's uterus (see Figure 10-9 ■). The normal length of time for a pregnancy (**gestation**) is 40 weeks. If a baby is born before completing at least 37 weeks of gestation, it is considered **premature**.

What's In A Name?
Look for these word parts:
-al = pertaining to
pre- = before

During pregnancy, the female body undergoes many changes. In fact, all of the body systems become involved in the development of a healthy infant. From

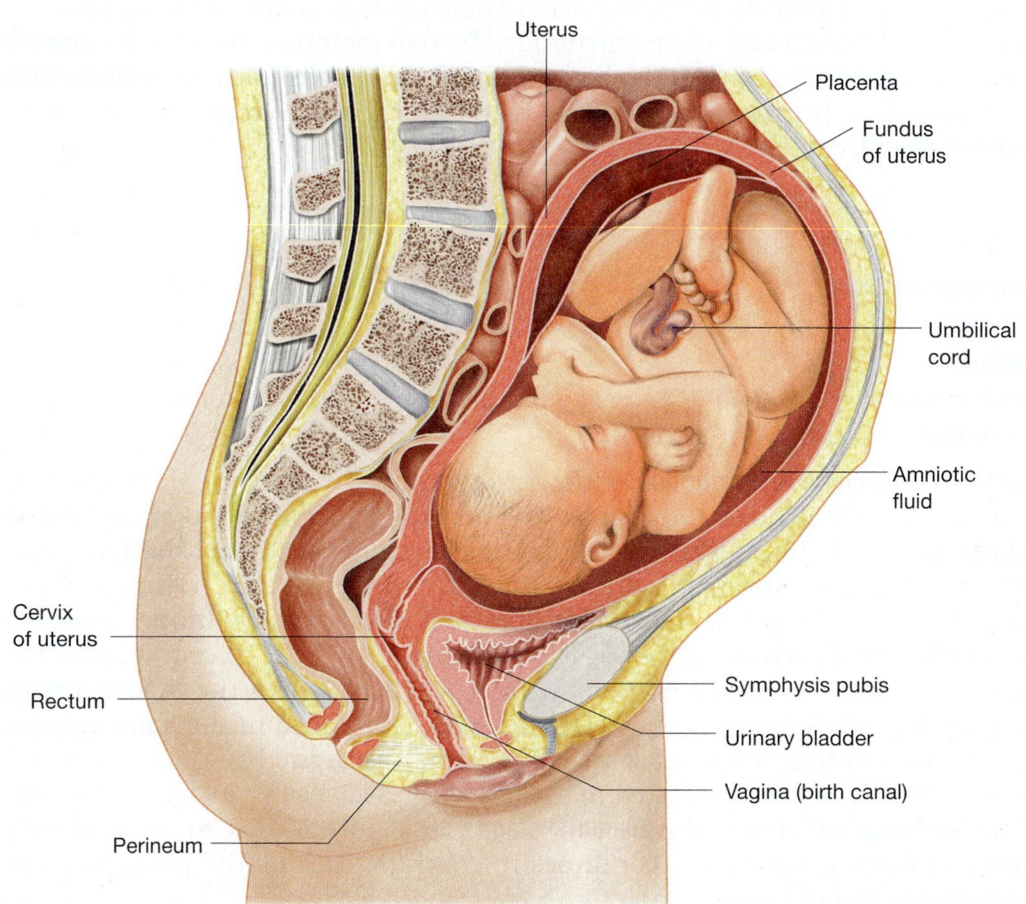

■ **Figure 10-9** A full-term pregnancy. Image illustrates position of the fetus and the structures associated with pregnancy.

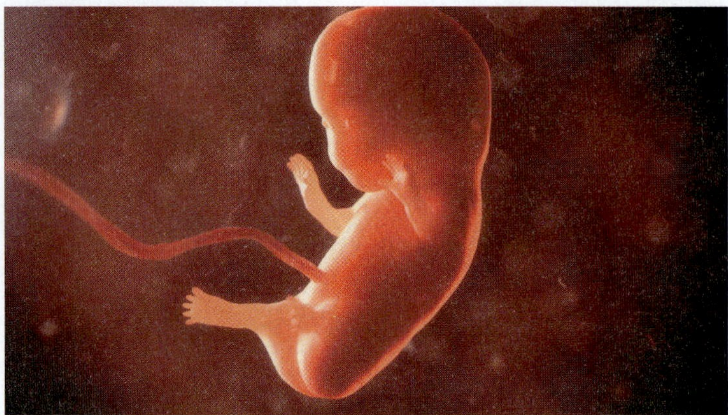

■ **Figure 10-10** Computer rendering illustrating the development of an embryo. *(u3d/Shutterstock)*

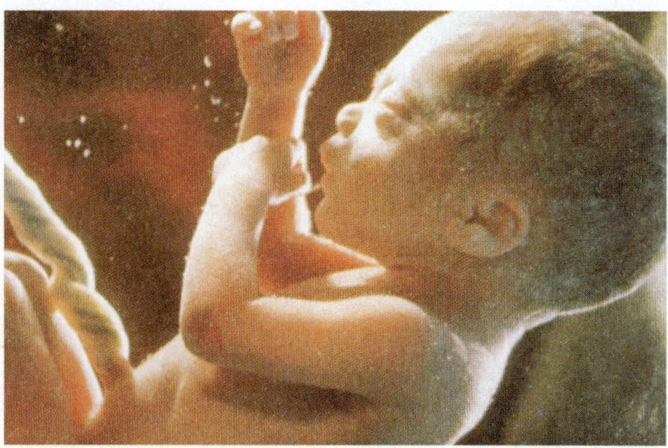

■ **Figure 10-11** Photograph illustrating the development of a fetus. *(Petit Format/Science Source)*

Med Term Tip

During the embryo stage of gestation, the organs and organ systems of the body are formed. Therefore, this is a very common time for *congenital anomalies*, or birth defects, to occur. This may happen before the woman is even aware of being pregnant.

Med Term Tip

The term *placenta* comes from the Latin word meaning *a flat cake*. This refers to the appearance of the placenta, which is a solid mass, flattened along the inner wall of the uterus.

the time the fertilized egg implants in the uterus until approximately the end of the eighth week, the infant is referred to as an **embryo** (see Figure 10-10 ■). During this period all the major organs and body systems are formed. Following the embryo stage and lasting until birth, the infant is called a **fetus** (see Figure 10-11 ■). During this time, the longest period of gestation, the organs mature and begin to function.

The fetus receives nourishment from its mother by way of the **placenta**, which is a spongy, blood-filled organ that forms in the uterus next to the fetus. The placenta is commonly referred to as the afterbirth because it is delivered through the birth canal after the birth of a baby. The fetus is attached to the placenta by way of the **umbilical cord** and is surrounded by two membranous sacs, the **amnion** and the **chorion**. The amnion is the innermost sac, and it holds the **amniotic fluid** in which the fetus floats. The chorion is an outer, protective sac and also forms part of the placenta.

Labor and Delivery

breech presentation
crowning
delivery
dilation stage (dye-LAY-shun)
effacement (eh-FAYS-ment)
expulsion stage (eks-PUL-shun)
labor
parturition (par-tyoo-RISH-un)
placental stage (plah-SEN-tal)

What's In A Name?

Look for these word parts:
dilat/o = to widen
-al = pertaining to
ex- = outward

Labor and **delivery**, or **parturition**, is the actual process of expelling the fetus from the uterus and through the vagina. The first stage is referred to as the **dilation stage**, in which the uterine muscle contracts strongly to expel the fetus (see Figure 10-12A ■). During this process the fetus presses on the cervix and causes it to dilate or expand. As the cervix dilates, it also becomes thinner, referred to as **effacement**. When the cervix is completely dilated to 10 centimeters, the second stage of labor begins (see Figure 10-12B ■). This is the **expulsion stage** and ends with delivery of the baby. Generally, the head of the baby appears first, which is referred to as **crowning**. In some cases, the baby's buttocks will appear first, and this is referred to as a **breech presentation** (see Figure 10-13 ■). The last stage of labor is the **placental stage** (see Figure 10-12C ■). Immediately after childbirth, the uterus continues to contract, causing the placenta to be expelled through the vagina.

A

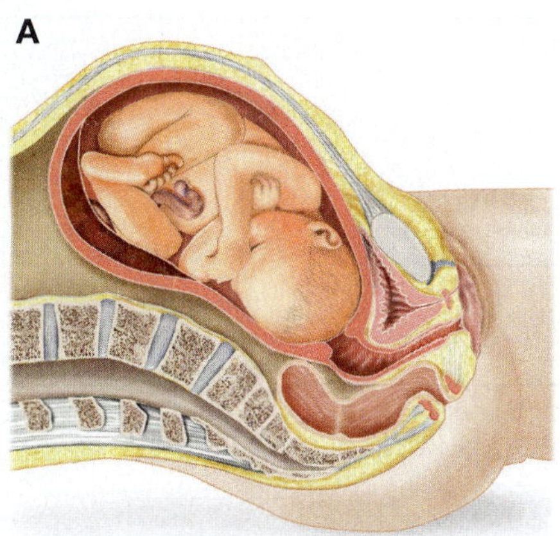

B

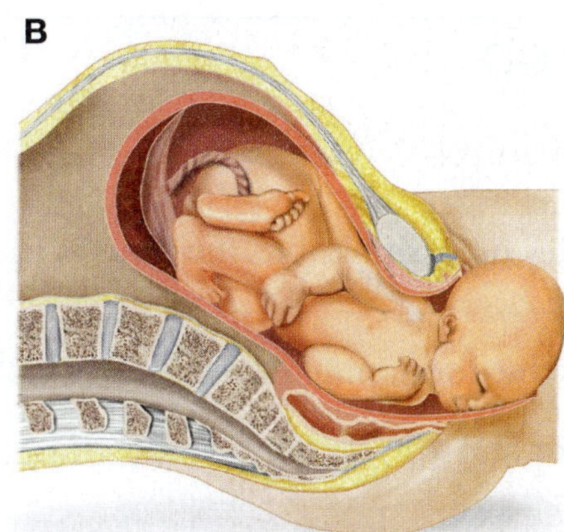

C

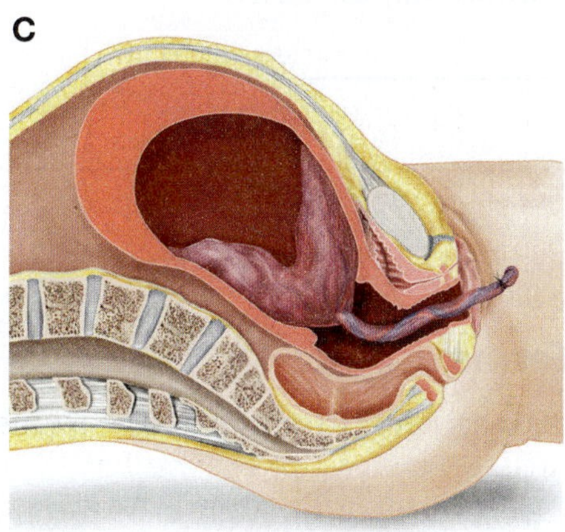

■ Figure 10-12 The stages of labor and delivery. A) During the dilation stage the cervix thins and dilates to 10 cm. B) During the expulsion stage the infant is delivered. C) During the placental stage the placenta is delivered.

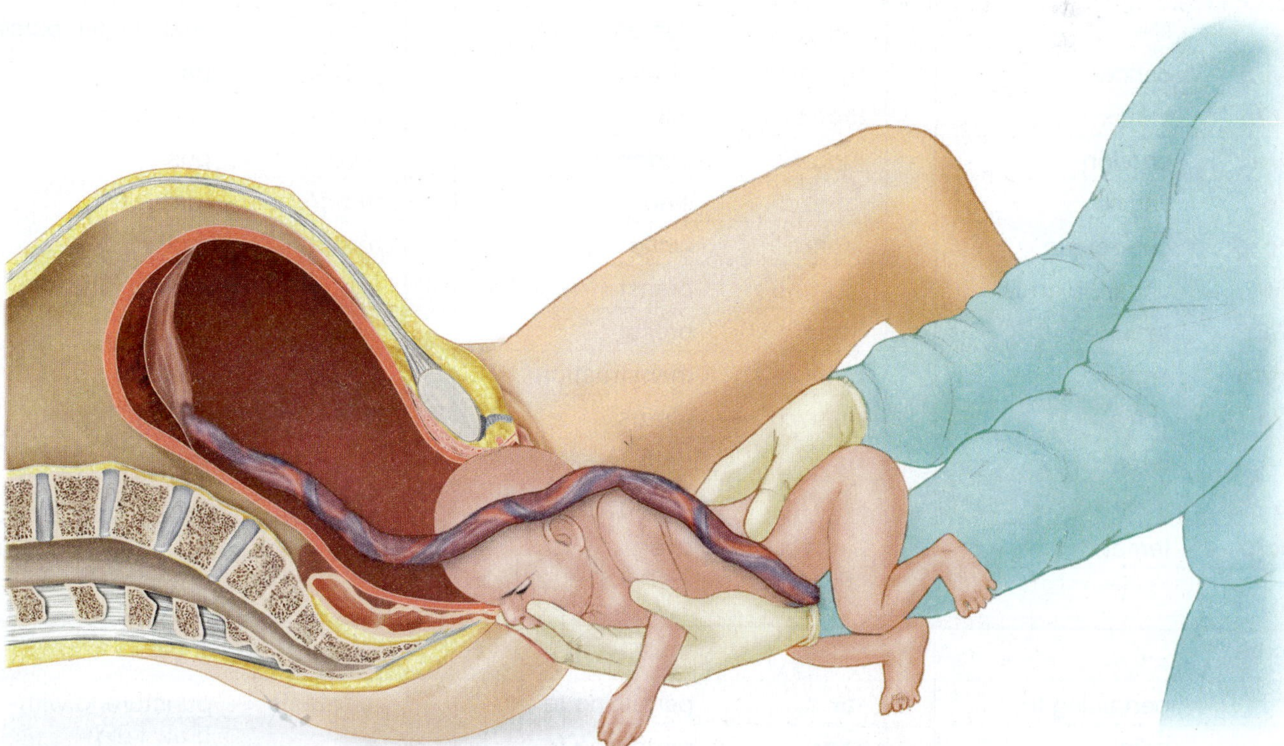

■ Figure 10-13 A breech birth. This image illustrates a newborn that has been delivered buttocks first.

PRACTICE AS YOU GO

B. Complete the Statement

1. The organ that provides nourishment to the fetus is the ____________________. The fetus is attached to it by the ____________________.
2. The time required for the development of a fetus is called ____________________.
3. The three stages of labor and delivery are the ____________________ stage, the ____________________ stage, and the ____________________ stage.
4. ____________________ refers to the head of the infant appearing in the birth canal.
5. In a(n) ____________________ presentation, the buttocks of the infant appear first.
6. The two membranous sacs surrounding the fetus are the ____________________ and ____________________.

Terminology

Word Parts Used to Build Female Reproductive System Terms

The following lists contain the combining forms, suffixes, and prefixes used to build terms in the remaining sections of this chapter.

Combining Forms

abdomin/o	abdomen
amni/o	amnion
bi/o	life
carcin/o	cancer
cervic/o	cervix
chori/o	chorion
colp/o	vagina
culd/o	cul-de-sac
cyst/o	urinary bladder
dilat/o	to widen
embry/o	embryo
episi/o	vulva
fet/o	fetus
fibr/o	fibers
gynec/o	female
hem/o	blood
hemat/o	blood
hymen/o	hymen
hyster/o	uterus
lact/o	milk
lapar/o	abdomen
later/o	side
leuk/o	white
mamm/o	breast
mast/o	breast
men/o	menstruation
metr/o	uterus
nat/o	birth
olig/o	scanty
oophor/o	ovary
or/o	mouth
ovari/o	ovary
pareun/o	sexual intercourse
pelv/o	pelvis
perine/o	perineum
py/o	pus
radic/o	root
rect/o	rectum
salping/o	uterine tube
son/o	sound
tox/o	poison
uter/o	uterus
vagin/o	vagina
vulv/o	vulva

Suffixes

-al	pertaining to
-algia	pain
-an	pertaining to
-ar	pertaining to
-ary	pertaining to
-cele	protrusion
-centesis	puncture to withdraw fluid
-cyesis	pregnancy

Suffixes (continued)

-ectomy	surgical removal	-lytic	destruction	-rrhagia	abnormal flow condition
-emesis	vomiting	-nic	pertaining to	-rrhaphy	suture
-gram	record	-oid	resembling	-rrhea	discharge
-graphy	process of recording	-oma	tumor	-rrhexis	rupture
-gravida	pregnant woman	-opsy	view of	-salpinx	uterine tube
-ia	condition	-osis	abnormal condition	-scope	instrument for viewing
-iasis	abnormal condition	-otomy	cutting into	-scopy	process of viewing
-ic	pertaining to	-ous	pertaining to	-tic	pertaining to
-ine	pertaining to	-para	to bear	-tocia	labor and childbirth
-itis	inflammation	-partum	childbirth		
-logy	study of	-pexy	surgical fixation		
		-plasty	surgical repair		

Prefixes

a-	without	hyper-	excessive	peri-	around
ante-	before	in-	not	post-	after
bi-	two	intra-	within	pre-	before
contra-	against	multi-	many	primi-	first
dys-	painful	neo-	new	pseudo-	false
endo-	inner, within	nulli-	none	ultra-	beyond

Adjective Forms of Anatomical Terms

Term	Word Parts	Definition
amniotic (am-nee-OT-ik)	amni/o = amnion -tic = pertaining to	Pertaining to amnion
cervical (SER-vih-kal)	cervic/o = cervix -al = pertaining to	Pertaining to cervix
chorionic (kor-ee-ON-ik)	chori/o = chorion -nic = pertaining to	Pertaining to chorion
embryonic (em-bree-ON-ik)	embry/o = embryo -nic = pertaining to	Pertaining to embryo
endometrial (en-doh-MEE-tree-al)	endo- = inner metr/o = uterus -al = pertaining to **Word Watch** Extra caution must be used in spelling terms containing **metr/o**. This combining form often uses an "**i**" for its combining vowel instead of the more common "**o**."	Pertaining to inner lining of uterus
fetal (FEE-tal)	fet/o = fetus -al = pertaining to	Pertaining to fetus
fibrous (FYE-bruss)	fibr/o = fibers -ous = pertaining to	Pertaining to having fibers

Adjective Forms of Anatomical Terms (continued)

Term	Word Parts	Definition
lactic (LAK-tik)	lact/o = milk -ic = pertaining to	Pertaining to milk
mammary (MAM-ah-ree)	mamm/o = breast -ary = pertaining to	Pertaining to breast
ovarian (oh-VAIR-ee-an)	ovari/o = ovary -an = pertaining to	Pertaining to ovary
perineal (pair-ih-NEE-al)	perine/o = perineum -al = pertaining to	Pertaining to perineum
uterine (YOO-ter-in)	uter/o = uterus -ine = pertaining to	Pertaining to uterus
vaginal (VAJ-in-al)	vagin/o = vagina -al = pertaining to	Pertaining to vagina
vulvar (VUL-var)	vulv/o = vulva -ar = pertaining to	Pertaining to vulva

PRACTICE AS YOU GO

C. Give the adjective form for each anatomical structure.

1. The embryo ______
2. The fetus ______
3. The uterus ______
4. An ovary ______
5. A breast ______
6. The vagina ______

Pregnancy Terms

Term	Word Parts	Definition
antepartum (an-tee-PAR-tum)	ante- = before -partum = childbirth	Period of time before birth
colostrum (kuh-LOS-trum)		Thin fluid first secreted by the breast after delivery; does not contain much protein, but is rich in antibodies
fraternal twins	-al = pertaining to	Twins that develop from two different ova fertilized by two different sperm; although twins, these siblings do not have identical DNA
identical twins	-al = pertaining to	Twins that develop from splitting of one fertilized ovum, these siblings have exactly the same DNA
meconium (meh-KOH-nee-um)		First bowel movement of newborn; greenish-black in color and consists of mucus and bile

Pregnancy Terms (continued)

Term	Word Parts	Definition
multigravida (mull-tih-GRAV-ih-dah)	multi- = many -gravida = pregnant woman	Woman who has been pregnant many (two or more) times
multipara (mull-TIP-ah-rah)	multi- = many -para = to bear	Woman who has given birth to live infant many (two or more) times
neonate (NEE-oh-nayt)	neo- = new nat/o = birth	Term for newborn baby
nulligravida (null-ih-GRAV-ih-dah)	nulli- = none -gravida = pregnant woman	Woman who has not been pregnant
nullipara (null-IP-ah-rah)	nulli- = none -para = to bear	Woman who has not given birth to a live infant
postpartum (post-PAR-tum)	post- = after -partum = childbirth	Period of time shortly after birth
primigravida (GI, grav I) (prye-mih-GRAV-ih-dah)	primi- = first -gravida = pregnant woman	Woman who is pregnant for the first time
primipara (PI, para I) (prye-MIP-ah-rah)	primi- = first -para = to bear	Woman who has given birth to a live infant once

Pathology

Term	Word Parts	Definition
Medical Specialties		
gynecology (GYN, gyn) (gigh-neh-KALL-oh-jee)	gynec/o = female -logy = study of	Branch of medicine specializing in diagnosis and treatment of conditions of the female reproductive system; physician is called a *gynecologist*
neonatology (nee-oh-nay-TALL-oh-jee)	neo- = new nat/o = birth -logy = study of	Branch of medicine specializing in diagnosis and treatment of conditions involving newborns; physician is called a *neonatologist*
obstetrics (OB) (ob-STET-riks)		Branch of medicine specializing in diagnosis and treatment of women during pregnancy and childbirth and immediately after childbirth; physician is called an *obstetrician*
Signs and Symptoms		
amenorrhea (ah-men-oh-REE-ah)	a- = without men/o = menstruation -rrhea = flow	Condition of having no menstrual flow
amniorrhea (am-nee-oh-REE-ah)	amni/o = amnion -rrhea = flow	Flow of amniotic fluid when amnion ruptures
dysmenorrhea (dis-men-oh-REE-ah)	dys- = painful men/o = menstruation -rrhea = flow	Condition of having painful menstrual flow
dyspareunia (dis-pah-ROO-nee-ah)	dys- = painful pareun/o = sexual intercourse -ia = condition	Condition of having painful sexual intercourse
dystocia (dis-TOH-see-ah)	dys- = abnormal, difficult -tocia = labor and childbirth	Difficult labor and childbirth

Pathology (continued)

Term	Word Parts	Definition
hematosalpinx (hee-mah-toh-SAL-pinks)	**hemat/o** = blood **-salpinx** = uterine tube	Presence of blood in a uterine tube
leukorrhea (loo-koh-REE-ah)	**leuk/o** = white **-rrhea** = discharge	Whitish or yellowish vaginal discharge; may be caused by vaginal infection
mastalgia (mas-TAL-jee-ah)	**mast/o** = breast **-algia** = pain	Breast pain
menorrhagia (men-oh-RAY-jee-ah)	**men/o** = menstruation **-rrhagia** = abnormal flow condition	Condition of having abnormally heavy menstrual flow during normal menstruation time
metrorrhagia (mee-troh-RAY-jee-ah)	**metr/o** = uterus **-rrhagia** = abnormal flow condition	Term used to describe uterine bleeding between menstrual periods
metrorrhea (mee-troh-REE-ah)	**metr/o** = uterus **-rrhea** = discharge	Having discharge (such as mucus or pus) from the uterus that is not the menstrual flow
oligomenorrhea (ol-ih-goh-men-oh-REE-ah)	**olig/o** = scanty **men/o** = menstruation **-rrhea** = flow	Condition of having light menstrual flow
Ovary		
oophoritis (oh-of-or-EYE-tis)	**oophor/o** = ovary **-itis** = inflammation	Inflammation of the ovary
ovarian carcinoma (oh-VAIR-ee-an / kar-sih-NOH-mah)	**ovari/o** = ovary **-an** = pertaining to **carcin/o** = cancer **-oma** = tumor	Cancer of the ovary
ovarian cyst (oh-VAIR-ee-an / SIST)	**ovari/o** = ovary **-an** = pertaining to	Cyst that develops within the ovary; may be multiple cysts and may rupture, causing pain and bleeding
Uterine Tubes		
pyosalpinx (pye-oh-SAL-pinks)	**py/o** = pus **-salpinx** = uterine tube	Presence of pus in a uterine tube
salpingitis (sal-pin-JIGH-tis)	**salping/o** = uterine tube **-itis** = inflammation	Inflammation of a uterine tube
Uterus		
cervical cancer (SER-vih-kal)	**cervic/o** = cervix **-al** = pertaining to	Malignant growth in the cervix; main cause is infection by *human papillomavirus* (HPV), a sexually transmitted virus for which there is now a vaccine; Pap smear tests have helped to detect early cervical cancer
endocervicitis (en-doh-ser-vih-SIGH-tis)	**endo-** = within **cervic/o** = cervix **-itis** = inflammation	Inflammation that occurs within the cervix
endometrial cancer (en-doh-MEE-tree-al)	**endo-** = inner **metr/o** = uterus **-al** = pertaining to	Cancer of endometrial lining of the uterus
endometritis (en-doh-meh-TRYE-tis)	**endo-** = inner **metr/o** = uterus **-itis** = inflammation	Inflammation of endometrium (inner layer of the uterine wall)

Word Watch

Be careful when using the combining form **metr/o** meaning *uterus* and the suffix **-metry** meaning *process of measuring.*

Pathology (continued)

Term	Word Parts	Definition
fibroid tumor (FIGH-broyd / TOO-mer)	fibr/o = fibers -oid = resembling	Benign tumor or growth that contains fiberlike tissue; uterine fibroid tumors are the most common benign tumors in women of childbearing age
hysterorrhexis (hiss-ter-oh-REK-sis)	hyster/o = uterus -rrhexis = rupture	Rupture of the uterus; may occur during labor
menometrorrhagia (men-oh-mee-troh-RAY-jee-ah)	men/o = menstruation metr/o = uterus -rrhagia = abnormal flow condition	Excessive bleeding during menstrual period and at intervals between menstrual periods
premenstrual syndrome (PMS) (pree-MEN-stroo-al / SIN-drohm)	pre- = before men/o = menstruation -al = pertaining to	Symptoms that develop just prior to onset of a menstrual period, which can include irritability, headache, tender breasts, and anxiety
prolapsed uterus (proh-LAPST / YOO-ter-us)		Fallen uterus that can cause the cervix to protrude through the vaginal opening; generally caused by weakened muscles from vaginal delivery or as a result of pelvic tumors pressing down
Vagina		
candidiasis (kan-dih-DYE-ah-sis)	-iasis = abnormal condition	Yeast infection of the skin and mucous membranes that can result in white plaques on tongue and vagina
cystocele (SIS-toh-seel)	cyst/o = urinary bladder -cele = protrusion	Hernia or outpouching of the bladder that protrudes into the vagina; may cause urinary frequency and urgency
rectocele (REK-toh-seel)	rect/o = rectum -cele = protrusion	Protrusion or herniation of the rectum into the vagina
toxic shock syndrome (TSS)	tox/o = poison -ic = pertaining to	Rare and sometimes fatal staphylococcus infection that generally occurs in menstruating women; initial infection occurs in vagina and associated with prolonged wearing of super-absorbent tampon; toxins secreted by bacteria then enter bloodstream

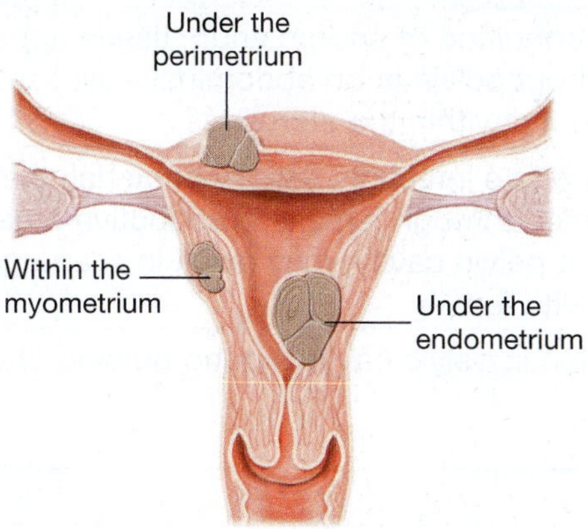

Under the perimetrium

Within the myometrium

Under the endometrium

Figure 10-14 Common sites for the development of fibroid tumors.

Med Term Tip

The term *candida* comes from a Latin term meaning *dazzling white.* Candida is the scientific name for yeast and refers to the very white discharge that is the hallmark of a yeast infection.

Pathology (continued)

Term	Word Parts	Definition
vaginitis (vaj-ih-NIGH-tis)	**vagin/o** = vagina **-itis** = inflammation	Inflammation of the vagina
Pelvic Cavity		
endometriosis (en-doh-mee-tree-OH-sis)	**endo-** = within **metr/o** = uterus **-osis** = abnormal condition	Abnormal condition of endometrium tissue appearing throughout pelvis or on abdominal wall; tissue normally found within the uterus
pelvic inflammatory disease (PID) (PEL-vik / in-FLAM-ah-tor-ee)	**pelv/o** = pelvis **-ic** = pertaining to	Chronic or acute infection, usually bacterial, that has ascended through female reproductive organs and out into pelvic cavity; may result in scarring that interferes with fertility
perimetritis (pair-ih-meh-TRYE-tis)	**peri-** = around **metr/o** = uterus **-itis** = inflammation	Inflammation in pelvic cavity around outside of the uterus
Breast		
breast cancer		Malignant tumor of the breast; usually forms in milk-producing gland tissue or lining of the milk ducts

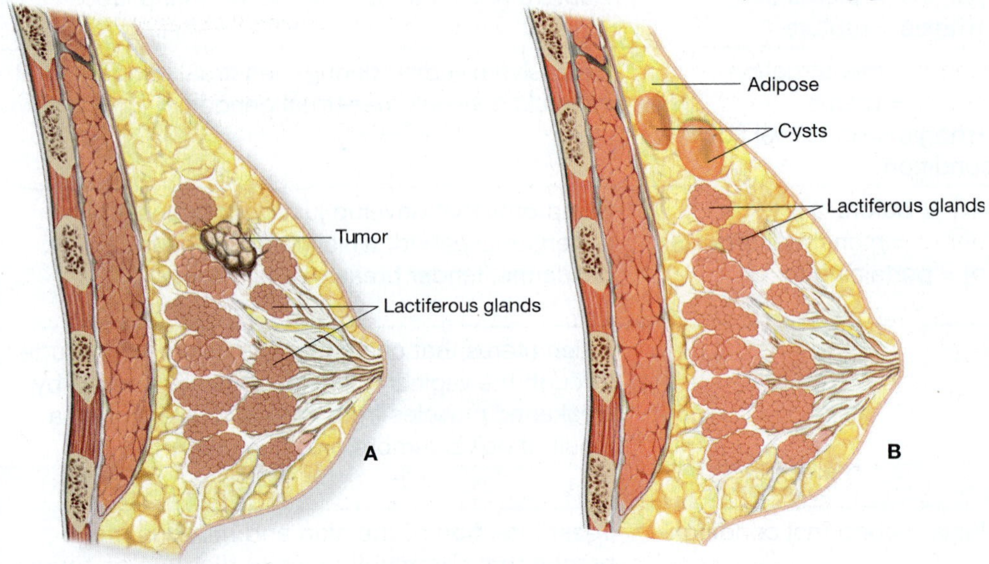

■ **Figure 10-15** Comparison of breast cancer and fibrocystic disease. A) Breast with a malignant tumor growing in the lactiferous gland and duct. B) The location of a fibrocystic lump in the adipose tissue covering the breast.

Term	Word Parts	Definition
fibrocystic breast disease (figh-broh-SIS-tik)	**fibr/o** = fibers **cyst/o** = pouch **-ic** = pertaining to	Benign cysts forming in the breast (see Figure 10-15B ■)
lactorrhea (lak-toh-REE-ah)	**lact/o** = milk **-rrhea** = discharge	Discharge of milk from the breast other than normal lactation; any white discharge from a nipple
mastitis (mas-TYE-tis)	**mast/o** = breast **-itis** = inflammation	Inflammation of the breast
Pregnancy		
abruptio placentae (ah-BRUP-shee-oh / plah-SEN-tee)		Emergency condition in which the placenta tears away from uterine wall prior to delivery of infant; requires immediate delivery of baby
eclampsia (eh-KLAMP-see-ah)	**-ia** = condition	Further worsening of preeclampsia symptoms with addition of seizures and coma; may occur between 20th week of pregnancy and up to six weeks postpartum

Pathology (continued)

Term	Word Parts	Definition
hemolytic disease of the newborn (HDN) (hee-moh-LIT-ik)	hem/o = blood -lytic = destruction	Condition developing in baby when mother's blood type is Rh-negative and baby's blood is Rh-positive; antibodies in mother's blood enter fetus' bloodstream through placenta and destroy fetus' red blood cells, causing anemia, jaundice, and enlargement of liver and spleen; treatment is early diagnosis and blood transfusion; also called *erythroblastosis fetalis*
hyperemesis gravidarum (high-per-EM-eh-sis / grav-ih-DAIR-um) **Med Term Tip** This term uses *gravidarum* as a free-standing word rather than a suffix. It also uses the plural form meaning *pregnant women* (rather than the singular *gravida*).	hyper- = excessive -emesis = vomiting	Severe nausea and vomiting during pregnancy; may cause dangerous level of dehydration and weight loss; may require hospitalization
infertility	in- = not	Inability to produce children; generally defined as no pregnancy after properly timed intercourse for one year
placenta previa (plah-SEN-tah / PREE-vee-ah) Umbilical cord Fetus Placenta Severe bleeding ■ **Figure 10-16** Placenta previa, longitudinal section showing the placenta growing over the opening into the cervix.		A placenta that is implanted in lower portion of the uterus and, in turn, blocks birth canal
preeclampsia (pree-eh-KLAMP-see-ah)	pre- = before	Metabolic disease of pregnancy; if untreated, may progress to eclampsia; symptoms include hypertension, headaches, albumin in urine, and edema; may occur between 20th week of pregnancy and up to six weeks postpartum; also called *toxemia* or *pregnancy-induced hypertension* (PIH)
prolapsed umbilical cord (proh-LAPST / um-BIL-ih-kal)		When the umbilical cord of baby is expelled first during delivery and is squeezed between baby's head and vaginal wall; presents emergency situation since baby's circulation is compromised
pseudocyesis (soo-doh-sigh-EE-sis)	pseudo- = false -cyesis = pregnancy	Condition in which body reacts as if there is a pregnancy (especially hormonal changes), but there is no pregnancy

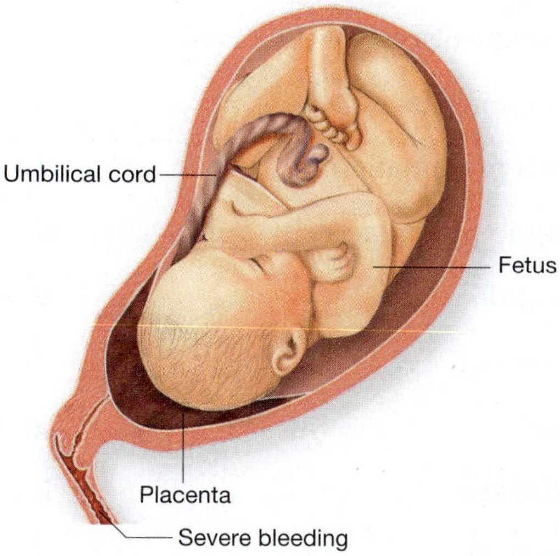

Pathology (continued)

Term	Word Parts	Definition
salpingocyesis (sal-ping-goh-sigh-EE-sis)	salping/o = uterine tube -cyesis = pregnancy	Pregnancy that occurs in the uterine tube instead of in the uterus
spontaneous abortion **Med Term Tip** The term *abortion* (AB) has different meanings for medical professionals and the general population. The general population equates the term *abortion* specifically with the planned termination of a pregnancy. However, to the medical community, *abortion* is a broader medical term meaning that a pregnancy has ended before a fetus is *viable*, meaning before it can live on its own.		Unplanned loss of a pregnancy due to death of embryo or fetus before time it is viable, commonly referred to as *miscarriage*
stillbirth		Birth in which a viable-aged fetus dies shortly before or at the time of delivery

PRACTICE AS YOU GO

D. Terminology Matching

Match each term to its definition.

1. ________ hemolytic disease of the newborn
2. ________ dysmenorrhea
3. ________ breech presentation
4. ________ abruptio placentae
5. ________ eclampsia
6. ________ pyosalpinx
7. ________ fibroid
8. ________ candidiasis
9. ________ lactorrhea
10. ________ neonate

a. seizures and coma during pregnancy
b. erythroblastosis fetalis
c. detached placenta
d. yeast infection
e. abnormal discharge from breast
f. newborn
g. buttocks first to appear in birth canal
h. painful menstruation
i. pus in the uterine tube
j. benign tumor

Diagnostic Procedures

Term	Word Parts	Definition
Clinical Laboratory Tests		
human papillomavirus (HPV) **DNA test** (pap-ih-LOH-mah-vigh-russ)		Examination of sample of cervical tissue, obtained by swabbing or scraping cervix, to determine infection by virus responsible for cervical cancer

Diagnostic Procedures (continued)

Term	Word Parts	Definition
Pap (Papanicolaou) **smear** (pap-ah-NIK-oh-lao)		Test for early detection of cancer of the cervix named after developer of test, George Papanicolaou, a Greek physician; a scraping of cells is removed from the cervix for examination under microscope
pregnancy test (PREG-nan-see)		Chemical test that can determine pregnancy during first few weeks; can be performed in physician's office or with home-testing kit
vaginal smear wet mount (VAJ-in-al)	vagin/o = vagina -al = pertaining to	Microscopic examination of cells obtained by swabbing vaginal wall; used to diagnose candidiasis
Diagnostic Imaging		
hysterosalpingography (HSG) (hiss-ter-oh-sal-pin-GOG-rah-fee)	hyster/o = uterus salping/o = uterine tube -graphy = process of recording	Taking of X-ray after injecting radiopaque material into uterus and uterine tubes
mammogram (MAM-oh-gram)	mamm/o = breast -gram = record	X-ray record of the breast
mammography (mam-OG-rah-fee)	mamm/o = breast -graphy = process of recording	X-ray to diagnose breast disease, especially breast cancer
pelvic ultrasonography (PEL-vik / ul-trah-son-OG-rah-fee)	pelv/o = pelvis -ic = pertaining to ultra- = beyond son/o = sound -graphy = process of recording	Use of high-frequency sound waves to produce image or photograph of an organ, such as uterus, ovaries, or fetus
Endoscopic Procedures		
colposcope (KOL-poh-skohp)	colp/o = vagina -scope = instrument for viewing	Instrument used to view inside the vagina
colposcopy (kol-POS-koh-pee)	colp/o = vagina -scopy = process of viewing	Examination of vagina using instrument called *colposcope*
culdoscopy (kul-DOS-koh-pee)	culd/o = cul-de-sac -scopy = process of viewing	Examination of a blind pouch-like area of the female pelvic cavity located posterior to the uterus, by introducing endoscope through wall of the vagina
laparoscope (LAP-ah-roh-skohp)	lapar/o = abdomen -scope = instrument for viewing	Instrument used to view inside abdomen
laparoscopy (lap-ar-OSS-koh-pee)	lapar/o = abdomen -scopy = process of viewing	Examination of peritoneal cavity using an instrument called a *laparoscope*; instrument is passed through small incision made by surgeon into abdominopelvic cavity

Figure 10-17 Illustration depicting a laparoscopic examination of the uterus, ovaries, and uterine tubes. *(Medical Art Inc/Shutterstock)*

Diagnostic Procedures (continued)

Term	Word Parts	Definition
Obstetrical Diagnostic Procedures		
amniocentesis (am-nee-oh-sen-TEE-sis)	amni/o = amnion -centesis = puncture to withdraw fluid	Puncturing of amniotic sac using needle and syringe for purpose of withdrawing amniotic fluid for testing; can assist in determining fetal maturity, development, and genetic disorders
Apgar score (AP-gar)		Evaluation of neonate's adjustment to outside world; observes color, heart rate, muscle tone, respiratory rate, and response to stimulus at one minute and five minutes after birth
chorionic villus sampling (CVS) (kor-ee-ON-ik / VILL-us)	chori/o = chorion -nic = pertaining to	Removal of a small piece of chorion for genetic analysis; may be done at earlier stage of pregnancy than amniocentesis
fetal monitoring (FEE-tal)	fet/o = fetus -al = pertaining to	Using electronic equipment placed on mother's abdomen or fetus' scalp to check fetal heart rate (FHR) (also called fetal heart tone [FHT]) during labor; normal heart rate of fetus is rapid, ranging from 120 to 160 beats per minute; a drop in fetal heart rate indicates fetus is in distress
Additional Diagnostic Procedures		
cervical biopsy (SER-vih-kal / BYE-op-see)	cervic/o = cervix -al = pertaining to bi/o = life -opsy = view of	Taking a sample of tissue from the cervix to test for presence of cancer cells
endometrial biopsy (EMB) (en-doh-MEE-tree-al / BYE-op-see)	endo- = inner metr/o = uterus -al = pertaining to bi/o = life -opsy = view of	Taking a sample of tissue from lining of the uterus to test for abnormalities
pelvic examination (PEL-vik)	pelv/o = pelvis -ic = pertaining to	Physical examination of the vagina and adjacent organs performed by physician placing fingers of one hand into the vagina in order to visually examine vagina and cervix and to obtain cervical cells for Pap smear; instrument called *speculum* is used to open the vagina

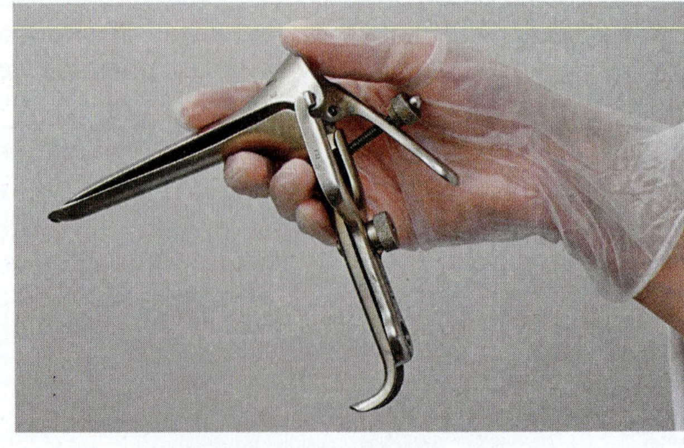

Figure 10-18 A speculum used to hold the vagina open in order to visualize the cervix. *(Patrick Watson/Pearson Education, Inc.)*

Therapeutic Procedures

Term	Word Parts	Definition
Medical Procedures		
barrier contraception (kon-trah-SEP-shun)	contra- = against	Prevention of pregnancy using a device to prevent sperm from meeting an ovum; examples include condoms, diaphragms, and cervical caps
hormonal contraception	-al = pertaining to contra- = against	Use of hormones to block ovulation and prevent conception; may be in form of a pill, a patch, an implant under the skin, or an injection
intrauterine device (IUD) (in-trah-YOO-ter-in)	intra- = within uter/o = uterus -ine = pertaining to	Device inserted into the uterus by physician for purpose of contraception

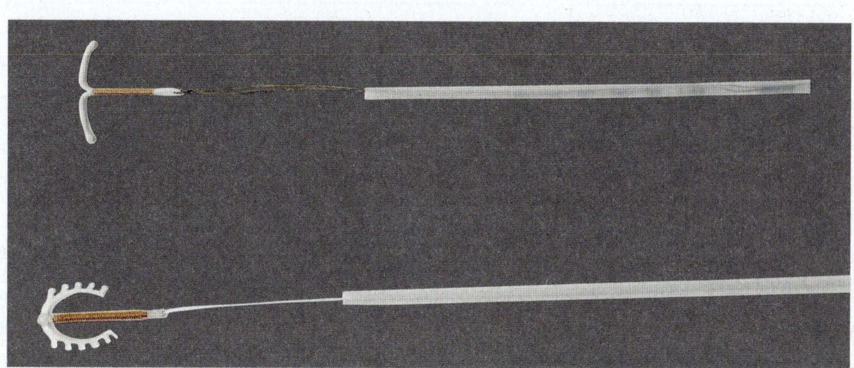

■ **Figure 10-19** Photograph illustrating the shape of two different intrauterine devices (IUDs). The intrauterine portion is approximately 1–1/4 inches long. The thin thread attached to the end of the device extends through the cervix into the vagina. This allows a woman to check that the IUD remains properly in place. *(Jules Selmes and Debi Treloar/Dorling Kindersley Media Library)*

Term	Word Parts	Definition
Surgical Procedures		
amniotomy (am-nee-OT-oh-mee)	amni/o = amnion -otomy = cutting into	Surgically cutting open the amnion; commonly referred to as *breaking the water*
cervicectomy (ser-vih-SEK-toh-mee)	cervic/o = cervix -ectomy = surgical removal	Surgical removal of the cervix
cesarean section (CS, C-section) (seh-SAIR-ee-an)		Surgical delivery of baby through incision into abdominal and uterine walls; legend has it that Roman emperor Julius Caesar was first person born by this method
conization (kon-ih-ZAY-shun)		Surgical removal of a core of cervical tissue; also refers to partial removal of the cervix
dilation and curettage (D&C) (dye-LAY-shun / kyoo-reh-TAZH)	dilat/o = to widen	Surgical procedure in which opening of the cervix is dilated and the uterus is scraped or suctioned of its lining or tissue; often performed after spontaneous abortion and to stop excessive bleeding from other causes
elective abortion		Legal termination of a pregnancy for nonmedical reasons
episiorrhaphy (eh-peez-ee-OR-ah-fee)	episi/o = vulva -rrhaphy = suture	To suture the perineum; postpartum procedure to repair episiotomy or any tearing of the perineum that occurred during birth; note that combining form **episi/o** is used even though the perineum is not part of the vulva
episiotomy (eh-peez-ee-OT-oh-mee)	episi/o = vulva -otomy = cutting into	Surgical incision of the perineum to facilitate delivery process; can prevent irregular tearing of tissue during birth; note that combining form **episi/o** is used even though the perineum is not part of the vulva

Therapeutic Procedures (continued)

Term	Word Parts	Definition
hymenectomy (high-men-EK-toh-mee)	hymen/o = hymen -ectomy = surgical removal	Surgical removal of the hymen
hysterectomy (hiss-ter-EK-toh-mee)	hyster/o = uterus -ectomy = surgical removal	Surgical removal of the uterus
hysteropexy (HISS-ter-oh-pek-see)	hyster/o = uterus -pexy = surgical fixation	To surgically anchor the uterus to its proper location in pelvic cavity; treatment for prolapsed uterus
laparotomy (lap-ah-ROT-oh-mee)	lapar/o = abdomen -otomy = cutting into	To cut open abdomen; performed in order to complete other surgical procedures inside abdomen or performed during a C-section
lumpectomy (lum-PEK-toh-mee)	-ectomy = surgical removal	Removal of only a breast tumor and tissue immediately surrounding it
mammoplasty (MAM-oh-plas-tee)	mamm/o = breast -plasty = surgical repair	Surgical repair or reconstruction of the breast
mastectomy (mas-TEK-toh-mee)	mast/o = breast -ectomy = surgical removal	Surgical removal of the breast
oophorectomy (oh-of-or-EK-toh-mee)	oophor/o = ovary -ectomy = surgical removal	Surgical removal of the ovary
radical mastectomy (mas-TEK-toh-mee)	radic/o = root -al = pertaining to mast/o = breast -ectomy = surgical removal	Surgical removal of breast tissue plus chest muscles and axillary lymph nodes; term *radical* is used to describe extensive surgical procedures designed to remove root cause of disease
salpingectomy (sal-pin-JEK-toh-mee)	salping/o = uterine tube -ectomy = surgical removal	Surgical removal of a uterine tube
simple mastectomy (mas-TEK-toh-mee)	mast/o = breast -ectomy = surgical removal	Surgical removal of only breast tissue; all underlying tissue is left intact
therapeutic abortion		Termination of a pregnancy for health of mother or another medical reason
total abdominal hysterectomy—bilateral salpingo-oophorectomy (TAH-BSO) (hiss-ter-EK-toh-mee / sal-ping-goh / oh-of-or-EK-toh-mee)	abdomin/o = abdomen -al = pertaining to hyster/o = uterus -ectomy = surgical removal bi- = two later/o = side -al = pertaining to salping/o = uterine tube oophor/o = ovary -ectomy = surgical removal	Removal of entire uterus, cervix, both ovaries, and both uterine tubes
tubal ligation (TOO-bal / lye-GAY-shun)	-al = pertaining to	Surgical tying-off of uterine tubes to prevent conception from taking place; results in sterilization of female
vaginal hysterectomy (VAJ-in-al / hiss-ter-EK-toh-mee)	vagin/o = vagina -al = pertaining to hyster/o = uterus -ectomy = surgical removal	Removal of the uterus through the vagina rather than through abdominal incision

PRACTICE AS YOU GO

E. Terminology Matching

Match each term to its definition.

1. ________ Pap smear
2. ________ intrauterine device
3. ________ colposcopy
4. ________ Apgar
5. ________ chorionic villus sampling
6. ________ lumpectomy
7. ________ episiotomy
8. ________ tubal ligation

a. measures newborn's adjustment to outside world
b. widens birth canal; facilitates delivery
c. removes only tumor and tissue around it
d. visually examines vagina
e. test for cervical cancer
f. sterilization procedure
g. birth control method
h. obtains cells for genetic testing

Pharmacology

Classification	Word Parts	Action	Examples
abortifacient (ah-bor-tih-FAY-shent)		Terminates a pregnancy	mifepristone, Mifeprex; dinoprostone, Prostin E2
fertility drug		Triggers ovulation; also called *ovulation stimulant*	clomiphene, Clomid; follitropin alfa, Gonal-F
hormone replacement therapy (HRT)		Replaces hormones missing from menopause or lost ovaries, which can result in lack of estrogen production; replacing this hormone may prevent some consequences of menopause, especially in younger women who have surgically lost their ovaries	conjugated estrogens, Cenestin, Premarin
oral contraceptive pills (OCPs) (kon-trah-SEP-tiv)	or/o = mouth -al = pertaining to contra- = against	Form of birth control that uses low doses of female hormones to prevent conception by blocking ovulation	desogestrel/ethinyl estradiol, Ortho-Cept; ethinyl estradiol/norgestrel, Lo/Ovral
oxytocin (ok-see-TOH-sin)		Natural hormone that begins or improves uterine contractions during labor and delivery	oxytocin, Pitocin, Syntocinon

Abbreviations

AB	abortion	**HPV**	human papillomavirus
AI	artificial insemination	**HRT**	hormone replacement therapy
BSE	breast self-examination	**HSG**	hysterosalpingography
CS, C-section	cesarean section	**IUD**	intrauterine device
CVS	chorionic villus sampling	**IVF**	*in vitro* fertilization
Cx	cervix	**LBW**	low birth weight
D&C	dilation and curettage	**LH**	luteinizing hormone
EDD	estimated date of delivery	**LMP**	last menstrual period
EMB	endometrial biopsy	**NB**	newborn
ERT	estrogen replacement therapy	**OB**	obstetrics
FEKG	fetal electrocardiogram	**OCPs**	oral contraceptive pills
FHR	fetal heart rate	**Pap**	Papanicolaou test
FHT	fetal heart tone	**PI, para I**	first delivery
FSH	follicle-stimulating hormone	**PID**	pelvic inflammatory disease
FTND	full-term normal delivery	**PIH**	pregnancy-induced hypertension
GI, grav I	first pregnancy	**PMS**	premenstrual syndrome
GYN, gyn	gynecology	**TAH-BSO**	total abdominal hysterectomy–bilateral salpingo-oophorectomy
HCG, hCG	human chorionic gonadotropin	**TSS**	toxic shock syndrome
HDN	hemolytic disease of the newborn	**UC**	uterine contractions

PRACTICE AS YOU GO

F. What's the Abbreviation?

1. first pregnancy ____________________
2. artificial insemination ____________________
3. uterine contractions ____________________
4. full-term normal delivery ____________________
5. intrauterine device ____________________
6. dilation and curettage ____________________
7. hormone replacement therapy ____________________
8. gynecology ____________________
9. abortion ____________________
10. oral contraceptive pills ____________________

SECTION II: MALE REPRODUCTIVE SYSTEM

AT A GLANCE

Function

Similar to the female reproductive system, the male reproductive system is responsible for producing sperm, the male reproductive cell, secreting the male sex hormones, and delivering sperm to the female reproductive tract.

Organs

The primary structures that comprise the male reproductive system:

testes
epididymis
penis
vas deferens
seminal vesicles
prostate gland
bulbourethral glands

Word Parts

Presented here are the most common word parts (with their meanings) used to build male reproductive system terms. For a more comprehensive list, refer to the Terminology section of this chapter.

Combining Forms

andr/o	male
balan/o	glans penis
crypt/o	hidden
epididym/o	epididymis
orch/o	testis
orchi/o	testis
orchid/o	testis
pen/o	penis
prostat/o	prostate gland
spermat/o	sperm
testicul/o	testes
vas/o	vas deferens
vesicul/o	seminal vesicle

Suffixes

-cide	to kill
-plasia	formation of cells
-spermia	condition of sperm

Male Reproductive System Illustrated

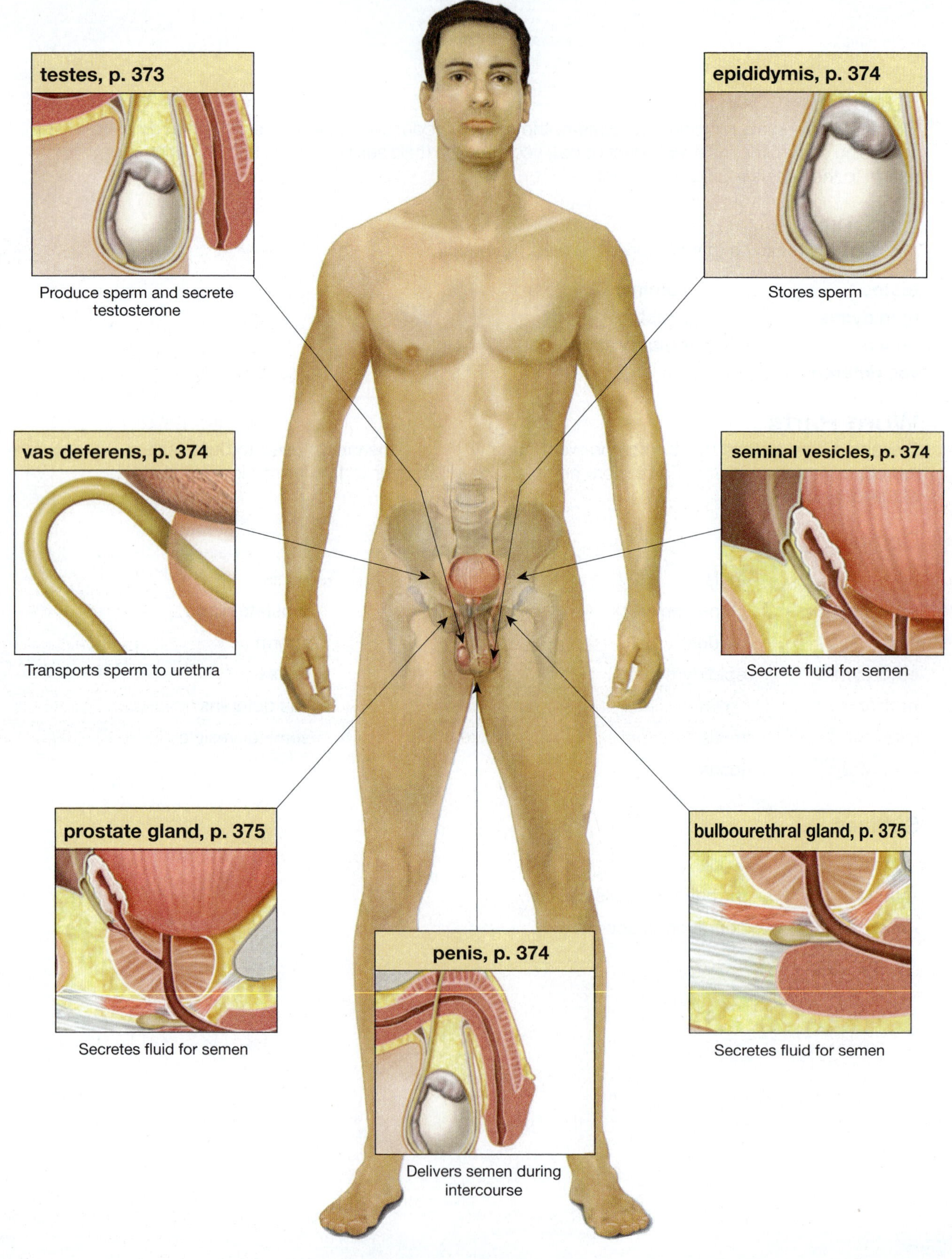

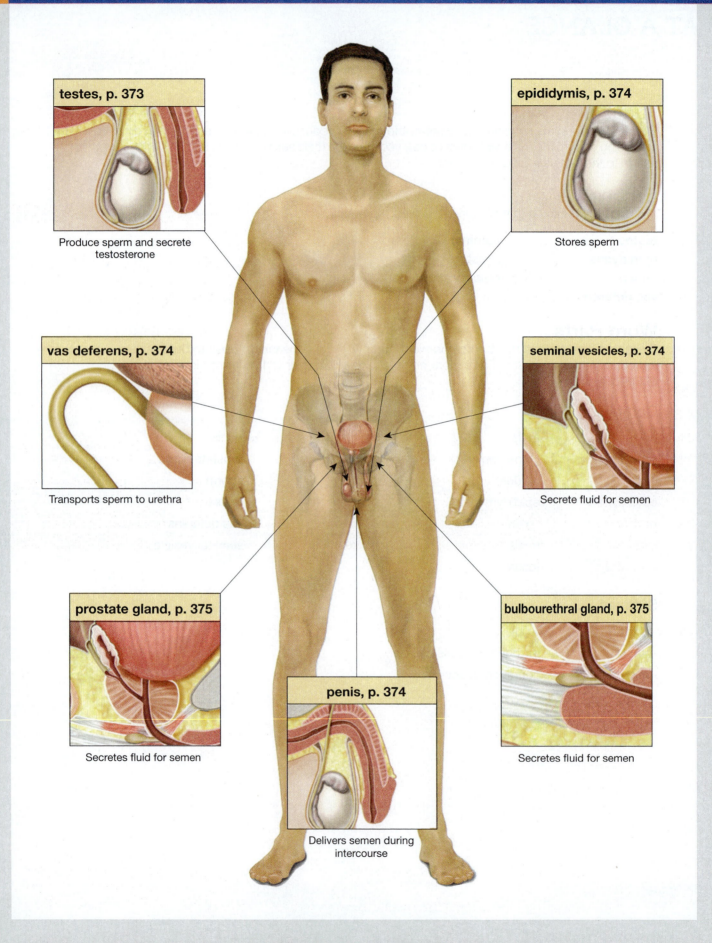

Anatomy and Physiology of the Male Reproductive System

bulbourethral glands (buhl-boh-yoo-REE-thral)
epididymis (ep-ih-DID-ih-mis)
genitourinary system (jen-ih-toh-YOO-rih-nair-ee)
penis (PEE-nis)
prostate gland (PROSS-tayt)
semen (SEE-men)
seminal vesicles (SEM-ih-nal / VES-ih-kls)
sex hormones
sperm
testes (TESS-teez)
vas deferens (VAS / DEF-er-enz)

The male reproductive system has two main functions. The first is to produce **sperm**, the male reproductive cell; the second is to secrete the male **sex hormones**. In the male, the major organs of reproduction are located outside the body: the **penis** and the two **testes**, each with an **epididymis** (see Figure 10-20 ■). The penis contains the urethra, which carries both urine and **semen** to the outside of the body. For this reason, this system is sometimes referred to as the **genitourinary (GU) system**.

The internal organs of reproduction include two **seminal vesicles**, two **vas deferens**, the **prostate gland**, and two **bulbourethral glands**.

> **What's In A Name?**
> Look for these word parts:
> **genit/o** = genitals
> **urethr/o** = urethra
> **urin/o** = urine
> **-al** = pertaining to
> **-ary** = pertaining to

External Organs of Reproduction

Testes

androgen (AN-droh-jen)
perineum
scrotum (SKROH-tum)
seminiferous tubules (sem-ih-NIF-er-us / TOO-byools)
spermatogenesis (sper-mat-oh-JEN-eh-sis)
testicles (TESS-tih-kls)
testosterone (tess-TAHS-ter-ohn)

> **What's In A Name?**
> Look for these word parts:
> **andr/o** = male
> **spermat/o** = sperm
> **-gen** = that which produces
> **-genesis** = produces
> **-ous** = pertaining to

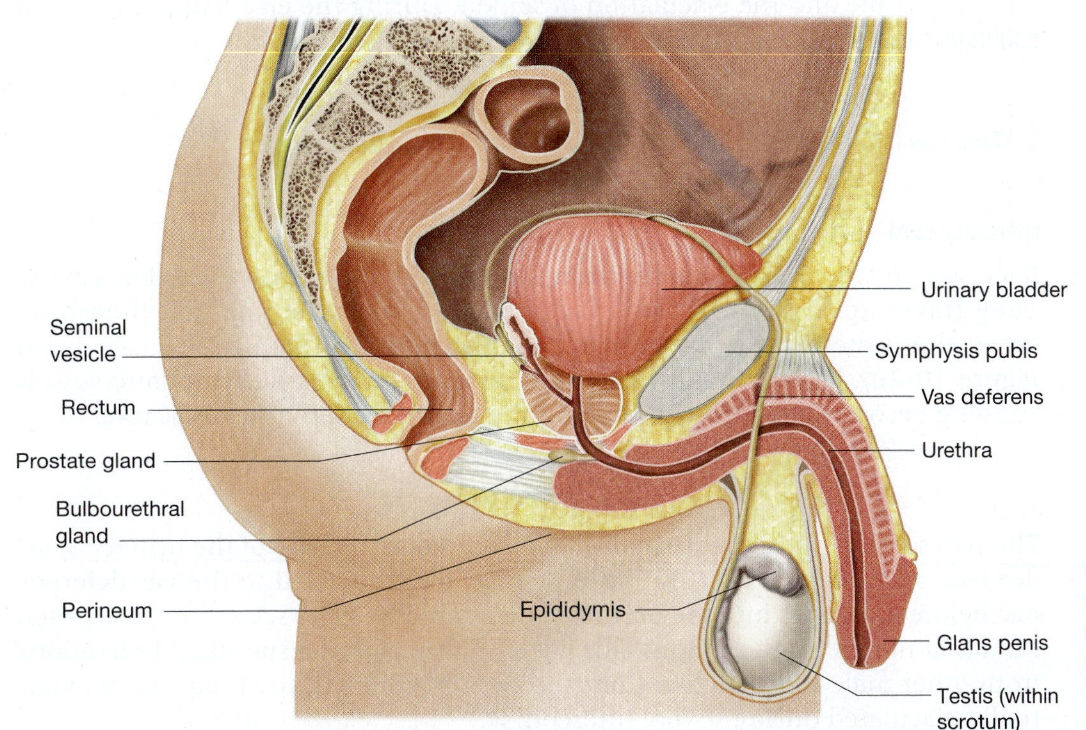

■ **Figure 10-20** The male reproductive system, sagittal section showing the organs of the system and their relation to the urinary bladder and rectum.

Med Term Tip

Spermatozoon and its plural form, *spermatozoa*, are other terms that mean *sperm*. You have no doubt realized that there can be several terms with the same meaning in medical terminology. You must continue to remain flexible when working with these terms in your career. In some cases, one term will be more commonly used, depending on the type of medical specialty or even in what part of the country you are located.

The testes (singular is *testis*) or **testicles** are oval in shape and are responsible for the production of sperm (see again Figure 10-20). This process, called **spermatogenesis**, takes place within the **seminiferous tubules** that make up the insides of the testes (see Figure 10-21 ■). The testes must be maintained at the proper temperature for the sperm to survive. This lower temperature level is achieved by the placement of the testes suspended in the **scrotum**, a sac outside the body. The **perineum** of the male is similar to that in the female and is the area between the scrotum and the anus. The chief **androgen** (male sex hormone) is **testosterone**, which is responsible for the development of the male reproductive organs, sperm, and secondary sex characteristics, and is also produced by the testes.

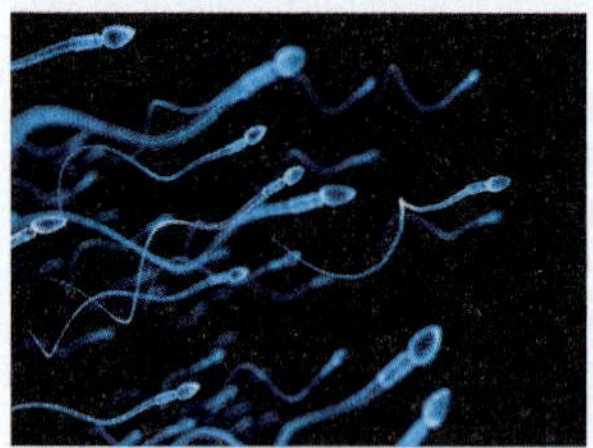

■ **Figure 10-21** Illustration of human sperm structure. *(Sebastian Kaulitzki/Shutterstock)*

Epididymis

Each epididymis is a coiled tubule that lies on top of the testes within the scrotum (see again Figure 10-20). This elongated structure serves as the location for sperm maturation and storage until they are ready to be released into the vas deferens.

Penis

circumcision (ser-kum-SIH-zhun)
ejaculation (ee-jak-yoo-LAY-shun)
erectile tissue (ee-REK-tile)
glans penis (GLANS / PEE-nis)
prepuce (PREE-pyoos)
sphincter (SFINGK-ter)
urinary meatus (YOO-rih-nair-ee / mee-AY-tus)

What's In A Name?

Look for these word parts:
urin/o = urine
-ary = pertaining to
-ile = pertaining to
circum- = around

The penis is the male sex organ containing **erectile tissue** that is encased in skin (see again Figure 10-20). This organ delivers semen into the female vagina. The soft tip of the penis is referred to as the **glans penis**. It is protected by a covering called the **prepuce** or foreskin. It is this covering of skin that is removed during the procedure known as **circumcision**. The penis becomes erect during sexual stimulation, which allows it to be placed within the female for the **ejaculation** of semen. The male urethra extends from the urinary bladder to the external opening in the penis, the **urinary meatus**, and serves a dual function: the elimination of urine and the ejaculation of semen. During the ejaculation process, a **sphincter** closes to keep urine from escaping.

Med Term Tip

During sexual intercourse, which is also referred to as *coitus*, the male can eject up to 100 million sperm cells. The adult male produces nearly 200 million sperm daily.

Internal Organs of Reproduction

Vas Deferens

spermatic cord (sper-MAT-ik)

Each vas deferens carries sperm from the epididymis up into the pelvic cavity. They travel up in front of the urinary bladder, over the top, and then back down the posterior side of the bladder to empty into the urethra (see again Figure 10-20). They, along with nerves, arteries, veins, and lymphatic vessels running between the pelvic cavity and the testes, form the **spermatic cord**.

Seminal Vesicles

The two seminal vesicles are small glands located at the base of the urinary bladder (see again Figure 10-20). These vesicles are connected to the vas deferens just before it empties into the urethra. The seminal vesicles secrete a glucose-rich fluid that nourishes the sperm. This liquid, along with the sperm and secretions from other male reproductive glands, constitutes semen, the fluid that is eventually ejaculated during sexual intercourse.

Prostate Gland

The single prostate gland is located just below the urinary bladder (see again Figure 10-20). It surrounds the urethra and when enlarged can cause difficulty in urination. The prostate is important for the reproductive process as it secretes an alkaline fluid that assists in keeping the sperm alive by neutralizing the pH of the urethra and female vagina.

Bulbourethral Glands

Cowper's glands (KOW-perz)

The bulbourethral glands, also known as **Cowper's glands**, are two small glands located on either side of the urethra just below the prostate (see again Figure 10-20). They produce a mucuslike lubricating fluid that joins with semen to become a part of the ejaculate.

PRACTICE AS YOU GO

G. Complete the Statement

1. The male reproductive system is a combination of the ____________________ and ____________________ systems.
2. The male's external organs of reproduction consist of the ____________________, ____________________, and ____________________.
3. Another term for the prepuce is the ____________________.
4. The organs responsible for developing the sperm cells are the ____________________.
5. The glands of lubrication and fluid production at each side of the male urethra are the ____________________.
6. The male sex hormone is ____________________.
7. The area between the scrotum and the anus is called the ____________________.

Terminology

Word Parts Used to Build Male Reproductive System Terms

The following lists contain the combining forms, suffixes, and prefixes used to build terms in the remaining sections of this chapter.

Combining Forms

andr/o	male	genit/o	genital	orchi/o	testis
balan/o	glans penis	hydr/o	water	orchid/o	testis
carcin/o	cancer	immun/o	protection	pen/o	penis
crypt/o	hidden	olig/o	scanty	prostat/o	prostate gland
epididym/o	epididymis	orch/o	testis	rect/o	rectum

Combining Forms (continued)

spermat/o	sperm	**urethr/o**	urethra	**vas/o**	vas deferens
testicul/o	testes	**varic/o**	dilated vein	**vesicul/o**	seminal vesicle
ur/o	urine				

Suffixes

-al	pertaining to	**-ile**	pertaining to	**-ostomy**	surgically create an opening
-ar	pertaining to	**-ism**	state of	**-otomy**	cutting into
-cele	protrusion	**-itis**	inflammation	**-pexy**	surgical fixation
-cide	to kill	**-logy**	study of	**-plasia**	formation of cells
-ectomy	surgical removal	**-lysis**	to destroy	**-plasty**	surgical repair
-gen	that which produces	**-oid**	resembling	**-rrhea**	discharge
-iasis	abnormal condition	**-oma**	tumor	**-spermia**	sperm condition
-ic	pertaining to	**-osis**	abnormal condition		

Prefixes

a-	without	**dys-**	abnormal	**hypo-**	below
an-	without	**epi-**	above	**trans-**	across
anti-	against	**hyper-**	excessive		

Adjective Forms of Anatomical Terms

Term	Word Parts	Definition
balanic (buh-LAN-ik)	**balan/o** = glans penis **-ic** = pertaining to	Pertaining to the glans penis
epididymal (ep-ih-DID-ih-mal)	**epididym/o** = epididymis **-al** = pertaining to	Pertaining to the epididymis
penile (PEE-nile)	**pen/o** = penis **-ile** = pertaining to	Pertaining to the penis
prostatic (pross-TAT-ik)	**prostat/o** = prostate gland **-ic** = pertaining to	Pertaining to the prostate gland
spermatic (sper-MAT-ik)	**spermat/o** = sperm **-ic** = pertaining to	Pertaining to sperm
testicular (tess-TIK-yoo-lar)	**testicul/o** = testes **-ar** = pertaining to	Pertaining to the testes
vasal (VAY-sal)	**vas/o** = vas deferens **-al** = pertaining to	Pertaining to the vas deferens
vesicular (veh-SIK-yoo-lar)	**vesicul/o** = seminal vesicle **-ar** = pertaining to	Pertaining to the seminal vesicle

Word Watch

Be careful using the combining forms **vesic/o** meaning *bladder* and **vesicul/o** meaning *seminal vesicle.*

PRACTICE AS YOU GO

H. Give the adjective form for each anatomical structure.

1. A testis ______________________
2. Sperm ______________________
3. A seminal vesicle ______________________
4. The penis ______________________
5. The prostate gland ______________________

Pathology

Term	Word Parts	Definition
Medical Specialties		
urology (yoo-RALL-oh-jee)	ur/o = urine -logy = study of	Branch of medicine involved in diagnosis and treatment of diseases and disorders of urinary system and male reproductive system; physician is a *urologist*
Signs and Symptoms		
aspermia (ah-SPER-mee-ah)	a- = without -spermia = sperm condition	Condition of having no sperm
balanorrhea (bah-lah-noh-REE-ah)	balan/o = glans penis -rrhea = discharge	Discharge from the glans penis
oligospermia (ol-ih-goh-SPER-mee-ah)	olig/o = scanty -spermia = sperm condition	Condition of having too few sperm, making chances of fertilization very low
spermatolysis (sper-mah-TALL-ih-sis)	spermat/o = sperm -lysis = to destroy	Term that refers to anything that destroys sperm
Testes		
anorchism (an-OR-kizm)	an- = without orch/o = testis -ism = state of	Absence of testes; may be congenital or as result of accident or surgery
cryptorchidism (kript-OR-kid-izm)	crypt/o = hidden orchid/o = testis -ism = state of	Failure of the testes to descend into scrotal sac before birth; usually, the testes will descend before birth; surgical procedure called *orchidopexy* may be required to bring the testes down into the scrotum permanently; failure of the testes to descend could result in sterility in male or increased risk of testicular cancer
hydrocele (HIGH-droh-seel)	hydr/o = water -cele = protrusion	Accumulation of fluid around the testes or along the spermatic cord; common in infants
orchitis (or-KIGH-tis)	orch/o = testis -itis = inflammation	Inflammation of one or both testes
sterility		Inability to father children due to problem with spermatogenesis
testicular carcinoma (kar-sih-NOH-mah)	testicul/o = testes -ar = pertaining to carcin/o = cancer -oma = tumor	Cancer of one or both testicles; most common cancer in men under age 40
testicular torsion	testicul/o = testes -ar = pertaining to	Twisting of the spermatic cord

Pathology (continued)

Term	Word Parts	Definition
varicocele (VAIR-ih-koh-seel)	**varic/o** = dilated vein **-cele** = protrusion	Enlargement of veins of the spermatic cord that commonly occurs on left side of adolescent males
Epididymis		
epididymitis (ep-ih-did-ih-MY-tis)	**epididym/o** = epididymis **-itis** = inflammation	Inflammation of the epididymis
Prostate Gland		
benign prostatic hyperplasia (BPH) (bee-NINE / pross-TAT-ik / high-per-PLAY-zha)	**prostat/o** = prostate gland **-ic** = pertaining to **hyper-** = excessive **-plasia** = formation of cells	Noncancerous enlargement of the prostate gland commonly seen in males over age 50; formerly called *benign prostatic hypertrophy*
prostate cancer (PROSS-tayt)		Slow-growing cancer that affects a large number of males after age 50; prostate-specific antigen (PSA) test is used to assist in early detection of disease
prostatitis (pross-tah-TYE-tis)	**prostat/o** = prostate gland **-itis** = inflammation	Inflammation of the prostate gland
Penis		
balanitis (bal-ah-NYE-tis)	**balan/o** = glans penis **-itis** = inflammation	Inflammation of the glans penis
epispadias (ep-ih-SPAY-dee-as)	**epi-** = above	Congenital opening of the urethra on dorsal surface of the penis
erectile dysfunction (ED) (ee-REK-tile)	**-ile** = pertaining to **dys-** = abnormal, difficult	Inability to engage in sexual intercourse due to inability to maintain erection; also called *impotence*
hypospadias (high-poh-SPAY-dee-as)	**hypo-** = below	Congenital opening of male urethra on underside of the penis
phimosis (fye-MOH-sis)	**-osis** = abnormal condition	Narrowing of foreskin over the glans penis resulting in difficulty with hygiene; condition can lead to infection or difficulty with urination; treated with circumcision, surgical removal of the foreskin
priapism (PRYE-ah-pizm)	**-ism** = state of	Persistent and painful erection due to pathological causes, not sexual arousal
Sexually Transmitted Diseases		
chancroid (SHANG-kroyd)	**-oid** = resembling	Highly infectious nonsyphilitic venereal ulcer

■ **Figure 10-22** Photograph showing a chancroid on the glans penis. *(Joe Miller/Centers for Disease Control and Prevention)*

Pathology (continued)

Term	Word Parts	Definition
chlamydia (klah-MID-ee-ah)		Bacterial infection causing genital inflammation in males and females; can lead to pelvic inflammatory disease in females and eventual infertility
genital herpes (JEN-ih-tal / HER-peez)	genit/o = genital -al = pertaining to	Spreading skin disease that can appear like a blister or vesicle on genital region of males and females; may spread to other areas of body; caused by sexually transmitted virus
genital warts (JEN-ih-tal)	genit/o = genital -al = pertaining to	Growth of warts on genitalia of both males and females that can lead to cancer of the cervix in females; caused by sexual transmission of human papillomavirus (HPV)
gonorrhea (GC) (gon-oh-REE-ah)	-rrhea = discharge	Sexually transmitted bacterial infection of mucous membranes of either sex; can be passed on to infant during birth process
human immunodeficiency virus (HIV)	immun/o = protection	Sexually transmitted virus that attacks immune system
sexually transmitted disease		Disease usually acquired as result of sexual intercourse; also called *sexually transmitted infection* (STI); formerly referred to as *venereal disease* (VD)
syphilis (SIF-ih-lis)		Infectious, chronic, bacterial sexually transmitted infection that can involve any organ; may exist for years without symptoms, but is fatal if untreated; treated with antibiotic penicillin
trichomoniasis (trik-oh-moh-NYE-ah-sis)	-iasis = abnormal condition	Genitourinary infection caused by single-cell protozoan parasite that is usually without symptoms (asymptomatic) in both males and females; in women disease can produce itching and/or burning, foul-smelling discharge, and result in vaginitis

PRACTICE AS YOU GO

I. Terminology Matching

Match each term to its definition.

1. ________ aspermia	**a.** inflammation of glans penis
2. ________ phimosis	**b.** having no sperm
3. ________ balanitis	**c.** venereal ulcer
4. ________ chancroid	**d.** having too few sperm
5. ________ varicocele	**e.** narrowing of foreskin
6. ________ oligospermia	**f.** enlarged spermatic cord veins

Diagnostic Procedures

Term	Word Parts	Definition
Clinical Laboratory Tests		
prostate-specific antigen (PSA) (PROSS-tayt-specific / AN-tih-jen)	**anti-** = against **-gen** = that which produces	Blood test to screen for prostate cancer; elevated blood levels of PSA are associated with prostate cancer
semen analysis (SEE-men / ah-NAL-ih-sis)		Procedure used when performing fertility workup to determine if male is able to produce sperm; semen is collected by patient after abstaining from sexual intercourse for a period of three to five days; sperm in semen are analyzed for number, swimming strength, and shape; also used to determine if vasectomy has been successful; after a period of six weeks, no further sperm should be present in a sample from patient
Additional Diagnostic Procedures		
digital rectal exam (DRE) (DIJ-ih-tal / REK-tal)	**rect/o** = rectum **-al** = pertaining to	Manual examination for an enlarged prostate gland performed by palpating (feeling) the prostate gland through wall of the rectum

Therapeutic Procedures

Term	Word Parts	Definition
Surgical Procedures		
balanoplasty (BAL-ah-noh-plas-tee)	**balan/o** = glans penis **-plasty** = surgical repair	Surgical repair of the glans penis
castration (kass-TRAY-shun)		Removal of the testicles in male or the ovaries in female
circumcision (ser-kum-SIH-zhun)		Surgical removal of the prepuce, or foreskin, of the penis; generally performed on newborn male at request of parents; primary reason is for ease of hygiene; circumcision is also a ritual practice in some religions
epididymectomy (ep-ih-did-ih-MEK-toh-mee)	**epididym/o** = epididymis **-ectomy** = surgical removal	Surgical removal of the epididymis
orchidectomy (or-kih-DEK-toh-mee)	**orchid/o** = testis **-ectomy** = surgical removal	Surgical removal of one or both testes
orchidopexy (OR-kid-oh-pek-see)	**orchid/o** = testis **-pexy** = surgical fixation	Surgical fixation to move undescended testes into the scrotum and to attach them to prevent retraction; used to treat cryptorchidism
orchiectomy (or-kee-EK-toh-mee)	**orchi/o** = testis **-ectomy** = surgical removal	Surgical removal of one or both testes
orchiotomy (or-kee-OT-oh-mee)	**orchi/o** = testis **-otomy** = cutting into	To cut into the testes
orchioplasty (OR-kee-oh-plas-tee)	**orchi/o** = testis **-plasty** = surgical repair	Surgical repair of the testes
prostatectomy (pross-tah-TEK-toh-mee)	**prostat/o** = prostate gland **-ectomy** = surgical removal	Surgical removal of the prostate gland
sterilization (stair-ih-lih-ZAY-shun)		Process of rendering a male or female sterile or unable to conceive children
transurethral resection of the prostate (TUR, TURP) (trans-yoo-REE-thral / ree-SEK-shun / PROSS-tayt)	**trans-** = across **urethr/o** = urethra **-al** = pertaining to	Surgical removal of part of the prostate gland that is blocking urine flow by inserting a device through the urethra and removing prostate tissue

Therapeutic Procedures (continued)

Term	Word Parts	Definition
vasectomy (vah-SEK-toh-mee)	**vas/o** = vas deferens **-ectomy** = surgical removal	Removal of a segment or all of the vas deferens to prevent sperm from leaving male body; used for contraception purposes

Med Term Tip

The vas deferens is the tubing that is severed during a procedure called a *vasectomy.* A vasectomy results in the sterilization of the male since the sperm are no longer able to travel into the urethra and out of the penis during sexual intercourse. The surgical procedure to reverse a vasectomy is a *vasovasostomy.* A new opening is created in order to reconnect one section of the vas deferens to another section of the vas deferens, thereby reestablishing an open tube for sperm to travel through.

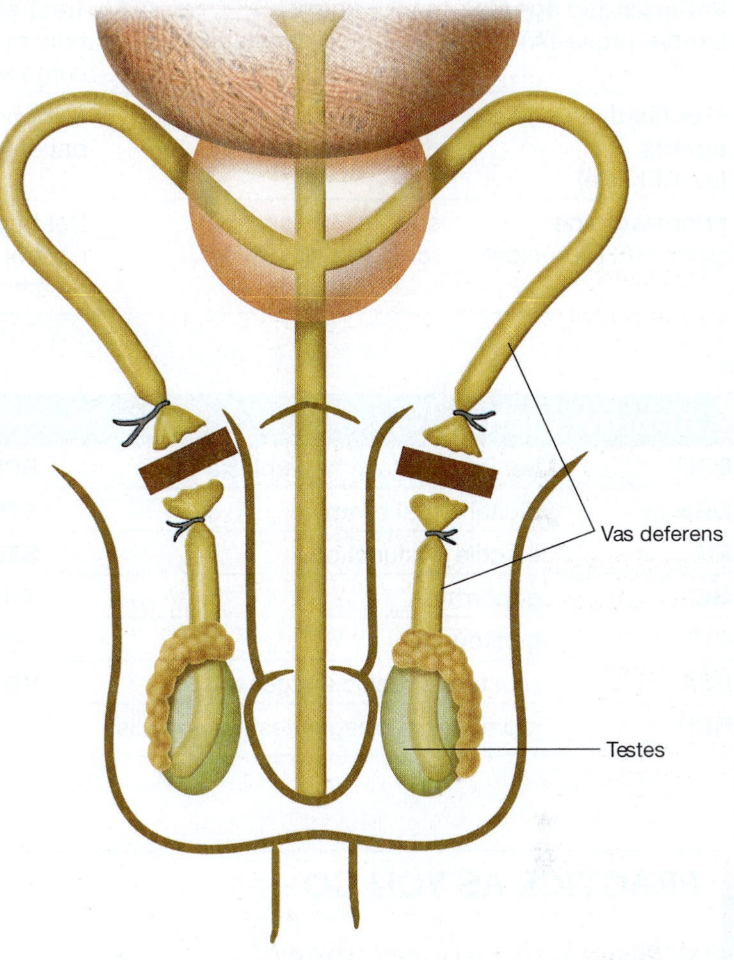

■ **Figure 10-23** A vasectomy, showing how each vas deferens is tied off in two places and then a section is removed from the middle. This prevents sperm from traveling through the vas deferens during ejaculation.

Term	Word Parts	Definition
vasovasostomy (vay-soh-vah-SOS-tah-mee)	**vas/o** = vas deferens **-ostomy** = surgically create an opening	Surgical procedure to reconnect the vas deferens to reverse a vasectomy

PRACTICE AS YOU GO

J. Procedure Matching

Match each procedure to its definition.

1. ________ digital rectal exam — **a.** removes prepuce

2. ________ circumcision — **b.** surgical fixation of testis

3. ________ vasectomy — **c.** examination for enlarged prostate

4. ________ orchidopexy — **d.** sterilization procedure

5. ________ semen analysis — **e.** part of a fertility workup

Pharmacology

Classification	Word Parts	Action	Examples
androgen therapy (AN-droh-jen)	andr/o = male -gen = that which produces	Replaces male hormones to treat patients who produce insufficient hormone naturally	testosterone cypionate, Andronate, depAndro
antiprostatic agents (an-tye-pross-TAT-ik)	anti- = against prostat/o = prostate gland -ic = pertaining to	Treat early cases of benign prostatic hyperplasia; may prevent surgery for mild cases	finasteride, Proscar; dutasteride, Avodart
erectile dysfunction agents (ee-REK-tile)	-ile = pertaining to dys- = abnormal	Temporarily produce erection in patients with erectile dysfunction	sildenafil citrate, Viagra; tadalafil, Cialis
spermatocide (sper-MAH-toh-side)	spermat/o = sperm -cide = to kill	Destroys sperm; one form of birth control is use of spermatolytic creams	octoxynol 9, Semicid, Ortho-Gynol

Abbreviations

BPH	benign prostatic hyperplasia	**SPP**	suprapubic prostatectomy
DRE	digital rectal exam	**STD**	sexually transmitted disease
ED	erectile dysfunction	**STI**	sexually transmitted infection
GC	gonorrhea	**TUR**	transurethral resection
GU	genitourinary	**TURP**	transurethral resection of the prostate
PSA	prostate-specific antigen	**VD**	venereal disease
RPR	rapid plasma reagin (test for syphilis)		

PRACTICE AS YOU GO

K. What's the Abbreviation?

1. erectile dysfunction ______________________
2. gonorrhea ______________________
3. digital rectal exam ______________________
4. transurethral resection of the prostate ______________________
5. sexually transmitted infection ______________________

Chapter Review

Real-World Applications

Medical Record Analysis

This High-Risk Obstetrics Consultation Report contains 12 medical terms. Underline each term and write it in the list below the report. Then explain each term as you would to a nonmedical person.

High-Risk Obstetrics Consultation Report

Reason for Consultation:	High-risk pregnancy with late-term bleeding
History of Present Illness:	Patient is 23 years old. She is currently estimated to be at 175 days' gestation. Amniocentesis at 20 weeks shows a normally developing male fetus. She noticed a moderate degree of bleeding this morning but denies any cramping or pelvic pain. She immediately saw her obstetrician who referred her for high-risk evaluation.
Past Medical History:	This patient is multigravida but nullipara with three early miscarriages without obvious cause.
Results of Physical Examination:	Patient appears well nourished and abdominal girth appears consistent with length of gestation. Pelvic ultrasound indicates placenta previa with placenta almost completely overlying cervix. However, there is no evidence of abruptio placentae at this time. Fetal size estimate is consistent with 25 weeks' gestation. The fetal heartbeat is strong with a rate of 130 beats/minute.
Recommendations:	Fetus appears to be developing well and in no distress at this time. The placenta appears to be well attached on ultrasound, but the bleeding is cause for concern. With the extremely low position of the placenta, this patient is at very high risk for abruptio placentae. She will require C-section at onset of labor.

	Term	Explanation
1.	______________	______________________________
2.	______________	______________________________
3.	______________	______________________________
4.	______________	______________________________
5.	______________	______________________________
6.	______________	______________________________
7.	______________	______________________________
8.	______________	______________________________
9.	______________	______________________________
10.	______________	______________________________
11.	______________	______________________________
12.	______________	______________________________

Chart Note Transcription

The chart note below contains 10 phrases that can be reworded with a medical term presented in this chapter. Each phrase is identified with an underline. Determine the medical term and write your answers in the space provided.

Pearson General Hospital Consultation Report

Task Edit View Time Scale Options Help Download Archive Date: 17 May 2017

Current Complaint:	Patient is a 77-year-old male seen by the urologist with complaints of nocturia and difficulty with the release of semen from the urethra. **1**
Past History:	Medical history revealed that the patient had failure of the testes to descend into the scrotum **2** at birth, which was repaired by surgical fixation of the testes. **3** He had also undergone elective sterilization by removal of a segment of the vas deferens **4** at the age of 41.
Signs and Symptoms:	Patient states he first noted these symptoms about five years ago. They have become increasingly severe and now he is not able to sleep without waking to urinate up to 20 times a night. He has difficulty with release of semen. **5** Palpation of the prostate gland through the rectum **6** revealed multiple round, firm nodules in prostate gland. A needle biopsy was negative for slow-growing cancer that frequently affects males over age 50 **7** and a blood test for prostate cancer **8** was normal.
Diagnosis:	Noncancerous enlargement of the prostate gland **9**
Treatment:	Patient was scheduled for a surgical removal of prostate tissue through the urethra. **10**

1. ______________________

2. ______________________

3. ______________________

4. ______________________

5. ______________________

6. ______________________

7. ______________________

8. ______________________

9. ______________________

10. ______________________

Case Study

Below is a case study presentation of a patient with a condition discussed in this chapter. Read the case study and answer the questions below. Some questions will ask for information not included within this chapter. Use your text, a medical dictionary, or any other reference material you choose to answer these questions.

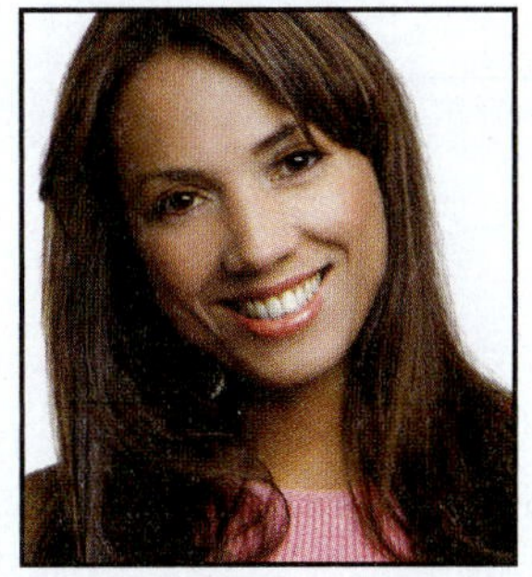

(Jason Stitt/Shutterstock)

A 22-year-old female has come into the gynecologist's office complaining of fever, malaise, dysuria, and vaginal leukorrhea. Upon examination the physician observes fluid-filled vesicles on her cervix, vulva, and perineum. Several have ruptured into ulcers with marked erythema and edema. Palpation revealed painful and enlarged inguinal lymph nodes. She also has an extragenital lesion on her mouth.

Her diagnosis is genital herpes.

Questions

1. What pathological condition does this patient have? Look this condition up in a reference source and include a short description of it.

____

____

2. List and define each of the patient's presenting symptoms in your own words.

____

____

3. Describe the results of the physician's examination in your own words.

____

____

4. Explain what *extragenital lesion* means.

____

____

5. Explain what *palpation* means.

____

____

6. What is the potential effect of having this virus present in open genital lesions on the patient's future pregnancy and childbirth?

____

____

Practice Exercises

A. Using Abbreviations

Fill in each blank with the appropriate abbreviation.

1. A(n) ________ specializes in treating conditions of the female reproductive system and a(n) ________ specializes in treating pregnant women.
2. ________ always develops symptoms just prior to the menstrual period.
3. ________ is also called erythroblastosis fetalis.
4. A(n) ________ can be performed at an earlier stage of the pregnancy than an amniocentesis.
5. When she stopped taking ________, Natasha had a(n) ________ inserted into her uterus for contraception.
6. Some cases of cervical cancer are caused by a(n) ________ infection.
7. ________ were formerly referred to as VD.
8. The ________ is an important screening tool for prostate cancer.
9. A(n) ________ is performed when the prostate gland is blocking urine flow from the bladder.
10. ________ is associated with prolonged wearing of a super-absorbent tampon.

B. Define the Term

1. spermatogenesis ________________________________
2. hydrocele ________________________________
3. transurethral resection of the prostate (TURP) ________________________________
4. sterility ________________________________
5. orchiectomy ________________________________
6. vasectomy ________________________________
7. castration ________________________________
8. gestation ________________________________
9. meconium ________________________________
10. nulligravida ________________________________
11. dystocia ________________________________
12. metrorrhea ________________________________
13. fibroid tumor ________________________________
14. fibrocystic disease ________________________________
15. placenta previa ________________________________

C. Word Building Practice

The combining form **colp/o** refers to the *vagina*. Use it to write a term that means:

1. visual examination of the vagina ________________________________
2. instrument used to examine the vagina ________________________________

The combining form **cervic/o** refers to the *cervix*. Use it to write a term that means:

3. removal of the cervix ________________________________

4. inflammation of the cervix ____________________

The combining form **hyster/o** also refers to the *uterus*. Use it to write a term that means:

5. surgical fixation of the uterus ____________________
6. removal of the uterus ____________________
7. rupture of the uterus ____________________

The combining form **oophor/o** refers to the *ovaries*. Use it to write a term that means:

8. inflammation of an ovary ____________________
9. removal of an ovary ____________________

The combining form **mamm/o** refers to the *breasts*. Use it to write a term that means:

10. record of breast ____________________
11. surgical repair of breast ____________________

The combining form **amni/o** refers to the *amnion*. Use it to write a term that means:

12. cutting into amnion ____________________
13. flow from amnion ____________________

The combining form **prostat/o** refers to the *prostate*. Use this to write a term that means:

14. removal of prostate ____________________
15. inflammation of the prostate ____________________

The combining form **orchi/o** refers to the *testis*. Use this to write a term that means:

16. removal of the testes ____________________
17. surgical repair of the testes ____________________
18. incision into the testes ____________________

The suffix **-spermia** refers to a *sperm condition*. Use this to write a term that means:

19. condition of being without sperm ____________________
20. condition of having too few (scanty) sperm ____________________

The combining form **spermat/o** refers to *sperm*. Use this to write a term that means:

21. sperm forming ____________________
22. to destroy sperm ____________________

D. Complete the Term

For each definition given below, fill in the blank with the word part that completes the term.

Definition	Term
1. surgical repair of glans penis	____________plasty
2. excessive formation of cells	hyper____________
3. state of hidden testes	____________ism
4. dilated vein protrusion	____________cele
5. scanty sperm condition	oligo____________

Definition	Term
6. surgical removal of ovary	________ectomy
7. instrument for viewing vagina	________scope
8. tubal pregnancy	________cyesis
9. milk flow	________rrhea
10. abnormal condition within the uterus	endo________osis
11. pus in the uterine tube	pyo________
12. study of new birth	neo________logy
13. menstruation abnormal flow condition	________rrhagia
14. first pregnancy	primi________
15. uterus rupture	________rrhexis

E. Fill in the Blank

premenstrual syndrome	**stillbirth**	**conization**	**laparoscopy**
D&C	**puberty**	**endometriosis**	**eclampsia**
fibroid tumor	**cesarean section**		

1. Kesha had a core of tissue from her cervix removed for testing. This is called ________.
2. Joan delivered a baby that had died while still in the uterus. She had a(n) ________.
3. Ashley has just started her first menstrual cycle. She is said to have entered ________.
4. Kimberly is experiencing tender breasts, headaches, and some irritability just prior to her monthly menstrual cycle. This may be ________.
5. Ana has been scheduled for an examination in which her physician will use an instrument to observe her abdominal cavity to rule out the diagnosis of severe endometriosis. The physician will insert the instrument through a small incision. This procedure is called a(n) ________.
6. Lenora is scheduled to have a hysterectomy as a result of a long history of large benign growths in her uterus that have caused pain and bleeding. Lenora has a(n) ________.
7. Tiffany's physician has recommended that she have a uterine scraping to stop excessive bleeding after a miscarriage. She will be scheduled for a(n) ________.
8. Stacey is having frequent prenatal checkups to prevent the serious condition of pregnancy called ________.
9. Marion has experienced painful menstrual periods as a result of the lining of her uterus being displaced into her pelvic cavity. This is called ________.
10. Because her cervix was not dilating, Shataundra was informed that she will probably require a(n) ________ for her baby's delivery.

F. Terminology Matching

Match each term to its definition.

1. ______ gonorrhea	a. also called STD
2. ______ genital herpes	b. may lead to pelvic inflammatory disease in females
3. ______ human immunodeficiency virus	c. treated with penicillin

4. ________ syphilis		d.	caused by human papillomavirus
5. ________ venereal disease		e.	can pass to infant during birth
6. ________ genital warts		f.	caused by protozoan parasite
7. ________ chancroid		g.	venereal ulcer
8. ________ chlamydia		h.	attacks the immune system
9. ________ trichomoniasis		i.	skin disease with vesicles

G. Pharmacology Challenge

Fill in the classification for each drug description, then match the brand name.

Drug Description	Classification	Brand Name
1. ________ replacement male hormone	________________	a. Pitocin
2. ________ improves uterine contractions	________________	b. Avodart
3. ________ treats early BPH	________________	c. Clomid
4. ________ blocks ovulation	________________	d. Semicid
5. ________ kills sperm	________________	e. Mifeprex
6. ________ produces an erection	________________	f. Andronate
7. ________ replaces estrogen	________________	g. Ortho-Cept
8. ________ terminates a pregnancy	________________	h. Viagra
9. ________ triggers ovulation	________________	i. Premarin

H. Anatomical Adjectives

Fill in the blank with the missing noun or adjective.

Noun	Adjective
1. amnion	________________
2. cervix	________________
3. embryo	________________
4. ________________	endometrial
5. breast	________________
6. ________________	ovarian
7. ________________	uterine
8. ________________	fetal
9. seminal vesicle	________________
10. ________________	spermatic
11. testes	________________
12. ________________	balanic
13. epididymis	________________
14. ________________	prostatic
15. penis	________________

I. Spelling Practice

Some of the following terms are misspelled. Identify the incorrect terms and spell them correctly in the blank provided.

1. spermatolysis ______________________
2. epispadius ______________________
3. chlamydia ______________________
4. circumsicion ______________________
5. salpingectomy ______________________
6. cesarean ______________________
7. mamogram ______________________
8. preclampsia ______________________
9. menometrorrhagia ______________________
10. premenstral ______________________

J. Complete the Statement

1. The two anterior pituitary hormones that target the ovaries are ______________ and ______________.

   The two ovarian hormones that target the uterus are ______________ and ______________.
2. During ______________, an ovum is released from an ovary.
3. Fertilization typically occurs in the ______________.
4. The process that produces milk is called ______________.
5. The major organs are formed during the ______________ period of gestation.
6. The infant is delivered during the ______________ stage of labor and delivery.
7. ______________ takes place in the seminiferous tubules.
8. The ______________ is located at the base of the urinary bladder.

Labeling Exercises

Image A

Write the labels for this figure on the numbered lines provided.

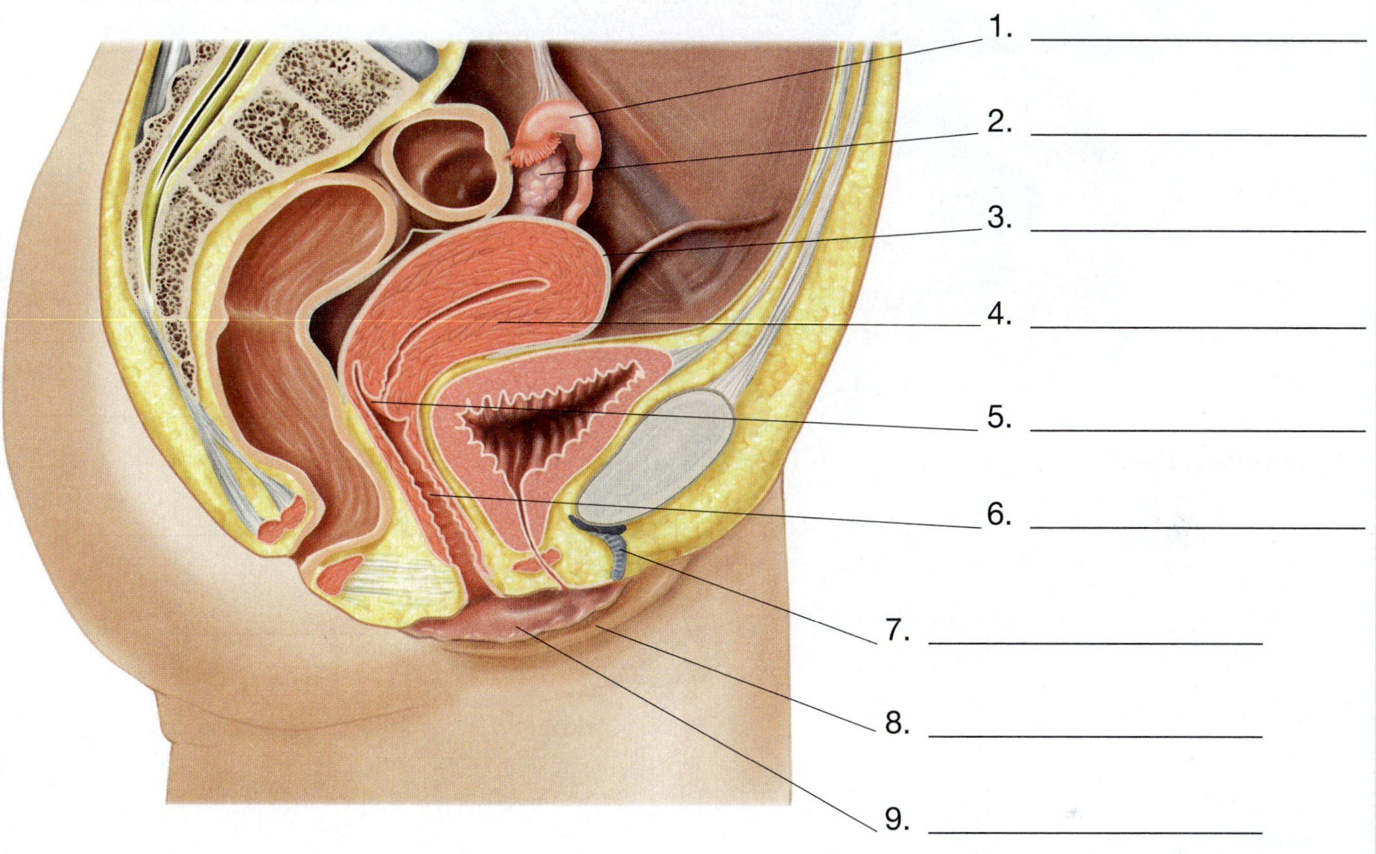

Image B

Write the labels for this figure on the numbered lines provided.

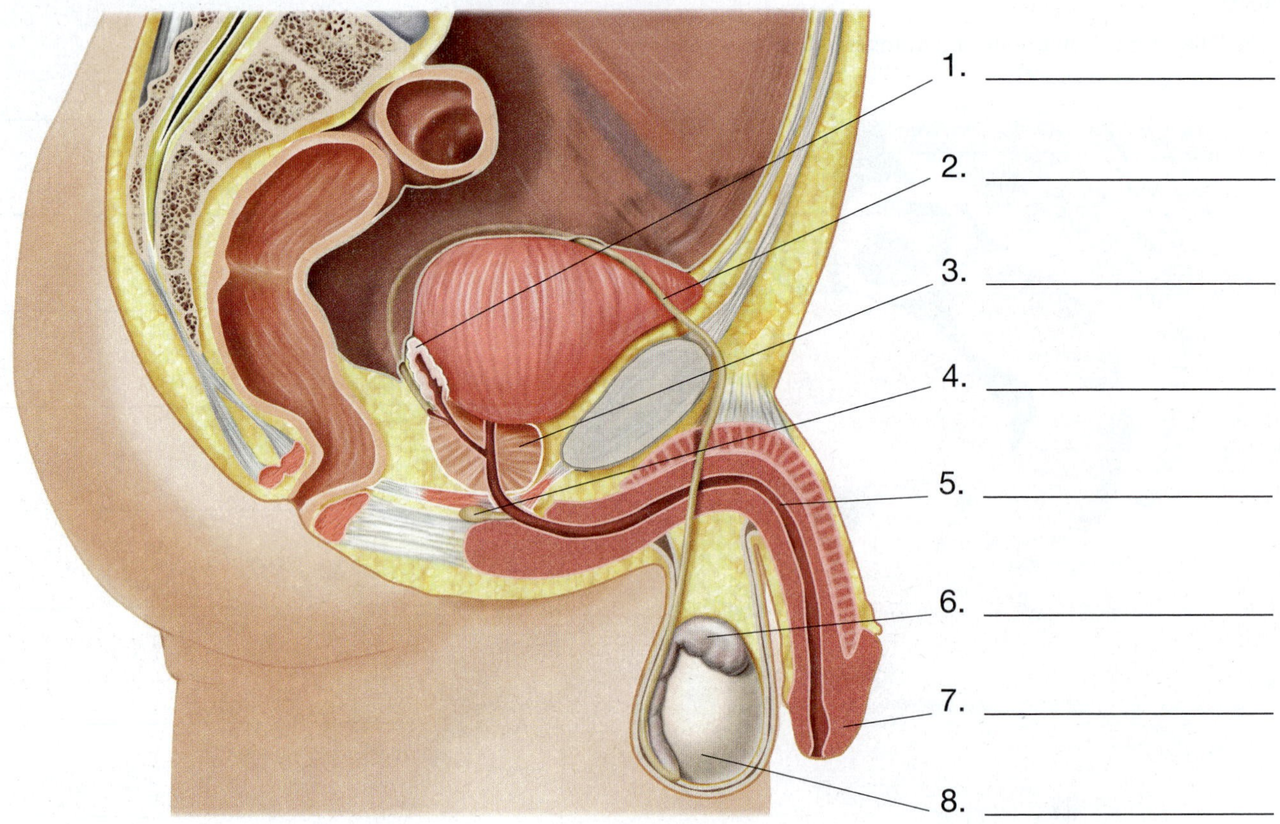

Image C

Write the labels for this figure on the numbered lines provided.

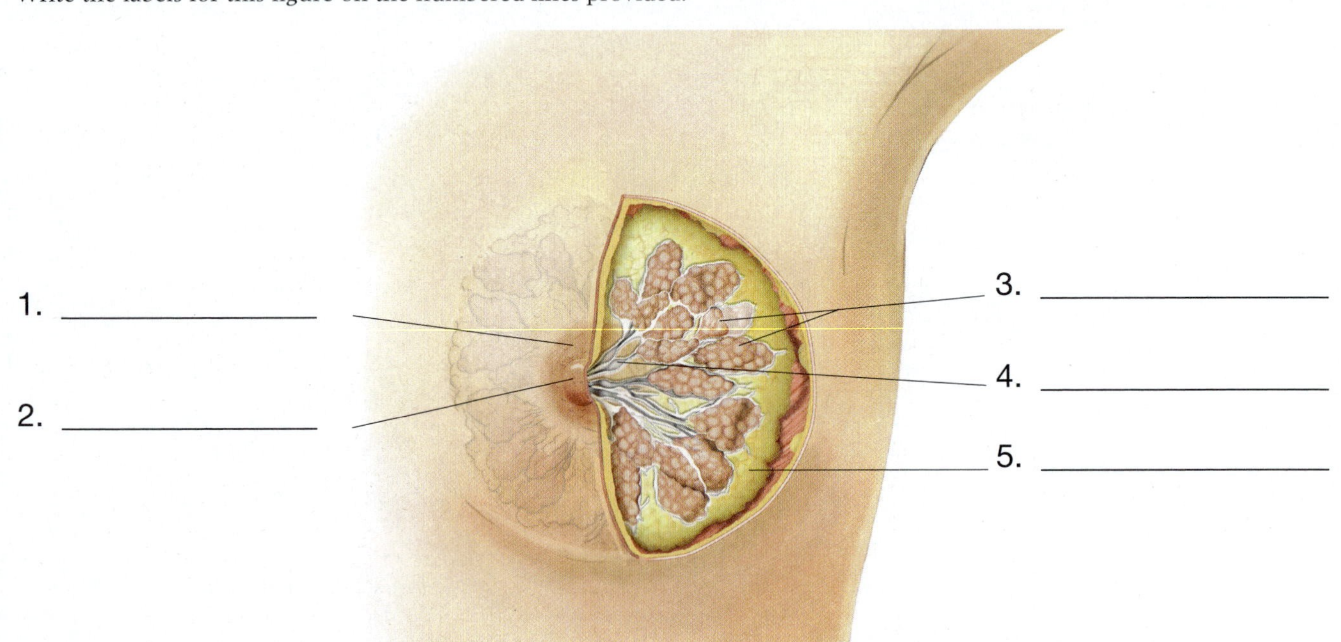

Chapter 11

Endocrine System

Learning Objectives

Upon completion of this chapter, you will be able to

1. Identify and define the combining forms and suffixes introduced in this chapter.
2. Correctly spell and pronounce medical terms and major anatomical structures relating to the endocrine system.
3. Locate and describe the major organs of the endocrine system and their functions.
4. List the major hormones secreted by each endocrine gland and describe their functions.
5. Identify and define endocrine system anatomical terms.
6. Identify and define selected endocrine system pathology terms.
7. Identify and define selected endocrine system diagnostic procedures.
8. Identify and define selected endocrine system therapeutic procedures.
9. Identify and define selected medications relating to the endocrine system.
10. Define selected abbreviations associated with the endocrine system.

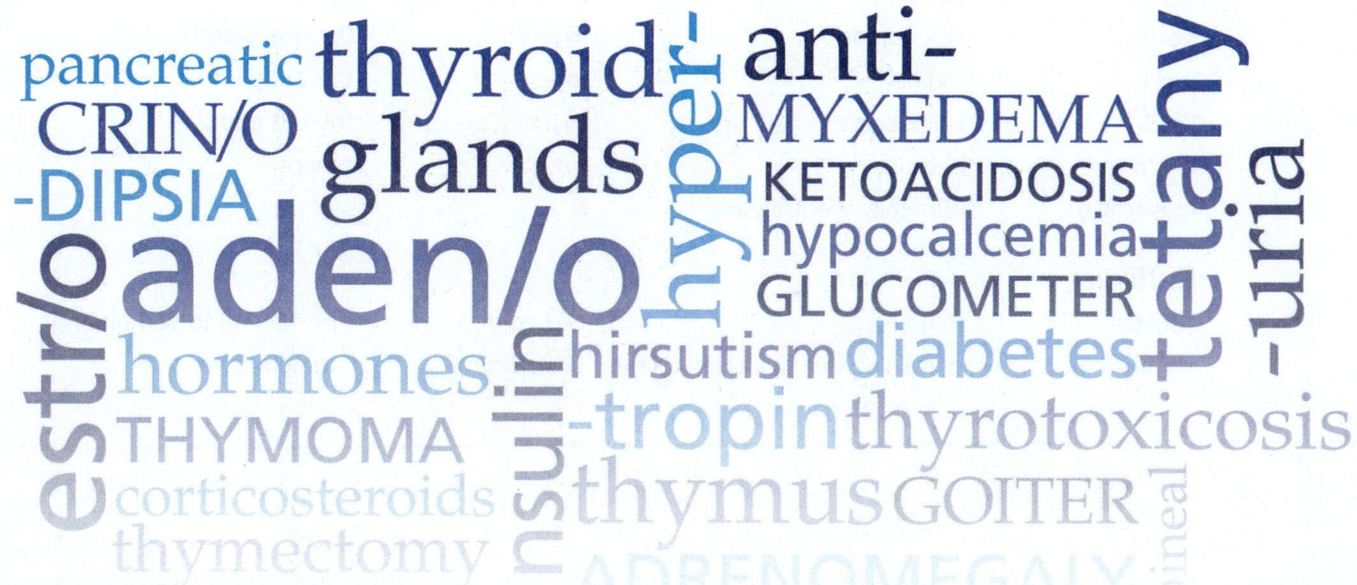

(Pearson Education, Inc.)

ENDOCRINE SYSTEM

AT A GLANCE

Function

Endocrine glands secrete hormones that regulate many body activities such as metabolic rate, water and mineral balance, immune system reactions, and sexual functioning.

Organs

The primary structures that comprise the endocrine system:

adrenal glands
ovaries
pancreas (islets of Langerhans)
parathyroid glands
pineal gland
pituitary gland
testes
thymus gland
thyroid gland

Word Parts

Presented here are the most common word parts used to build endocrine system terms. For a more comprehensive list, refer to the Terminology section of this chapter.

Combining Forms

acr/o	extremities
aden/o	gland
adren/o	adrenal glands
adrenal/o	adrenal glands
andr/o	male
calc/o	calcium
crin/o	to secrete
estr/o	female
gluc/o	glucose
glyc/o	sugar
gonad/o	sex glands
iod/o	iodine
kal/i	potassium
ket/o	ketones
mineral/o	minerals, electrolytes
natr/o	sodium
ovari/o	ovary
pancreat/o	pancreas
parathyroid/o	parathyroid gland
pineal/o	pineal gland
pituit/o	pituitary gland
pituitar/o	pituitary gland
radi/o	ray
somat/o	body
testicul/o	testes
thym/o	thymus gland
thyr/o	thyroid gland
thyroid/o	thyroid gland
toxic/o	poison

Suffixes

-dipsia	thirst
-emic	pertaining to a blood condition
-tropic	pertaining to stimulating
-tropin	to stimulate

Endocrine System Illustrated

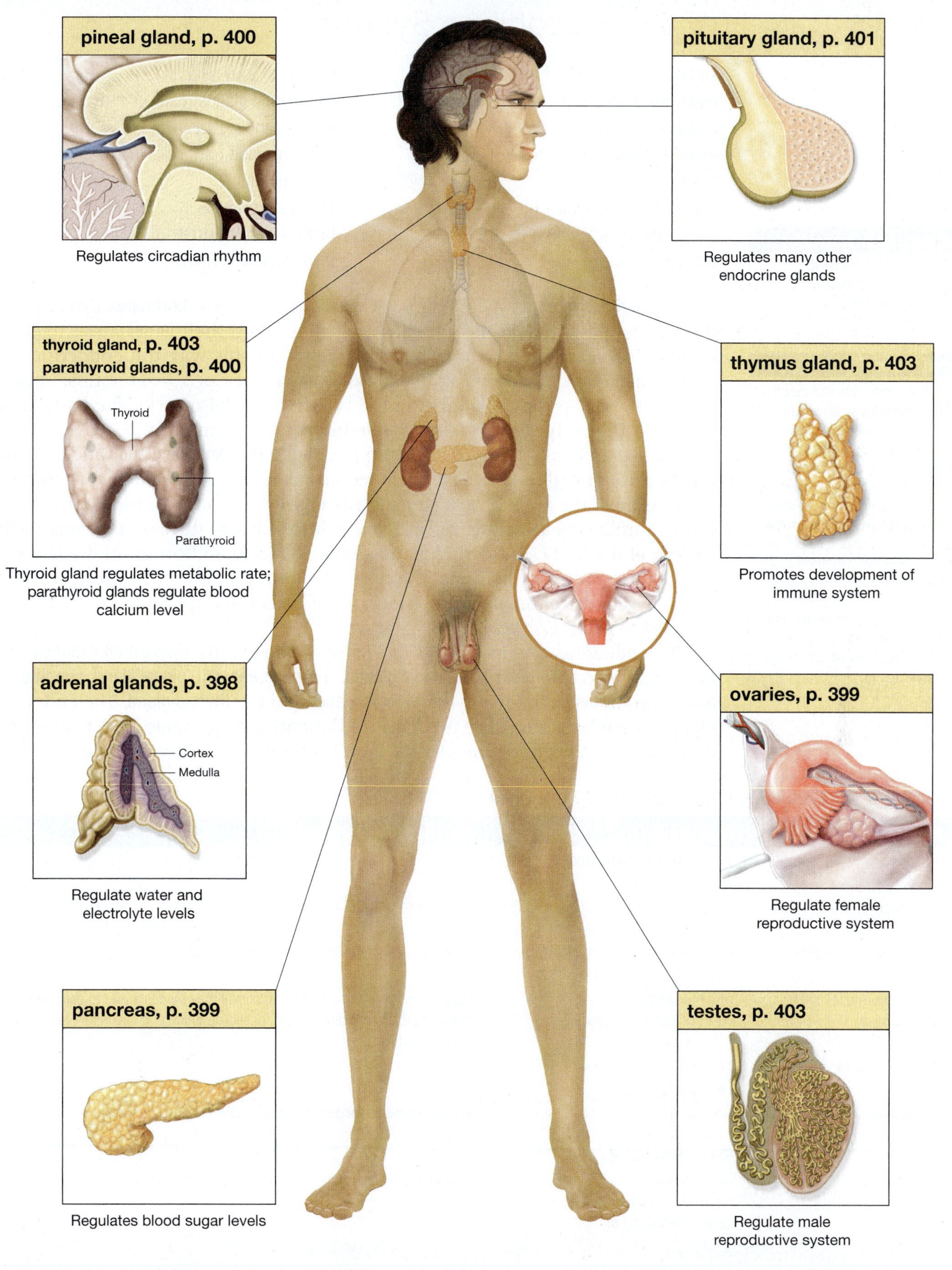

pineal gland, p. 400
Regulates circadian rhythm
pituitary gland, p. 401
Regulates many other endocrine glands
thyroid gland, p. 403
parathyroid glands, p. 400
Thyroid
Parathyroid
Thyroid gland regulates metabolic rate; parathyroid glands regulate blood calcium level
thymus gland, p. 403
Promotes development of immune system
adrenal glands, p. 398
Cortex
Medulla
Regulate water and electrolyte levels
ovaries, p. 399
Regulate female reproductive system
pancreas, p. 399
Regulates blood sugar levels
testes, p. 403
Regulate male reproductive system

Anatomy and Physiology of the Endocrine System

adrenal glands (ah-DREE-nal)
endocrine glands (EN-doh-krin)
endocrine system
exocrine glands (EKS-oh-krin)
glands
homeostasis (hoh-mee-oh-STAY-sis)
hormones (HOR-mohnz)
ovaries (OH-vah-reez)
pancreas (PAN-kree-as)
parathyroid glands (pair-ah-THIGH-royd)
pineal gland (PIN-ee-al)
pituitary gland (pih-TOO-ih-tair-ee)
target organs
testes (TESS-teez)
thymus gland (THIGH-mus)
thyroid gland (THIGH-royd)

What's In A Name?
Look for these word parts:
home/o = sameness
-stasis = standing still

Med Term Tip
The terms *endocrine* and *exocrine* were constructed to reflect the function of each type of gland. As glands, they both secrete, indicated by the combining form **crin/o**. The prefix **exo-**, meaning *external* or *outward*, tells us that exocrine gland secretions are carried to the outside of the body or to a passageway connected to the outside of the body. However, the prefix **endo-**, meaning *within* or *internal*, indicates that endocrine gland secretions are carried to other internal body structures by the bloodstream.

The **endocrine system** is a collection of **glands** that secrete **hormones** directly into the bloodstream. Hormones are chemicals that act on their **target organs** to either increase or decrease the target's activity level. In this way the endocrine system is instrumental in maintaining **homeostasis** (**home/o** = sameness; **-stasis** = standing still)—that is, adjusting the activity level of most of the tissues and organs of the body to maintain a stable internal environment.

The body actually has two distinct types of glands: **exocrine glands** and **endocrine glands**. Exocrine glands release their secretions into a duct that carries them to the outside of the body or to a passageway connected to the outside of the body. For example, sweat glands release sweat into a sweat duct that travels to the surface of the body. Endocrine glands, however, release hormones directly into the bloodstream. For example, the thyroid gland secretes its hormones directly into the bloodstream. Because endocrine glands have no ducts, they are also referred to as *ductless glands*.

The endocrine system consists of the following glands: two **adrenal glands**, two **ovaries** in the female, four **parathyroid glands**, the **pancreas**, the **pineal gland**, the **pituitary gland**, two **testes** in the male, the **thymus gland**, and the **thyroid gland**. The endocrine glands as a whole affect the functions of the entire body. Table 11-1 ■ presents a description of the endocrine glands, their hormones, and their functions.

■ TABLE 11-1 Endocrine Glands and Their Hormones

Gland and Hormone	Word Parts	Function
Adrenal cortex	**adren/o** = adrenal gland **-al** = pertaining to	
Glucocorticoids such as cortisol	**gluc/o** = glucose **cortic/o** = outer layer	Regulate carbohydrate levels in body
Mineralocorticoids such as aldosterone	**mineral/o** = minerals, electrolytes **cortic/o** = outer layer	Regulate electrolytes and fluid volume in body
Steroid sex hormones such as androgen	**andr/o** = male **-gen** = that which produces	Male sex hormones from adrenal cortex may be converted to estrogens in the bloodstream; responsible for reproduction and secondary sexual characteristics
Adrenal medulla	**adren/o** = adrenal gland **-al** = pertaining to	
Epinephrine (adrenaline)	**epi-** = above **nephr/o** = kidney **-ine** = pertaining to	Intensifies response during stress; "fight-or-flight" response
Norepinephrine	**epi-** = above **nephr/o** = kidney **-ine** = pertaining to	Chiefly a vasoconstrictor
Ovaries		
Estrogen	**estr/o** = female **-gen** = that which produces	Stimulates development of secondary sex characteristics in females; regulates menstrual cycle

TABLE 11-1 Endocrine Glands and Their Hormones (continued)

Gland and Hormone	Word Parts	Function
Progesterone	**pro-** = before **estr/o** = female	Prepares for conditions of pregnancy
Pancreas		
Glucagon		Stimulates liver to release glucose into the blood
Insulin		Regulates and promotes entry of glucose into cells
Parathyroid glands	**para-** = beside	
Parathyroid hormone (PTH)	**para-** = beside	Stimulates bone breakdown; regulates calcium level in the blood
Pineal gland	**pineal/o** = pineal gland **-al** = pertaining to	
Melatonin		Regulates circadian rhythm
Pituitary anterior lobe	**pituit/o** = pituitary gland **-ary** = pertaining to **anter/o** = front **-ior** = pertaining to	
Adrenocorticotropic hormone (ACTH)	**adren/o** = adrenal gland **cortic/o** = outer layer **-tropic** = pertaining to stimulating	Regulates secretion of some adrenal cortex hormones
Gonadotropins	**gonad/o** = gonads **-tropin** = to stimulate	Consists of two hormones, follicle-stimulating hormone and luteinizing hormone
Follicle-stimulating hormone (FSH)		Stimulates growth of eggs in females and sperm in males
Luteinizing hormone (LH)		Regulates function of male and female gonads and plays role in releasing ova in females
Growth hormone (GH)		Stimulates growth of body
Melanocyte-stimulating hormone (MSH)	**melan/o** = black **-cyte** = cell	Stimulates pigment production in skin
Prolactin (PRL)	**pro-** = before **lact/o** = milk	Stimulates milk production
Thyroid-stimulating hormone (TSH)		Regulates function of thyroid gland
Pituitary posterior lobe	**pituit/o** = pituitary gland **-ary** = pertaining to **poster/o** = back **-ior** = pertaining to	
Antidiuretic hormone (ADH)	**anti-** = against **-tic** = pertaining to	Stimulates reabsorption of water by the kidneys
Oxytocin		Stimulates uterine contractions and releases milk into ducts
Testes		
Testosterone		Promotes sperm production and development of secondary sex characteristics in males
Thymus		
Thymosin	**thym/o** = thymus gland	Promotes development of cells in immune system
Thyroid gland		
Calcitonin (CT)		Stimulates deposition of calcium into bone
Thyroxine (T_4)	**thyr/o** = thyroid gland **-ine** = pertaining to	Stimulates metabolism in cells
Triiodothyronine (T_3)	**tri-** = three **iod/o** = iodine **thyr/o** = thyroid gland **-ine** = pertaining to	Stimulates metabolism in cells

PRACTICE AS YOU GO

A. Match Glands and Hormones

_______	1. epinephrine	a.	pancreas
_______	2. oxytocin	b.	pineal gland
_______	3. testosterone	c.	thyroid gland
_______	4. insulin	d.	adrenal medulla
_______	5. cortisol	e.	ovaries
_______	6. melatonin	f.	anterior pituitary gland
_______	7. estrogen	g.	posterior pituitary gland
_______	8. growth hormone	h.	thymus gland
_______	9. thymosin	i.	testes
_______	10. thyroxine	j.	adrenal cortex

Adrenal Glands

What's In A Name?

Look for these word parts:
adrenal/o = adrenal gland
-ine = pertaining to

Med Term Tip

The term *adrenal* contains the word part **ren/o**, meaning *kidney*. Likewise, the term *epinephrine* contains another word part meaning *kidney*, **nephr/o**. But neither the adrenal gland nor epinephrine have anything to do with the kidney. Both received their names because the adrenal glands sit on top of the kidney, but have no connection to it.

Med Term Tip

The term *cortex* is frequently used in anatomy to indicate the outer layer of an organ such as the adrenal gland or the kidney. The term *cortex* means *bark*, as in the bark of a tree. The term *medulla* means *marrow*. Because marrow is found in the inner cavity of bones, the term came to stand for the middle of an organ.

adrenal cortex (KOR-teks)
adrenal medulla (meh-DULL-ah)
adrenaline (ah-DREN-ah-lin)
aldosterone (al-DOSS-ter-ohn)
androgens (AN-droh-jenz)
corticosteroids (kor-tih-koh-STAIR-oydz)
cortisol (KOR-tih-zawl)
epinephrine (ep-ih-NEF-rin)
glucocorticoids (gloo-koh-KOR-tih-koydz)
mineralocorticoids (min-er-al-oh-KOR-tih-koydz)
norepinephrine (nor-ep-ih-NEF-rin)
steroid sex hormones (STAIR-oyd)

The two adrenal glands are located above each of the kidneys (see Figure 11-1 ■). Each gland is composed of two sections: **adrenal cortex** and **adrenal medulla**.

The outer adrenal cortex manufactures several different families of hormones: **mineralocorticoids**, **glucocorticoids**, and **steroid sex hormones** (see again Table 11-1). However, because they are all produced by the cortex, they are collectively referred to as **corticosteroids**. The mineralocorticoid hormone, **aldosterone**, regulates sodium (Na^+) and potassium (K^+) levels in the body. The glucocorticoid

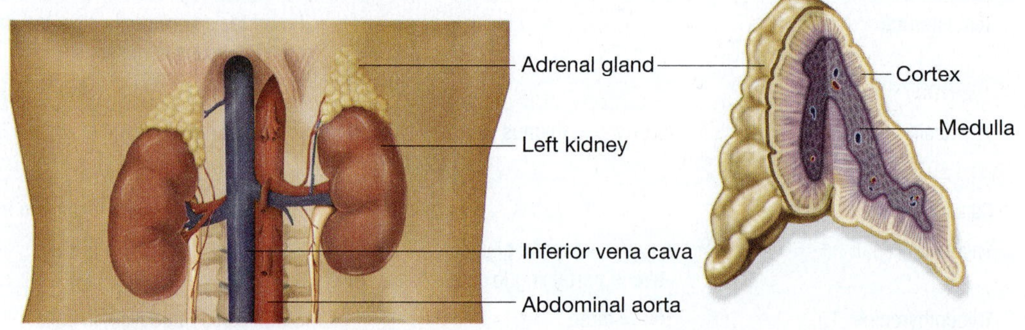

■ **Figure 11-1** The adrenal glands. These glands sit on top of each kidney. Each adrenal is subdivided into an outer cortex and an inner medulla. Each region secretes different hormones.

hormone, **cortisol**, regulates carbohydrates in the body. The adrenal cortex of both men and women secretes steroid sex hormones, **androgens** (which may be converted to estrogen once released into the bloodstream). These hormones regulate secondary sexual characteristics. All hormones secreted by the adrenal cortex are steroid hormones.

The inner adrenal medulla is responsible for secreting the hormones **epinephrine**, also called **adrenaline**, and **norepinephrine**. These hormones are critical during emergency situations because they increase blood pressure, heart rate, and respiration levels. This helps the body perform better during emergencies or otherwise stressful times.

Ovaries

estrogen (ESS-troh-gen)
gametes (GAM-eets)
gonads (GOH-nadz)
menstrual cycle (MEN-stroo-al)
ova
progesterone (proh-JES-ter-ohn)

The two ovaries are located in the lower abdominopelvic cavity of the female (see Figure 11-2 ■). They are the female **gonads**. Gonads are organs that produce **gametes** or the reproductive sex cells. In the case of females, the gametes are the **ova**. Of importance to the endocrine system, the ovaries produce the female sex hormones, **estrogen** and **progesterone** (see again Table 11-1). Estrogen is responsible for the appearance of the female sexual characteristics and regulation of the **menstrual cycle**. Progesterone helps to maintain a suitable uterine environment for pregnancy.

What's In A Name?
Look for these word parts:
men/o = menses, menstruation
-al = pertaining to

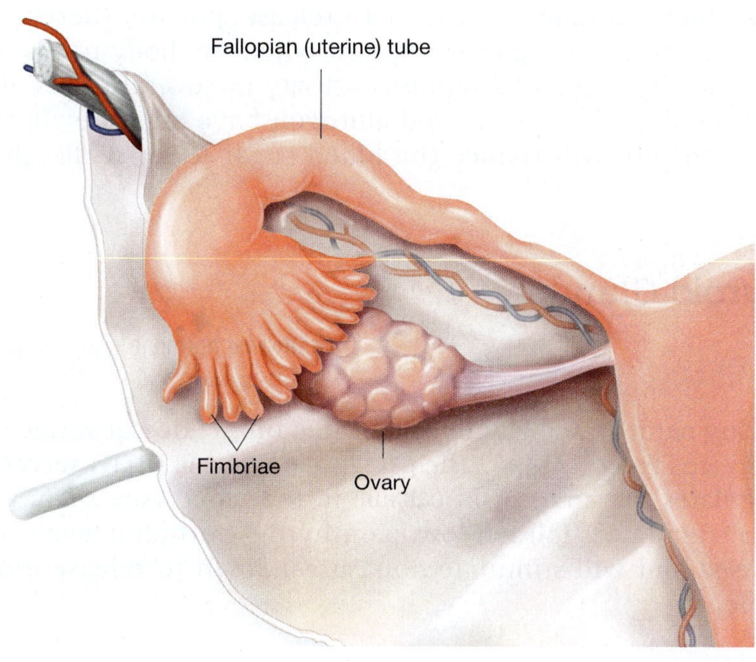

■ **Figure 11-2** The right ovary. In addition to producing ova, each ovary secretes the female sex hormones, estrogen and progesterone.

Pancreas

glucagon (GLOO-kuh-gon)
insulin (IN-suh-lin)
islets of Langerhans (EYE-lets / of / LAHNG-er-hahnz)
pancreatic islets (pan-kree-AT-ik / EYE-lets)

The pancreas is located along the lower curvature of the stomach (see Figure 11-3A ■). It is the only organ in the body that has both endocrine and

■ Figure 11-3 The pancreas. This organ sits just below the stomach and is both an exocrine and an endocrine gland. The endocrine regions of the pancreas are called the islets of Langerhans and they secrete insulin and glucagon.

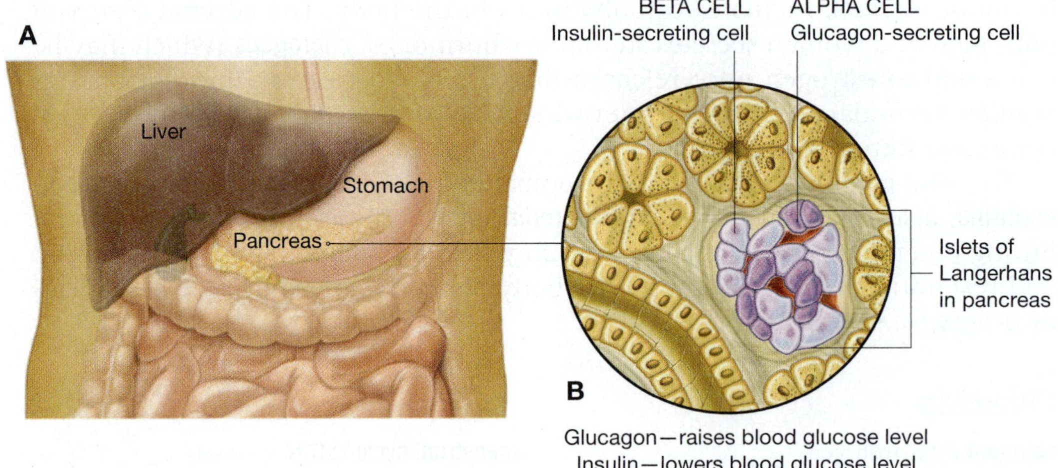

exocrine functions. The exocrine portion of the pancreas releases digestive enzymes through a duct into the duodenum of the small intestine. The endocrine sections of the pancreas are the **pancreatic islets** or **islets of Langerhans** (see Figure 11-3B ■). The islets cells produce two different hormones: **insulin** and **glucagon** (see again Table 11-1). Insulin, produced by beta (β) islet cells, stimulates the cells of the body to take in glucose from the bloodstream, lowering the body's blood sugar level. This occurs after a meal has been eaten and the carbohydrates are absorbed into the bloodstream. In this way the cells obtain the glucose they need for cellular respiration.

Another set of islet cells, the alpha (α) cells, secrete a different hormone, glucagon, which stimulates the liver to release glucose, thereby raising the blood glucose level. Glucagon is released when the body needs more sugar, such as at the beginning of strenuous activity or several hours after the last meal has been digested. Insulin and glucagon have opposite effects on blood sugar level. Insulin will reduce the blood sugar level, while glucagon will increase it.

Parathyroid Glands

calcium

parathyroid hormone (pair-ah-THIGH-royd / HOR-mohn)

> **Med Term Tip**
>
> A calcium deficiency in the system can result in a condition called *tetany*, or muscle excitability and tremors. If the parathyroid glands are removed during thyroid surgery, calcium replacement in the body is often necessary.

The four tiny parathyroid glands are located on the dorsal surface of the thyroid gland (see Figure 11-4 ■). The **parathyroid hormone** (PTH) secreted by these glands regulates the amount of **calcium** in the blood (see again Table 11-1). If blood calcium levels fall too low, parathyroid hormone levels in the blood are increased and will stimulate bone breakdown to release more calcium into the blood.

Pineal Gland

circadian rhythm (ser-KAY-dee-an)

melatonin (mel-ah-TOH-nin)

thalamus (THAL-ah-mus)

> **Med Term Tip**
>
> The pineal gland is an example of an organ named for its shape. *Pineal* means *shaped like a pine cone.*

The pineal gland is a small pine cone–shaped organ that is part of the **thalamus** region of the brain (see Figure 11-5 ■). The pineal gland secretes **melatonin**, which plays a role in regulating the body's **circadian rhythm** (see again Table 11-1). This is the 24-hour clock that governs periods of wakefulness and sleepiness.

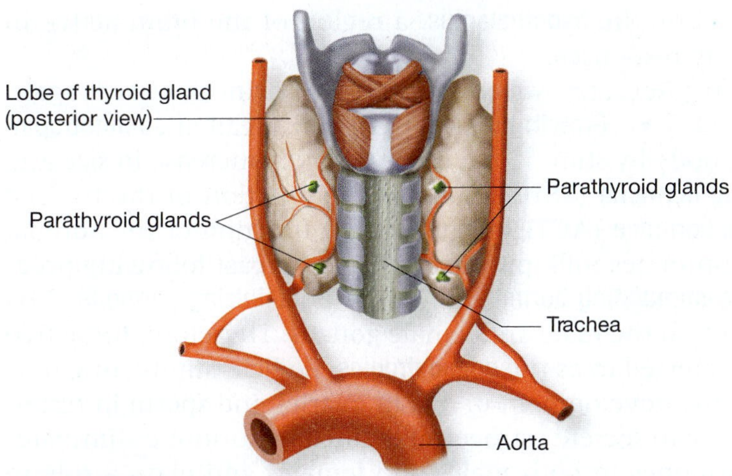

■ **Figure 11-4** The parathyroid glands. These four glands are located on the posterior side of the thyroid gland. They secrete parathyroid hormone.

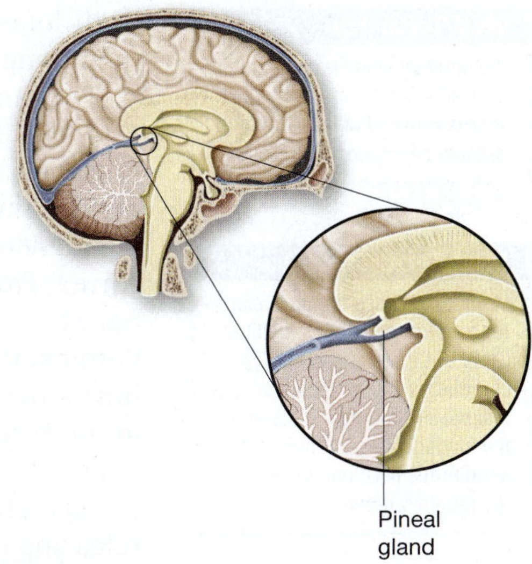

■ **Figure 11-5** The pineal gland is a part of the thalamus region of the brain. It secretes melatonin.

Pituitary Gland

adrenocorticotropic hormone (ah-dree-noh-kor-tih-koh-TROH-pik)
anterior lobe
antidiuretic hormone (an-tye-dye-yoo-RET-ik)
follicle-stimulating hormone (FALL-ih-kl / STIM-yoo-lay-ting)
gonadotropins (goh-nad-oh-TROH-pins)
growth hormone
hypothalamus (high-poh-THAL-ah-mus)
luteinizing hormone (LOO-teh-nigh-zing)
melanocyte-stimulating hormone
oxytocin (ok-see-TOH-sin)
posterior lobe
prolactin (proh-LAK-tin)
somatotropin (soh-mat-oh-TROH-pin)
thyroid-stimulating hormone

What's In A Name?
Look for these word parts:
somat/o = body
-tropin = to stimulate
hypo- = below

The pituitary gland is located underneath the brain (see Figure 11-6 ■). The small marble-shaped organ is divided into an **anterior lobe** and a **posterior lobe**.

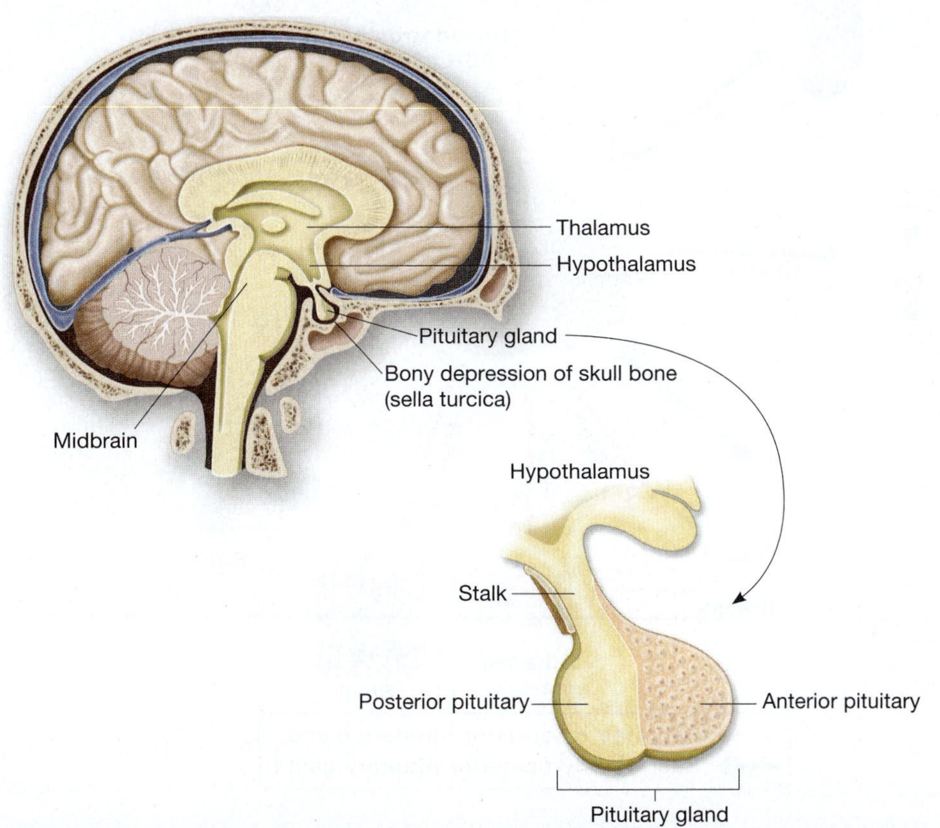

■ **Figure 11-6** The pituitary gland lies just underneath the brain. It is subdivided into anterior and posterior lobes. Each lobe secretes different hormones.

Med Term Tip

The pituitary gland is sometimes referred to as the *master gland* because several of its secretions regulate other endocrine glands.

Med Term Tip

Many people use the term *diabetes* to refer to diabetes mellitus (DM). But there is another type of diabetes, called *diabetes insipidus* (DI), that is a result of the inadequate secretion of the antidiuretic hormone (ADH) from the pituitary gland.

Both lobes are controlled by the **hypothalamus**, a region of the brain active in regulating automatic body responses.

The anterior pituitary secretes several different hormones (see again Table 11-1 and Figure 11-7 ■). **Growth hormone** (GH), also called **somatotropin**, promotes growth of the body by stimulating cells to rapidly increase in size and divide. **Thyroid-stimulating hormone** (TSH) regulates the function of the thyroid gland. **Adrenocorticotropic hormone** (ACTH) regulates the function of the adrenal cortex. **Prolactin** (PRL) stimulates milk production in the breast following pregnancy and birth. **Follicle-stimulating hormone** (FSH) and **luteinizing hormone** (LH) both exert their influence on the male and female gonads. Therefore, these two hormones together are referred to as the **gonadotropins**. Follicle-stimulating hormone is responsible for the development of ova in ovaries and sperm in testes. It also stimulates the ovary to secrete estrogen. Luteinizing hormone stimulates the secretion of sex hormones in both males and females and plays a role in releasing ova in females. **Melanocyte-stimulating hormone** (MSH) stimulates melanocytes to produce more melanin, thereby darkening the skin.

The posterior pituitary secretes two hormones, **antidiuretic hormone** (ADH) and **oxytocin** (see again Table 11-1). Antidiuretic hormone promotes water reabsorption by the kidney tubules. Oxytocin stimulates uterine contractions during labor and delivery and, after birth, the release of milk from the mammary glands.

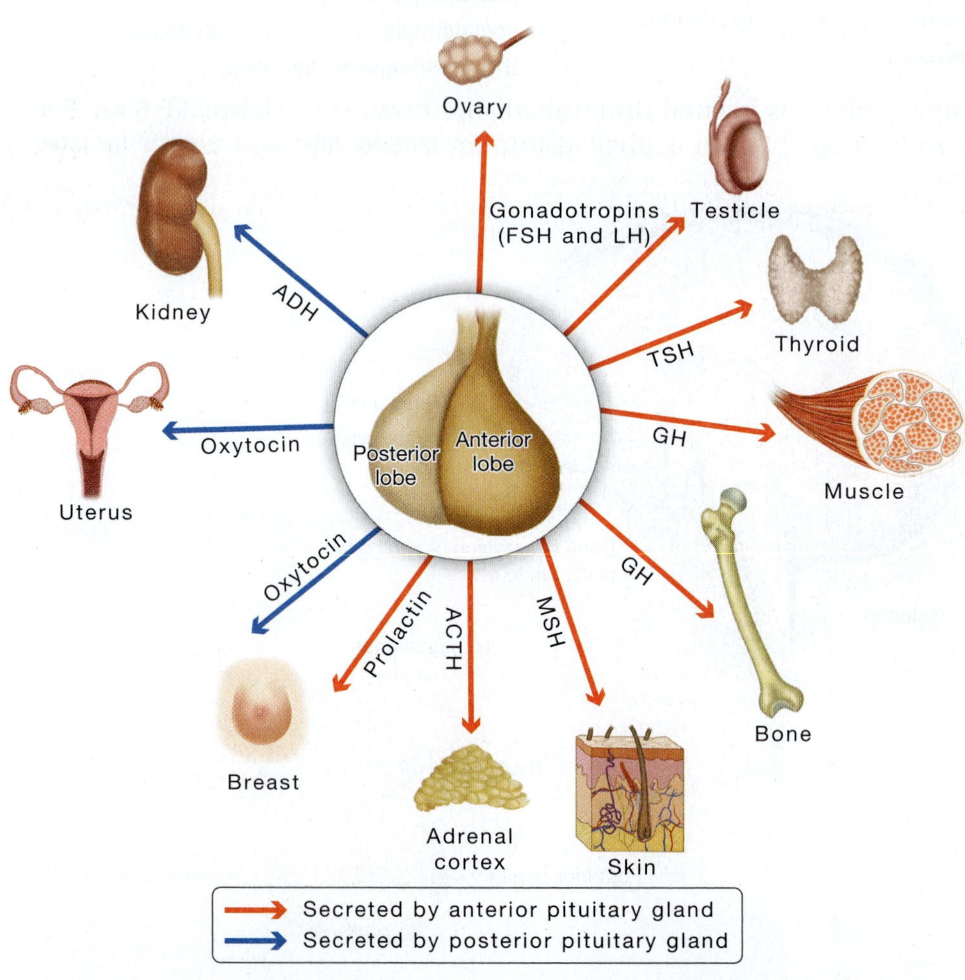

■ **Figure 11-7** The pituitary gland is sometimes called the master gland because it secretes many hormones that regulate other glands. This figure illustrates the different hormones and target tissues for the pituitary gland. *(Pearson Education, Inc.)*

Testes

sperm **testosterone** (tess-TAHS-ter-ohn)

The testes are two oval glands located in the scrotal sac of the male (see Figure 11-8 ■). They are the male gonads, which produce the male gametes, **sperm**, and the male sex hormone, **testosterone** (see again Table 11-1). Testosterone produces the male secondary sexual characteristics and regulates sperm production.

Thymus Gland

T cells **thymosin** (THIGH-moh-sin)

In addition to its role as part of the immune system, the thymus is also one of the endocrine glands because it secretes the hormone **thymosin** (see again Table 11-1). Thymosin, like the rest of the thymus gland, is important for proper development of the immune system. The thymus gland is located in the mediastinal cavity anterior and superior to the heart (see Figure 11-9 ■). The thymus is present at birth and grows to its largest size during puberty. At puberty it begins to shrink and eventually is replaced with connective and adipose tissue.

The most important function of the thymus is its role in the development of the immune system in the newborn. It is essential to the growth and development of thymic lymphocytes or **T cells**, which are critical for the body's immune system.

Thyroid Gland

basal metabolic rate
calcitonin (kal-sih-TOH-nin)
iodine (EYE-oh-dine)
thyroxine (thigh-ROKS-in)
triiodothyronine (trye-eye-oh-doh-THIGH-roh-neen)

What's In A Name?
Look for these word parts:
bas/o = base
-al = pertaining to
-ic = pertaining to

The thyroid gland, which resembles a butterfly in shape, has right and left lobes (see Figure 11-10 ■). It is located on either side of the trachea and larynx. The

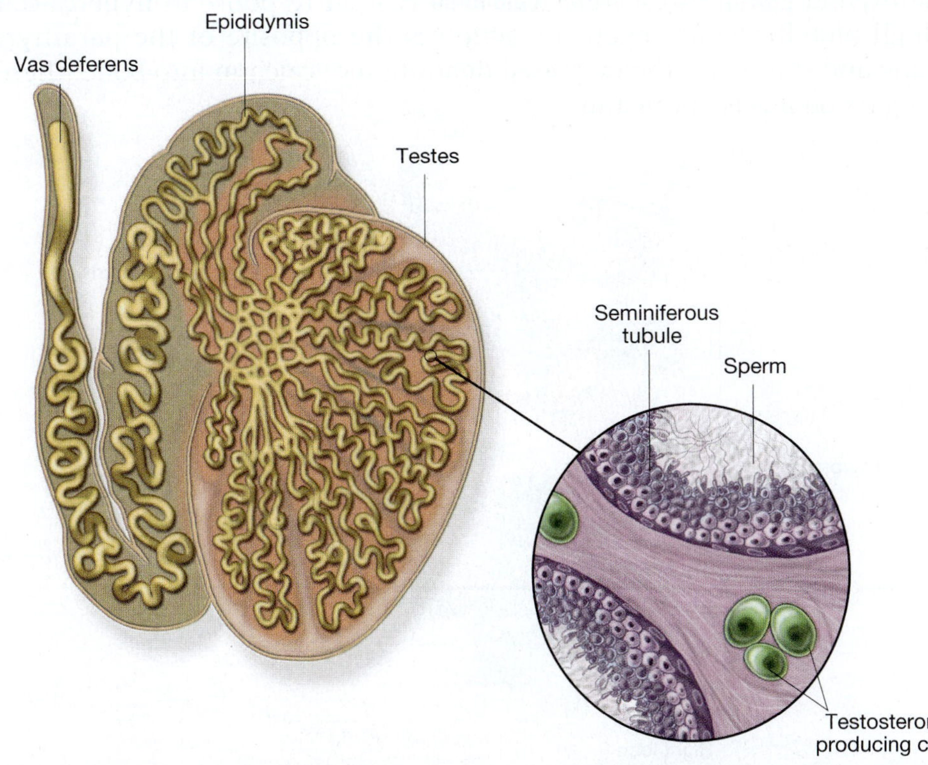

■ **Figure 11-8** A testis. In addition to producing sperm, each testis secretes the male sex hormones, primarily testosterone.

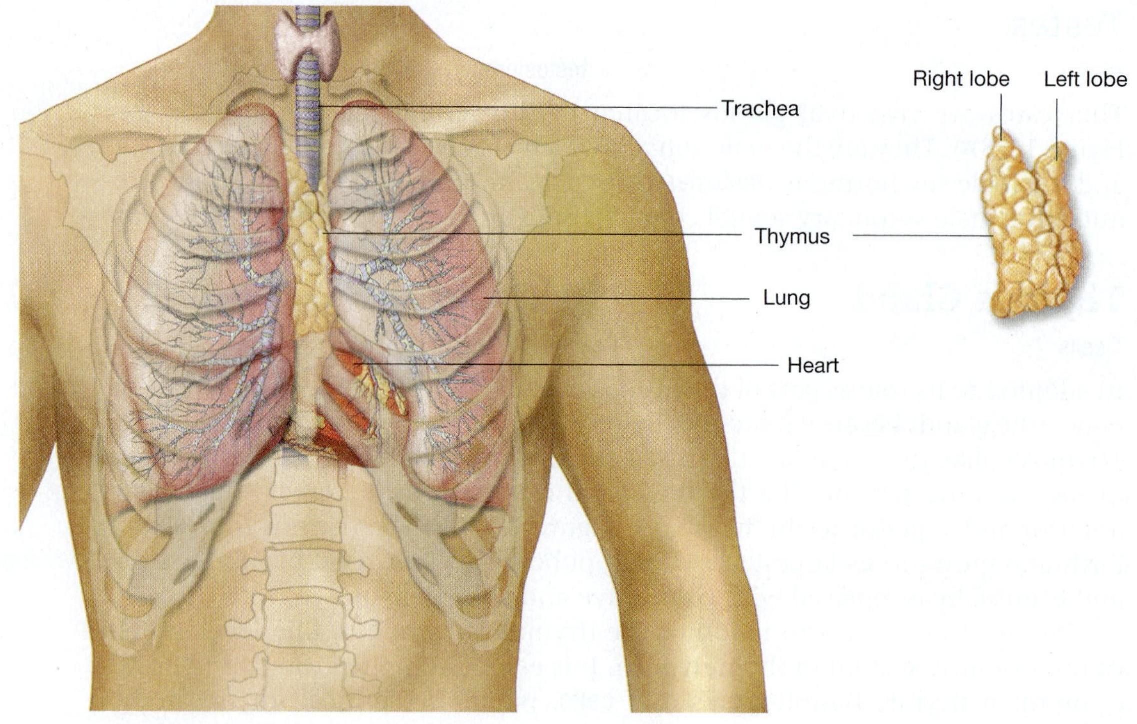

■ **Figure 11-9** The thymus gland. This gland lies in the mediastinum of the thoracic cavity, just above the heart. It secretes thymosin.

Med Term Tip

Iodine is found in many foods, including vegetables and seafood. It is also present in iodized salt, which is one of the best sources of iodine for people living in the Goiter Belt, composed of states located away from saltwater. A lack of iodine in the diet can lead to thyroid disorders, including *goiter*.

thyroid cartilage, or Adam's apple, is located just above the thyroid gland. This gland produces the hormones **thyroxine** (T_4) and **triiodothyronine** (T_3) (see again Table 11-1). These hormones are produced in the thyroid gland using the mineral **iodine**. Thyroxine and triiodothyronine help to regulate the production of energy and heat in the body to adjust the body's metabolic rate. The minimum rate of metabolism necessary to support the function of the body at rest is called the **basal metabolic rate** (BMR).

The thyroid gland also secretes **calcitonin** (CT) in response to hypercalcemia (too high blood calcium level). Its action is the opposite of the parathyroid hormone and stimulates the increased deposition of calcium into bone, thereby lowering blood levels of calcium.

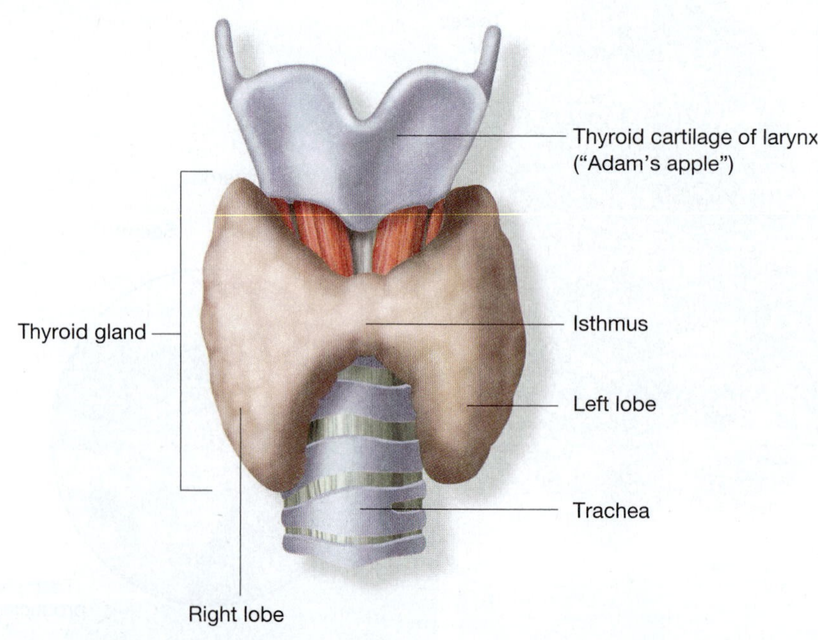

■ **Figure 11-10** The thyroid gland is subdivided into two lobes, one on each side of the trachea.

PRACTICE AS YOU GO

B. Complete the Statement

1. The study of the endocrine system is called ________________.
2. The master endocrine gland is the ________________.
3. ________________ is a general term for the sexual organs that produce gametes.
4. The term for the hormones produced by the outer layer of the adrenal cortex is ________________.
5. The ________________ is the body's 24-hour clock that governs periods of wakefulness and sleepiness.
6. Thyroxine and triiodothyronine are produced using the mineral ________________.
7. ________________ and ________________ work to regulate the level of glucose in the bloodstream.
8. The endocrine gland associated with the immune system is the ________________.

Terminology

Word Parts Used to Build Endocrine System Terms

The following lists contain the combining forms, suffixes, and prefixes used to build terms in the remaining sections of this chapter.

Combining Forms

acr/o	extremities
aden/o	gland
adren/o	adrenal gland
adrenal/o	adrenal gland
calc/o	calcium
carcin/o	cancer
chem/o	drug
cortic/o	outer layer
crin/o	to secrete
cyt/o	cell
gluc/o	glucose
glyc/o	sugar
glycos/o	sugar
gynec/o	female
immun/o	protection
kal/i	potassium
ket/o	ketones
lapar/o	abdomen
lob/o	lobe
mast/o	breast
natr/o	sodium
neur/o	nerve
ophthalm/o	eye
or/o	mouth
ovari/o	ovary
pancreat/o	pancreas
parathyroid/o	parathyroid gland
pineal/o	pineal gland
pituit/o	pituitary gland
pituitar/o	pituitary gland
radi/o	radiation
retin/o (see Chapter 13)	retina
testicul/o	testes
thym/o	thymus gland
thyr/o	thyroid gland
thyroid/o	thyroid gland
toxic/o	poison

Suffixes

-al	pertaining to
-an	pertaining to
-ar	pertaining to
-ary	pertaining to
-dipsia	thirst
-ectomy	surgical removal
-edema	swelling
-emia	blood condition
-emic	pertaining to a blood condition
-graphy	process of recording
-ia	condition
-ic	pertaining to
-ism	state of
-itis	inflammation
-logy	study of
-megaly	enlarged
-meter	instrument to measure
-oma	tumor
-osis	abnormal condition
-pathy	disease
-prandial	pertaining to a meal
-scopic	pertaining to visually examining
-tic	pertaining to
-uria	urine condition

Prefixes

anti-	against
endo-	within
ex-	outward
hyper-	excessive
hypo-	insufficient
pan-	all
poly-	many
post-	after

Adjective Forms of Anatomical Terms

Term	Word Parts	Definition
adrenal (ah-DREE-nal)	adren/o = adrenal gland -al = pertaining to	Pertaining to adrenal glands
ovarian (oh-VAIR-ee-an)	ovari/o = ovary -an = pertaining to	Pertaining to ovary
pancreatic (pan-kree-AT-ik)	pancreat/o = pancreas -ic = pertaining to	Pertaining to pancreas
parathyroidal (pair-ah-thigh-ROYD-al)	parathyroid/o = parathyroid gland -al = pertaining to	Pertaining to parathyroid gland
pineal (PIN-ee-al)	pineal/o = pineal gland -al = pertaining to **Word Watch** Note the atypical way in which the term *pineal* is formed. More of the letters from the combining form are dropped before adding the suffix.	Pertaining to pineal gland
pituitary (pih-TOO-ih-tair-ee)	pituit/o = pituitary gland -ary = pertaining to	Pertaining to pituitary gland
testicular (tess-TIK-yoo-lar)	testicul/o = testes -ar = pertaining to	Pertaining to testes
thymic (THIGH-mik)	thym/o = thymus gland -ic = pertaining to	Pertaining to thymus gland
thyroidal (thigh-ROYD-al)	thyroid/o = thyroid gland -al = pertaining to	Pertaining to thyroid gland

PRACTICE AS YOU GO

C. Give the adjective form for each anatomical structure.

1. The thymus gland ____________________
2. The pancreas ____________________
3. The thyroid gland ____________________
4. An ovary ____________________
5. A testis ____________________

Pathology

Term	Word Parts	Definition
Medical Specialties		
endocrinology (en-doh-krin-ALL-oh-jee)	endo- = within crin/o = to secrete -logy = study of	Branch of medicine involving diagnosis and treatment of conditions and diseases of endocrine glands; physician is *endocrinologist*
Signs and Symptoms		
adrenomegaly (ah-dree-noh-MEG-ah-lee)	adren/o = adrenal gland -megaly = enlarged	Having one or both adrenal glands enlarged
adrenopathy (ad-ren-OP-ah-thee)	adren/o = adrenal gland -pathy = disease	General term for adrenal gland disease
edema (eh-DEE-mah)	**Word Watch** Watch how the term *edema* is used in this condition. It may also appear as the suffix **-edema**.	Condition in which body tissues contain excessive amounts of fluid
endocrinopathy (en-doh-krin-OP-ah-thee)	endo- = within crin/o = to secrete -pathy = disease	General term for diseases of the endocrine system
exophthalmos (eks-off-THAL-muss)	ex- = outward ophthalm/o = eye	Condition in which the eyeballs protrude, such as in Graves' disease; generally caused by overproduction of thyroid hormone
glycosuria (gly-kohs-YOO-ree-ah)	glycos/o = sugar -uria = urine condition	Having a high level of sugar excreted in urine
gynecomastia (gigh-neh-koh-MAST-ee-ah)	gynec/o = female mast/o = breast -ia = condition	Development of breast tissue in males; may be symptom of adrenal feminization
hirsutism (HER-soo-tizm)	-ism = state of	Condition of having excessive amount of hair; generally used to describe females who have adult male pattern of hair growth; can be result of hormonal imbalance

Pathology (continued)

Term	Word Parts	Definition
hypercalcemia (high-per-kal-SEE-mee-ah)	hyper- = excessive calc/o = calcium -emia = blood condition	Condition of having high level of calcium in the blood; associated with hypersecretion of parathyroid hormone
hyperglycemia (high-per-gly-SEE-mee-ah)	hyper- = excessive glyc/o = sugar -emia = blood condition	Condition of having high level of sugar in the blood; associated with diabetes mellitus
hyperkalemia (high-per-kuh-LEE-mee-ah)	hyper- = excessive kal/i = potassium -emia = blood condition	Condition of having high level of potassium in the blood
hypersecretion	hyper- = excessive	Excessive hormone production by an endocrine gland
hypocalcemia (high-poh-kal-SEE-mee-ah)	hypo- = insufficient calc/o = calcium -emia = blood condition	Condition of having low level of calcium in the blood; associated with hyposecretion of parathyroid hormone; hypocalcemia may result in tetany
hypoglycemia (high-poh-gly-SEE-mee-ah)	hypo- = insufficient glyc/o = sugar -emia = blood condition	Condition of having low level of sugar in the blood
hyponatremia (high-poh-nuh-TREE-mee-ah)	hypo- = insufficient natr/o = sodium -emia = blood condition	Condition of having low level of sodium in the blood
hyposecretion	hypo- = insufficient	Deficient hormone production by an endocrine gland
obesity (oh-BEE-sih-tee)		Having abnormal amount of fat in the body
polydipsia (pol-ee-DIP-see-ah)	poly- = many -dipsia = thirst	Excessive feeling of thirst
polyuria (pol-ee-YOO-ree-ah)	poly- = many -uria = urine condition	Condition of producing excessive amount of urine
syndrome (SIN-drohm)		Group of symptoms and signs that, when combined, present clinical picture of disease or condition
thyromegaly (thigh-roh-MEG-ah-lee)	thyr/o = thyroid gland -megaly = enlarged	Having enlarged thyroid gland
Adrenal Glands		
Addison's disease (AD-ih-sons)		Disease named for British physician Thomas Addison; results from deficiency in adrenocortical hormones; there may be increased pigmentation of skin, generalized weakness, and weight loss
adrenal feminization (ah-DREE-nal / fem-ih-nih-ZAY-shun)	adren/o = adrenal gland -al = pertaining to	Development of female secondary sexual characteristics (such as breasts) in a male; often as result of increased estrogen secretion by the adrenal cortex
adrenal virilism (ah-DREE-nal / VIR-ill-izm)	adren/o = adrenal gland -al = pertaining to -ism = state of	Development of male secondary sexual characteristics (such as deeper voice and facial hair) in a female; often as result of increased androgen secretion by the adrenal cortex

Pathology (continued)

Term	Word Parts	Definition
adrenalitis (ah-dree-nal-EYE-tis)	adrenal/o = adrenal gland -itis = inflammation	Inflammation of one or both adrenal glands
Cushing's syndrome (KUSH-ings / SIN-drohm)		Set of symptoms caused by excessive levels of cortisol due to high doses of corticosteroid drugs and adrenal tumors; syndrome may present symptoms of weakness, edema, excess hair growth, skin discoloration, and osteoporosis
pheochromocytoma (fee-oh-kroh-moh-sigh-TOH-mah)	cyt/o = cell -oma = tumor	Usually benign tumor of the adrenal medulla that secretes epinephrine; symptoms include anxiety, heart palpitations, dyspnea, profuse sweating, headache, and nausea
Pancreas		
diabetes mellitus (DM) (dye-ah-BEE-teez / MEL-ih-tus)		Chronic disorder of carbohydrate metabolism resulting in hyperglycemia and glycosuria; there are two distinct forms of diabetes mellitus: *insulin-dependent diabetes mellitus* (IDDM) or *type 1*, and *non-insulin-dependent diabetes mellitus* (NIDDM) or *type 2*
diabetic retinopathy (dye-ah-BET-ik / ret-in-OP-ah-thee)	-tic = pertaining to retin/o = retina -pathy = disease	Secondary complication of diabetes that affects blood vessels of the retina, resulting in visual changes and even blindness
insulin-dependent diabetes mellitus (IDDM) (dye-ah-BEE-teez / MEL-ih-tus)		Also called *type 1 diabetes mellitus*; develops early in life when the pancreas stops insulin production; patient must take daily insulin injections
insulinoma (in-soo-lin-OH-mah)	-oma = tumor	Tumor of the islets of Langerhans cells of the pancreas that secretes excessive amount of insulin
ketoacidosis (kee-toh-ass-ih-DOH-sis)	ket/o = ketones -osis = abnormal condition	Acidosis due to excess of acidic ketone bodies (waste products); serious condition requiring immediate treatment as it may result in death for diabetic patient if not reversed; also called *diabetic acidosis*
non-insulin-dependent diabetes mellitus (NIDDM) (dye-ah-BEE-teez / MEL-ih-tus)		Also called *type 2 diabetes mellitus*; typically develops later in life; the pancreas produces normal to high levels of insulin, but cells fail to respond to it; patients may take oral hypoglycemics to improve insulin function or may eventually have to take insulin
peripheral neuropathy (per-IF-eh-ral / noo-ROP-ah-thee)	-al = pertaining to neur/o = nerve -pathy = disease	Damage to nerves in lower legs and hands as result of diabetes mellitus; symptoms include either extreme sensitivity or numbness and tingling
Parathyroid Glands		
hyperparathyroidism (high-per-pair-ah-THIGH-royd-izm)	hyper- = excessive parathyroid/o = parathyroid gland -ism = state of	Hypersecretion of parathyroid hormone; may result in hypercalcemia and Recklinghausen disease
hypoparathyroidism (high-poh-pair-ah-THIGH-royd-izm)	hypo- = insufficient parathyroid/o = parathyroid gland -ism = state of	Hyposecretion of parathyroid hormone; may result in hypocalcemia and tetany

Pathology (continued)

Term	Word Parts	Definition
Recklinghausen disease (REK-ling-how-zen)		Excessive production of parathyroid hormone resulting in degeneration of bones
tetany (TET-ah-nee)		Nerve irritability and painful muscle cramps resulting from hypocalcemia; hypoparathyroidism is one cause of tetany
Pituitary Gland		
acromegaly (ak-roh-MEG-ah-lee)	acr/o = extremities -megaly = enlarged	Chronic disease of adults that results in elongation and enlargement of bones of head and extremities; can also be mood changes; due to excessive amount of growth hormone in adult
diabetes insipidus (DI) (dye-ah-BEE-teez / in-SIP-ih-dus)		Disorder caused by inadequate secretion of antidiuretic hormone by posterior lobe of the pituitary gland; may be polyuria and polydipsia
dwarfism (DWARF-izm)	-ism = state of	Condition of being abnormally short in height; may be result of hereditary condition or lack of growth hormone
gigantism (JYE-gan-tizm)	-ism = state of	Excessive development of body due to overproduction of growth hormone by the pituitary gland in child or teenager; opposite of *dwarfism*
hyperpituitarism (high-per-pih-TOO-ih-tuh-rizm)	hyper- = excessive pituitar/o = pituitary gland -ism = state of	Hypersecretion of one or more pituitary gland hormones
hypopituitarism (high-poh-pih-TOO-ih-tuh-rizm)	hypo- = insufficient pituitar/o = pituitary gland -ism = state of	Hyposecretion of one or more pituitary gland hormones
panhypopituitarism (pan-high-poh-pih-TOO-ih-tuh-rizm)	pan- = all hypo- = insufficient pituitar/o = pituitary gland -ism = state of	Deficiency in all hormones secreted by the pituitary gland; often recognized because of problems with glands regulated by the pituitary—adrenal cortex, thyroid, ovaries, and testes
Thymus Gland		
thymitis (thigh-MY-tis)	thym/o = thymus gland -itis = inflammation	Inflammation of the thymus gland

Figure 11-11 Skull X-ray (lateral view) of person with acromegaly showing abnormally enlarged mandible. *(Zephyr/Science Source)*

Pathology (continued)

Term	Word Parts	Definition
thymoma (thigh-MOH-mah)	thym/o = thymus gland -oma = tumor	Tumor in the thymus gland
Thyroid Gland		
congenital hypothyroidism (high-poh-THIGH-royd-izm)	hypo- = insufficient thyroid/o = thyroid gland -ism = state of	Congenital condition in which lack of thyroid hormones may result in arrested physical and mental development; formerly called *cretinism*
goiter (GOY-ter) ■ **Figure 11-12** Goiter. A photograph of a male with an extreme goiter or enlarged thyroid gland. *(Eugene Gordon/ Pearson Education, Inc.)*		Enlargement of the thyroid gland
Graves' disease		Condition named for Irish physician Robert Graves that results in overactivity of the thyroid gland and can cause a crisis situation; symptoms include exophthalmos and goiter; a type of *hyperthyroidism*
Hashimoto's thyroiditis (hash-ee-MOH-tohz / thigh-roy-DYE-tis)	thyroid/o = thyroid gland -itis = inflammation	Chronic autoimmune form of thyroiditis; results in hyposecretion of thyroid hormones
hyperthyroidism (high-per-THIGH-royd-izm)	hyper- = excessive thyroid/o = thyroid gland -ism = state of	Hypersecretion of thyroid gland hormones
hypothyroidism (high-poh-THIGH-royd-izm)	hypo- = insufficient thyroid/o = thyroid gland -ism = state of	Hyposecretion of thyroid gland hormones
myxedema (miks-eh-DEE-mah)	-edema = swelling	Condition resulting from hyposecretion of the thyroid gland in adult; symptoms can include swollen facial features, edematous skin, anemia, slow speech, drowsiness, and mental lethargy
thyrotoxicosis (thigh-roh-tok-sih-KOH-sis)	thyr/o = thyroid gland toxic/o = poison -osis = abnormal condition	Condition resulting from marked overproduction of the thyroid gland; symptoms include rapid heart action, tremors, enlarged thyroid gland, exophthalmos, and weight loss
All Glands		
adenocarcinoma (ad-eh-noh-kar-sih-NOH-mah)	aden/o = gland carcin/o = cancer -oma = tumor	Cancerous tumor in gland that is capable of producing hormones secreted by that gland; one cause of hypersecretion pathologies

PRACTICE AS YOU GO

D. Terminology Matching

Match each term to its definition.

1. ________ Cushing's syndrome
2. ________ goiter
3. ________ acromegaly
4. ________ gigantism
5. ________ myxedema
6. ________ diabetes mellitus
7. ________ diabetes insipidus
8. ________ Hashimoto's thyroiditis
9. ________ Graves' disease
10. ________ Addison's disease

a. enlarged thyroid
b. overactive adrenal cortex
c. hyperthyroidism
d. underactive adrenal cortex
e. enlarged bones of head and extremities
f. may cause polyuria and polydipsia
g. an autoimmune disease
h. excessive growth hormone in a child
i. disorder of carbohydrate metabolism
j. insufficient thyroid hormone in an adult

Diagnostic Procedures

Term	Word Parts	Definition
Clinical Laboratory Tests		
blood serum test		Blood test to measure level of substances such as calcium, electrolytes, testosterone, insulin, and glucose; used to assist in determining function of various endocrine glands
fasting blood sugar (FBS)		Blood test to measure amount of sugar circulating throughout body after 12-hour fast
glucose tolerance test (GTT) (GLOO-kohs)		Test to determine blood sugar level; measured dose of glucose is given to a patient either orally or intravenously; blood samples are then drawn at certain intervals to determine ability of patient to use glucose; used for diabetic patients to determine insulin response to glucose
protein-bound iodine (PBI) **test**		Blood test to measure concentration of thyroxine (T_4) circulating in bloodstream; iodine becomes bound to protein in blood and can be measured; useful in establishing thyroid function
radioimmunoassay (RIA) (ray-dee-oh-im-yoo-noh-ASS-ay)	radi/o = ray immun/o = protection	Blood test that uses radioactively tagged hormones and antibodies to measure quantity of hormone in the plasma
thyroid function test (TFT) (THIGH-royd)		Blood test used to measure levels of thyroxine, triiodothyronine, and thyroid-stimulating hormone in bloodstream to assist in determining thyroid function

Diagnostic Procedures (continued)

Term	Word Parts	Definition
total calcium		Blood test to measure total amount of calcium to assist in detecting parathyroid and bone disorders
two-hour postprandial glucose tolerance test (post-PRAN-dee-al)	post- = after -prandial = pertaining to a meal	Blood test to assist in evaluating glucose metabolism; patient eats high-carbohydrate diet and then fasts overnight before test; then blood sample is taken two hours after a meal
Diagnostic Imaging		
thyroid echography (THIGH-royd / eh-KOG-rah-fee)	-graphy = process of recording	Ultrasound examination of thyroid that can assist in distinguishing a thyroid nodule from a cyst
thyroid scan (THIGH-royd)		Test in which radioactive iodine is administered that localizes in the thyroid gland; gland can then be visualized with scanning device to detect pathology such as tumors

Therapeutic Procedures

Term	Word Parts	Definition
Medical Procedures		
adrenalectomy (ah-dree-nal-EK-toh-mee)	adrenal/o = adrenal gland -ectomy = surgical removal	Surgical removal of one or both adrenal glands
chemical thyroidectomy (thigh-royd-EK-toh-mee)	chem/o = drug -al = pertaining to thyroid/o = thyroid gland -ectomy = surgical removal	Large dose of radioactive iodine (RAI) is given in order to kill thyroid gland cells without having to actually do surgery
glucometer (gloo-KOM-eh-ter)	gluc/o = glucose -meter = instrument to measure	Device designed for diabetic to use at home to measure level of glucose in bloodstream
hormone replacement therapy (HRT)		Artificial replacement of hormones in patients with hyposecretion disorders; may be oral pills, injections, or adhesive skin patches
laparoscopic adrenalectomy (lap-ar-oh-SKOP-ik / ah-dree-nal-EK-toh-mee)	lapar/o = abdomen -scopic = pertaining to visually examining adrenal/o = adrenal gland -ectomy = surgical removal	Removal of the adrenal gland through small incision in abdomen and using endoscopic instruments
lobectomy (loh-BEK-toh-mee)	lob/o = lobe -ectomy = surgical removal	Removal of a lobe from an organ; for example, one lobe of the thyroid gland
parathyroidectomy (pair-ah-thigh-royd-EK-toh-mee)	parathyroid/o = parathyroid gland -ectomy = surgical removal	Surgical removal of one or more of the parathyroid glands
pinealectomy (pin-ee-ah-LEK-toh-mee)	pineal/o = pineal gland -ectomy = surgical removal	Surgical removal of the pineal gland
thymectomy (thigh-MEK-toh-mee)	thym/o = thymus gland -ectomy = surgical removal	Surgical removal of the thymus gland
thyroidectomy (thigh-royd-EK-toh-mee)	thyroid/o = thyroid gland -ectomy = surgical removal	Surgical removal of the thyroid gland

PRACTICE AS YOU GO

E. Procedure Matching

Match each procedure term with its definition.

1. ________ protein-bound iodine test
2. ________ fasting blood sugar
3. ________ radioimmunoassay
4. ________ thyroid scan
5. ________ two-hour postprandial glucose tolerance test
6. ________ glucose tolerance test
7. ________ glucometer
8. ________ chemical thyroidectomy

a. measures levels of hormones in the blood
b. determines glucose metabolism after patient receives a measured dose of glucose
c. test of glucose metabolism two hours after eating a meal
d. measures blood sugar level after 12-hour fast
e. measures T_4 concentration in the blood
f. uses radioactive iodine
g. used instead of a surgical procedure
h. instrument to measure blood glucose

Pharmacology

Classification	Word Parts	Action	Examples
antithyroid agents	anti- = against	Block production of thyroid hormones in patients with hypersecretion disorders	methimazole, Tapazole; propylthiouracil
aquaretics (ak-wuh-RET-iks)	*Aqua* is the Latin term for *water*	Inserts aquaporins (water channels) in the nephron to treat hyponatremia; increases water excretion by kidney without increasing sodium excretion	conivaptan, Vaprisol; tolvaptan, Samsca
corticosteroids (kor-tih-koh-STAIR-oydz)	cortic/o = outer layer	Although function of these hormones in body is to regulate carbohydrate metabolism, they also have strong anti-inflammatory action; therefore are used to treat severe chronic inflammatory diseases such as rheumatoid arthritis; long-term use has adverse side effects such as osteoporosis and symptoms of Cushing's syndrome; also used to treat adrenal cortex hyposecretion disorders such as Addison's disease	prednisone, Deltasone
human growth hormone therapy		Hormone replacement therapy with human growth hormone in order to stimulate skeletal growth; used to treat children with abnormally short stature	somatropin, Genotropin; somatrem, Protropin
insulin (IN-suh-lin)		Replaces insulin for type 1 diabetics or treats severe type 2 diabetics	human insulin, Humulin
oral hypoglycemic agents (high-poh-gly-SEE-mik)	or/o = mouth -al = pertaining to hypo- = insufficient glyc/o = sugar -emic = pertaining to a blood condition	Taken by mouth to cause decrease in blood sugar; not used for insulin-dependent patients	metformin, Glucophage; glipizide, Glucotrol

Pharmacology (continued)

Classification	Word Parts	Action	Examples
thyroid replacement hormone		Hormone replacement therapy for patients with hypothyroidism or who have had a thyroidectomy	levothyroxine, Levo-T; liothyronine, Cytomel

Abbreviations

α	alpha	**MSH**	melanocyte-stimulating hormone
ACTH	adrenocorticotropic hormone	**Na^+**	sodium
ADH	antidiuretic hormone	**NIDDM**	non-insulin-dependent diabetes mellitus
aq	aqueous	**NPH**	neutral protamine Hagedorn (insulin)
β	beta	**od**	overdose
BMR	basal metabolic rate	**PBI**	protein-bound iodine
cap(s)	capsule(s)	**PRL**	prolactin
CT	calcitonin	**PTH**	parathyroid hormone
DI	diabetes insipidus	**RAI**	radioactive iodine
DM	diabetes mellitus	**RIA**	radioimmunoassay
FBS	fasting blood sugar	**sol**	solution
FSH	follicle-stimulating hormone	**susp**	suspension
GH	growth hormone	**syr**	syrup
GTT	glucose tolerance test	**T_3**	triiodothyronine
HRT	hormone replacement therapy	**T_4**	thyroxine
IDDM	insulin-dependent diabetes mellitus	**tab(s)**	tablet(s)
inj	injection	**TFT**	thyroid function test
K^+	potassium	**TSH**	thyroid-stimulating hormone
LH	luteinizing hormone		

PRACTICE AS YOU GO

F. What's the Abbreviation?

1. non-insulin-dependent diabetes mellitus ____________________
2. insulin-dependent diabetes mellitus ____________________
3. adrenocorticotropic hormone ____________________
4. parathyroid hormone ____________________
5. triiodothyronine ____________________
6. thyroid-stimulating hormone ____________________
7. fasting blood sugar ____________________
8. prolactin ____________________

Chapter Review

Real-World Applications

Medical Record Analysis

This Discharge Summary below contains 10 medical terms. Underline each term and write it in the list below the report. Then explain each term as you would to a nonmedical person.

Discharge Summary

Admitting Diagnosis:	Hyperglycemia, ketoacidosis, glycosuria
Final Diagnosis:	New-onset type 1 diabetes mellitus
History of Present Illness:	A 12-year-old female patient presented to her physician's office with a two-month history of weight loss, fatigue, polyuria, and polydipsia. Her family history is significant for a grandfather, mother, and older brother with type 1 diabetes mellitus. The pediatrician found hyperglycemia with a fasting blood sugar and glycosuria with a urine dipstick. She is being admitted at this time for management of new-onset diabetes mellitus.
Summary of Hospital Course:	At the time of admission, the FBS was 300 mg/100 mL and she was in ketoacidosis. She rapidly improved after receiving insulin; her blood glucose level normalized. The next day a glucose tolerance test confirmed the diagnosis of diabetes mellitus. The patient was started on insulin injections. Patient and family were instructed on diabetes mellitus, insulin, diet, exercise, and long-term complications.
Discharge Plans:	Patient was discharged to home with her parents. Her parents are to check her blood glucose levels twice daily and call the office for insulin dosage. She is to return to the office in two weeks.

	Term	Explanation
1.	______________	______________________________
2.	______________	______________________________
3.	______________	______________________________
4.	______________	______________________________
5.	______________	______________________________
6.	______________	______________________________
7.	______________	______________________________
8.	______________	______________________________
9.	______________	______________________________
10.	______________	______________________________

Chart Note Transcription

The chart note below contains 11 phrases that can be reworded with a medical term presented in this chapter. Each phrase is identified with an underline. Determine the medical term and write your answers in the space provided.

Pearson General Hospital Consultation Report

Task Edit View Time Scale Options Help Download Archive Date: 17 May 2017

Current Complaint:	A 56-year-old female was referred to the specialist in the treatment of diseases of the endocrine glands **1** for evaluation of weakness, edema, an abnormal amount of fat in the body, **2** and an excessive amount of hair for a female. **3**
Past History:	Patient reports she has been overweight most of her life in spite of a healthy diet and regular exercise. She was diagnosed with osteoporosis after incurring a pathological rib fracture following a coughing attack.
Signs and Symptoms:	Patient has moderate edema in bilateral feet and lower legs as well as a puffy face and an upper lip moustache. She is 100 lbs. over normal body weight for her age and height. She moves slowly and appears generally lethargic. A test to measure the hormone levels in the blood plasma **4** reports increased steroid hormone that regulates carbohydrates in the body. **5** A CT scan demonstrates a gland tumor **6** in the right outer layer of the adrenal gland. **7**
Diagnosis:	A group of symptoms associated with hypersecretion of the adrenal cortex **8** secondary to a gland tumor **9** in the right outer layer of the adrenal gland **10**
Treatment:	Surgical removal of the right adrenal gland **11**

1. ____________________

2. ____________________

3. ____________________

4. ____________________

5. ____________________

6. ____________________

7. ____________________

8. ____________________

9. ____________________

10. ____________________

11. ____________________

Case Study

Below is a case study presentation of a patient with a condition discussed in this chapter. Read the case study and answer the questions below. Some questions will ask for information not included within this chapter. Use your text, a medical dictionary, or any other reference material you choose to answer these questions.

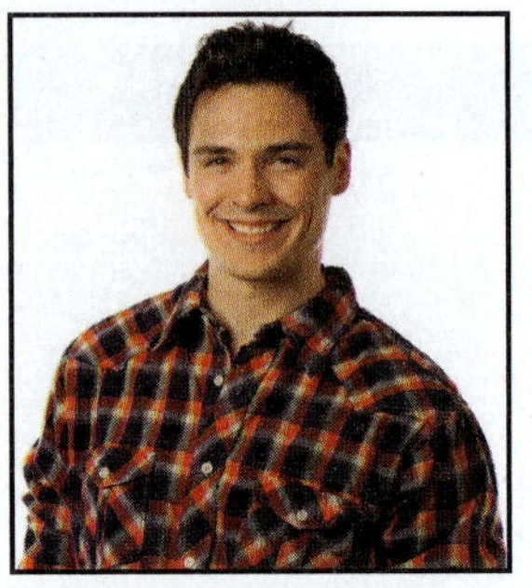

(Flashon Studio/Shutterstock)

A 22-year-old college student was admitted to the emergency room after his friends called an ambulance when he passed out in a bar. He had become confused, developed slurred speech, and had difficulty walking after having only consumed one beer. In the ER he was noted to have diaphoresis, rapid respirations and pulse, and was disoriented. Upon examination, needle marks were found on his abdomen and outer thighs. The physician ordered blood serum tests that revealed hyperglycemia and ketoacidosis. Unknown to his friends, this young man has had diabetes mellitus since early childhood. The patient quickly recovered following an insulin injection.

Questions

1. What pathological condition has this patient had since childhood? Look this condition up in a reference source and include a short description of it.

   ____

   ____

2. List and define each symptom noted in the ER in your own words.

   ____

   ____

3. What diagnostic test was performed? Describe it in your own words.

   ____

   ____

4. Explain the results of the test.

   ____

   ____

5. What specific type of diabetes does this young man probably have? Justify your answer.

   ____

   ____

6. Describe the other type of diabetes mellitus that this young man did not have.

   ____

   ____

Practice Exercises

A. Word Building Practice

The combining form **thyroid/o** refers to the *thyroid*. Use it to write a term that means:

1. removal of the thyroid ______
2. pertaining to the thyroid ______
3. state of excessive thyroid ______

The combining form **pancreat/o** refers to the *pancreas*. Use it to write a term that means:

4. pertaining to the pancreas ______
5. inflammation of the pancreas ______
6. removal of the pancreas ______
7. cutting into the pancreas ______

The combining form **adren/o** refers to the *adrenal glands*. Use it to write a term that means:

8. pertaining to the adrenal glands ______
9. enlargement of an adrenal gland ______
10. adrenal gland disease ______

The combining form **thym/o** refers to the *thymus gland*. Use it to write a term that means:

11. tumor of the thymus gland ______
12. removal of the thymus gland ______
13. pertaining to the thymus gland ______
14. inflammation of the thymus gland ______

B. Complete the Term

For each definition given below, fill in the blank with the word part that completes the term.

Definition	Term
1. surgical removal of thyroid gland	______ectomy
2. instrument to measure glucose	______meter
3. relating to after a meal	post______
4. state of insufficient thyroid gland	hypo______ism
5. state of excessive pituitary gland	hyper______ism
6. enlarged extremities	______megaly
7. blood condition of insufficient sodium	hypo______emia
8. many (abnormally great) thirst	poly______
9. inflammation of adrenal gland	______itis
10. blood condition of excessive calcium	hyper______emia
11. sugar urine condition	______uria
12. tumor of thymus gland	______oma

C. Using Abbreviations

Fill in each blank with the appropriate abbreviation.

1. Due to low estrogen levels following early menopause, she received ____________________.
2. ____________________ is a test using radioactively tagged hormones and antibodies to measure hormone levels.
3. A(n) ____________________ measures the level of glucose in the blood after a 12-hour fast.
4. ____________________ may be either insulin-dependent or non-insulin-dependent.
5. The two gonadotropins are ____________________ and ____________________.
6. ____________________ is the only hormone secreted by the parathyroid gland.
7. ____________________ is secreted by the anterior pituitary and regulates secretion of some adrenal cortex hormones.
8. ____________________ regulates function of the thyroid gland.
9. ____________________ stimulates reabsorption of water by the kidneys.
10. ____________________ and ____________________ are secreted by the thyroid gland and stimulate metabolism in the cells.

D. Define the Term

1. corticosteroid ____________________
2. hirsutism ____________________
3. tetany ____________________
4. diabetic retinopathy ____________________
5. hyperglycemia ____________________
6. hypoglycemia ____________________
7. adrenaline ____________________
8. insulin ____________________
9. thyrotoxicosis ____________________
10. hypersecretion ____________________

E. Fill in the Blank

insulinoma	ketoacidosis	pheochromocytoma
gynecomastia	panhypopituitarism	Hashimoto's thyroiditis

1. The doctor found that Marsha's high level of insulin and hypoglycemia were caused by a(n) ________________.
2. Kevin developed ________________ as a result of his diabetes mellitus and required emergency treatment.
3. It was determined that Karen had ________________________________ when doctors realized she had problems with her thyroid gland, adrenal cortex, and ovaries.
4. Luke's high epinephrine level was caused by a(n) ________________.
5. When it was determined that Carl's thyroiditis was an autoimmune condition, it became obvious that he had ________________.
6. Excessive sex hormones caused Jack to develop ________________.

F. Pharmacology Challenge

Fill in the classification for each drug description, then match the brand name.

	Drug Description	Classification	Brand Name
1.	________ strong anti-inflammatory	________________	a. Genotropin
2.	________ stimulates skeletal growth	________________	b. Levo-T
3.	________ treats type 2 diabetes mellitus	________________	c. Tapazole
4.	________ blocks production of thyroid hormone	________________	d. Glucophage
5.	________ treats type 1 diabetes mellitus	________________	e. Deltasone
6.	________ treatment for hypothyroidism	________________	f. Humulin

G. Terminology Matching

Match each term to its definition.

1.	________ calcitonin	a. a severe condition for diabetics
2.	________ exophthalmos	b. elongation and enlargement of bones of head and limbs
3.	________ ketoacidosis	c. caused by excessive levels of cortisol
4.	________ Cushing's syndrome	d. regulates circadian rhythm
5.	________ tetany	e. enlarged thyroid gland
6.	________ goiter	f. secreted by thyroid gland
7.	________ acromegaly	g. stimulates pigment in the skin
8.	________ MSH	h. determines blood sugar level
9.	________ melatonin	i. bulging eyeballs
10.	________ GTT	j. nerve irritability

H. Spelling Practice

Some of the following terms are misspelled. Identify the incorrect terms and spell them correctly in the blank provided.

1. endocrinopathy ________________________________
2. glycouria ________________________________
3. hypocalcemia ________________________________
4. adrenallitis ________________________________
5. pheochromocytoma ________________________________
6. ketoacidosis ________________________________
7. Reklinghausen ________________________________
8. hyperpituitarianism ________________________________
9. myxedema ________________________________
10. radioimunoassay ________________________________

I. Anatomical Adjectives

Fill in the blank with the adjective for each anatomical structure.

Noun	Adjective
1. ovary	____________________
2. pancreas	____________________
3. testes	____________________
4. thymus gland	____________________
5. thyroid gland	____________________
6. parathyroid gland	____________________

J. Complete the Statement

1. The endocrine system is instrumental in maintaining ____________________ to maintain a stable internal environment.
2. ____________________ glands release their secretions into a duct; ____________________ glands release their secretions into the bloodstream.
3. The ____________________ glands are located above each kidney.
4. The pancreatic ____________________ cells secrete ____________________ and ____________________.
5. Parathyroid hormone regulates the level of ____________________ in the bloodstream.
6. The ____________________ gland is sometimes called the "master gland."
7. ____________________ is a hormone instrumental in the proper development of the immune system.
8. The minimum rate of metabolism necessary to support the function of the body is the ____________________.

Labeling Exercises

Image A

Write the labels for this figure on the numbered lines provided.

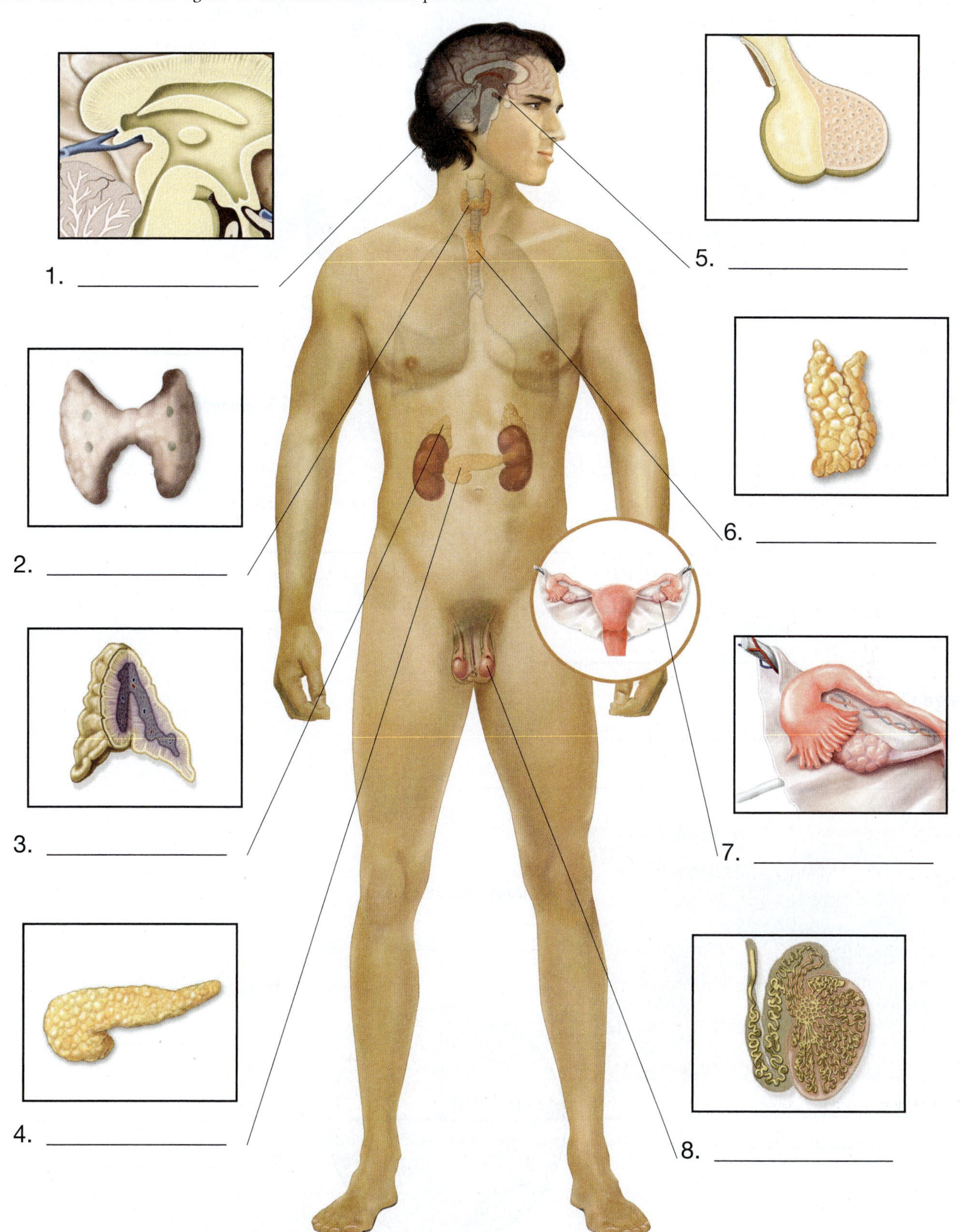

Image B

Write the labels for this figure on the numbered lines provided.

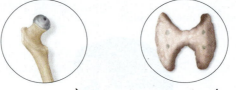

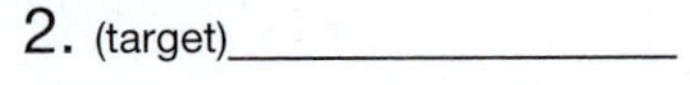
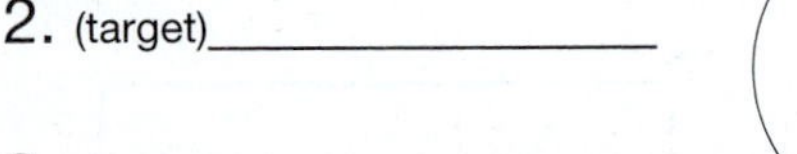
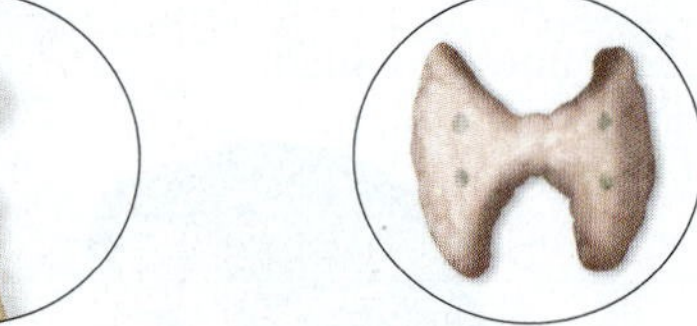

2. (target)________________

3. (hormone)________________

8. (target)________________

9. (hormone)________________

1. ________________

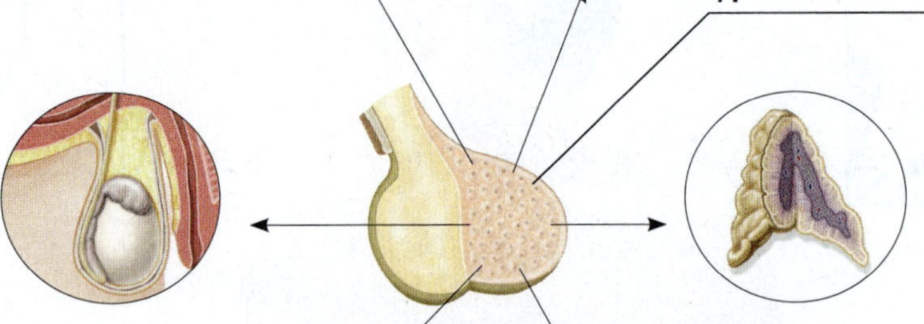

4. (target)________________

5. (hormones)________________, ________________

10. (target)________________

11. (hormone)________________

6. (target)________________

7. (hormones)________________, ________________

12. (target)________________

13. (hormone)________________

Image C

Write the labels for this figure on the numbered lines provided.

1. ________________

2. ________________

3. ________________

4. Insulin-secreting cell ________________

5. Glucagon-secreting cell ________________

6. ________________

Chapter 12

Nervous System and Mental Health

Learning Objectives

Upon completion of this chapter, you will be able to

1. Identify and define the combining forms and suffixes introduced in this chapter.
2. Correctly spell and pronounce medical terms and major anatomical structures relating to the nervous system.
3. Locate and describe the major organs of the nervous system and their functions.
4. Describe the components of a neuron.
5. Distinguish between the central nervous system, peripheral nervous system, and autonomic nervous system.
6. Identify and define nervous system anatomical terms.
7. Identify and define selected nervous system pathology terms.
8. Identify and define selected nervous system diagnostic procedures.
9. Identify and define selected nervous system therapeutic procedures.
10. Identify and define selected medications relating to the nervous system.
11. Define selected abbreviations associated with the nervous system.
12. Define the classifications of mental disorders as defined in the *Diagnostic and Statistical Manual of Mental Disorders,* 5th edition.
13. Describe examples of each classification of mental disorders.
14. Identify and define selected mental health therapeutic procedures.
15. Define selected abbreviations associated with mental health.

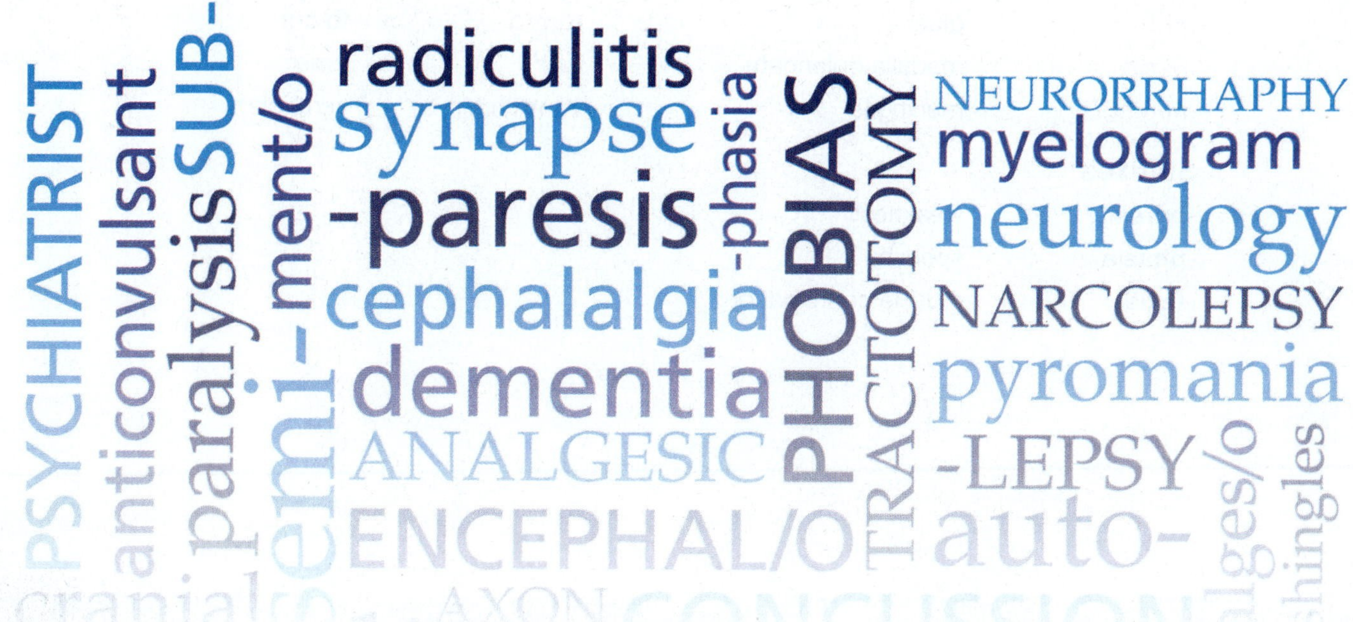

(Pearson Education, Inc.)

SECTION I: NERVOUS SYSTEM

AT A GLANCE

Function

The nervous system coordinates and controls body functions. It receives sensory input, makes decisions, and then orders body responses.

Organs

The primary structures that comprise the nervous system:

brain

spinal cord

nerves

Word Parts

Presented here are the most common word parts (with their meanings) used to build nervous system terms. For a more comprehensive list, refer to the Terminology section of this chapter.

Combining Forms

alges/o	sense of pain	**meningi/o**	meninges
astr/o	star	**ment/o**	mind
centr/o	center	**myel/o**	spinal cord
cerebell/o	cerebellum	**neur/o**	nerve
cerebr/o	cerebrum	**peripher/o**	away from center
clon/o	rapid contracting and relaxing	**poli/o**	gray matter
concuss/o	to shake violently	**pont/o**	pons
dur/o	dura mater	**radicul/o**	nerve root
encephal/o	brain	**thalam/o**	thalamus
esthesi/o	sensation, feeling	**thec/o**	sheath (meninges)
gli/o	glue	**tom/o**	to cut
medull/o	medulla oblongata	**ton/o**	tone
mening/o	meninges	**ventricul/o**	ventricle

Suffixes

-paresis	weakness
-phasia	speech
-taxia	muscle coordination

Nervous System Illustrated

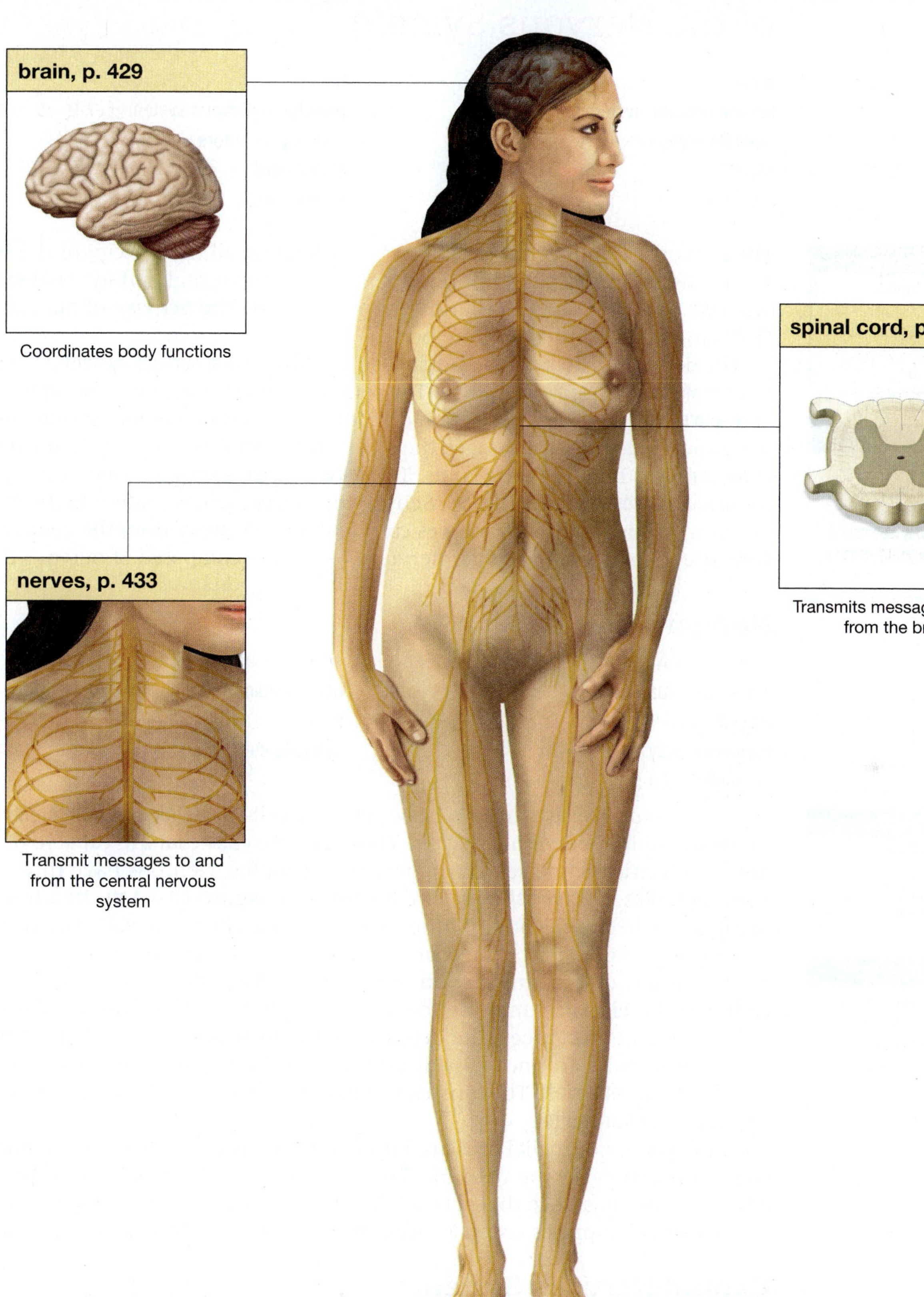

Anatomy and Physiology of the Nervous System

brain
central nervous system
cranial nerves (KRAY-nee-al)
glands
muscles
nerves
peripheral nervous system (per-IF-eh-ral)
sensory receptors
spinal cord
spinal nerves

What's In A Name?
Look for these word parts:
centr/o = center
peripher/o = away from center
-al = pertaining to
-ory = pertaining to

Med Term Tip
Neuroglial tissue received its name as a result of its function. This tissue holds neurons together. Therefore, it was called *neuroglial*, a term literally meaning *nerve glue*.

The nervous system is responsible for coordinating all the activity of the body. To do this, it first receives information from both external and internal **sensory receptors** and then uses that information to adjust the activity of **muscles** and **glands** to match the needs of the body.

The nervous system can be subdivided into the **central nervous system** (CNS) and the **peripheral nervous system** (PNS). The central nervous system consists of the **brain** and **spinal cord**. Sensory information comes into the central nervous system, where it is processed. Motor messages then exit the central nervous system carrying commands to muscles and glands. The **nerves** of the peripheral nervous system are **cranial nerves** and **spinal nerves**. Sensory nerves carry information to the central nervous system, and motor nerves carry commands away from the central nervous system. All portions of the nervous system are composed of nervous tissue.

Nervous Tissue

axon (AK-son)
dendrites (DEN-drights)
myelin (MY-eh-lin)
nerve cell body
neuroglial cells (noo-ROG-lee-al)
neuron (NOO-ron)
neurotransmitter (noo-roh-TRANS-mit-ter)
synapse (SIN-aps)
synaptic cleft (sih-NAP-tik)

What's In A Name?
Look for these word parts:
neur/o = nerve
-tic = pertaining to

Med Term Tip
A synapse is the point at which two nerves contact each other. The term *synapse* comes from the Greek word meaning *connection*.

Nervous tissue consists of two basic types of cells: **neurons** and **neuroglial cells**. Neurons are individual nerve cells. These are the cells that are capable of conducting electrical impulses in response to a stimulus. Neurons have three basic parts: **dendrites**, a **nerve cell body**, and an **axon** (see Figure 12-1A ■). Dendrites are highly branched projections that receive impulses. The nerve cell body contains the nucleus and many of the other organelles of the cell (see Figure 12-1B ■). A neuron has only a single axon, a projection from the nerve cell body that conducts the electrical impulse toward its destination. The point at which the axon of one neuron meets the dendrite of the next neuron is called a **synapse**. Electrical impulses cannot pass directly across the gap between two neurons, called the **synaptic cleft**. They instead require the help of a chemical messenger, called a **neurotransmitter**.

A variety of neuroglial cells are found in nervous tissue. Each has a different support function for the neurons. For example, some neuroglial cells produce **myelin**, a fatty substance that acts as insulation for many axons so that they conduct electrical impulses faster. Neuroglial cells *do not* conduct electrical impulses.

Central Nervous System

gray matter
meninges (men-IN-jeez)
myelinated (MY-eh-lih-nayt-ed)
tracts
white matter

Because the central nervous system is a combination of the brain and spinal cord, it is able to receive impulses from all over the body, process this information, and

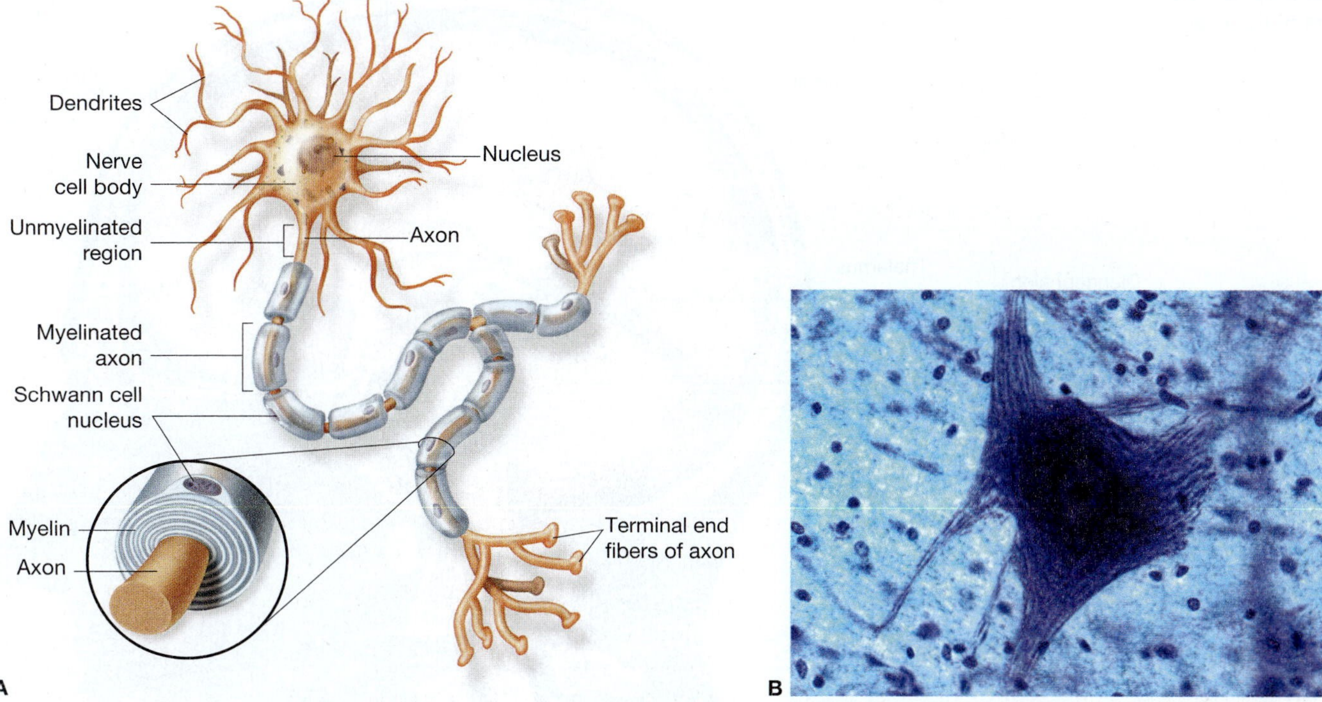

■ **Figure 12-1** A) The structure of a neuron, showing the dendrites, nerve cell body, and axon. B) Photomicrograph of typical neuron showing the nerve cell body, nucleus, and dendrites. *(Christopher Meade/Shutterstock)*

then respond with an action. This system consists of both **gray matter** and **white matter**. Gray matter is comprised of unsheathed or uncovered cell bodies and dendrites. White matter is **myelinated** nerve fibers. The myelin sheath makes the nervous tissue appear white. Bundles of nerve fibers interconnecting different parts of the central nervous system are called **tracts**. The central nervous system is encased and protected by three membranes known as the **meninges**.

Med Term Tip

Myelin is a lipid and a very white molecule. This is why myelinated neurons are called *white matter*.

Brain

brainstem
cerebellum (sair-eh-BELL-um)
cerebral cortex (seh-REE-bral / KOR-teks)
cerebral hemisphere
cerebrospinal fluid (seh-ree-broh-SPY-nal)
cerebrum (seh-REE-brum)
diencephalon (dye-en-SEFF-ah-lon)
frontal lobe
gyri (JYE-rye)
hypothalamus (high-poh-THAL-ah-mus)
medulla oblongata (meh-DULL-ah / ob-long-GAH-tah)
midbrain
occipital lobe (ok-SIP-ih-tal)
parietal lobe (pah-RYE-eh-tal)
pons (PONZ)
sulci (SULL-sigh)
temporal lobe (TEM-por-al)
thalamus (THAL-ah-mus)
ventricles (VEN-trih-kulz)

What's In A Name?

Look for these word parts:
encephal/o = brain
-al = pertaining to
hypo- = below

The brain is one of the largest organs in the body and coordinates most body activities. It is the center for all thought, memory, judgment, and emotion. Each part of the brain is responsible for controlling different body functions, such as temperature regulation, blood pressure, and breathing. There are four sections to the brain: the **cerebrum**, **cerebellum**, **diencephalon**, and **brainstem** (see Figure 12-2 ■).

Located in the upper portion of the brain is the largest section called the cerebrum. It is this area that processes thoughts, judgment, memory, problem solving, and language. The outer layer of the cerebrum is the **cerebral cortex**, which is composed of folds of gray matter. The elevated portions of the cerebrum, or

■ **Figure 12-2** The regions of the brain.

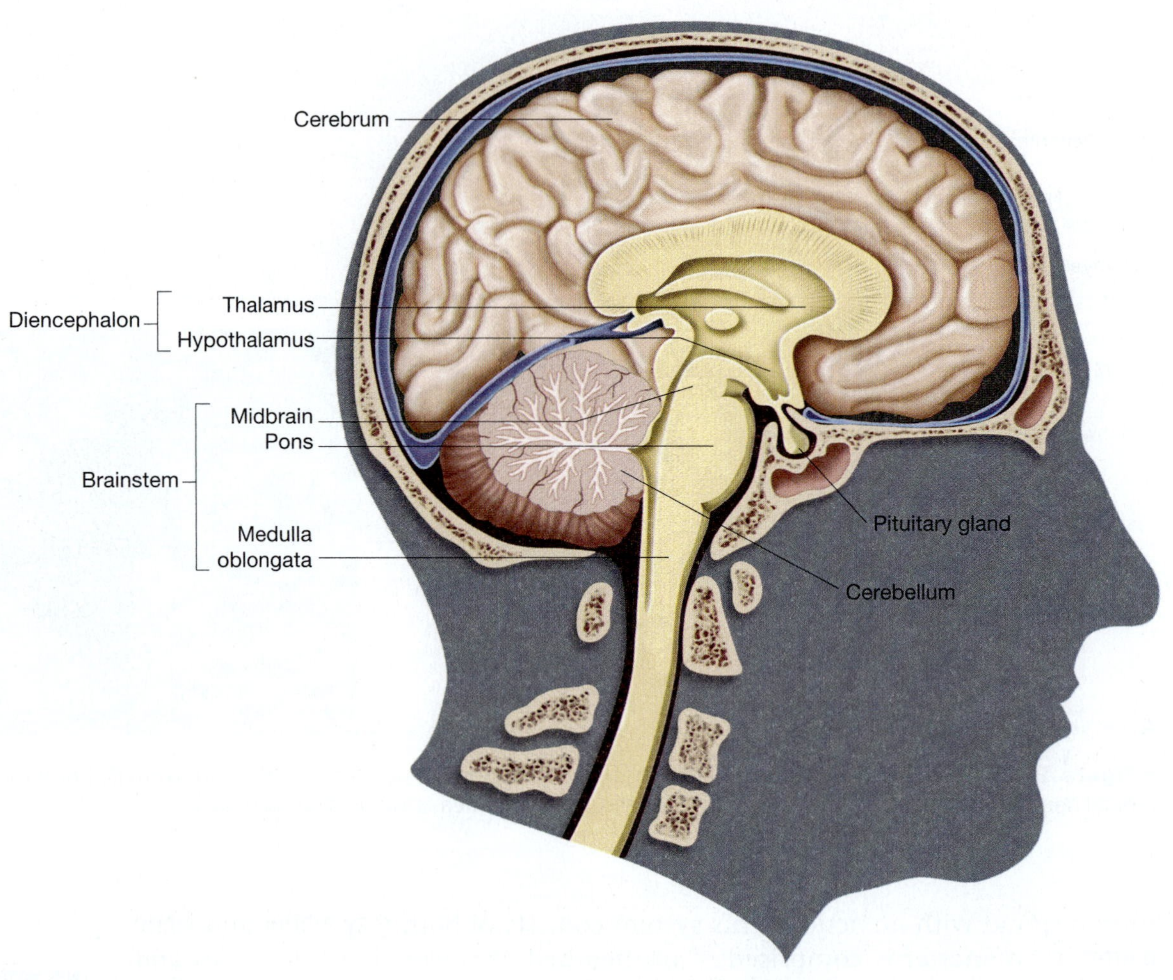

convolutions, are called **gyri** and are separated by fissures, or valleys, called **sulci**. The cerebrum is subdivided into left and right halves called **cerebral hemispheres**. Each hemisphere has four lobes. The lobes and their locations and functions are (see Figure 12-3 ■):

1. **Frontal lobe:** Most anterior portion of the cerebrum; controls motor function, personality, and speech
2. **Parietal lobe:** Most superior portion of the cerebrum; receives and interprets nerve impulses from sensory receptors and interprets language
3. **Occipital lobe:** Most posterior portion of the cerebrum; controls vision
4. **Temporal lobe:** Left and right lateral portion of the cerebrum; controls hearing and smell

The diencephalon, located below the cerebrum, contains two of the most critical areas of the brain, the **thalamus** and the **hypothalamus**. The thalamus is composed of gray matter and acts as a center for relaying impulses from the eyes, ears, and skin to the cerebrum. Pain perception is controlled by the thalamus. The hypothalamus, located just below the thalamus, controls body temperature, appetite, sleep, sexual desire, and emotions. The hypothalamus is actually responsible for controlling the autonomic nervous system, cardiovascular system, digestive system, and the release of hormones from the pituitary gland.

The cerebellum, the second largest portion of the brain, is located beneath the posterior part of the cerebrum. This part of the brain aids in coordinating voluntary body movements and maintaining balance and equilibrium. The cerebellum refines the muscular movement that is initiated in the cerebrum.

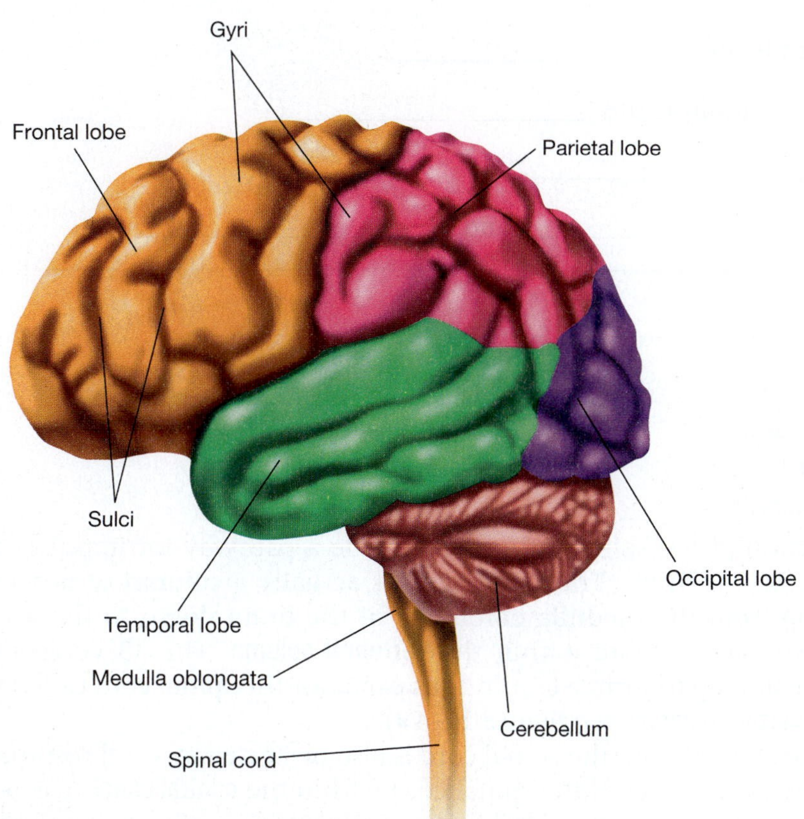

■ **Figure 12-3** The brain; colors indicate the different cerebral lobes. *(Lightspring/Shutterstock)*

The final portion of the brain is the brainstem, which has three components: **midbrain**, **pons**, and **medulla oblongata**. The midbrain acts as a pathway for impulses to be conducted between the brain and the spinal cord. The pons—a term meaning *bridge*—connects the cerebellum to the rest of the brain. The medulla oblongata is the most inferior positioned portion of the brain; it connects the brain to the spinal cord. However, this vital area contains the centers that control respiration, heart rate, temperature, and blood pressure. Additionally, this is the site where nerve tracts cross from one side of the brain to control functions and movement on the other side of the body. In other words, with few exceptions, the left side of the brain controls the right side of the body and vice versa.

The brain has four interconnected cavities called **ventricles**: one in each cerebral hemisphere, one in the thalamus, and one in front of the cerebellum. These contain **cerebrospinal fluid** (CSF), which is the watery, clear fluid that provides protection from shock or sudden motion to the brain and spinal cord.

PRACTICE AS YOU GO

A. Complete the Statement

1. The organs of the central nervous system are the ____________________ and ____________________.
2. The nerves of the peripheral nervous system are either ____________________ nerves or ____________________ nerves.
3. The three basic parts of a neuron are ____________________, ____________________, and ____________________.
4. ____________________ is a fatty substance that insulates some axons.

5. The largest portion of the brain is the ____________________.

6. The second largest portion of the brain is the ____________________.

7. The occipital lobe controls ____________________.

8. The temporal lobe controls ____________________ and ____________________.

Spinal Cord

ascending tracts
central canal
descending tracts
spinal cavity
vertebral canal
vertebral column

> **Med Term Tip**
> Certain disease processes attack the gray matter and the white matter of the central nervous system. For instance, *poliomyelitis* is a viral infection of the gray matter of the spinal cord. The combining term **poli/o** means *gray matter*. This disease has almost been eradicated, due to the polio vaccine.

The function of the spinal cord is to provide a pathway for impulses traveling to and from the brain. The spinal cord is actually a column of nervous tissue extending from the medulla oblongata of the brain down to the level of the second lumbar vertebra within the **vertebral column**. The 33 vertebrae of the backbone line up to form a continuous canal for the spinal cord called the **spinal cavity** or **vertebral canal** (see Figure 12-4 ■).

Similar to the brain, the spinal cord is also protected by cerebrospinal fluid. It flows down the center of the spinal cord within the **central canal**. The inner core of the spinal cord consists of cell bodies and dendrites of peripheral nerves and therefore is gray matter. The outer portion of the spinal cord is myelinated white

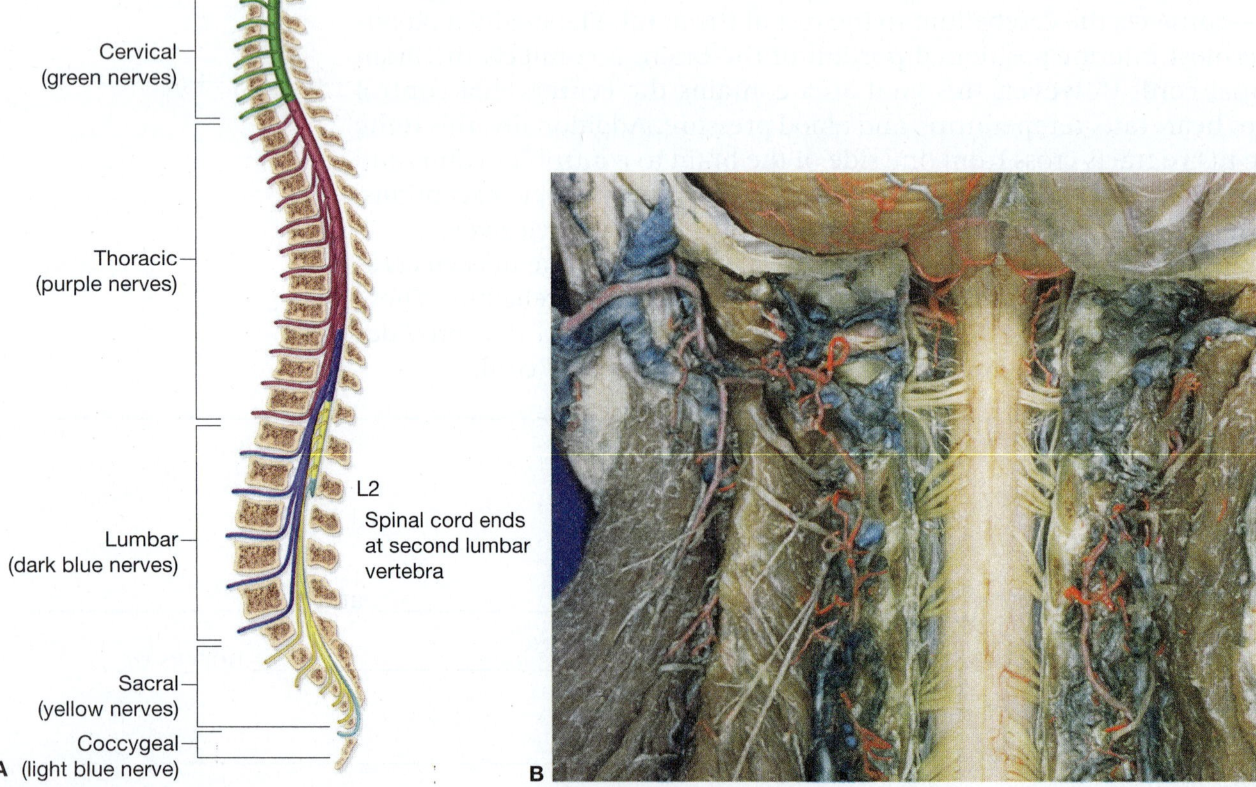

■ **Figure 12-4** A) The levels of the spinal cord and spinal nerves. B) Photograph of the spinal cord as it descends from the brain. The spinal nerve roots are clearly visible branching off from the spinal cord. *(VideoSurgery/Science Source)*

matter. The white matter is either **ascending tracts** carrying sensory information up to the brain or **descending tracts** carrying motor commands down from the brain to a peripheral nerve.

Meninges

arachnoid layer (ah-RAK-noyd)
dura mater (DOO-rah / MAH-ter)
pia mater (PEE-ah / MAH-ter)
subarachnoid space (sub-ah-RAK-noyd)
subdural space (sub-DOO-ral)

What's In A Name?

Look for these word parts:
-oid = resembling
sub- = under

The meninges are three layers of connective tissue membranes surrounding the brain and spinal cord (see Figure 12-5■). Moving from external to internal, the meninges are:

1. **Dura mater:** Meaning *tough mother*; it forms a tough, fibrous sac around the central nervous system
2. **Subdural space:** Actual space between the dura mater and arachnoid layer
3. **Arachnoid layer:** Meaning *spiderlike*; it is a thin, delicate layer attached to the pia mater by weblike filaments
4. **Subarachnoid space:** Space between the arachnoid layer and the pia mater; it contains cerebrospinal fluid that cushions the brain from the outside
5. **Pia mater:** Meaning *soft mother*; it is the innermost membrane layer and is applied directly to the surface of the brain and spinal cord

Peripheral Nervous System

afferent neurons (AF-er-ent)
autonomic nervous system (aw-toh-NOM-ik)
efferent neurons (EF-er-ent)
ganglion (GANG-lee-on)
motor neurons
nerve root
sensory neurons
somatic nerves

What's In A Name?

Look for these word parts:
somat/o = body
-ic = pertaining to
auto- = self

The peripheral nervous system (PNS) includes both the 12 pairs of cranial nerves and the 31 pairs of spinal nerves. A nerve is a group or bundle of axon fibers located outside the central nervous system that carries messages between the central nervous system and the various parts of the body. Whether a nerve is

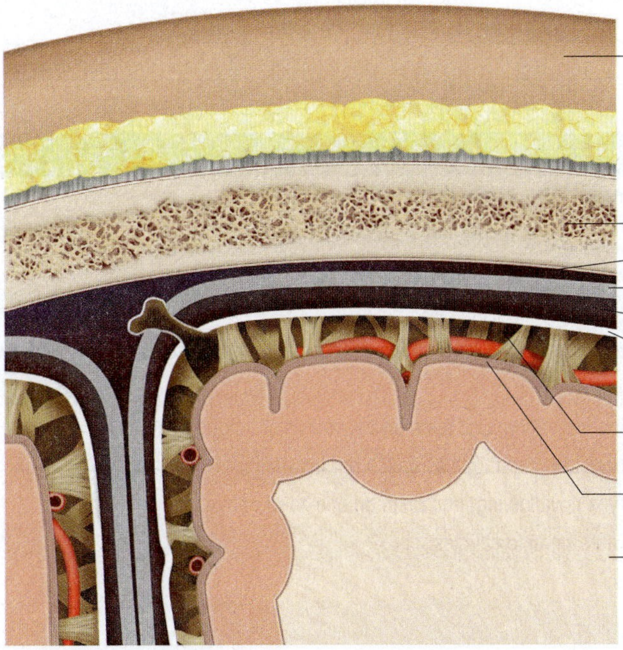

■ **Figure 12-5** The meninges. This figure illustrates the location and structure of each layer of the meninges and their relationship to the skull and brain.

cranial or spinal is determined by where the nerve originates. Cranial nerves arise from the brain, mainly at the medulla oblongata. Spinal nerves split off from the spinal cord, and one pair (a left and a right) exits between each pair of vertebrae. The point where either type of nerve is attached to the central nervous system is called the **nerve root**. The names of most nerves reflect either the organ the nerve serves or the portion of the body the nerve is traveling through. The entire list of cranial nerves is found in Table 12-1 ■. Figure 12-6 ■ illustrates some of the major spinal nerves in the human body.

Med Term Tip

Because nerve tracts cross from one side of the body to the other side of the brain, damage to one side of the brain results in symptoms appearing on the opposite side of the body. Since nerve cells that control the movement of the right side of the body are located in the left side of the medulla oblongata, a stroke that paralyzed the right side of the body would actually have occurred in the left side of the brain.

Although most nerves carry information to and from the central nervous system, individual neurons carry information in only one direction. **Afferent neurons**, also called **sensory neurons**, carry sensory information from a sensory receptor to the central nervous system. **Efferent neurons**, also called **motor neurons**, carry activity instructions from the central nervous system to muscles or glands out in the body (see Figure 12-7 ■). The nerve cell bodies of the neurons forming the nerve are grouped together in a knot-like mass, called a **ganglion**, located outside the central nervous system.

The nerves of the peripheral nervous system are subdivided into two divisions, the **autonomic nervous system** (ANS) and **somatic nerves**, each serving a different area of the body.

Autonomic Nervous System

parasympathetic branch (pair-ah-sim-pah-THET-ik)

sympathetic branch (sim-pah-THET-ik)

Med Term Tip

The term *autonomic* comes from the Latin word *autonomia*, meaning *independent*.

What's In A Name?

Look for these word parts:
-ic = pertaining to
para- = beside

The autonomic nervous system is involved with the control of involuntary or unconscious bodily functions. It may increase or decrease the activity of the smooth muscle found in viscera and blood vessels, cardiac muscle, and glands. The autonomic nervous system is divided into two branches: **sympathetic branch** and **parasympathetic branch**. The sympathetic nerves control the "fight-or-flight" reaction during times of stress and crisis. These nerves increase heart rate, dilate airways, increase blood pressure, inhibit digestion, and stimulate the production of adrenaline during a crisis. The parasympathetic nerves serve as a counterbalance for the sympathetic nerves, the "rest-and-digest" reaction. Therefore, they cause heart rate to slow down, lower blood pressure, and stimulate digestion.

■ **TABLE 12-1** Cranial Nerves

Number	Name	Function
I	Olfactory	Transports impulses for sense of smell
II	Optic	Carries impulses for sense of sight
III	Oculomotor	Motor impulses for eye muscle movement and the pupil of the eye
IV	Trochlear	Controls superior oblique muscle of eye on each side
V	Trigeminal	Carries sensory facial impulses and controls muscles for chewing; branches into eyes, forehead, upper and lower jaw
VI	Abducens	Controls eyeball muscle to turn eye to side
VII	Facial	Controls facial muscles for expression, salivation, and taste on two-thirds of tongue (anterior)
VIII	Vestibulocochlear	Responsible for impulses of equilibrium and hearing; also called *auditory nerve*
IX	Glossopharyngeal	Carries sensory impulses from pharynx (swallowing) and taste on one-third of tongue
X	Vagus	Supplies most organs in abdominal and thoracic cavities
XI	Accessory	Controls neck and shoulder muscles
XII	Hypoglossal	Controls tongue muscles

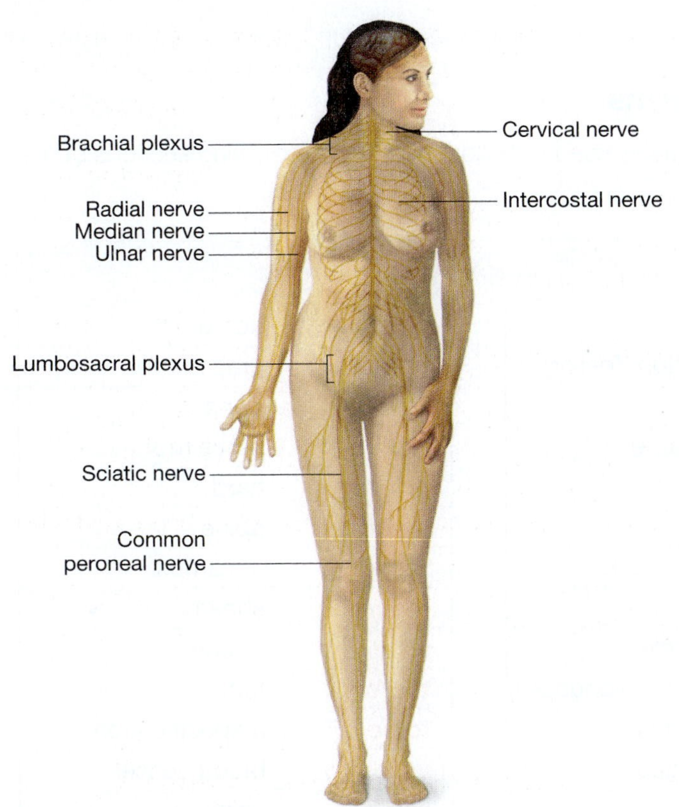

Figure 12-6 The major spinal nerves.

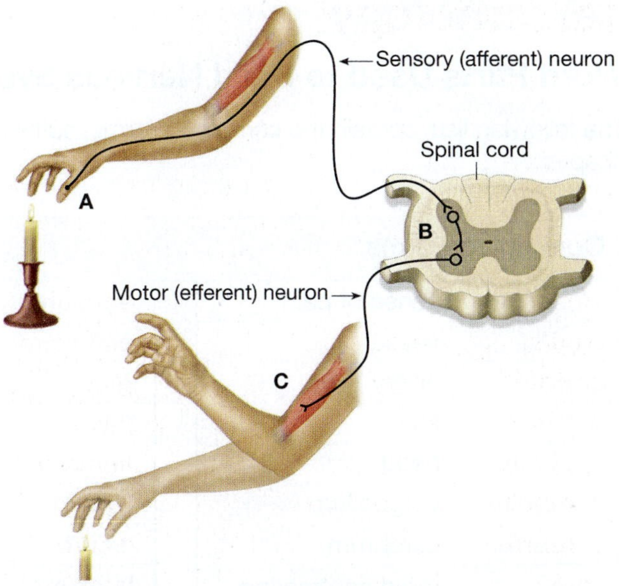

Figure 12-7 The functional structure of the peripheral nervous system. A) Afferent or sensory neurons carry sensory information to the spinal cord. B) The spinal cord receives incoming sensory information and delivers motor messages. C) Efferent or motor neurons deliver motor commands to muscles and glands.

Somatic Nerves

Somatic nerves serve the skin and skeletal muscles and are mainly involved with the conscious and voluntary activities of the body. The large variety of sensory receptors found in the dermis layer of the skin use somatic nerves to send their information, such as touch, temperature, pressure, and pain, to the brain. These are also the nerves that carry motor commands to skeletal muscles.

PRACTICE AS YOU GO

B. Complete the Statement

1. ____________________ tracts of the spinal cord carry sensory information. ____________________ tracts carry motor commands.
2. The neurons that carry impulses away from the brain and spinal cord are called ____________________ neurons and the neurons that carry impulses to the brain and spinal cord are called ____________________ neurons.
3. The tough outer meninges is the ____________________. The spiderlike middle meninges is the ____________________. The delicate inner meninges is the ____________________.
4. The two divisions of the autonomic nervous system are the ____________________ and ____________________.
5. ____________________ nerves serve the skin and skeletal muscles.

Terminology

Word Parts Used to Build Nervous System Terms

The following lists contain the combining forms, suffixes, and prefixes used to build terms in the remaining sections of this chapter.

Combining Forms

Combining Form	Meaning	Combining Form	Meaning	Combining Form	Meaning
alges/o	sense of pain	**encephal/o**	brain	**neur/o**	nerve
angi/o	vessel	**esthesi/o**	sensation, feeling	**poli/o**	gray matter
arteri/o	artery	**gli/o**	glue	**pont/o**	pons
astr/o	star	**hal/o**	to breathe	**radicul/o**	nerve root
cephal/o	head	**hemat/o**	blood	**scler/o**	hard
cerebell/o	cerebellum	**hydr/o**	water	**spin/o**	spine
cerebr/o	cerebrum	**isch/o**	to hold back	**thalam/o**	thalamus
clon/o	rapid contracting and relaxing	**later/o**	side	**thec/o**	sheath
concuss/o	to shake violently	**lumb/o**	low back	**tom/o**	to cut
crani/o	skull	**medull/o**	medulla oblongata	**ton/o**	tone
cutane/o	skin	**mening/o**	meninges	**topic/o**	a specific area
cyt/o	cell	**meningi/o**	meninges	**vascul/o**	blood vessel
dur/o	dura mater	**ment/o**	mind	**ven/o**	vein
electr/o	electricity	**my/o**	muscle	**ventricul/o**	ventricle
		myel/o	spinal cord	**vertebr/o**	vertebra

Suffixes

Suffix	Meaning	Suffix	Meaning	Suffix	Meaning
-al	pertaining to	**-ia**	condition	**-ous**	pertaining to
-algia	pain	**-ic**	pertaining to	**-paresis**	weakness
-ar	pertaining to	**-ical**	pertaining to	**-pathy**	disease
-ary	pertaining to	**-ine**	pertaining to	**-phasia**	speech
-asthenia	weakness	**-ion**	action	**-plasty**	surgical repair
-cele	protrusion	**-itis**	inflammation	**-plegia**	paralysis
-eal	pertaining to	**-logy**	study of	**-rrhaphy**	suture
-ectomy	surgical removal	**-nic**	pertaining to	**-taxia**	muscle coordination
-emic	pertaining to a blood condition	**-oma**	tumor, mass	**-tic**	pertaining to
-gram	record	**-osis**	abnormal condition	**-trophic**	pertaining to development
-graphy	process of recording	**-otomy**	cutting into		

Prefixes

Prefix	Meaning	Prefix	Meaning	Prefix	Meaning
a-	without	**dys-**	abnormal, difficult	**in-**	inward
an-	without	**endo-**	within	**intra-**	within
anti-	against	**epi-**	above	**mono-**	one
bi-	two	**hemi-**	half	**para-**	abnormal, two like parts of a pair
de-	without	**hyper-**	excessive		

Prefixes (continued)

poly-	many
quadri-	four
semi-	partial
sub-	under
trans-	across
tri-	three
un-	not

Adjective Forms of Anatomical Terms

Term	Word Parts	Definition
cephalic (seh-FAL-ik)	**cephal/o** = head **-ic** = pertaining to	Pertaining to head
cerebellar (sair-eh-BELL-ar)	**cerebell/o** = cerebellum **-ar** = pertaining to	Pertaining to cerebellum
cerebral (seh-REE-bral)	**cerebr/o** = cerebrum **-al** = pertaining to	Pertaining to cerebrum
cerebrospinal (seh-ree-broh-SPY-nal)	**cerebr/o** = cerebrum **spin/o** = spine **-al** = pertaining to	Pertaining to cerebrum and spine
cranial (KRAY-nee-al)	**crani/o** = skull **-al** = pertaining to	Pertaining to skull
encephalic (en-seh-FAL-ik)	**encephal/o** = brain **-ic** = pertaining to	Pertaining to brain
intracranial (in-trah-KRAY-nee-al)	**intra-** = within **crani/o** = skull **-al** = pertaining to	Pertaining to within the skull
intrathecal (in-trah-THEE-kal)	**intra-** = within **thec/o** = sheath **-al** = pertaining to	Pertaining to within the meninges (sheath encasing central nervous system), specifically the subdural or subarachnoid space
medullary (MED-yoo-lair-ee)	**medull/o** = medulla oblongata **-ary** = pertaining to	Pertaining to medulla oblongata
meningeal (meh-NIN-jee-al)	**mening/o** = meninges **-eal** = pertaining to	Pertaining to meninges
myelonic (my-eh-LON-ik)	**myel/o** = spinal cord **-nic** = pertaining to	Pertaining to spinal cord
neural (NOO-ral)	**neur/o** = nerve **-al** = pertaining to	Pertaining to nerves
neuroglial (noo-ROG-lee-al)	**neur/o** = nerve **gli/o** = glue **-al** = pertaining to	Pertaining to glial cells that surround and support neurons
pontine (PON-teen)	**pont/o** = pons **-ine** = pertaining to	Pertaining to pons
spinal (SPY-nal)	**spin/o** = spine **-al** = pertaining to	Pertaining to spine
subdural (sub-DOO-ral)	**sub-** = under **dur/o** = dura mater **-al** = pertaining to	Pertaining to under dura mater
thalamic (thah-LAM-ik)	**thalam/o** = thalamus **-ic** = pertaining to	Pertaining to thalamus
ventricular (ven-TRIK-yoo-lar)	**ventricul/o** = ventricle **-ar** = pertaining to	Pertaining to ventricles
vertebral (VER-teh-bral)	**vertebr/o** = vertebra **-al** = pertaining to	Pertaining to vertebrae

PRACTICE AS YOU GO

C. Give the adjective form for each anatomical structure.

1. The cerebrum and spinal cord ____________
2. The meninges ____________
3. Under the dura mater ____________
4. The brain ____________
5. A nerve ____________
6. Within the skull ____________

Pathology

Term	Word Parts	Definition
Medical Specialties		
anesthesiology (an-es-thee-zee-ALL-oh-jee)	an- = without esthesi/o = sensation, feeling -logy = study of	Branch of medicine specializing in all aspects of anesthesia, including for surgical procedures, resuscitation measures, and management of acute and chronic pain; physician is *anesthesiologist*
neurology (noo-RALL-oh-jee)	neur/o = nerve -logy = study of	Branch of medicine concerned with diagnosis and treatment of diseases and conditions of the nervous system; physician is *neurologist*
neurosurgery (noo-roh-SER-jer-ee)	neur/o = nerve	Branch of medicine concerned with treating conditions and diseases of the nervous system by surgical means; physician is *neurosurgeon*
Signs and Symptoms		
absence seizure		Type of epileptic seizure that lasts only a few seconds to half a minute, characterized by loss of awareness and absence of activity; also known as *petit mal seizure*
analgesia (an-al-JEE-zee-ah)	an- = without alges/o = sense of pain -ia = condition	Absence of pain
anesthesia (an-es-THEE-zha)	an- = without esthesi/o = feeling, sensation -ia = condition	Condition in which there is lack of feeling or sensation
aphasia (ah-FAY-zee-ah)	a- = without -phasia = speech	Inability to communicate verbally or in writing due to damage of speech or language centers in the brain
ataxia (ah-TAK-see-ah)	a- = without -taxia = muscle coordination	Lack of muscle coordination
aura (AW-ruh)		Sensations, such as seeing colors or smelling an unusual odor, that occur just prior to epileptic seizure or migraine headache

Pathology (continued)

Term	Word Parts	Definition
cephalalgia (seff-al-AL-jee-ah)	cephal/o = head -algia = pain	Headache (HA)
coma (KOH-mah)		Profound unconsciousness resulting from illness or injury
conscious (KON-shus)		Condition of being awake and aware of surroundings
convulsion (kon-VUL-shun)		Severe involuntary muscle contractions and relaxations; have a variety of causes, such as epilepsy, fever, and toxic conditions
delirium (deh-LEER-ee-um)	de- = without	Abnormal mental state characterized by confusion, disorientation, and agitation
dementia (deh-MEN-sha)	de- = without ment/o = mind -ia = condition	Progressive impairment of intellectual function that interferes with performing activities of daily living; patients have little awareness of their condition; found in disorders such as Alzheimer's
dysphasia (dis-FAY-zee-ah)	dys- = abnormal, difficult -phasia = speech	Difficulty communicating verbally or in writing due to damage of speech or language centers in the brain
focal seizure (FOH-kal)	-al = pertaining to	Localized seizure often affecting one limb
hemiparesis (hem-ee-pah-REE-sis)	hemi- = half -paresis = weakness	Weakness or loss of motion on one side of the body
hemiplegia (hem-ee-PLEE-jee-ah)	hemi- = half -plegia = paralysis	Paralysis on only one side of the body
hyperesthesia (high-per-es-THEE-zee-ah)	hyper- = excessive esthesi/o = feeling, sensation -ia = condition	Condition of abnormally heightened sense of feeling, sense of pain, or sensitivity to touch
monoparesis (mon-oh-pah-REE-sis)	mono- = one -paresis = weakness	Muscle weakness in one limb
monoplegia (mon-oh-PLEE-jee-ah)	mono- = one -plegia = paralysis	Paralysis of one limb
neuralgia (noo-RAL-jee-ah)	neur/o = nerve -algia = pain	Nerve pain
palsy (PAWL-zee)		Temporary or permanent loss of ability to control movement
paralysis (pah-RAL-ih-sis)		Temporary or permanent loss of function or voluntary movement
paraplegia (pair-ah-PLEE-jee-ah)	para- = two like parts of a pair -plegia = paralysis	Paralysis of lower portion of the body and both legs (the two like parts of a pair)
paresthesia (pair-es-THEE-zee-ah)	para- = abnormal esthesi/o = sensation, feeling -ia = condition	Abnormal sensation such as burning or tingling
quadriplegia (kwod-rih-PLEE-jee-ah)	quadri- = four -plegia = paralysis	Paralysis of all four limbs
seizure (SEE-zyoor)		Sudden, uncontrollable onset of symptoms, such as in epileptic seizure

Pathology (continued)

Term	Word Parts	Definition
semiconscious (sem-ee-KON-shus)	semi- = partial	State of being aware of surroundings and responding to stimuli only part of the time
syncope (SIN-koh-pee)		Fainting
tonic-clonic seizure	ton/o = tone clon/o = rapid contracting and relaxing -ic = pertaining to	Type of severe epileptic seizure characterized by loss of consciousness and convulsions; seizure alternates between strong continuous muscle spasms (tonic) and rhythmic muscle contraction and relaxation (clonic); also known as *grand mal seizure*
tremor (TREM-or)		Involuntary, repetitive, alternating movement of a part of the body
unconscious (un-KON-shus)	un- = not	State of being unaware of surroundings, with the inability to respond to stimuli
Brain		
Alzheimer's disease (AD) (ALTS-high-merz)		Chronic, organic mental disorder consisting of dementia, which is more prevalent in adults after age 65; involves progressive disorientation, apathy, speech and gait disturbances, and loss of memory; named for German neurologist Alois Alzheimer
anencephaly (an-en-SEFF-ah-lee)	an- = without encephal/o = brain	Congenital defect in which portions of the brain (usually the cerebrum) do not develop; child born with condition is missing a portion of the brain, cranium, and scalp; condition usually fatal within a few hours of birth
astrocytoma (ass-troh-sigh-TOH-mah)	astr/o = star cyt/o = cell -oma = tumor	Tumor of brain or spinal cord composed of astrocytes, one type of neuroglial cells that has arms projecting off it like a star
brain tumor ■ **Figure 12-8** CT scan showing large malignant tumor in left hemisphere of the brain. *(Puwadol Jaturawutthichai/Shutterstock)*		Intracranial mass, either benign or malignant; benign tumor of the brain can still be fatal since it will grow and cause pressure on normal brain tissue
cerebellitis (sair-eh-bell-EYE-tis)	cerebell/o = cerebellum -itis = inflammation	Inflammation of the cerebellum
cerebral aneurysm (AN-yoo-rizm)	cerebr/o = cerebrum -al = pertaining to	Localized abnormal dilation of blood vessel, usually artery; result of congenital defect or weakness in wall of vessel; ruptured aneurysm is common cause of hemorrhagic cerebrovascular accident (see Figure 12-9■)

Pathology (continued)

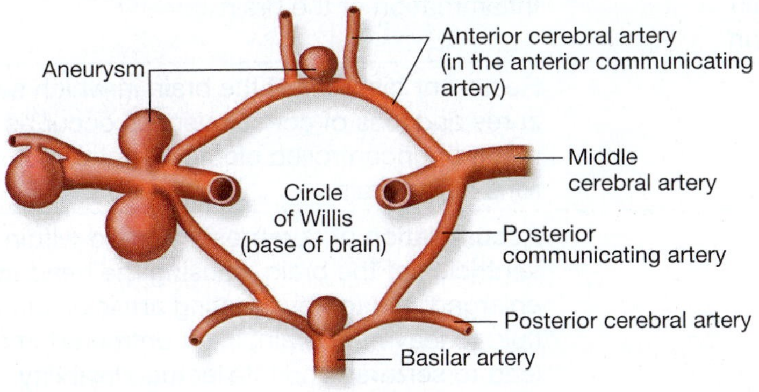

Term	Word Parts	Definition
Aneurysm; Anterior cerebral artery (in the anterior communicating artery); Middle cerebral artery; Circle of Willis (base of brain); Posterior communicating artery; Posterior cerebral artery; Basilar artery		■ **Figure 12-9** Common locations for cerebral artery aneurysms in the Circle of Willis, also called the *cerebral arterial circle*.
cerebral contusion (kon-TOO-zhun)	cerebr/o = cerebrum -al = pertaining to	Bruising of the brain from blow or impact
cerebral palsy (CP) (seh-REE-bral / PAWL-zee)	cerebr/o = cerebrum -al = pertaining to	Brain damage resulting from defect, trauma, infection, or lack of oxygen before, during, or shortly after birth
cerebrovascular accident (CVA) (seh-ree-broh-VAS-kyoo-lar)	cerebr/o = cerebrum vascul/o = blood vessel -ar = pertaining to	Development of infarct due to loss in blood supply to area of the brain; blood flow can be interrupted by ruptured blood vessel (hemorrhage), floating clot (embolus), stationary clot (thrombosis), or compression; extent of damage depends on size and location of infarct and often includes dysphasia and hemiplegia; commonly called *stroke*
Cerebral hemorrhage: Cerebral artery ruptures and bleeds into brain tissue. Cerebral thrombosis: Blood clot forms in cerebral artery and blocks blood flow.	Cerebral embolism: Embolus from another area lodges in cerebral artery and blocks blood flow. Compression: Pressure from tumor squeezes adjacent blood vessel and blocks blood flow.	■ **Figure 12-10** The four common causes of cerebrovascular accidents.
chronic traumatic encephalopathy (CTE) (en-seff-ah-LOP-ah-thee)	encephal/o = brain -pathy = disease	Condition characterized by severe blow or repeated less severe blows to the head resulting in progressive degeneration of brain tissue; initially recognized only in boxing, has now been identified in athletes of all contact sports
concussion (kon-KUSH-un)	concuss/o = to shake violently -ion = action	Injury to the brain resulting from the brain being shaken inside the skull from blow or impact; symptoms vary and may include headache, blurred vision, nausea or vomiting, dizziness, and balance problems; also called *mild traumatic brain injury (TBI)*

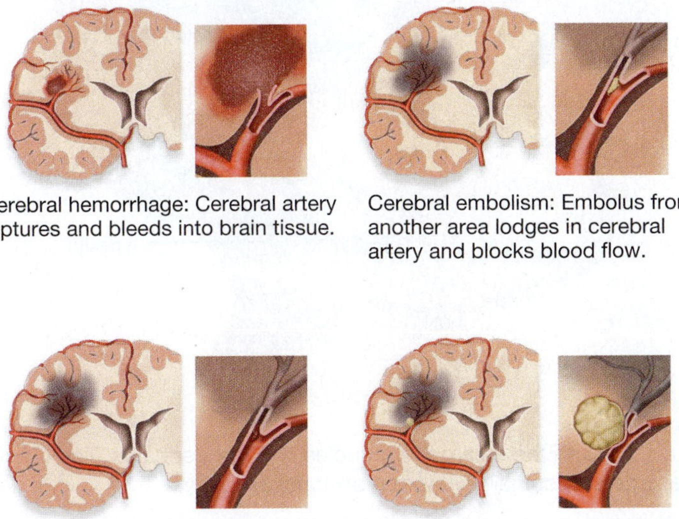

Pathology (continued)

Term	Word Parts	Definition
encephalitis (en-seff-ah-LYE-tis)	encephal/o = brain -itis = inflammation	Inflammation of the brain
epilepsy (EP-ih-lep-see)		Recurrent disorder of the brain in which seizures and loss of consciousness occur as result of uncontrolled electrical activity of neurons in the brain
hydrocephalus (high-droh-SEFF-ah-lus)	hydr/o = water cephal/o = head	Accumulation of cerebrospinal fluid within ventricles of the brain, causing the head to be enlarged; treated by creating artificial shunt for fluid to leave the brain; if left untreated, may lead to seizures and intellectual disability

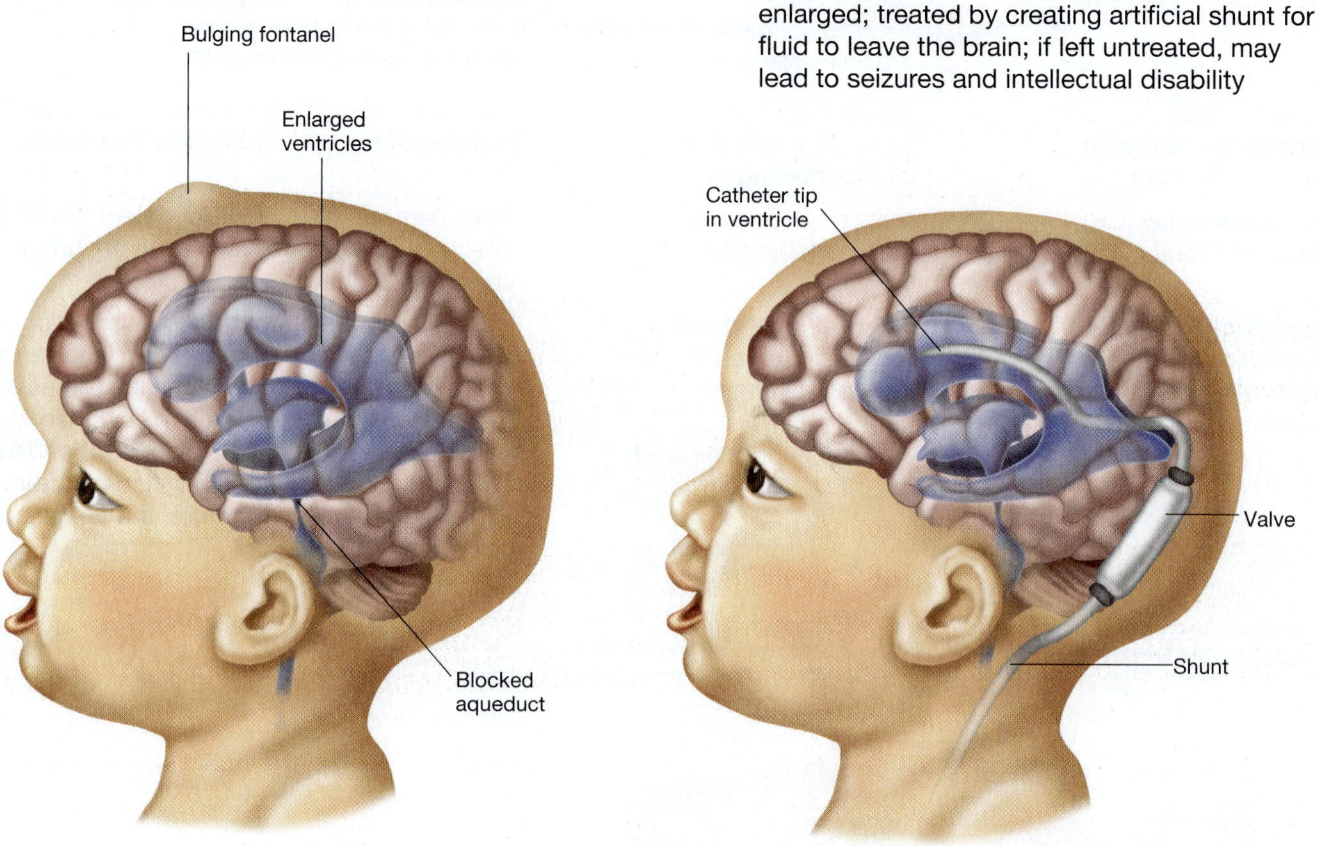

Figure 12-11 Hydrocephalus. The figure on the left is a child with the enlarged ventricles of hydrocephalus. The figure on the right is the same child with a shunt to send the excess cerebrospinal fluid to the abdominal cavity.

Term	Word Parts	Definition
migraine (MY-grain)		Specific type of headache characterized by severe head pain, sensitivity to light, dizziness, and nausea
Parkinson's disease (PARK-in-sons)		Chronic disorder of the nervous system with fine tremors, muscular weakness, rigidity, and shuffling gait; named for British physician James Parkinson
Reye's syndrome (RISE / SIN-drohm)		Combination of symptoms first recognized by Australian pathologist R. D. K. Reye that includes acute encephalopathy and damage to various organs, especially the liver; occurs in children under age 15 who have had a viral infection; also associated with taking aspirin; for this reason, it's not recommended for children to use aspirin

Pathology (continued)

Term	Word Parts	Definition
shaken baby syndrome (SBS)		Caused by violent shaking of infant or toddler; symptoms may include subdural hematoma, brain swelling, and bleeding in retina of the eyes; usually no evidence of external trauma; also called *abusive head trauma (AHT)*
transient ischemic attack (TIA) (TRAN-zee-ent / iss-KEEM-ik)	isch/o = to hold back -emic = pertaining to a blood condition	Temporary interference with blood supply to the brain, causing neurological symptoms such as dizziness, numbness, and hemiparesis; may eventually lead to full-blown stroke (cerebrovascular accident)
traumatic brain injury (TBI)	-tic = pertaining to	Damage to the brain resulting from impact (such as car accident), blast waves (such as an explosion), or penetrating projectile (such as a bullet); symptoms may be mild, moderate, or severe and may include loss of consciousness, headache, vomiting, loss of motor coordination, and dizziness
Spinal Cord		
amyotrophic lateral sclerosis (ALS) (ay-my-oh-TROH-fik / LAT-er-al / skleh-ROH-sis)	a- = without my/o = muscle -trophic = pertaining to development later/o = side -al = pertaining to scler/o = hard -osis = abnormal condition	Condition with muscular weakness and atrophy due to degeneration of motor neurons of the spinal cord; also called *Lou Gehrig's disease*, after New York Yankees baseball player who died from this disease
meningocele (meh-NIN-goh-seel)	mening/o = meninges -cele = protrusion	Congenital condition in which the meninges protrude through opening in the vertebral column (see Figure 12-12A ■); see *spina bifida*
myelitis (my-eh-LYE-tis)	myel/o = spinal cord -itis = inflammation	Inflammation of the spinal cord
myelomeningocele (my-eh-loh-meh-NIN-goh-seel)	myel/o = spinal cord mening/o = meninges -cele = protrusion	Congenital condition in which meninges and spinal cord protrude through opening in the vertebral column (see Figure 12-12B ■); see *spina bifida*
poliomyelitis (poh-lee-oh-my-eh-LYE-tis)	poli/o = gray matter myel/o = spinal cord -itis = inflammation	Viral inflammation of gray matter of the spinal cord; results in varying degrees of paralysis; may be mild and reversible or may be severe and permanent; disease has been almost eliminated due to discovery of vaccine in the 1950s
spina bifida (SPY-nah / BIF-ih-dah)	spin/o = spine bi- = two	Congenital defect in walls of the spinal canal in which laminae of the vertebra do not meet or close (see Figure 12-12C ■); may result in meningocele or myelomeningocele—meninges or the spinal cord being pushed through opening

Pathology (continued)

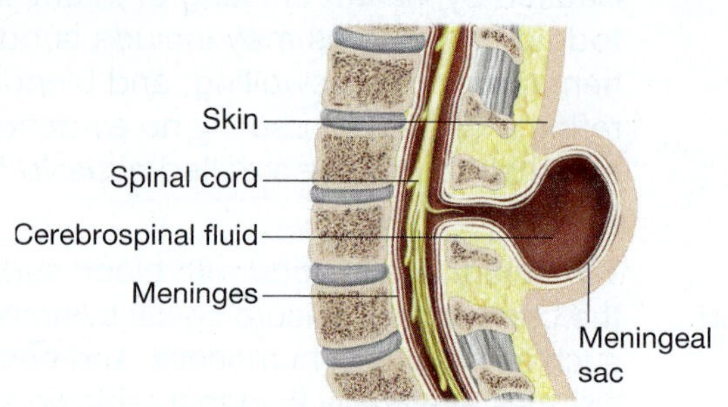

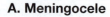

Skin
Spinal cord
Cerebrospinal fluid
Spinal cord and spinal nerves in meningeal sac
B. Myelomeningocele

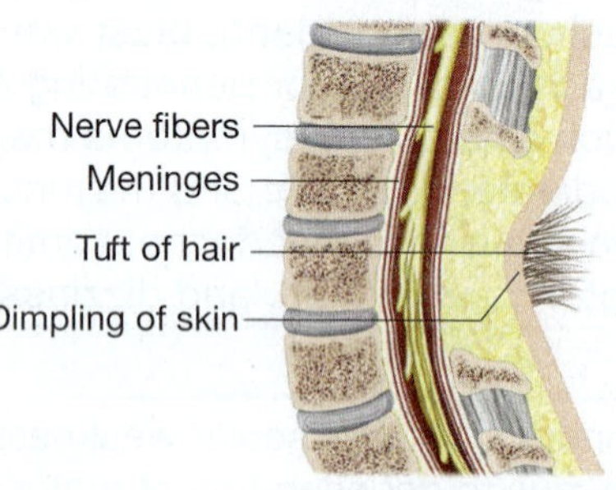

■ Figure 12-12 A) Meningocele, the meninges sac protrudes through the opening in the vertebra.
B) Myelomeningocele, the meninges sac and spinal cord protrude through the opening in the vertebra.
C) Spina bifida occulta, the vertebra is not complete, but there is no protrusion of nervous system structures.

Term	Word Parts	Definition
spinal cord injury (SCI)	**spin/o** = spine **-al** = pertaining to	Damage to the spinal cord as result of trauma; spinal cord may be bruised or completely severed
Nerves		
Bell's palsy (BELLZ / PAWL-zee)		One-sided facial paralysis due to inflammation of facial nerve, probably viral in nature; patient cannot control salivation, tearing of the eyes, or expression, but most will eventually recover
Guillain-Barré syndrome (GHEE-yan / bah-RAY)		Disease of the nervous system in which nerves lose their myelin covering; may be caused by autoimmune reaction; characterized by loss of sensation and/or muscle control starting in the legs; symptoms then move toward trunk and may even result in paralysis of the diaphragm
multiple sclerosis (MS) (MULL-tih-pl / skleh-ROH-sis)	**scler/o** = hard **-osis** = abnormal condition	Inflammatory disease of the central nervous system in which there is extreme weakness and numbness due to loss of myelin insulation from around nerves that result in "hard" patches called plaques to appear
myasthenia gravis (my-as-THEE-nee-ah / GRAV-iss)	**my/o** = muscle **-asthenia** = weakness	Disease with severe muscular weakness and fatigue due to insufficient neurotransmitter at a synapse
neuroma (noo-ROH-mah)	**neur/o** = nerve **-oma** = tumor	Nerve tumor or tumor of connective tissue sheath around a nerve
neuropathy (noo-ROP-ah-thee)	**neur/o** = nerve **-pathy** = disease	General term for disease or damage to a nerve

Pathology (continued)

Term	Word Parts	Definition
polyneuritis (pol-ee-noo-RYE-tis)	poly- = many neur/o = nerve -itis = inflammation	Inflammation of two or more nerves
radiculitis (rah-dik-yoo-LYE-tis)	radicul/o = nerve root -itis = inflammation	Inflammation of a nerve root; may be caused by herniated nucleus pulposus
radiculopathy (rah-dik-yoo-LOP-ah-thee)	radicul/o = nerve root -pathy = disease	Refers to condition that occurs when a herniated nucleus pulposus puts pressure on a nerve root; symptoms include pain and numbness along path of affected nerve
shingles (SHING-lz)		Eruption of painful blisters on body along a nerve path caused by *Herpes zoster* virus infection of nerve root; virus initially introduced into body during chickenpox infection but becomes dormant in nerve cells; reactivation of virus later in life results in shingles **Figure 12-13** Photograph of the skin eruptions associated with shingles. *(Stephen VanHorn/Shutterstock)*
trigeminal neuralgia (trye-JEM-ih-nal / noo-RAL-jee-ah)	tri- = three -al = pertaining to neur/o = nerve -algia = pain	Chronic disorder characterized by sudden, sharp pain on one side of face in area served by the trigeminal cranial nerve; usually caused by pressure on and irritation of nerve or may be sign of multiple sclerosis; also called *tic douloureux*
Meninges		
epidural hematoma (ep-ih-DOO-ral / hee-mah-TOH-mah)	epi- = above dur/o = dura mater -al = pertaining to hemat/o = blood -oma = mass	Mass of blood in space outside the dura mater of the brain and spinal cord
meningioma (meh-nin-jee-OH-mah)	meningi/o = meninges -oma = tumor	Tumor in the meninges
meningitis (men-in-JYE-tis)	mening/o = meninges -itis = inflammation	Inflammation of the meninges around brain or spinal cord caused by bacterial or viral infection; symptoms include fever, headache, neck stiffness, lethargy, vomiting, irritability, and photophobia

Pathology (continued)

Term	Word Parts	Definition
subdural hematoma (sub-DOO-ral / hee-mah-TOH-mah)	sub- = under dur/o = dura mater -al = pertaining to hemat/o = blood -oma = mass	Mass of blood forming beneath the dura mater if the meninges are torn by trauma; may exert fatal pressure on the brain if hematoma not drained by surgery

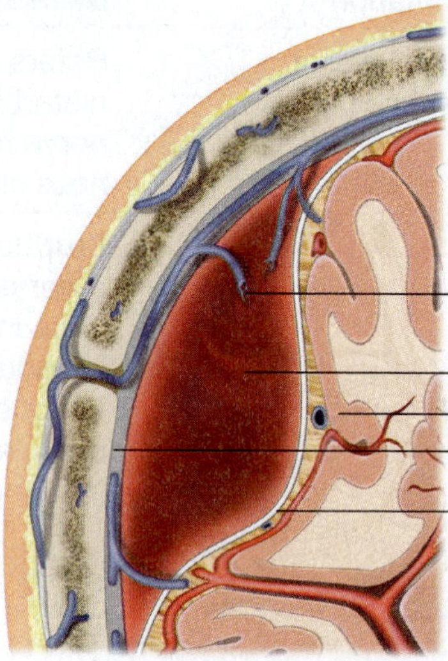

■ **Figure 12-14** A subdural hematoma. A meningeal vein is ruptured and blood has accumulated in the subdural space, producing pressure on the brain.

PRACTICE AS YOU GO

D. Pathology Matching

Match each pathology term to its definition.

1. ________ aura

2. ________ meningitis

3. ________ coma

4. ________ shingles

5. ________ syncope

6. ________ palsy

7. ________ absence seizure

8. ________ tonic-clonic seizure

9. ________ meningocele

10. ________ concussion

a. mild traumatic brain injury

b. sensations before a seizure

c. seizure with convulsions

d. congenital hernia of meninges

e. seizure without convulsion

f. inflammation of meninges

g. profound unconsciousness

h. *Herpes zoster* infection

i. fainting

j. loss of ability to control movement

Diagnostic Procedures

Term	Word Parts	Definition
Clinical Laboratory Tests		
cerebrospinal fluid analysis (seh-ree-broh-SPY-nal / ah-NAL-ih-sis)	cerebr/o = cerebrum spin/o = spine -al = pertaining to	Laboratory examination of clear, watery, colorless fluid from within brain and spinal cord; infections and abnormal presence of blood can be detected in this test
Diagnostic Imaging		
brain scan		Image of the brain taken after injection of radioactive isotopes into circulation
cerebral angiography (seh-REE-bral / an-jee-OG-rah-fee)	cerebr/o = cerebrum -al = pertaining to angi/o = vessel -graphy = process of recording	X-ray of blood vessels of the brain after injection of radiopaque dye
computed tomography scan (CT scan) (toh-MOG-rah-fee)	tom/o = to cut -graphy = process of recording	Imaging technique able to produce cross-sectional view of body; X-ray pictures are taken at multiple angles through body; computer then uses these images to construct composite cross-section; see again Figure 12-8 for example of CT scan showing brain tumor
echoencephalography (ek-oh-en-seff-ah-LOG-rah-fee)	encephal/o = brain -graphy = process of recording	Recording of ultrasonic echoes of the brain; useful in determining abnormal patterns of shifting in the brain
myelogram (MY-eh-loh-gram)	myel/o = spinal cord -gram = record	X-ray record of the spinal cord
myelography (my-eh-LOG-rah-fee)	myel/o = spinal cord -graphy = process of recording	Injection of radiopaque dye into the spinal canal; X-ray is then taken to examine normal and abnormal outlines made by dye
positron emission tomography (PET) (POZ-ih-tron / ee-MISH-un / toh-MOG-rah-fee)	tom/o = to cut -graphy = process of recording	Image of the brain cut along a plane produced by measuring gamma rays emitted from the brain after injecting glucose tagged with positively charged isotopes; measurement of glucose uptake by brain tissue indicates measurement of metabolic activity
Additional Diagnostic Tests		
Babinski's reflex (bah-BIN-skeez)		Reflex test developed by French neurologist Joseph Babinski to determine lesions and abnormalities in the nervous system; Babinski's reflex is present if great toe extends instead of flexes when lateral sole of the foot is stroked; normal response to this stimulation is flexion of the toe
electroencephalogram (EEG) (ee-lek-troh-en-SEFF-ah-loh-gram)	electr/o = electricity encephal/o = brain -gram = record	Record of the brain's electrical patterns
electroencephalography (EEG) (ee-lek-troh-en-seff-ah-LOG-rah-fee)	electr/o = electricity encephal/o = brain -graphy = process of recording	Recording electrical activity of the brain by placing electrodes at various positions on the scalp; also used in sleep studies to determine if there is a normal pattern of activity during sleep

Diagnostic Procedures (continued)

Term	Word Parts	Definition
lumbar puncture (LP) (LUM-bar / PUNK-chur)	**lumb/o** = low back **-ar** = pertaining to	Puncture with needle into lumbar area (usually fourth intervertebral space) to withdraw fluid for examination and for injection of anesthesia; also called *spinal puncture* or *spinal tap*
nerve conduction velocity		Test to determine if nerves have been damaged by recording rate an electrical impulse is able to travel along a nerve; if nerve is damaged, velocity will be decreased

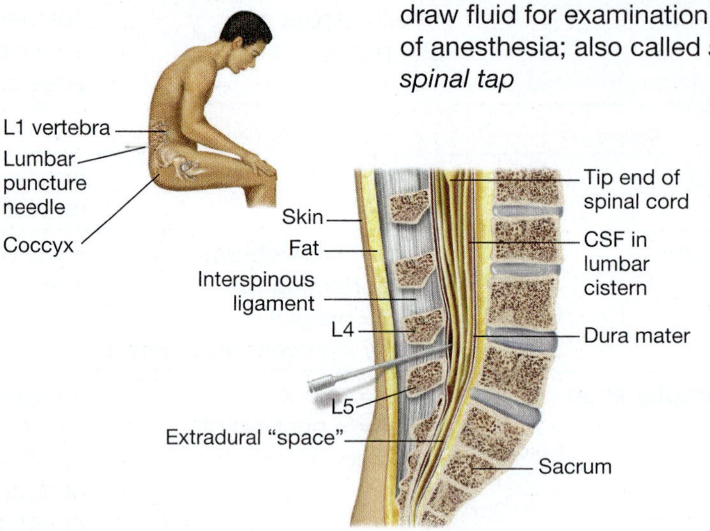

■ **Figure 12-15**
A lumbar puncture. The needle is inserted between the lumbar vertebrae and into the spinal canal.

Therapeutic Procedures

Term	Word Parts	Definition
Anesthesia		
anesthesia (an-es-THEE-zha)	**an-** = without **esthesi/o** = sensation, feeling **-ia** = condition	Administering medication to produce loss of feeling or sensation
general anesthesia (GA) (an-es-THEE-zha)		Produces loss of consciousness including absence of pain sensation; patient's vital signs (VS)—heart rate, breathing rate, pulse, and blood pressure—are carefully monitored when using general anesthetic
inhalation anesthesia (in-hah-LAY-shun / an-es-THEE-zha)	**in-** = inward **hal/o** = to breathe	Route for administering general anesthesia by breathing it in
intravenous (IV) **anesthesia** (in-trah-VEE-nus / an-es-THEE-zha)	**intra-** = within **ven/o** = vein **-ous** = pertaining to	Route for administering general anesthesia via injection into vein
local anesthesia (an-es-THEE-zha)	**-al** = pertaining to	Produces loss of sensation in one localized part of body; patient remains conscious
regional anesthesia (an-es-THEE-zha)	**-al** = pertaining to	Interrupts patient's pain sensation in region of body, such as the arm; anesthetic is injected near nerve that will be blocked from sensation; also called *nerve block*

Therapeutic Procedures (continued)

Term	Word Parts	Definition
subcutaneous anesthesia (sub-kyoo-TAY-nee-us / an-es-THEE-zha)	**sub-** = under **cutane/o** = skin **-ous** = pertaining to	Method of applying local anesthesia involving injecting anesthetic under the skin; for example, used to deaden skin prior to suturing a laceration
topical anesthesia (TOP-ih-kal / an-es-THEE-zha)	**topic/o** = a specific area **-al** = pertaining to	Method of applying local anesthesia involving placing liquid or gel directly onto specific area of skin; for example, used on the skin, cornea, or gums
Medical Procedures		
nerve block		Injection of regional anesthetic to stop passage of sensory or pain impulses along a nerve path
transcutaneous electrical nerve stimulation (TENS) (trans-kyoo-TAY-nee-us)	**trans-** = across **cutane/o** = skin **-ous** = pertaining to **electr/o** = electricity **-ical** = pertaining to	Application of mild electrical current by device with electrodes placed on skin over a painful area; relieves pain by interfering with nerve signal to the brain on pain nerve
Surgical Procedures		
carotid endarterectomy (kah-ROT-id / end-ar-teh-REK-toh-mee)	**endo-** = within **arteri/o** = artery **-ectomy** = surgical removal	Surgical procedure for removing obstruction within carotid artery, a major artery in the neck that carries oxygenated blood to the brain; developed to prevent strokes, but is found to be useful only in severe stenosis with transient ischemic attack
cerebrospinal fluid shunt (seh-ree-broh-SPY-nal)	**cerebr/o** = cerebrum **spin/o** = spine **-al** = pertaining to	Surgical procedure in which bypass is created to drain cerebrospinal fluid; used to treat hydrocephalus by draining excess cerebrospinal fluid from the brain and diverting it to abdominal cavity
laminectomy (lam-ih-NEK-toh-mee)	**-ectomy** = surgical removal	Removal of a portion of a vertebra, called the *lamina*, in order to relieve pressure on spinal nerve
neurectomy (noo-REK-toh-mee)	**neur/o** = nerve **-ectomy** = surgical removal	Surgical removal of a nerve
neuroplasty (NOOR-oh-plas-tee)	**neur/o** = nerve **-plasty** = surgical repair	Surgical repair of a nerve
neurorrhaphy (noo-ROR-ah-fee)	**neur/o** = nerve **-rrhaphy** = suture	To suture a nerve back together; actually refers to suturing connective tissue sheath around the nerve
tractotomy (trak-TOT-oh-mee)	**-otomy** = cutting into	Precision cutting of a nerve tract in the spinal cord; used to treat intractable pain or muscle spasms

PRACTICE AS YOU GO

E. Procedure Matching

Match each procedure term with its definition.

1. ________ brain scan
2. ________ lumbar puncture
3. ________ cerebral angiography
4. ________ EEG
5. ________ PET scan
6. ________ nerve block
7. ________ neurorrhaphy
8. ________ myelogram

a. image made by measuring gamma rays
b. record of brain's electrical activity
c. obtains CSF from around spinal cord
d. regional injection of anesthetic
e. diagnostic image made with radioactive isotopes
f. X-ray of spinal cord
g. X-ray of brain's blood vessels
h. suture together sheath around a nerve

Pharmacology

Classification	Word Parts	Action	Examples
analgesic (an-al-JEE-zik)	an- = without alges/o = sense of pain -ic = pertaining to	Treats minor to moderate pain without loss of consciousness	aspirin, Bayer, Ecotrin; acetaminophen, Tylenol; ibuprofen, Motrin
anesthetic (an-es-THET-ik)	an- = without esthesi/o = feeling, sensation -tic = pertaining to	Produces loss of sensation or loss of consciousness	lidocaine, Xylocaine; pentobarbital, Nembutal; propofol, Diprivan; procaine, Novocain
anticonvulsant (an-tye-kon-VUL-sant)	anti- = against	Reduces excitability of neurons and therefore prevents uncontrolled neuron activity associated with seizures	carbamazepine, Tegretol; phenobarbital, Nembutal
dopaminergic drugs (doh-pah-men-ER-jik)	-ic = pertaining to	Treat Parkinson's disease by either replacing dopamine that is lacking or increasing strength of dopamine that is present	levodopa; L-dopa, Larodopa; levodopa/carbidopa, Sinemet
hypnotic (hip-NOT-ik)	-ic = pertaining to	Promotes sleep	secobarbital, Seconal; temazepam, Restoril
narcotic analgesic (nar-KOT-ik)	-ic = pertaining to an- = without alges/o = sense of pain -ic = pertaining to	Treats severe pain; has potential to be habit forming if taken for prolonged time; also called *opiate*	morphine, MS Contin; oxycodone, OxyContin; meperidine, Demerol
sedative (SED-ah-tiv)		Has relaxing or calming effect	amobarbital, Amytal; butabarbital, Butisol

Abbreviations

AD	Alzheimer's disease	**ICP**	intracranial pressure
AHT	abusive head trauma	**IV**	intravenous
ALS	amyotrophic lateral sclerosis	**LP**	lumbar puncture
ANS	autonomic nervous system	**MS**	multiple sclerosis
CNS	central nervous system	**PET**	positron emission tomography
CP	cerebral palsy	**PNS**	peripheral nervous system
CSF	cerebrospinal fluid	**SBS**	shaken baby syndrome
CTE	chronic traumatic encephalopathy	**SCI**	spinal cord injury
CVA	cerebrovascular accident	**TBI**	traumatic brain injury
CVD	cerebrovascular disease	**TENS**	transcutaneous electrical nerve stimulation
EEG	electroencephalogram, electroencephalography	**TIA**	transient ischemic attack
GA	general anesthesia	**VS**	vital signs
HA	headache		

PRACTICE AS YOU GO

F. What's the Abbreviation?

1. cerebrospinal fluid __________
2. cerebrovascular disease __________
3. electroencephalogram __________
4. intracranial pressure __________
5. positron emission tomography __________
6. cerebrovascular accident __________
7. autonomic nervous system __________

SECTION II: MENTAL HEALTH

AT A GLANCE

Word Parts

Presented here are the most common word parts (with their meanings) used to build mental health terms.

Combining Forms

amnes/o	forgetfulness
anxi/o	fear, worry
compuls/o	drive, compel
delus/o	false belief
depress/o	to press down
hallucin/o	imagined perception
klept/o	to steal
ment/o	mind
narc/o	stupor, sleep
neur/o	nerve
obsess/o	besieged by thoughts
phob/o	irrational fear
phren/o	mind
psych/o	mind
pyr/o	fire
schiz/o	split
soci/o	society

Suffixes

-iatrist	physician
-iatry	medical treatment
-lepsy	seizure
-mania	frenzy
-phoria	condition to bear

Mental Health Disciplines

Psychology

abnormal psychology
clinical psychologist (sigh-KALL-oh-jist)
normal psychology
psychology (sigh-KALL-oh-jee)

Psychology is the study of human behavior and thought processes. This behavioral science is primarily concerned with understanding how human beings interact with their physical environment and with each other. Behavior can be divided into two categories: normal and abnormal. The study of **normal psychology** includes how the personality develops, how people handle stress, and the stages of mental development. In contrast, **abnormal psychology** studies and treats behaviors that are outside of normal and that are detrimental to the person or society. These maladaptive behaviors range from occasional difficulty coping with stress, to bizarre actions and beliefs, to total withdrawal. A **clinical psychologist**, though not a physician, is a specialist in evaluating and treating persons with mental and emotional disorders.

Med Term Tip

All social interactions pose some problems for some people. These problems are not necessarily abnormal. One means of judging if behavior is abnormal is to compare one person's behavior with others in the community. Also, if a person's behavior interferes with the activities of daily living, it is often considered abnormal.

Psychiatry

psychiatric nurse (sigh-kee-AT-rik)
psychiatric social worker
psychiatrist (sigh-KIGH-ah-trist)
psychiatry (sigh-KIGH-ah-tree)

Psychiatry is the branch of medicine that deals with the diagnosis, treatment, and prevention of mental disorders. A **psychiatrist** is a medical physician specializing in the care of patients with mental, emotional, and behavioral disorders. Other health professions also have specialty areas in caring for clients with mental illness. Good examples are **psychiatric nurses** and **psychiatric social workers**.

What's In A Name?

Look for these word parts:
psych/o = mind
-iatric = pertaining to medical treatment
-iatrist = physician
-iatry = medical treatment
-logist = one who studies
-logy = study of

Pathology

The legal definition of mental disorder is "impaired judgment and lack of self-control." The guide for terminology and classifications relating to psychiatric disorders is the *Diagnostic and Statistical Manual of Mental Disorders, Fifth Edition* (DSM-5), which is published by the American Psychiatric Association (2013). The DSM organizes mental disorders into 19 major diagnostic categories of disorders. These categories and examples of conditions included in each are described below.

Med Term Tip

Mental disorders are sometimes more simply characterized by whether they are a *neurosis* or a *psychosis.* Neuroses are inappropriate coping mechanisms to handle stress, such as phobias and panic attacks. Psychoses involve extreme distortions of reality and disorganization of a person's thinking, including bizarre behaviors, hallucinations, and delusions. Schizophrenia is an example of a psychosis.

Term	Word Parts	Definition
Anxiety Disorders	**anxi/o** = fear, worry **dis-** = apart	Characterized by persistent worry and apprehension
general anxiety disorder (ang-ZYE-eh-tee)	**anxi/o** = fear, worry **dis-** = apart	Feeling of dread in absence of clearly identifiable stress trigger
panic disorder	**-ic** = pertaining to **dis-** = apart	Feeling of intense apprehension, terror, or sense of impending danger
phobias (FOH-bee-ahs)	**phob/o** = irrational fear **-ia** = condition	Irrational fear, such as *arachnophobia*, the fear of spiders

Pathology (continued)

Term	Word Parts	Definition
Bipolar and Related Disorders	bi- = two -ar = pertaining to dis- = apart	
bipolar disorder (BPD)	bi- = two -ar = pertaining to	Alternation between periods of deep depression and mania
Med Term Tip The healthcare professional must take all threats of suicide from patients seriously. Psychologists tell us that there is no clear suicide type, which means that we cannot predict who will actually take his or her own life. Always tell the physician caring for the person about any discussion a patient has concerning suicide. If you believe a patient is in danger of suicide, do not be afraid to ask, "Are you thinking about suicide?"		
Depressive Disorders	depress/o = to press down dis- = apart	Characterized by instability in mood
major depressive disorder	depress/o = to press down dis- = apart	Feelings of hopelessness, helplessness, worthlessness; lack of pleasure in any activity; potential for suicide
mania (MAY-nee-ah)	-mania = frenzy	Displaying extreme elation, hyperactivity, excessive talkativeness, impaired judgment, distractibility, and grandiose delusions
Disruptive, Impulse Control, and Conduct Disorders	dis- = apart	Inability to resist impulse to perform some act that is harmful to individual or others
explosive disorder	ex- = outward dis- = apart	Violent rages
kleptomania (klep-toh-MAY-nee-ah)	klept/o = to steal -mania = frenzy	Uncontrollable impulse to steal
pyromania (pye-roh-MAY-nee-ah)	pyr/o = fire -mania = frenzy	Uncontrollable impulse to set fires
Dissociative Disorders	dis- = apart soci/o = society	Disorders in which severe emotional conflict is so repressed that a split in personality may occur or person may lose memory
dissociative amnesia (dih-SOH-see-ah-tiv / am-NEE-zee-ah)	dis- = apart soci/o = society amnes/o = forgetfulness -ia = condition	Loss of memory
dissociative identity disorder	dis- = apart soci/o = society	Having two or more distinct personalities
Elimination Disorders	dis- = apart	
encopresis		Act of voiding feces in inappropriate places after toilet training
enuresis (en-yoo-REE-sis)		Act of voiding urine in inappropriate places after toilet training
Feeding and Eating Disorders		Abnormal behaviors related to eating

Pathology (continued)

Term	Word Parts	Definition
anorexia nervosa (an-oh-REK-see-ah / ner-VOH-sah)	an- = without -orexia = appetite	Disorder characterized by distorted body image, pathological fear of becoming fat, and severe weight loss due to excessive dieting
■ **Figure 12-16** Photograph of a young woman suffering from anorexia nervosa, posterior view. *(Den Rise/Shutterstock)*		
bulimia (boo-LEE-mee-ah)	-ia = condition	Condition of binge eating and intentional vomiting
Gender Dysphoria	dys- = abnormal -phoria = condition to bear	
gender dysphoria (dis-FOR-ee-ah)	dys- = abnormal -phoria = condition to bear	Occurs when birth gender is contrary to gender with which person identifies; includes both male to female (MTF) and female to male (FTM)
Neurocognitive Disorders	neur/o = nerve dis- = apart	Deterioration of mental functions due to temporary or permanent brain dysfunction
Alzheimer's disease (AD) (ALTS-high-merz)	dis- = apart	Degenerative brain disorder with gradual loss of cognitive abilities
dementia (deh-MEN-sha)	de- = without ment/o = mind -ia = condition	Progressive confusion and disorientation
Neurodevelopmental Disorders	neur/o = nerve -al = pertaining to dis- = apart	Impairment in growth or development of the central nervous system
attention-deficit/hyperactivity disorder (ADHD)	hyper- = excessive dis- = apart	Inattention and impulsive behavior
autism spectrum disorder (AW-tizm)	auto- = self -ism = state of dis- = apart	Range of conditions involving deficits in social interaction, communication skills, and restricted patterns of behavior
intellectual development disorder	-al = pertaining to dis- = apart	Below-average intellectual functioning
Obsessive–Compulsive and Related Disorders	dis- = apart	Characterized by obsessive preoccupations and repetitive behaviors
obsessive–compulsive disorder (OCD) (ob-SESS-iv / kom-PUHL-siv)	obsess/o = besieged by thoughts compuls/o = drive, compel dis- = apart	Performing repetitive rituals to reduce anxiety caused by persistent thoughts, ideas, or impulses

Pathology (continued)

Term	Word Parts	Definition
Paraphilic Disorders	para- = abnormal -philic = pertaining to being attracted to dis- = apart	Disorders include aberrant sexual activity and sexual dysfunction
pedophilic disorder (pee-doh-FILL-ik)	ped/o = child -philic = pertaining to being attracted to dis- = apart	Sexual interest in children
sexual masochism disorder (MAS-oh-kizm)	-al = pertaining to -ism = state of dis- = apart	Gratification derived from being hurt or abused
voyeuristic disorder (VOY-er-iss-tik)	-tic = pertaining to	Gratification derived from observing others engaged in sexual acts
Personality Disorders	dis- = apart	Inflexible or maladaptive behavior patterns that affect person's ability to function in society
antisocial personality disorder	anti- = against soci/o = society -al = pertaining to dis- = apart	Behaviors that are against legal or social norms
narcissistic personality disorder (nar-sih-SIS-tik)	dis- = apart	Abnormal sense of self-importance
paranoid personality disorder	dis- = apart	Exaggerated feelings of persecution
Schizophrenia Spectrum and Other Psychotic Disorders	schiz/o = split phren/o = mind -ia = condition	Mental disorders characterized by distortions of reality
delusional disorder (dee-LOO-zhun-al)	delus/o = false belief -al = pertaining to dis- = apart	False belief held even in face of contrary evidence
hallucination (hah-loo-sih-NAY-shun)	hallucin/o = imagined perception	Perceiving something that is not there
Sexual Dysfunctions	-al = pertaining to dys- = abnormal, difficult	Having difficulty during any stage of normal sexual activity that negatively impacts quality of life
erectile dysfunction	-ile = pertaining to dys- = difficult	Pertaining to difficulty achieving or maintaining erection
premature ejaculation	pre- = before	Ejaculation of semen before or shortly after penetration
Sleep–Wake Disorders	dis- = apart	Disorders relating to either sleeping or wakefulness
insomnia disorder (in-SOM-nee-ah)	in- = not somn/o = sleep -ia = condition	Condition of inability to sleep
narcolepsy (NAR-koh-lep-see)	narc/o = stupor, sleep -lepsy = seizure	Recurring episodes of sleeping during daytime and often difficulty sleeping at night
Somatic Symptom and Related Disorders	somat/o = body -ic = pertaining to dis- = apart	Patient has physical symptoms for which no physical disease can be determined
conversion disorder	vers/o = to turn dis- = apart	Anxiety is transformed into physical symptoms such as heart palpitations, paralysis, or blindness

Pathology (continued)

Term	Word Parts	Definition
somatic symptom disorder (SSD)	somat/o = body -ic = pertaining to dis- = apart	Having physical symptoms that cause distress and disrupt daily life; includes preoccupation with symptoms and behaviors based on symptoms
Substance Use and Addictive Disorders	dis- = apart	
gambling disorder	dis- = apart	Inability to stop gambling
substance use disorder	dis- = apart	Overindulgence or dependence on chemical substances including alcohol, illegal drugs, and prescription drugs
Trauma- and Stressor-Related Disorders	dis- = apart	
posttraumatic stress disorder (PTSD)	post- = after -ic = pertaining to dis- = apart	Results from exposure to actual or implied death, serious injury, or sexual violence; condition impairs person's social interactions and capacity to work

PRACTICE AS YOU GO

G. Pathology Matching

Match each term to its description.

______ **1.** panic disorder	**a.** type of feeding and eating disorder
______ **2.** autism spectrum disorder	**b.** type of disruptive, impulse control, and conduct disorder
______ **3.** dementia	**c.** type of sleep–wake disorder
______ **4.** anorexia nervosa	**d.** type of anxiety disorder
______ **5.** narcolepsy	**e.** type of substance use and addictive disorder
______ **6.** mania	**f.** type of somatic symptom and related disorder
______ **7.** conversion disorder	**g.** type of neurodevelopmental disorder
______ **8.** gambling disorder	**h.** type of elimination disorder
______ **9.** enuresis	**i.** type of depressive disorder
______ **10.** pyromania	**j.** type of neurocognitive disorder

Therapeutic Procedures

Term	Word Parts	Definition
electroconvulsive therapy (ECT) (ee-lek-troh-kon-VUL-siv)	electr/o = electricity	Procedure occasionally used for cases of prolonged major depression; once-controversial treatment involves placement of electrode on one or both sides of patient's head and a current is turned on, briefly causing convulsive seizure; low level of voltage is used in modern electroconvulsive therapy, and patient is administered muscle relaxant and anesthesia; when first introduced in the 1940s, was very primitive and convulsions were not controlled in any manner; advocates of treatment today correctly state that it is a more effective way to treat severe depression than using drugs; not effective with disorders other than depression, such as schizophrenia and alcoholism

Therapeutic Procedures (continued)

Term	Word Parts	Definition
Psychopharmacology (sigh-koh-far-mah-KALL-oh-jee)	psych/o = mind pharmac/o = drug -logy = study of	Study of effects of drugs on the mind and particularly use of drugs in treating mental disorders; main classes of drugs for treatment of mental disorders are:
antidepressant drugs	anti- = against depress/o = to press down	Classified as stimulants; alter patient's mood by affecting levels of neurotransmitters in the brain; antidepressants, such as serotonin norepinephrine reuptake inhibitors, are nonaddictive but can produce unpleasant side effects such as dry mouth, weight gain, blurred vision, and nausea
antipsychotic drugs	anti- = against psych/o = mind -tic = pertaining to	These major tranquilizers include chlorpromazine (Thorazine), haloperidol (Haldol), clozapine (Clozaril), and risperidone; these drugs have transformed treatment of patients with psychoses and schizophrenia by reducing patient agitation and panic and shortening schizophrenic episodes; one side effect of these drugs is involuntary muscle movements, which approximately one-fourth of all adults who take the drugs develop
lithium		Special category of drug used successfully to calm patients who suffer from bipolar disorder (depression alternating with manic excitement)
minor tranquilizers		Include Valium and Xanax; also classified as central nervous system depressants and are prescribed for anxiety
Psychotherapy (sigh-koh-THAIR-ah-pee)	psych/o = mind -therapy = treatment	Method of treating mental disorders by mental rather than chemical or physical means; includes:
family and group psychotherapy	psych/o = mind -therapy = treatment	Often described as solution focused, therapist places minimal emphasis on patient past history and strong emphasis on having patient state and discuss goals and then find a way to achieve them
humanistic psychotherapy	-tic = pertaining to psych/o = mind -therapy = treatment	Therapist does not delve into patients' past when using these methods; instead, it is believed that patients can learn how to use their own internal resources to deal with their problems; therapist creates therapeutic atmosphere, which builds patient self-esteem and encourages discussion of problems, thereby gaining insight in how to handle them; also called *client-centered* or *nondirective psychotherapy*
psychoanalysis	psych/o = mind	Method of obtaining detailed account of past and present emotional and mental experiences from patient to determine source of problem and eliminate effects; system developed by Sigmund Freud that encourages patient to discuss repressed, painful, or hidden experiences with hope of eliminating or minimizing problem

Abbreviations

AD	Alzheimer's disease	**MA**	mental age
ADD	attention-deficit disorder	**MMPI**	Minnesota Multiphasic Personality Inventory
ADHD	attention-deficit/hyperactivity disorder	**MTF**	male to female
BPD	bipolar disorder	**OCD**	obsessive–compulsive disorder
CA	chronological age	**PTSD**	posttraumatic stress disorder
DSM	*Diagnostic and Statistical Manual of Mental Disorders*	**SAD**	seasonal affective disorder
ECT	electroconvulsive therapy	**SSD**	somatic symptom disorder
FTM	female to male		

Chapter Review

Real-World Applications

Medical Record Analysis

This Discharge Summary contains 12 medical terms. Underline each term and write it in the list below the report. Then explain each term as you would to a nonmedical person.

Discharge Summary

Admitting Diagnosis:	Paraplegia following motorcycle accident
Final Diagnosis:	Comminuted L2 fracture with epidural hematoma and spinal cord injury resulting in complete paraplegia at the L2 level.
History of Present Illness:	Patient is a 23-year-old male who was involved in a motorcycle accident. He was unconscious for 35 minutes but was fully aware of his surroundings upon regaining consciousness. He was immediately aware of total anesthesia and paralysis below the waist.
Summary of Hospital Course:	CT scan revealed extensive bone destruction at the fracture site and that the spinal cord was severed. Patient was unable to voluntarily contract any lower extremity muscles and was not able to feel touch or pinpricks. Lumbar laminectomy with spinal fusion was performed to stabilize the fracture and remove the epidural hematoma. The immediate postoperative recovery period proceeded normally. Patient began physical therapy and occupational therapy. After two months, X-rays indicated full healing of the spinal fusion and patient was transferred to a rehabilitation institute.
Discharge Plans:	Patient was transferred to a rehabilitation institute to continue intensive PT and OT.

	Term	Explanation
1.	______________	______________________________
2.	______________	______________________________
3.	______________	______________________________
4.	______________	______________________________
5.	______________	______________________________
6.	______________	______________________________
7.	______________	______________________________
8.	______________	______________________________
9.	______________	______________________________
10.	______________	______________________________
11.	______________	______________________________
12.	______________	______________________________

Chart Note Transcription

The chart note below contains 11 phrases that can be reworded with a medical term presented in this chapter. Each phrase is identified with an underline. Determine the medical term and write your answers in the space provided.

Pearson General Hospital Consultation Report

Task Edit View Time Scale Options Help Download Archive Date: 17 May 2017

Current Complaint:	Patient is a 38-year-old female referred to the specialist in the treatment of diseases of the nervous system **1** by her family physician with complaints of difficulty with speech, **2** loss of motion on one side of the body, **3** and severe involuntary muscle contractions. **4**
Past History:	Patient is married and nulliparous. Has been healthy prior to current symptoms.
Signs and Symptoms:	Her husband reports he first noted loss of motion on one side of the body when she began to drag her left foot. It has progressed to involve both left upper and lower extremities, with approximately a 50% loss in control of left lower extremity and a 25% loss of control in left upper extremity. Difficulty with speech is mild and mainly with recalling the names of common objects. Severe involuntary muscle contractions appear to be triggered by stress and last approximately two minutes. Results of a recording of the electrical activity of the brain **5** and a puncture with a needle into the low back to withdraw fluid for examination **6** were normal. However, an injection with radioactive isotopes **7** revealed the presence of a mass in the right outer layer of the largest section of the brain. **8**
Diagnosis:	Astrocyte tumor **9** in the right outer layer of the largest section of the brain **8**
Treatment:	A right skull incision **10** was performed to permit the surgical use of extreme cold **11** to destroy the tumor. Patient experienced moderate improvement in loss of motion on one side of the body **3** and severe involuntary muscle contractions, **4** but difficulty with speech **2** was unchanged.

1. ____________________

2. ____________________

3. ____________________

4. ____________________

5. ____________________

6. ____________________

7. ____________________

8. ____________________

9. ____________________

10. ____________________

11. ____________________

Case Study

Below is a case study presentation of a patient with a condition discussed in this chapter. Read the case study and answer the questions below. Some questions will ask for information not included within this chapter. Use your text, a medical dictionary, or any other reference material you choose to answer these questions.

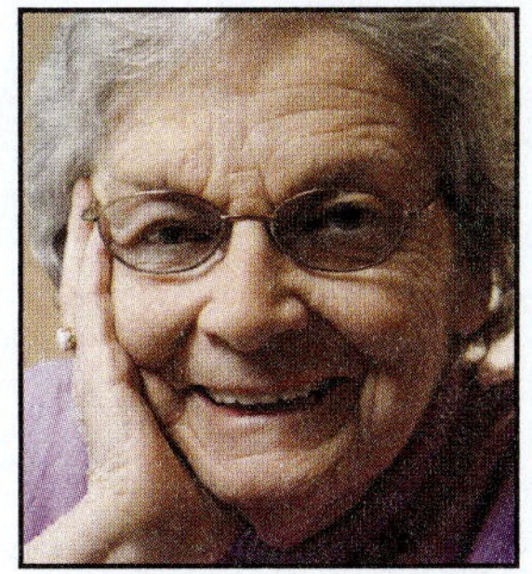
(Iofoto/Shutterstock)

Anna Moore, an 83-year-old female, is admitted to the ER with aphasia, hemiparesis on her left side, syncope, and delirium. Her daughter called the ambulance after discovering her mother in this condition at home. Mrs. Moore has a history of hypertension, atherosclerosis, and diabetes mellitus. She was admitted to the hospital after a brain scan revealed an infarct in the right cerebral hemisphere, leading to a diagnosis of CVA of the middle cerebral artery.

Questions

1. What pathological condition does Mrs. Moore have? Look this condition up in a reference source and include a short description of it.

____

____

2. List and define each of the patient's presenting symptoms in the ER.

____

____

3. The patient has a history of three significant conditions. Describe each in your own words.

____

____

4. What diagnostic test did the physician perform? Describe this test and the results in your own words.

____

____

5. What is an *infarct* and what causes it?

____

____

6. List and describe the four common causes of a CVA.

____

____

Practice Exercises

A. Terminology Matching

Match each cranial nerve to its function.

1. ________ olfactory	a. carries facial sensory impulses
2. ________ optic	b. turns eye to side
3. ________ oculomotor	c. controls tongue muscles
4. ________ trochlear	d. controls eye muscles and pupils
5. ________ trigeminal	e. swallowing
6. ________ abducens	f. controls facial muscles
7. ________ facial	g. controls oblique eye muscles
8. ________ vestibulocochlear	h. smell
9. ________ glossopharyngeal	i. controls neck and shoulder muscles
10. ________ vagus	j. hearing and equilibrium
11. ________ accessory	k. vision
12. ________ hypoglossal	l. supplies most organs in abdominal and thoracic cavities

B. Word Building Practice

The combining form **neur/o** refers to the *nerve*. Use it to write a term that means:

1. inflammation of the nerve ____________________
2. specialist in nerves ____________________
3. pain in the nerve ____________________
4. inflammation of many nerves ____________________
5. removal of a nerve ____________________
6. surgical repair of a nerve ____________________
7. nerve tumor ____________________
8. suture of a nerve ____________________

The combining form **mening/o** refers to the *meninges* or *membranes*. Use it to write a term that means:

9. inflammation of the meninges ____________________
10. protrusion of the meninges ____________________
11. protrusion of the spinal cord and the meninges ____________________

The combining form **encephal/o** refers to the *brain*. Use it to write a term that means:

12. X-ray record of the brain ____________________
13. disease of the brain ____________________
14. inflammation of the brain ____________________
15. protrusion of the brain ____________________

The combining form **cerebr/o** refers to the *cerebrum*. Use it to write a term that means:

16. pertaining to the cerebrum and spinal cord ____________________
17. pertaining to the cerebrum ____________________

C. Using Abbreviations

Fill in each blank with the appropriate abbreviation.

1. Joseph's inattention and impulsive behavior led to a diagnosis of ____________________.
2. Performing repetitive rituals to reduce anxiety is the hallmark of ____________________.
3. A(n) ____________________ is also called a *spinal tap*.
4. A(n) ____________________ measures the metabolic activity of tissue.
5. ____________________ is caused by the loss of the myelin sheath around nerves.
6. Juanita suffered a(n) ____________________ from an auto accident, but luckily the spinal cord was only bruised and not severed.
7. ____________________ is commonly called *Lou Gehrig's disease.*
8. In a(n) ____________________, the neurological symptoms are temporary.
9. The newborn has ____________________ resulting from lack of oxygen during a difficult delivery.
10. The brain damage from the ____________________ included hemiplegia and dysphasia.

D. Define the Procedures and Tests

1. myelography ____________________
2. cerebral angiography ____________________
3. Babinski's reflex ____________________
4. nerve conduction velocity ____________________
5. cerebrospinal fluid analysis ____________________
6. PET scan ____________________
7. echoencephalography ____________________
8. lumbar puncture ____________________

E. Complete the Term

For each definition given below, fill in the blank with the word part that completes the term.

Definition	Term
1. treatment of the mind	__________therapy
2. condition of being without a mind	de__________ia
3. pertaining to without sense of pain	an__________ic
4. record of the spinal cord	__________gram
5. process of recording electricity of the brain	electro__________graphy
6. pertaining to under the dura	sub__________al
7. inflammation of the meninges	__________itis
8. inflammation of many nerves	poly__________itis
9. abnormal hardened condition	__________osis
10. action of shaking violently	__________ion
11. nerve root disease	__________pathy
12. pertaining to without feeling/sensation	an__________tic
13. fire frenzy	pyro__________
14. condition of not sleeping	in__________ia

F. Define the Term

1. astrocytoma ____________________
2. epilepsy ____________________
3. anesthesia ____________________
4. hemiparesis ____________________
5. neurosurgeon ____________________
6. analgesia ____________________
7. focal seizure ____________________
8. quadriplegia ____________________
9. subdural hematoma ____________________
10. intrathecal ____________________

G. Terminology Matching

Match each term to its definition.

1. ________ neurologist	a. sudden attack
2. ________ cerebrovascular accident	b. type of severe headache
3. ________ concussion	c. loss of intellectual ability
4. ________ aphasia	d. physician who treats nerve problems
5. ________ migraine	e. stroke

6. ________ seizure — f. mild traumatic brain injury
7. ________ dementia — g. loss of ability to speak
8. ________ ataxia — h. congenital anomaly
9. ________ spina bifida — i. state of being unaware
10. ________ unconscious — j. lack of muscle coordination

H. Fill in the Blank

Parkinson's disease	transient ischemic attack	cerebral palsy	cerebrospinal fluid shunt
Bell's palsy	subdural hematoma	amyotrophic lateral sclerosis	nerve conduction velocity
delirium	cerebral aneurysm		

1. Dr. Martin noted that a 96-year-old patient suffered from ________________ when she determined that he was confused, disoriented, and agitated.
2. Lucinda's ________________ resulted in increasing muscle weakness as the motor neurons in her spinal cord degenerated.
3. The diagnosis of ________________ was correct because the weakness affected only one side of Charles's face.
4. A cerebral angiogram was ordered because Dr. Larson suspected Mrs. Constantine had a(n) ________________.
5. Roberta's symptoms included fine tremors, muscular weakness, rigidity, and a shuffling gait, leading to a diagnosis of ________________.
6. Matthew's hydrocephalus required the placement of a(n) ________________.
7. Because Mae's hemiparesis was temporary, the final diagnosis was ________________.
8. Following a car accident, a CT scan showed a(n) ________________ was putting pressure on the brain, necessitating immediate neurosurgery.
9. Birth trauma resulted in the newborn developing ________________.
10. A(n) ________________ test was performed in order to pinpoint the exact position of the nerve damage.

I. Pharmacology Challenge

Fill in the classification for each drug description, then match the brand name.

Drug Description	Classification	Brand Name
1. ________ produces loss of sensation	____________________	a. L-dopa
2. ________ treats Parkinson's disease	____________________	b. Amytal
3. ________ promotes sleep	____________________	c. OxyContin
4. ________ medication for mild pain	____________________	d. Seconal
5. ________ produces a calming effect	____________________	e. Xylocaine
6. ________ treats severe pain	____________________	f. Tegretol
7. ________ treats seizures	____________________	g. Motrin

J. Terminology Matching

Match each term to its clue.

1. ________ neurocognitive disorder
2. ________ elimination disorder
3. ________ dissociative disorder
4. ________ eating disorder
5. ________ sleep–wake disorder
6. ________ depressive disorder
7. ________ impulse control disorder
8. ________ somatic symptom disorder
9. ________ personality disorder
10. ________ paraphilic disorder
11. ________ anxiety disorder

a. conversion disorder
b. kleptomania
c. pedophilic disorder
d. narcissistic personality
e. insomnia
f. mania
g. panic attacks
h. amnesia
i. dementia
j. anorexia nervosa
k. enuresis

K. Name the Treatment

Identify each mental health treatment from its description.

1. depressant drugs prescribed for anxiety ________________
2. client-centered psychotherapy ________________
3. drug used to calm patients with bipolar disorder ________________
4. reduces patient agitation and panic and shortens schizophrenic episodes ________________
5. obtains a detailed account of the past and present emotional and mental experiences ________________
6. stimulants that alter the patient's mood by affecting neurotransmitter levels ________________

L. Name the Anesthesia

Identify the type of anesthesia for each description.

1. produces loss of consciousness and absence of pain ________________
2. produces loss of sensation in one localized part of the body ________________
3. anesthetic applied directly onto a specific skin area ________________
4. also referred to as a nerve block ________________

M. Anatomical Adjectives

Fill in the blank with the missing noun or adjective.

Noun	Adjective
1. cerebellum	______________
2. ______________	thalamic
3. ______________	cerebral
4. ______________	vertebral
5. within the skull	______________
6. ______________	spinal
7. brain	______________
8. pons	______________
9. medulla oblongata	______________
10. ______________	neural
11. meninges	______________
12. ______________	ventricular

N. Spelling Practice

Some of the following terms are misspelled. Identify the incorrect terms and spell them correctly in the blank provided.

1. anesthesiology ______________________________
2. cephalgia ______________________________
3. voyeuristic ______________________________
4. postraumatic ______________________________
5. hallucination ______________________________
6. hyperesthesia ______________________________
7. quadraplegia ______________________________
8. hydrocephalis ______________________________
9. amyotropic ______________________________
10. echoencephalography ______________________________

O. Complete the Statement

1. ____________________ is a behavioral science that studies human behavior and thought processes.

   ____________________ is a branch of medicine that diagnoses and treats mental disorders.
2. ____________________ nerves serve the skin and skeletal muscles.
3. The ____________________ nervous system is involved with the control of involuntary bodily functions.
4. ____________________ neurons are afferent neurons and ____________________ neurons are efferent neurons.
5. Cerebrospinal fluid is found in the ____________________ space.
6. The midbrain, pons, and medulla oblongata make up the ____________________.
7. The occipital lobe of the cerebrum controls ____________________.
8. ____________________ is a fatty substance that insulates some axons.

Labeling Exercises

Image A

Write the labels for this figure on the numbered lines provided.

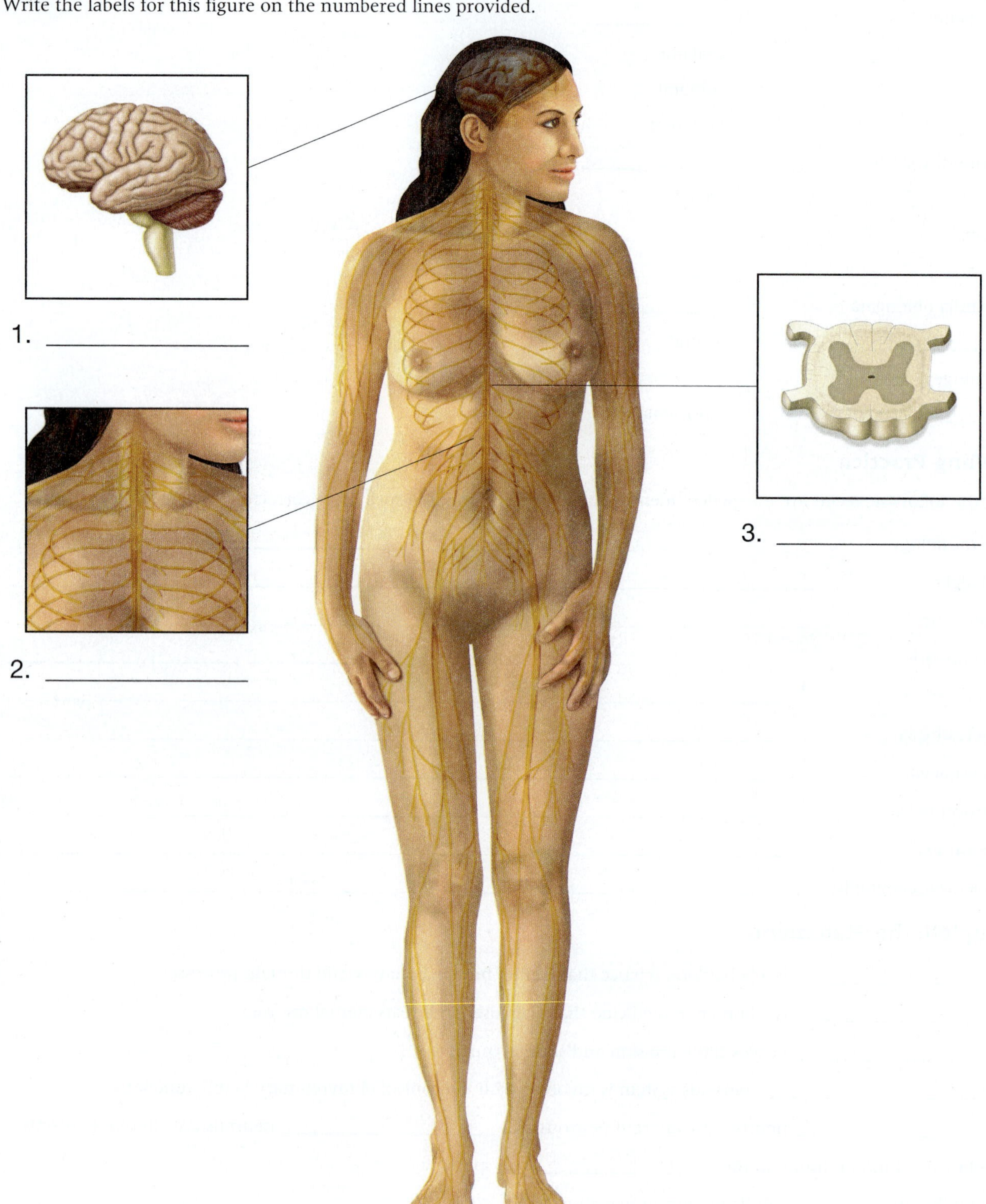

Image B

Write the labels for this figure on the numbered lines provided.

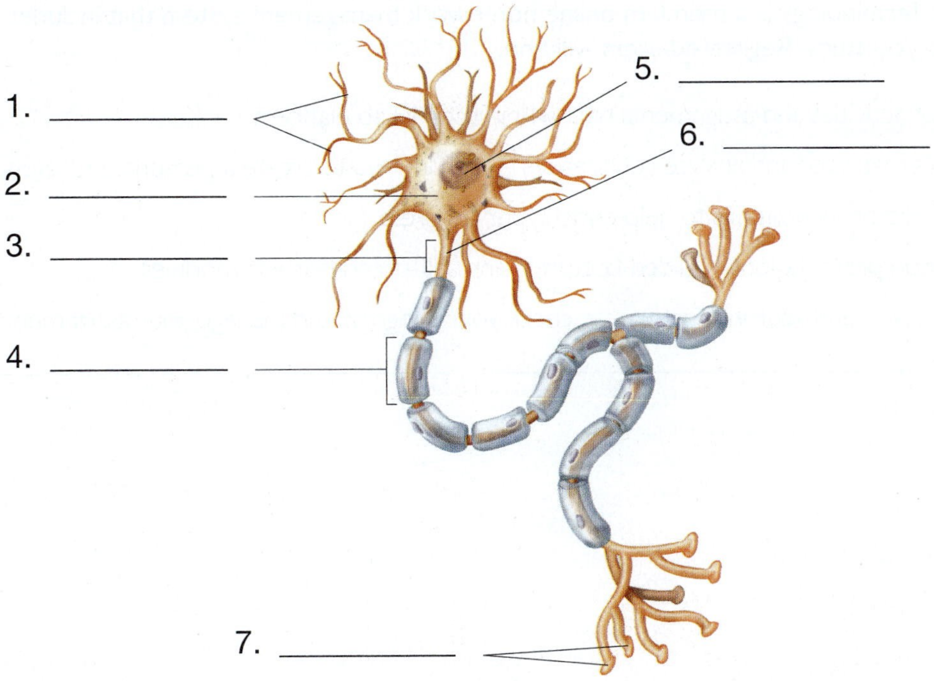

Image C

Write the labels for this figure on the numbered lines provided.

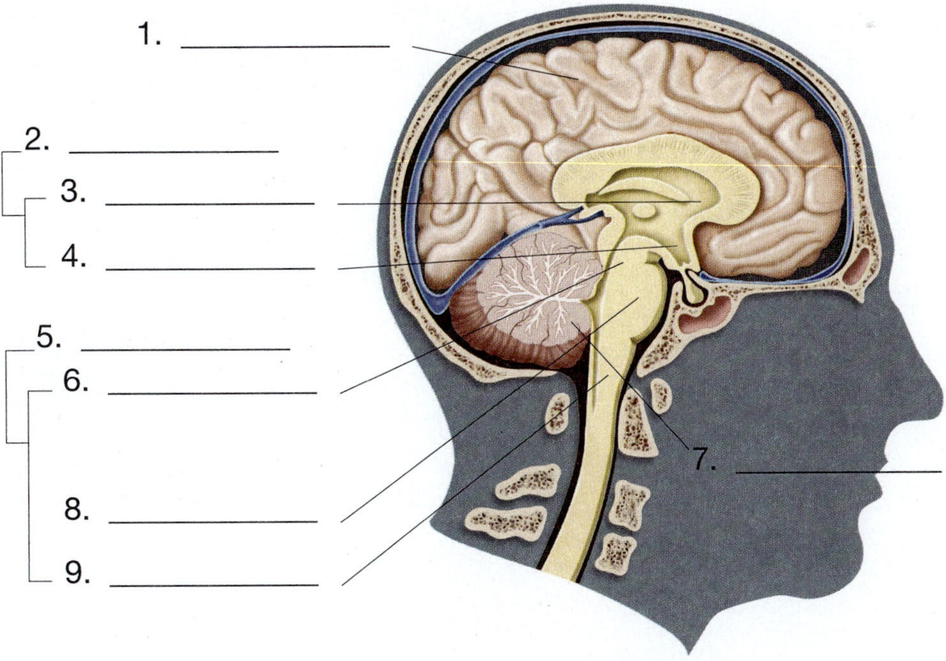

MyLab Medical Terminology™

MyLab Medical Terminology is a premium online homework management system that includes a host of features to help you study. Registered users will find:

- A multitude of activities and assignments built within the MyLab platform
- Powerful tools that track and analyze your results—allowing you to create a personalized learning experience
- Videos and audio pronunciations to help enrich your progress
- Streaming lesson presentations (Guided Lectures) and self-paced learning modules
- A space where you and your instructors can check your progress and manage your assignments

Chapter 13

Special Senses: The Eye and Ear

Learning Objectives

Upon completion of this chapter, you will be able to

1. Identify and define the combining forms, suffixes, and prefixes introduced in this chapter.
2. Correctly spell and pronounce medical terms and major anatomical structures relating to the eye and ear.
3. Locate and describe the major structures of the eye and ear and their functions.
4. Describe the process of vision.
5. Describe the path of sound vibration.
6. Identify and define eye and ear anatomical terms.
7. Identify and define selected eye and ear pathology terms.
8. Identify and define selected eye and ear diagnostic procedures.
9. Identify and define selected eye and ear therapeutic procedures.
10. Identify and define selected medications relating to the eye and ear.
11. Define selected abbreviations associated with the eye and ear.

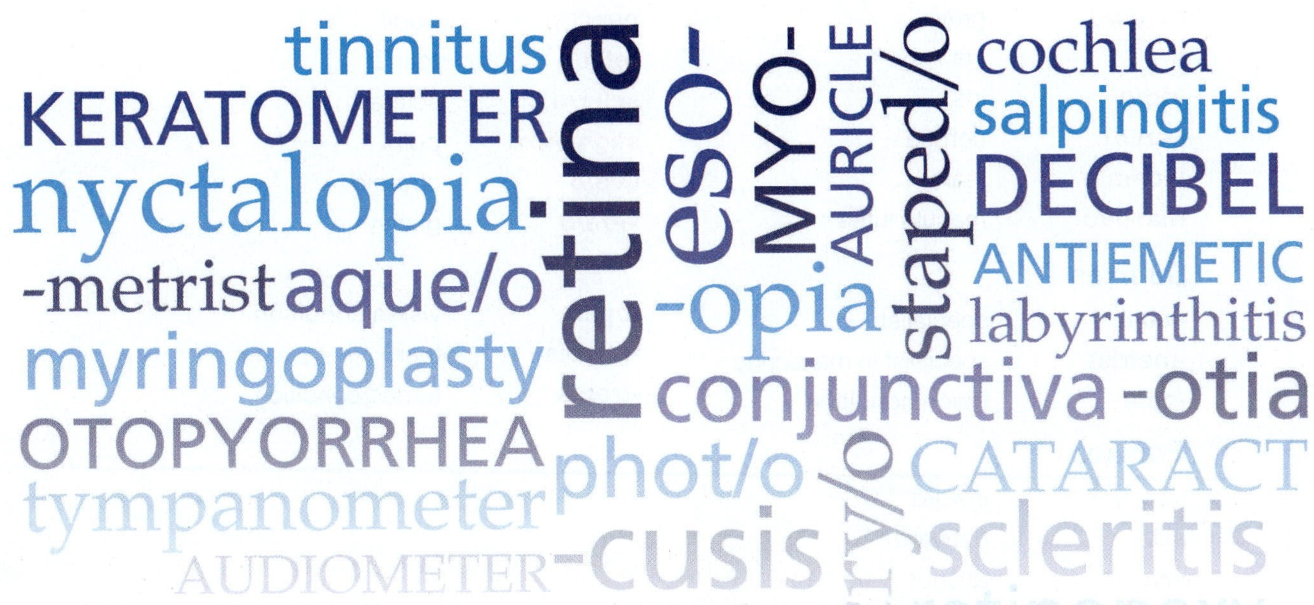

(Pearson Education, Inc.)

SECTION I: THE EYE

AT A GLANCE

Function

The eye contains the sensory receptor cells for vision.

Structures

The primary structures that comprise the eye:

eyeball	**eye muscles**
sclera	**eyelids**
choroid	**conjunctiva**
retina	**lacrimal apparatus**

Word Parts

Presented here are the most common word parts (with their meanings) used to build eye terms. For a more comprehensive list, refer to the Terminology section of this chapter.

Combining Forms

ambly/o	dull, dim	**mi/o**	lessening
aque/o	water	**mydr/i**	widening
blast/o	immature	**nyctal/o**	night
blephar/o	eyelid	**ocul/o**	eye
chromat/o	color	**ophthalm/o**	eye
conjunctiv/o	conjunctiva	**opt/o**	eye, vision
corne/o	cornea	**optic/o**	eye, vision
cycl/o	ciliary body	**papill/o**	optic disk
dacry/o	tears	**phac/o**	lens
dipl/o	double	**phot/o**	light
emmetr/o	correct, proper	**presby/o**	old age
glauc/o	gray	**pupill/o**	pupil
ir/o	iris	**retin/o**	retina
irid/o	iris	**scler/o**	sclera
kerat/o	cornea	**stigmat/o**	point
lacrim/o	tears	**uve/o**	choroid
macul/o	macula lutea	**vitre/o**	glassy

Suffixes

-ician	specialist	**-opsia**	vision condition
-metrist	specialist in measuring	**-phobia**	fear
-opia	vision condition	**-tropia**	turned condition

Prefixes

eso-	inward
exo-	outward
myo-	to shut

The Eye Illustrated

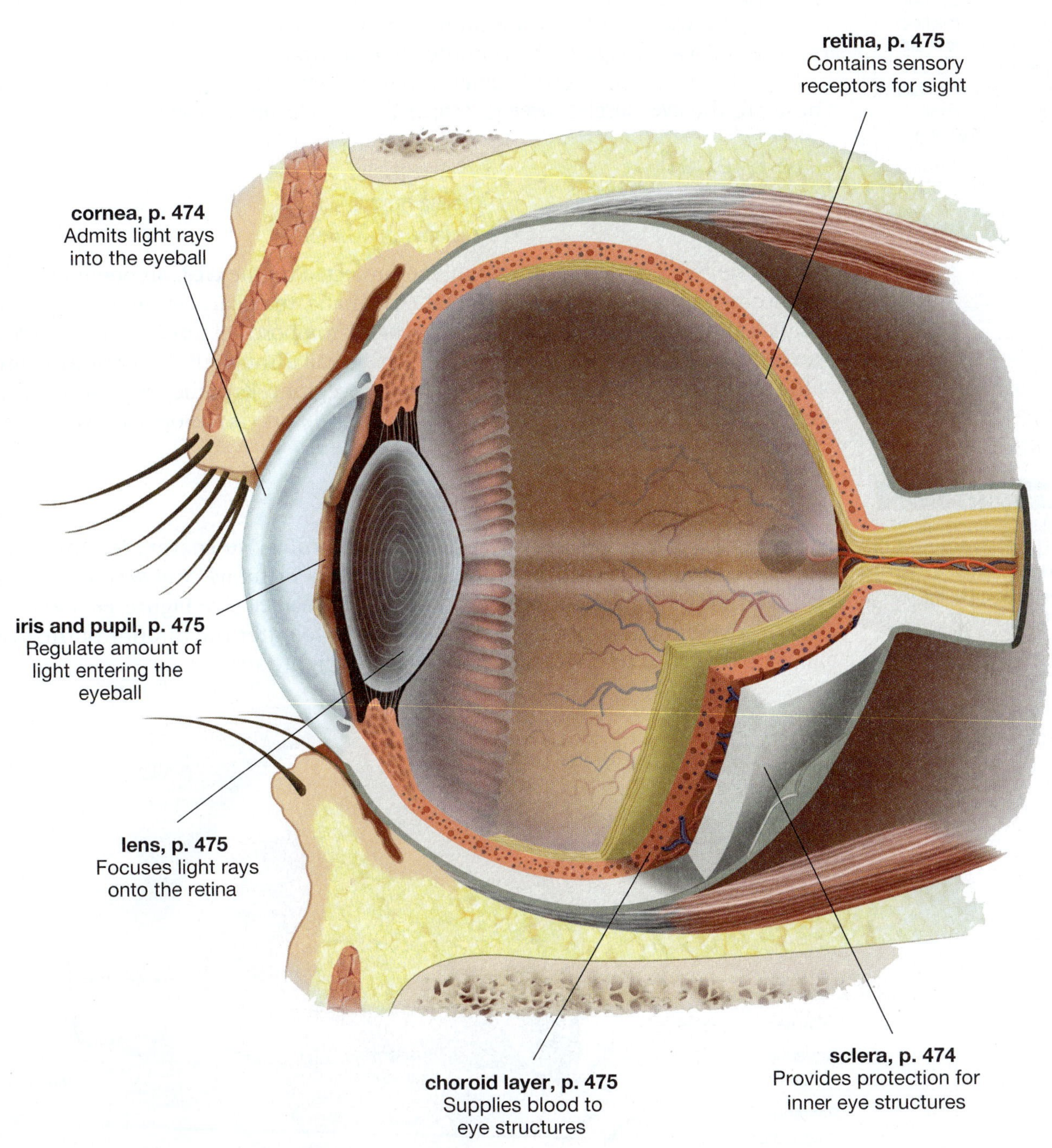

retina, p. 475
Contains sensory receptors for sight
cornea, p. 474
Admits light rays into the eyeball
iris and pupil, p. 475
Regulate amount of light entering the eyeball
lens, p. 475
Focuses light rays onto the retina
choroid layer, p. 475
Supplies blood to eye structures
sclera, p. 474
Provides protection for inner eye structures

Anatomy and Physiology of the Eye

conjunctiva (kon-junk-TYE-vah)
eye muscles
eyeball
eyelids
lacrimal apparatus (LAK-rim-al)
ophthalmology (off-thal-MALL-oh-jee)
optic nerve (OP-tik)

Med Term Tip

When studying the functions and terminology of the eye, it is helpful to know the meanings of the terms *opaque* and *transparent*. Opaque means that light is unable to pass through. Transparent, however, means that light is permitted through.

The study of the eye is known as **ophthalmology** (Ophth). The **eyeball** is the incredible organ of sight that transmits an external image by way of the nervous system—the **optic nerve**—to the brain. The brain then translates these sensory impulses into an image with computer-like accuracy.

In addition to the eyeball, several external structures play a role in vision. These are the **eye muscles**, **eyelids**, **conjunctiva**, and **lacrimal apparatus**.

The Eyeball

choroid (KOR-oyd)
orbit
retina (RET-ih-nah)
sclera (SKLAIR-ah)

Each of the two eyeballs is housed in and protected by the **orbit**, an opening in the skull formed by a portion of the frontal, zygomatic, maxillary, ethmoid, sphenoid, lacrimal, and palatine bones. The actual eyeball is composed of three layers: the **sclera**, the **choroid**, and the **retina**. Light rays enter the eyeball through the anterior structures of the sclera and are focused onto the sensory receptor cells of the retina where they are converted to electrical signals that travel to the brain via the optic nerve.

Med Term Tip

The color of the sclera can indicate the presence of disease. For instance, a yellowish cast to the sclera may be present in liver disease and certain anemias.

Sclera

cornea (KOR-nee-ah)
refracts

The outer layer, the sclera, provides a tough protective coating for the inner structures of the eye. Another term for the sclera is the *white of the eye*.

The anterior portion of the sclera is called the **cornea** (see Figure 13-1 ■). This clear, transparent area of the sclera allows light to enter the interior of the eyeball. The cornea actually bends, or **refracts**, the light rays.

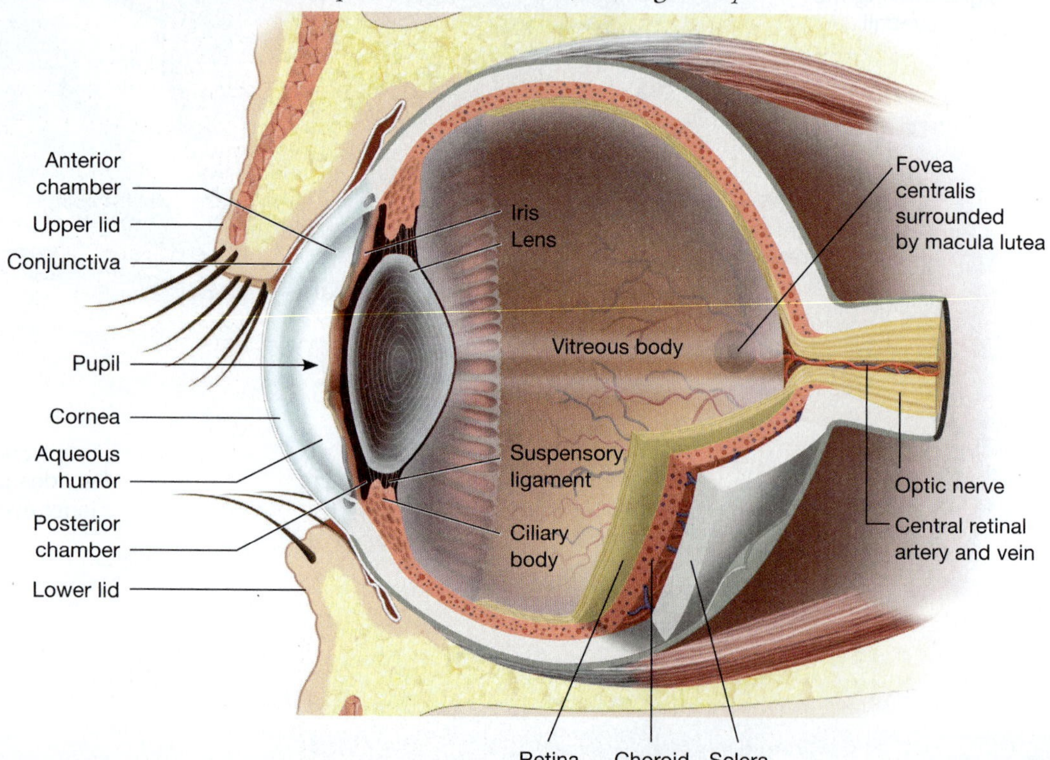

■ **Figure 13-1** The internal structures of the eye.

Choroid

ciliary body (SIL-ee-air-ee)
iris
lens
pupil

The second or middle layer of the eyeball is called the *choroid*. This opaque layer distributes the blood supply for the eye.

The anterior portion of the choroid layer consists of the **iris**, **pupil**, and **ciliary body** (see again Figure 13-1). The iris is the colored portion of the eye and contains smooth muscle. The pupil is the opening in the center of the iris that allows light rays to enter the eyeball. The iris muscles contract or relax to change the size of the pupil, thereby controlling how much light enters the interior of the eyeball. Immediately posterior to the iris is a ring of smooth muscle called the ciliary body. Sitting in the center of the ring is the **lens**. The lens is not actually part of the choroid layer, but it is attached to the ciliary body by many thin ligaments called *suspensory ligaments*. The muscular ciliary body contracts or relaxes to pull on the edge of the lens, changing the shape of the lens so it can focus incoming light onto the retina.

Med Term Tip

The term *ciliary* comes from the Latin word *cilium*, which is taken to refer to the eyelashes (or hair-like structures). In this case, the ciliary body received its name because of the many, very fine ligaments extending from it and attaching to the edge of the lens.

Retina

aqueous humor (AY-kwee-us)
cones
fovea centralis (FOH-vee-ah / sen-TRAH-lis)
macula lutea (MAK-yoo-lah / LOO-tee-ah)
optic disk
retinal blood vessels (RET-ih-nal)
rods
vitreous humor (VIT-ree-us)

The third and innermost layer of the eyeball is the retina. It contains the sensory receptor cells (**rods** and **cones**) that respond to light rays. Rods are active in dim light and help the eye to see in gray tones. Cones are active only in bright light and are responsible for color vision. When someone looks directly at an object, the image falls on an area called the **macula lutea**, or "yellow spot" (see again Figure 13-1). In the center of the macula lutea is a depression called the **fovea centralis**, meaning *central pit*. This pit contains a high concentration of sensory receptor cells and, therefore, is the point of clearest vision. Also visible on the retina is the **optic disk**. This is the point where the **retinal blood vessels** enter and exit the eyeball and where the optic nerve leaves the eyeball (see Figure 13-2 ■). There are no sensory receptor cells in the optic disk and therefore it causes a blind spot in each eye's field of vision. Because the blind spot of each eye is set to the side, one eye is able to cover for the missing information from the other. For this reason, a person is not generally aware of their existence. The interior spaces of the eyeball are not empty. The spaces between the cornea and lens are filled with **aqueous humor**, a watery fluid, and the large open area between the lens and retina contains **vitreous humor**, a semisolid gel.

What's In A Name?

Look for these word parts:
aque/o = water
centr/o = center
vitre/o = glassy
-ous = pertaining to

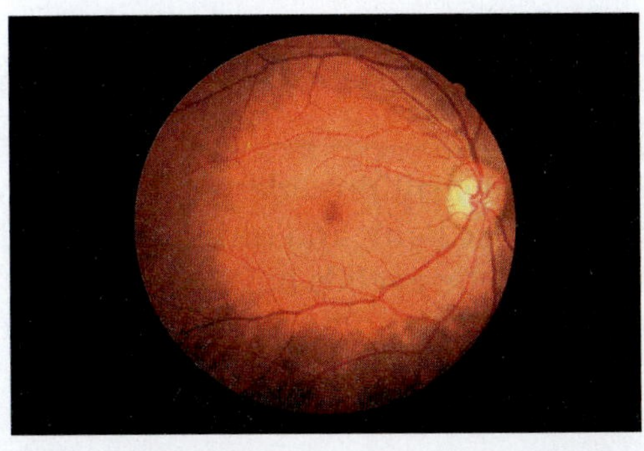

■ **Figure 13-2** Photograph of the retina of the eye. The optic disk appears yellow and the retinal arteries radiate out from it. The darker area in the center of the photo is the macula lutea. *(Left Handed Photography/Shutterstock)*

Muscles of the Eye

oblique muscles (oh-BLEEK) **rectus muscles** (REK-tus)

Med Term Tip

Like many other muscles, the names *rectus* and *oblique* provide clues regarding the direction of their fibers, or their *line of pull*. Rectus means *straight* and oblique means *slanted*. Rectus muscles have a straight line of pull. Because the fibers of an oblique muscle are slanted on an angle, they produce rotation.

Six muscles connect the actual eyeball to the skull (see Figure 13-3 ■). These muscles allow for change in the direction of each eye's sightline. In addition, they provide support for the eyeball in the eye socket. Children may be born with a weakness in some of these muscles and may require treatments such as eye exercises or even surgery to correct this problem, commonly referred to as crossed eyes or *strabismus* (see Figure 13-4 ■). The muscles involved are the four **rectus** and two **oblique muscles**. Rectus (meaning *straight*) muscles pull the eye up, down, left, or right in a straight line. Oblique muscles are on an angle and produce diagonal eye movement.

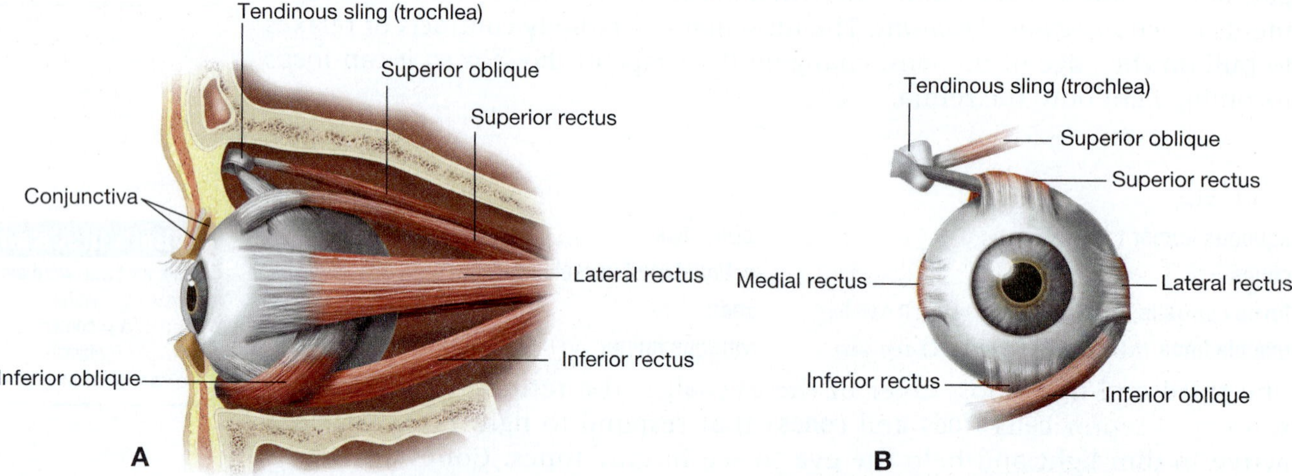

■ **Figure 13-3** The arrangement of the external eye muscles, A) lateral and B) anterior views.

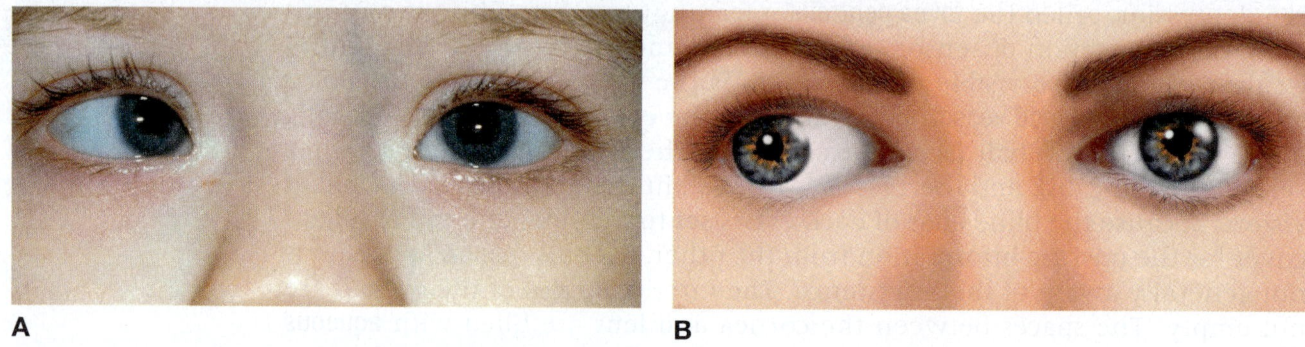

■ **Figure 13-4** Examples of common forms of strabismus. A) Esotropia with the right eye turning inward. *(Biophoto Associates/Science Source)* B) Exotropia with the right eye turning outward. *(Gwen Shockey/Science Source)*

The Eyelids

cilia (SIL-ee-ah) **sebaceous glands** (sih-BAY-shus)

eyelashes

What's In A Name?

Look for these word parts:
seb/o = oil
-ous = pertaining to

A pair of eyelids over each eyeball provides protection from foreign particles, injury from the sun and intense light, and trauma (see again Figure 13-1). Both the upper and lower edges of the eyelids have **eyelashes**, or **cilia**, that protect the eye from foreign particles. In addition, **sebaceous glands** located in the eyelids secrete lubricating oil onto the eyeball.

Conjunctiva

mucous membrane (MYOO-kus)

The conjunctiva of the eye is a **mucous membrane** lining. It forms a continuous covering on the underside of each eyelid and across the anterior surface of each eyeball (see again Figure 13-1). This serves as protection for the eye by sealing off the eyeball in the socket.

> **What's In A Name?**
> Look for these word parts:
> **muc/o** = mucus
> **-ous** = pertaining to

Lacrimal Apparatus

lacrimal canals
lacrimal gland
nasal cavity
nasolacrimal duct (nay-zoh-LAK-rim-al)
tears

The **lacrimal gland** is located under the outer upper corner of each eyelid. These glands produce **tears**. Tears serve the important function of washing and lubricating the anterior surface of the eyeball. **Lacrimal canals**, located in the inner corner of the eye socket, then collect the tears and drain them into the **nasolacrimal duct**. This duct ultimately drains the tears into the **nasal cavity** (see Figure 13-5 ■).

> **What's In A Name?**
> Look for these word parts:
> **lacrim/o** = tears
> **nas/o** = nose
> **-al** = pertaining to

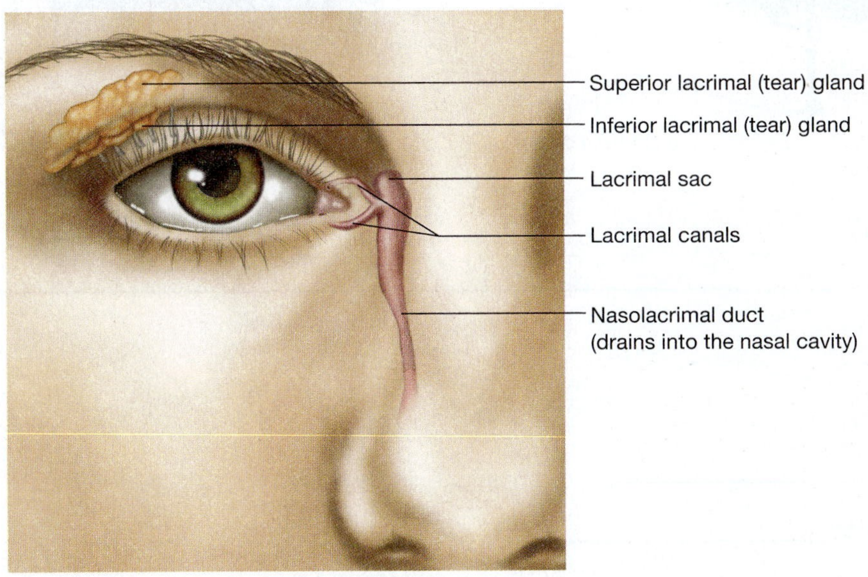

■ **Figure 13-5** The structure of the lacrimal apparatus.

How Vision Works

When light rays strike the eye, they first pass through the cornea, pupil, aqueous humor, lens, and vitreous humor (see Figure 13-6 ■). They then strike the retina and stimulate the rods and cones. When the light rays hit the retina, an upside-down image is sent along nerve impulses to the optic nerve (see Figure 13-7 ■). The optic nerve transmits these impulses to the brain, where the upside-down image is translated into the right-side-up image being looked at.

Vision requires proper functioning of four mechanisms:

1. Coordination of the external eye muscles so that both eyes move together.
2. The correct amount of light admitted by the pupil.
3. The correct focus of light on the retina by the lens.
4. The optic nerve transmitting sensory images to the brain.

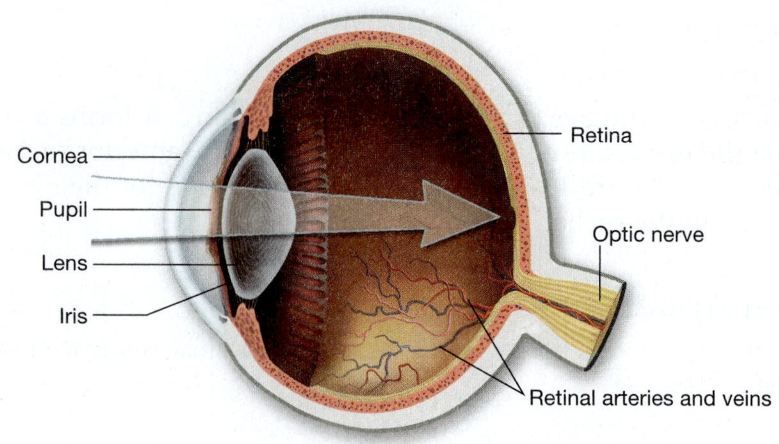

■ **Figure 13-6** The path of light through the cornea, iris, lens, and striking the retina.

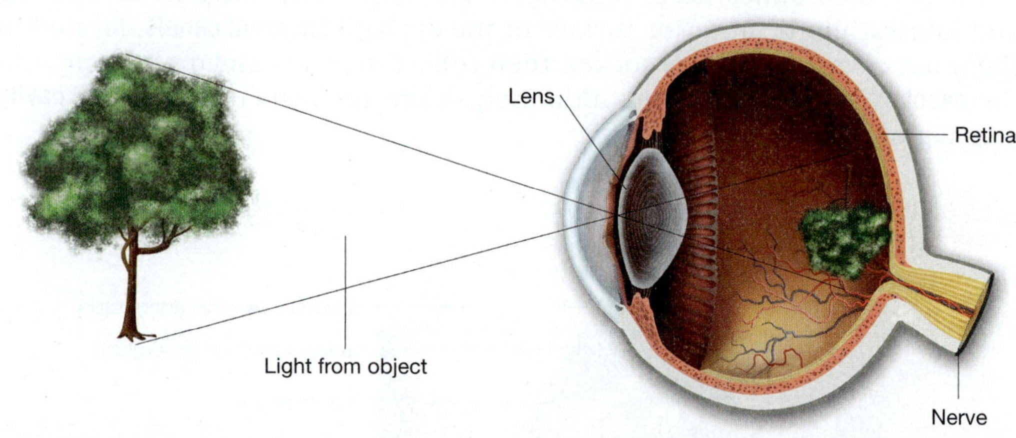

■ **Figure 13-7** The image formed on the retina is inverted. The brain rights the image as part of the interpretation process.

PRACTICE AS YOU GO

A. Complete the Statement

1. The study of the eye is ______________________.
2. Another term for eyelashes is ______________________.
3. The glands responsible for tears are called ______________________ glands.
4. The clear, transparent portion of the sclera is called the ______________________.
5. The innermost layer of the eye, which is composed of sensory receptors, is the __________________.
6. The pupil of the eye is actually a hole in the ______________________.
7. The ______________________ layer of the eyeball distributes the blood supply to the eyeball.
8. ______________________ are active in bright light and perceive color. ______________________ are active in dim light and see in gray tones.
9. ______________________ muscles pull the eyeball in a straight line, whereas ______________________ muscles produce diagonal eye movement.
10. The ______________________ is a mucous membrane covering the anterior surface of the eyeball.

Terminology

Word Parts Used to Build Eye Terms

The following lists contain the combining forms, suffixes, and prefixes used to build terms in the remaining sections of this chapter.

Combining Forms

aden/o	gland	**emmetr/o**	correct, proper	**opt/o**	eye, vision
ambly/o	dull, dim	**esthesi/o**	sensation, feeling	**optic/o**	eye, vision
angi/o	vessel	**glauc/o**	gray	**papill/o**	optic disk
bi/o	life	**ir/o**	iris	**phac/o**	lens
blast/o	immature	**irid/o**	iris	**phot/o**	light
blephar/o	eyelid	**kerat/o**	cornea	**pneum/o**	air
chromat/o	color	**lacrim/o**	tears	**presby/o**	old age
conjunctiv/o	conjunctiva	**macul/o**	macula lutea	**pupill/o**	pupil
corne/o	cornea	**mi/o**	lessening	**retin/o**	retina
cry/o	cold	**myc/o**	fungus	**scler/o**	sclera
cycl/o	ciliary body	**mydr/i**	widening	**stigmat/o**	point
cyst/o	sac	**nyctal/o**	night	**ton/o**	tone
dacry/o	tears	**ocul/o**	eye	**uve/o**	choroid
dipl/o	double	**ophthalm/o**	eye	**xer/o**	dry

Suffixes

-al	pertaining to	**-logy**	study of	**-pexy**	surgical fixation
-algia	pain	**-malacia**	abnormal softening	**-phobia**	fear
-ar	pertaining to	**-meter**	instrument to measure	**-plasty**	surgical repair
-ary	pertaining to	**-metrist**	specialist in measuring	**-plegia**	paralysis
-atic	pertaining to	**-metry**	process of measuring	**-ptosis**	drooping
-ectomy	surgical removal	**-oma**	tumor; mass	**-rrhagia**	abnormal flow condition
-edema	swelling	**-opia**	vision condition	**-scope**	instrument for viewing
-graphy	process of recording	**-opsia**	vision condition	**-scopy**	process of visually examining
-ia	condition	**-osis**	abnormal condition	**-tic**	pertaining to
-ic	pertaining to	**-otomy**	cutting into	**-tropia**	turned condition
-ician	specialist	**-pathy**	disease		
-ism	state of				
-itis	inflammation				

Prefixes

a-	without	**exo-**	outward	**intra-**	within
an-	without	**extra-**	outside of	**micro-**	small
anti-	against	**hemi-**	half	**mono-**	one
de-	without	**hyper-**	excessive	**myo-**	to shut
eso-	inward				

Adjective Forms of Anatomical Terms

Term	Word Parts	Definition
conjunctival (kon-junk-TYE-val)	conjunctiv/o = conjunctiva -al = pertaining to	Pertaining to conjunctiva
corneal (KOR-nee-al)	corne/o = cornea -al = pertaining to **Word Watch** Be careful using the combining forms **core/o** meaning *pupil* and **corne/o** meaning *cornea*.	Pertaining to cornea
extraocular (eks-trah-OK-yoo-lar)	extra- = outside of ocul/o = eye -ar = pertaining to	Pertaining to being outside the eyeball; for example, the extra-ocular eye muscles
intraocular (in-trah-OK-yoo-lar)	intra- = within ocul/o = eye -ar = pertaining to	Pertaining to within the eye
iridal (IR-id-al)	irid/o = iris -al = pertaining to	Pertaining to iris
lacrimal (LAK-rim-al)	lacrim/o = tears -al = pertaining to	Pertaining to tears
macular (MAK-yoo-lar)	macul/o = macula lutea -ar = pertaining to	Pertaining to macula lutea
ocular (OK-yoo-lar)	ocul/o = eye -ar = pertaining to	Pertaining to eye
ophthalmic (off-THAL-mik)	ophthalm/o = eye -ic = pertaining to	Pertaining to eye
optic (OP-tik)	opt/o = eye, vision -ic = pertaining to	Pertaining to eye or vision
optical (OP-tih-kal)	optic/o = eye, vision -al = pertaining to	Pertaining to eye or vision
pupillary (PYOO-pih-lair-ee)	pupill/o = pupil -ary = pertaining to	Pertaining to pupil
retinal (RET-ih-nal)	retin/o = retina -al = pertaining to	Pertaining to retina
scleral (SKLAIR-al)	scler/o = sclera -al = pertaining to	Pertaining to sclera
uveal (YOO-vee-al)	uve/o = choroid -al = pertaining to	Pertaining to choroid layer of eye

PRACTICE AS YOU GO

B. Give the adjective form for each term.

1. The pupil ______________________
2. The eye or vision ______________________ or ______________________
3. The retina ______________________

4. Tears ______________________________

5. Within the eye ______________________________

6. Outside of the eye ______________________________

Pathology

Term	Word Parts	Definition
Medical Specialties		
ophthalmology (Ophth) (off-thal-MALL-oh-jee)	**ophthalm/o** = eye **-logy** = study of	Branch of medicine involving diagnosis and treatment of conditions and diseases of the eye and surrounding structures; physician is *ophthalmologist*
optician (op-TISH-an)	**opt/o** = vision **-ician** = specialist	Vision specialist trained in grinding and fitting corrective lenses
optometrist (op-TOM-eh-trist)	**opt/o** = vision **-metrist** = specialist in measuring	Doctor of optometry
optometry (op-TOM-eh-tree)	**opt/o** = vision **-metry** = process of measuring	Medical profession specializing in examining the eyes, testing visual acuity, and prescribing corrective lenses
Signs and Symptoms		
blepharoptosis (blef-ah-rop-TOH-sis)	**blephar/o** = eyelid **-ptosis** = drooping	Drooping eyelid
cycloplegia (sigh-kloh-PLEE-jee-ah)	**cycl/o** = ciliary body **-plegia** = paralysis	Paralysis of ciliary body that, in turn, changes shape of lens and makes it difficult to bring images into focus
diplopia (dip-LOH-pee-ah)	**dipl/o** = double **-opia** = vision condition	Condition of seeing double
emmetropia (EM) (em-eh-TROH-pee-ah)	**emmetr/o** = correct, proper **-opia** = vision condition	State of normal vision
iridoplegia (ir-id-oh-PLEE-jee-ah)	**irid/o** = iris **-plegia** = paralysis	Paralysis of the iris that, in turn, changes size of the pupil and makes it difficult to regulate amount of light entering the eye
nyctalopia (nik-tah-LOH-pee-ah)	**nyctal/o** = night **-opia** = vision condition **Med Term Tip** The simple translation of *nyctalopia* is *night vision*. However, it is used to mean *night blindness*.	Difficulty seeing in dim light; also called *night blindness*; usually due to damaged rods
ophthalmalgia (off-thal-MAL-jee-ah)	**ophthalm/o** = eye **-algia** = pain	Eye pain
ophthalmoplegia (off-thal-moh-PLEE-jee-ah)	**ophthalm/o** = eye **-plegia** = paralysis	Paralysis of one or more of the extraocular eye muscles
ophthalmorrhagia (off-thal-moh-RAY-jee-ah)	**ophthalm/o** = eye **-rrhagia** = abnormal flow condition	Bleeding from the eye
papilledema (pap-il-eh-DEE-mah)	**papill/o** = optic disk **-edema** = swelling	Swelling of the optic disk; often as result of increased intraocular pressure; also called *choked disk*

Pathology (continued)

Term	Word Parts	Definition
photophobia (foh-toh-FOH-bee-ah)	phot/o = light -phobia = fear	Although term translates into *fear of light*, actually means strong sensitivity to bright light
presbyopia (prez-bee-OH-pee-ah)	presby/o = old age -opia = vision condition	Expected changes in vision due to normal aging process; resulting in difficulty in focusing for near vision (such as reading)
scleromalacia (sklair-oh-mah-LAY-shee-ah)	scler/o = sclera -malacia = abnormal softening	Softening of the sclera
xerophthalmia (zeer-off-THAL-mee-ah)	xer/o = dry ophthalm/o = eye -ia = condition	Condition of dry eyes
Eyeball		
achromatopsia (ah-kroh-mah-TOP-see-ah)	a- = without chromat/o = color -opsia = vision condition	Severe congenital deficiency in color vision; complete color blindness; more common in males
amblyopia (am-blee-OH-pee-ah)	ambly/o = dull, dim -opia = vision condition	Loss of vision not as result of eye pathology; usually occurs in patients who see two images; in order to see only one image, the brain will no longer recognize image being sent to it by one of the eyes; may occur if strabismus is not corrected; condition is not treatable with prescription lens; commonly referred to as *lazy eye*
astigmatism (Astigm) (ah-STIG-mah-tizm)	a- = without stigmat/o = point -ism = state of	Condition in which light rays are focused unevenly on the retina (no sharp point of focus), causing distorted image, due to abnormal curvature of the cornea
cataract (KAT-ah-rakt)		Development of an opaque or cloudy lens, resulting in diminished vision; most common causes are aging, eye trauma, or radiation (especially sunlight) exposure, but may be present at birth; treatment is usually surgical removal of lens with cataract and replacement with prosthetic lens
corneal abrasion	corne/o = cornea -al = pertaining to	Scraping injury to the cornea; if it does not heal, may develop into ulcer
glaucoma (glaw-KOH-mah)	glauc/o = gray -oma = mass	Increase in intraocular pressure, which, if untreated, may result in atrophy (wasting-away) of optic nerve and blindness; treated with medication and surgery; there is increased risk of developing glaucoma in persons over age 60, those of African ancestry, people who have sustained serious eye injury, or anyone with family history of diabetes or glaucoma

Med Term Tip

The term *cataract* comes from the Latin word meaning *waterfall*. This refers to how a person with a cataract sees the world—as if looking through a waterfall.

Figure 13-8 Photograph of a person with a cataract in the right eye. *(ARZTSAMUI/Shutterstock)*

Med Term Tip

The term *glaucoma* was first used by the ancient Greeks to describe the dull, glazed appearance of a blind eye, not an actual color change.

Pathology (continued)

Term	Word Parts	Definition
hyperopia (high-per-OH-pee-ah)	**hyper-** = excessive **-opia** = vision condition	With this condition person can see things in distance but has trouble reading material at close range; also known as *farsightedness;* condition is corrected with converging or biconvex lenses

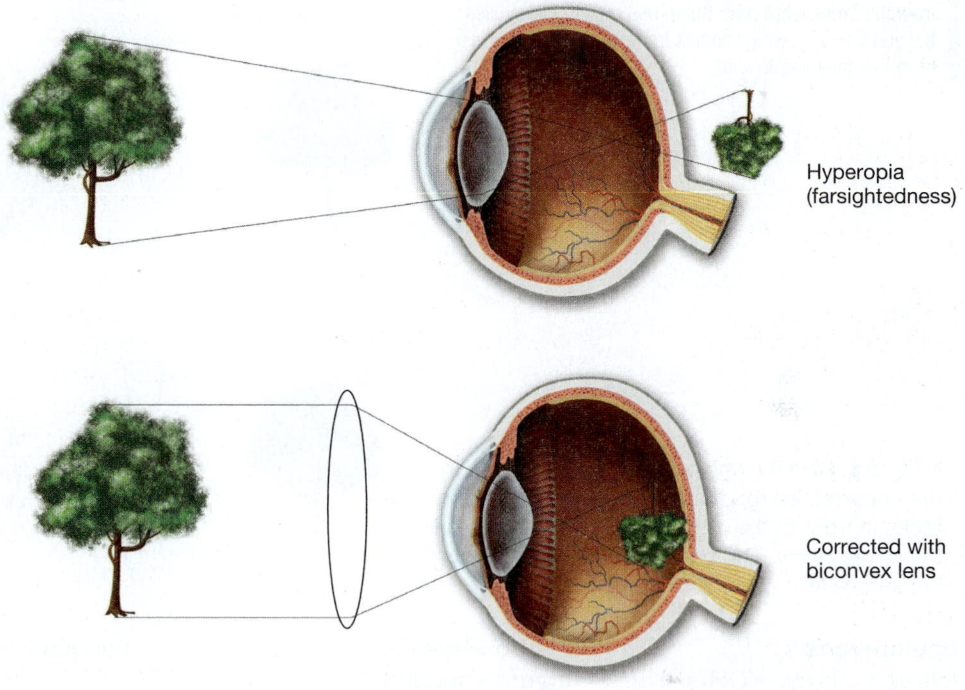

Hyperopia (farsightedness)

Corrected with biconvex lens

■ **Figure 13-9** Hyperopia (farsightedness). In the uncorrected top figure, the image would come into focus behind the retina, making the image on the retina blurry. The bottom image shows how a biconvex lens corrects this condition.

Term	Word Parts	Definition
iritis (eye-RYE-tis)	**ir/o** = iris **-itis** = inflammation	Inflammation of the iris
keratitis (kair-ah-TYE-tis)	**kerat/o** = cornea **-itis** = inflammation	Inflammation of the cornea

Word Watch

Be careful using the combining form **kerat/o**, which means both *cornea* and the hard protein *keratin*.

Term	Word Parts	Definition
legally blind		Describes person who has severely impaired vision; usually defined as having visual acuity of 20/200 that cannot be improved with corrective lenses or having visual field of less than 20 degrees
macular degeneration (MAK-yoo-lar)	**macul/o** = macula lutea **-ar** = pertaining to	Deterioration of macular area of the retina of the eye; may be treated with laser surgery to destroy blood vessels beneath the macula
monochromatism (mon-oh-KROH-mah-tizm)	**mono-** = one **chromat/o** = color **-ism** = state of	Unable to perceive one color

Pathology (continued)

Term	Word Parts	Definition
myopia (MY) (my-OH-pee-ah)	**myo-** = to shut **-opia** = vision condition	With this condition person can see things close up but distance vision is blurred; also known as *nearsightedness*; condition is corrected with diverging or biconcave lenses; named because persons with myopia often partially shut their eyes, squint, in order to see more clearly

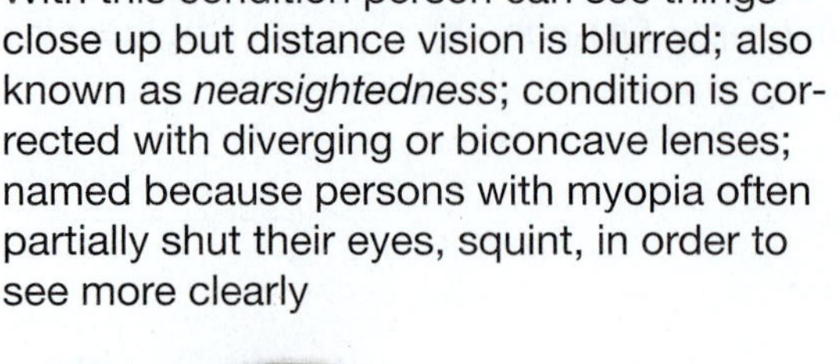

Med Term Tip

The term *myopia* appears to use the combining form **my/o**, which means *muscle*. This combining form comes from the Greek word *mys*. But in this case the term uses the prefix **myo-**, which comes from the Greek word *myo* or *myein*, meaning *to shut*.

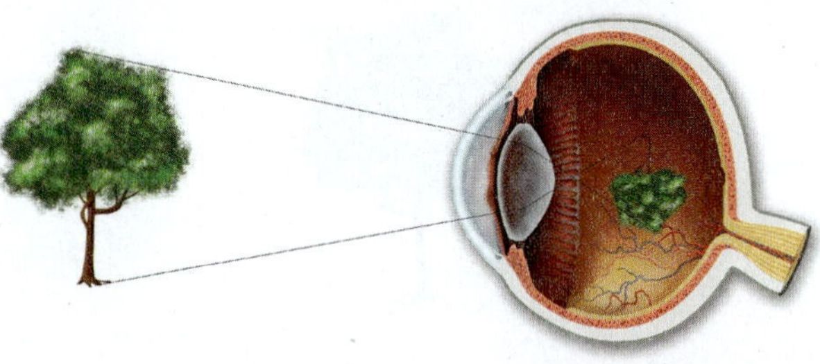

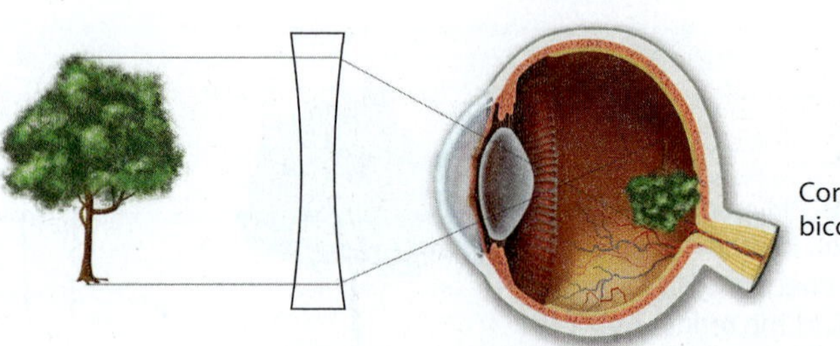

Figure 13-10 Myopia (nearsightedness). In the uncorrected top figure, the image comes into focus in front of the retina, making the image on the retina blurry. The bottom image shows how a biconcave lens corrects this condition.

Term	Word Parts	Definition
oculomycosis (ok-yoo-loh-my-KOH-sis)	**ocul/o** = eye **myc/o** = fungus **-osis** = abnormal condition	Fungus infection of the eye
retinal detachment (RET-ih-nal)	**retin/o** = retina **-al** = pertaining to	Occurs when the retina becomes separated from the choroid layer; separation seriously damages blood vessels and nerves, resulting in blindness; may be treated with surgical or medical procedures to stabilize the retina and prevent separation
retinitis pigmentosa (ret-ih-NYE-tis / pig-men-TOH-sah)	**retin/o** = retina **-itis** = inflammation	Progressive disease of the eye resulting in the retina becoming sclerosed (hard), pigmented (colored), and atrophied (wasting-away); no known cure for this condition
retinoblastoma (ret-ih-noh-blas-TOH-mah)	**retin/o** = retina **blast/o** = immature **-oma** = tumor	Malignant eye tumor occurring in children, usually under age 3; requires enucleation
retinopathy (ret-in-OP-ah-thee)	**retin/o** = retina **-pathy** = disease	General term for disease affecting the retina
scleritis (skler-EYE-tis)	**scler/o** = sclera **-itis** = inflammation	Inflammation of the sclera

Pathology (continued)

Term	Word Parts	Definition
uveitis (yoo-vee-EYE-tis)	**uve/o** = choroid **-itis** = inflammation	Inflammation of the choroid layer
Conjunctiva		
conjunctivitis (kon-junk-tih-VYE-tis)	**conjunctiv/o** = conjunctiva **-itis** = inflammation	Inflammation of the conjunctiva usually as result of bacterial infection, but may also be caused by viruses and allergens; commonly called *pinkeye*
pterygium (teh-RIJ-ee-um)		Hypertrophied conjunctival tissue in inner corner of the eye
Eyelids		
blepharitis (blef-ah-RYE-tis)	**blephar/o** = eyelid **-itis** = inflammation	Inflammation of the eyelid
hordeolum (hor-DEE-oh-lum)		Refers to a *stye* (or *sty*), a small purulent inflammatory infection of a sebaceous gland of the eyelid; treated with hot compresses and/or surgical incision
Lacrimal Apparatus		
dacryoadenitis (dak-ree-oh-ad-eh-NYE-tis)	**dacry/o** = tears **aden/o** = gland **-itis** = inflammation	Inflammation of the lacrimal gland
dacryocystitis (dak-ree-oh-sis-TYE-tis)	**dacry/o** = tears **cyst/o** = sac **-itis** = inflammation	Inflammation of the lacrimal sac
Eye Muscles		
esotropia (ET) (ess-oh-TROH-pee-ah)	**eso-** = inward **-tropia** = turned condition	Inward turning of the eye; also called *cross-eyed*; example of a form of strabismus (muscle weakness of the eye)
exotropia (XT) (eks-oh-TROH-pee-ah)	**exo-** = outward **-tropia** = turned condition	Outward turning of the eye; also called *wall-eyed*; also an example of strabismus (muscle weakness of the eye)
strabismus (strah-BIZ-mus)		Eye muscle weakness commonly seen in children resulting in eyes looking in different directions at the same time; may be corrected with glasses, eye exercises, and/or surgery
Brain-Related Vision Pathologies		
hemianopia (hem-ee-ah-NOH-pee-ah)	**hemi-** = half **an-** = without **-opia** = vision condition	Loss of vision in half of visual field; a stroke patient may suffer from this disorder
nystagmus (niss-TAG-mus)		Jerky-appearing involuntary eye movements, usually left and right; often an indication of brain injury

PRACTICE AS YOU GO

C. Pathology Matching

Match each pathology term to its definition.

1. ________	emmetropia	**a.**	opacity of the lens
2. ________	hyperopia	**b.**	a form of strabismus
3. ________	cataract	**c.**	nearsightedness
4. ________	astigmatism	**d.**	due to abnormal curvature of cornea
5. ________	esotropia	**e.**	lazy eye
6. ________	xerophthalmia	**f.**	involuntary movements of the eye
7. ________	myopia	**g.**	farsightedness
8. ________	nystagmus	**h.**	normal vision
9. ________	amblyopia	**i.**	dry eyes
10. ________	presbyopia	**j.**	vision loss due to normal aging

Diagnostic Procedures

Term	Word Parts	Definition
Eye Examination Tests		
color vision tests		Use of polychromic (multicolored) charts to determine ability of patient to recognize color; most common is Ishihara test for red-green color blindness
■ **Figure 13-11** An example of color blindness test. A person with red-green color blindness would not be able to distinguish the green 27 from the surrounding red circles.		
fluorescein angiography (floor-ESS-see-in / an-jee-OG-rah-fee)	angi/o = vessel -graphy = process of recording	Process of injecting dye (fluorescein) to observe movement of blood and detect lesions in macular area of the retina; used to determine if there is detachment of the retina
fluorescein staining (floor-ESS-see-in)		Application of dye eyedrops of bright green fluorescent color used to look for corneal abrasions or ulcers
keratometer (kair-ah-TOM-eh-ter)	kerat/o = cornea -meter = instrument to measure	Instrument used to measure curvature of the cornea

Diagnostic Procedures (continued)

Term	Word Parts	Definition
keratometry (kair-ah-TOM-eh-tree)	kerat/o = cornea -metry = process of measuring	Measurement of curvature of the cornea using instrument called *keratometer*
ophthalmoscope (off-THAL-moh-skohp)	ophthalm/o = eye -scope = instrument for viewing	Instrument used to examine inside of the eye through the pupil
ophthalmoscopy (off-thal-MOSS-koh-pee)	ophthalm/o = eye -scopy = process of visually examining	Examination of interior of the eyes using instrument called *ophthalmoscope*; pupil is dilated in order to see cornea, lens, and retina; used to identify abnormalities in blood vessels of the eye and some systemic diseases

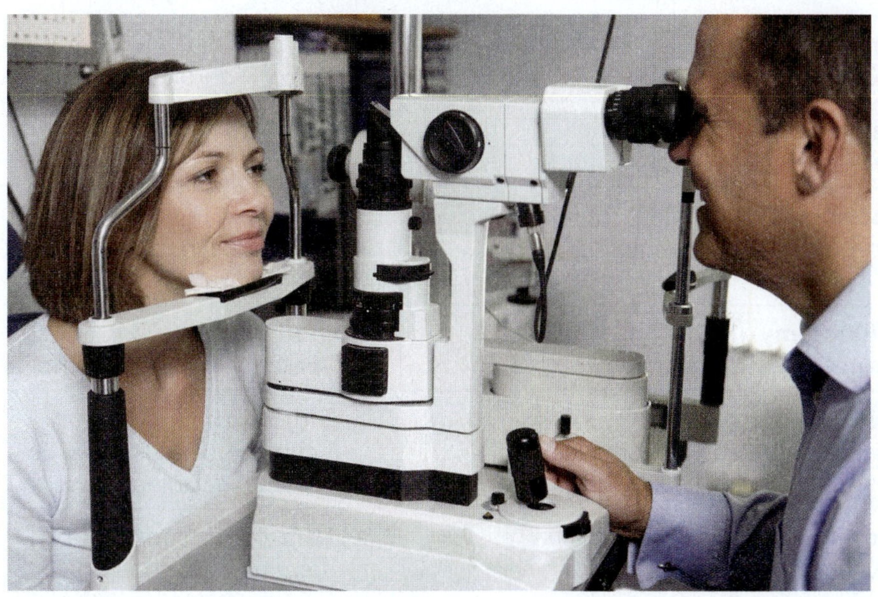

■ **Figure 13-12** Examination of the interior of the eye using an ophthalmoscope. *(Monkey Business Images/ Shutterstock)*

Term	Word Parts	Definition
optometer (op-TOM-eh-ter)	opt/o = vision -meter = instrument to measure	Instrument used to measure how well the eye is able to focus images clearly on the retina
refractive error test (ree-FRAK-tiv)		Vision test for defect in ability of the eye to accurately focus image that is hitting it; refractive errors result in myopia and hyperopia
slit lamp microscopy	micro- = small -scopy = process of visually examining	Process of visually examining conjunctiva, cornea, iris, and lens of the eye
Snellen chart (SNEL-en)		Chart used for testing distance vision named for Dutch ophthalmologist Herman Snellen; contains letters of varying sizes and is administered from a distance of 20 feet; person who can read at 20 feet what average person can read at this distance is said to have 20/20 vision
tonometry (tohn-OM-eh-tree)	ton/o = tone -metry = process of measuring	Measurement of intraocular pressure of the eye using *tonometer* to check for condition of glaucoma; generally part of normal eye exam for adults
visual acuity (VA) **test** (VIZH-oo-al / ah-KYOO-ih-tee)	-al = pertaining to	Measurement of sharpness of patient's vision; usually, Snellen chart is used for this test in which patient identifies letters from a distance of 20 feet

Therapeutic Procedures

Terms	Word Parts	Definition
Surgical Procedures		
blepharectomy (blef-ah-REK-toh-mee)	blephar/o = eyelid -ectomy = surgical removal	Surgical removal of all or part of the eyelid
blepharoplasty (BLEF-ah-roh-plas-tee)	blephar/o = eyelid -plasty = surgical repair	Surgical repair of the eyelid; common plastic surgery to correct blepharoptosis
conjunctivoplasty (kon-JUNK-tih-voh-plas-tee)	conjunctiv/o = conjunctiva -plasty = surgical repair	Surgical repair of the conjunctiva
cryopexy (KRY-oh-pek-see)	cry/o = cold -pexy = surgical fixation	Surgical fixation of the retina by using extreme cold
enucleation (ee-noo-klee-AY-shun)		Surgical removal of an eyeball
intraocular lens (IOL) **implant** (in-trah-OK-yoo-lar)	intra- = within ocul/o = eye -ar = pertaining to	Use of artificial lens to replace the lens removed during cataract surgery
iridectomy (ir-ih-DEK-toh-mee)	irid/o = iris -ectomy = surgical removal	Surgical removal of a small portion of the iris
iridosclerotomy (ir-ih-doh-skleh-ROT-oh-mee)	irid/o = iris scler/o = sclera -otomy = cutting into	To cut into iris and sclera
keratoplasty (KAIR-ah-toh-plas-tee)	kerat/o = cornea -plasty = surgical repair	Surgical repair of the cornea is simple translation of this term utilized to mean corneal transplant
laser-assisted in situ keratomileusis (LASIK) (in-SIGH-tyoo / kair-ah-toh-mih-LOO-sis) ■ **Figure 13-13** LASIK surgery uses a laser to reshape the cornea. *(Mehmetcan/Shutterstock)*	kerat/o = cornea	Correction of myopia using laser surgery to remove corneal tissue
laser photocoagulation (LAY-zer / foh-toh-koh-ag-yoo-LAY-shun)	phot/o = light	Use of laser beam to destroy very small precise areas of the retina; may be used to treat retinal detachment or macular degeneration

Therapeutic Procedures (continued)

Terms	Word Parts	Definition
phacoemulsification (fay-koh-ee-mull-sih-fih-KAY-shun)	phac/o = lens	Use of high-frequency sound waves to emulsify (liquefy) a lens with a cataract, which is then aspirated (removed by suction) with a needle
photorefractive keratectomy (PRK) (foh-toh-ree-FRAK-tiv / kair-ah-TEK-toh-mee)	phot/o = light kerat/o = cornea -ectomy = surgical removal	Surgical use of laser to reshape the cornea and correct errors of refraction
pneumatic retinopexy (noo-MAT-ik / ret-ih-noh-PEK-see)	pneum/o = air -atic = pertaining to retin/o = retina -pexy = surgical fixation	Surgical injection of gas bubble into the eye and positioning the head so that bubble presses against area of detached retina
radial keratotomy (RK) (RAY-dee-al / kair-ah-TOT-oh-mee)	-al = pertaining to kerat/o = cornea -otomy = cutting into	Spokelike incisions around the cornea that result in it becoming flatter; surgical treatment for myopia
retinopexy (ret-ih-noh-PEK-see)	retin/o = retina -pexy = surgical fixation	Surgical fixation of the retina; one treatment for a detaching retina
scleral buckling (SKLAIR-al)	scler/o = sclera -al = pertaining to	Placing a band of silicone around outside of the sclera that stabilizes a detaching retina
sclerotomy (skleh-ROT-oh-mee)	scler/o = sclera -otomy = cutting into	To cut into the sclera
strabotomy (strah-BOT-oh-mee)	-otomy = cutting into	Incision into the eye muscles in order to correct strabismus

PRACTICE AS YOU GO

D. Procedure Matching

Match each procedure term to its definition.

1. ______________ fluorescein staining
2. ______________ ophthalmoscopy
3. ______________ tonometry
4. ______________ enucleation
5. ______________ keratoplasty
6. ______________ phacoemulsification

a. examining the interior of the eyeball
b. corneal transplant
c. liquefies a cataract
d. looks for corneal abrasions or ulcers
e. surgical removal of an eyeball
f. measures intraocular pressure

Pharmacology

Classification	Word Parts	Action	Examples
anesthetic ophthalmic solution (off-THAL-mik)	an- = without esthesi/o = sensation, feeling -tic = pertaining to ophthalm/o = eye -ic = pertaining to	Eyedrops for pain relief associated with eye infections, corneal abrasions, or surgery	proparacain, Ak-Taine, Ocu-Caine; tetracaine, Opticaine, Pontocaine
antibiotic ophthalmic solution (off-THAL-mik)	anti- = against bi/o = life -tic = pertaining to ophthalm/o = eye -ic = pertaining to	Eyedrops for treatment of bacterial eye infections	erythromycin, Del-Mycin, Ilotycin Ophthalmic
antiglaucoma medications (an-tye-glaw-KOH-mah)	anti- = against glauc/o = gray -oma = mass	Reduce intraocular pressure by lowering amount of aqueous humor in the eyeball; may achieve this by either reducing production of aqueous humor or increasing its outflow	timolol, Betimol, Timoptic; acetazolamide, Ak-Zol, Dazamide; prostaglandin analogs, Lumigan, Xalatan
artificial tears		Medications, many of them over-the-counter, to treat dry eyes	buffered isotonic solutions, Akwa Tears, Refresh Plus, Moisture Eyes
miotic drops (my-OT-ik)	mi/o = lessening -tic = pertaining to	Any substance that causes the pupil to constrict (lessen); these medications may also be used to treat glaucoma	physostigmine, Eserine Sulfate, Isopto Eserine; carbachol, Carbastat, Miostat
mydriatic drops (mid-ree-AT-ik)	mydr/i = widening -atic = pertaining to	Any substance that causes the pupil to dilate (widen) by paralyzing iris and/or ciliary body muscles; particularly useful during eye examinations and eye surgery	atropine sulfate, Atropine-Care Ophthalmic, Atropisol Ophthalmic
ophthalmic decongestants	ophthalm/o = eye -ic = pertaining to de- = without	Over-the-counter medications that constrict the arterioles of the eye and reduce redness and itching of the conjunctiva	tetrahydrozoline, Visine, Murine

Abbreviations

ARMD	age-related macular degeneration	**LASIK**	laser-assisted in situ keratomileusis
Astigm	astigmatism	**MY**	myopia
c.gl.	correction with glasses	**Ophth**	ophthalmology
D	diopter (lens strength)	**PERRLA**	pupils equal, round, reactive to light and accommodation
DVA	distance visual acuity	**PRK**	photorefractive keratectomy
ECCE	extracapsular cataract extraction	**REM**	rapid eye movement
EENT	eyes, ears, nose, and throat	**RK**	radial keratotomy
EM	emmetropia	**s.gl.**	without correction or glasses
EOM	extraocular movement	**SMD**	senile macular degeneration
ET	esotropia	**VA**	visual acuity
ICCE	intracapsular cataract extraction	**VF**	visual field
IOL	intraocular lens	**XT**	exotropia
IOP	intraocular pressure		

PRACTICE AS YOU GO

E. What's the Abbreviation?

1. intraocular lens ________________
2. emmetropia ________________
3. exotropia ________________
4. myopia ________________
5. extraocular movement ________________
6. visual acuity ________________

SECTION II: THE EAR

AT A GLANCE

Function

The ear contains the sensory receptors for hearing and equilibrium (balance).

Structures

The primary structures that comprise the ear:

external ear	**middle ear**
auricle	**inner ear**

Word Parts

Presented here are the most common word parts (with their meanings) used to build ear terms. For a more comprehensive list, refer to the Terminology section of this chapter.

Combining Forms

acous/o	hearing	**labyrinth/o**	labyrinth (inner ear)
audi/o	hearing	**myring/o**	tympanic membrane
audit/o	hearing	**ot/o**	ear
aur/o	ear	**salping/o**	auditory tube (eustachian tube)
auricul/o	ear	**staped/o**	stapes
cerumin/o	cerumen	**tympan/o**	tympanic membrane
cochle/o	cochlea	**vestibul/o**	vestibule

Suffixes

-cusis	hearing
-otia	ear condition

The Ear Illustrated

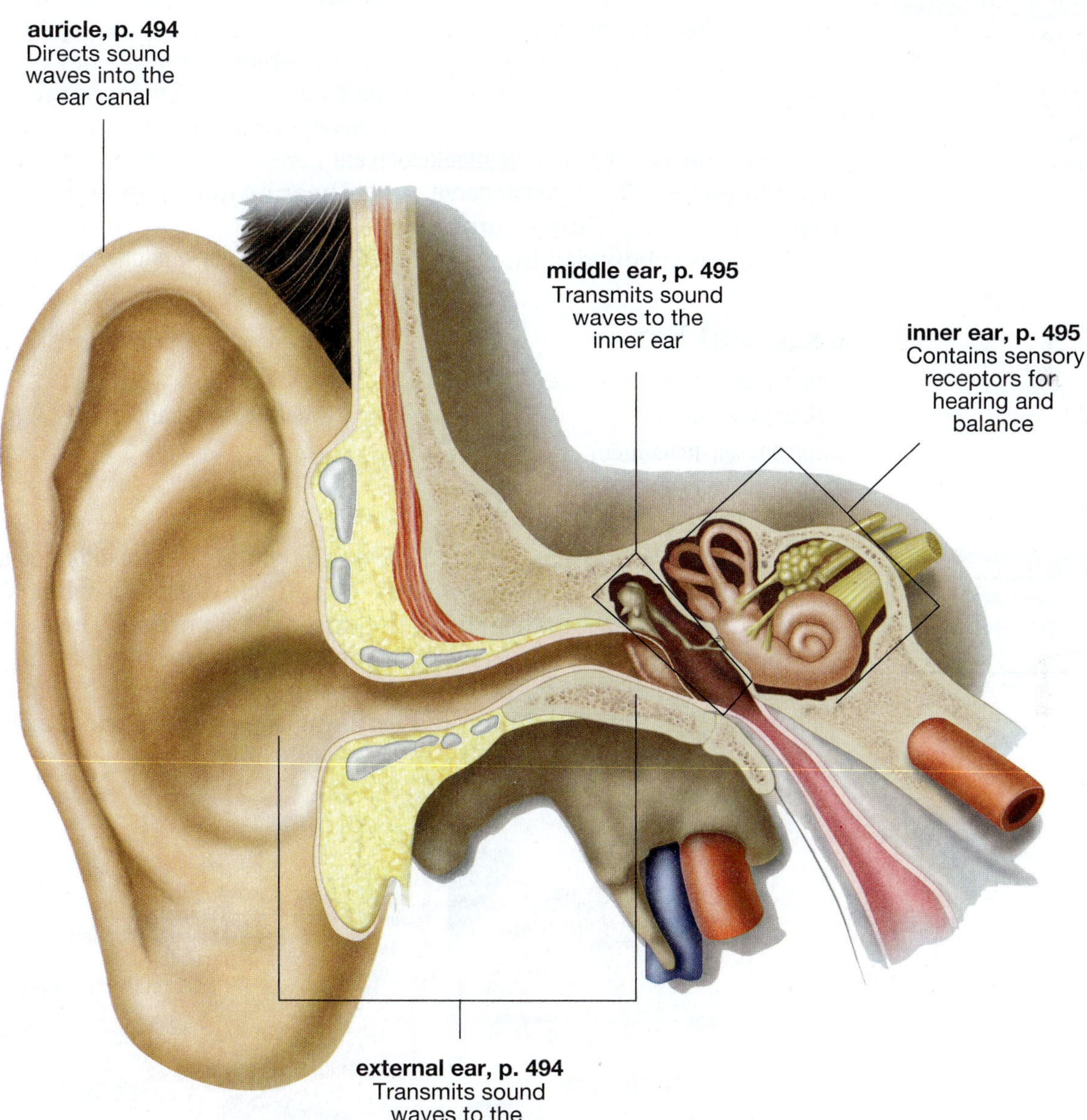

auricle, p. 494
Directs sound waves into the ear canal
middle ear, p. 495
Transmits sound waves to the inner ear
inner ear, p. 495
Contains sensory receptors for hearing and balance
external ear, p. 494
Transmits sound waves to the middle ear

Anatomy and Physiology of the Ear

audiology (aw-dee-ALL-oh-jee)
cochlear nerve (KOH-klee-ar)
equilibrium (ee-kwih-LIB-ree-um)
external ear
hearing
inner ear
middle ear
otology (oh-TALL-oh-jee)
vestibular nerve (ves-TIB-yoo-lar)
vestibulocochlear nerve (ves-tib-yoo-loh-KOH-klee-ar)

What's In A Name?
Look for these word parts:
cochle/o = cochlea
vestibul/o = vestibule
-al = pertaining to
-ar = pertaining to
ex- = outward

The study of the ear is referred to as **otology** (Oto), and the study of hearing disorders is called **audiology**. While there is a large amount of overlap between these two areas, there are also examples of ear problems that do not affect hearing. The ear is responsible for two senses: **hearing** and **equilibrium**, or the body's sense of balance. Hearing and equilibrium sensory information is carried to the brain by cranial nerve VIII, the **vestibulocochlear nerve**. This nerve is divided into two major branches. The **cochlear nerve** carries hearing information, and the **vestibular nerve** carries equilibrium information.

The ear is subdivided into three areas: **external ear**, **middle ear**, and **inner ear**.

External Ear

auditory canal (AW-dih-tor-ee)
auricle (AW-rih-kl)
cerumen (seh-ROO-men)
external auditory meatus (AW-dih-tor-ee / mee-AY-tus)
pinna (PIN-ah)
tympanic membrane (tim-PAN-ik)

What's In A Name?
Look for these word parts:
-al = pertaining to
ex- = outward

The external ear consists of three parts: the **auricle**, the **auditory canal**, and the **tympanic membrane** (see Figure 13-14■). The auricle or **pinna** is what is commonly referred to as the *ear* because this is the only visible portion. The auricle with its earlobe has a unique shape in each person and functions like a funnel to capture sound waves as they go past the outer ear and channel them through the **external auditory meatus**. The sound then moves along the auditory canal and causes the

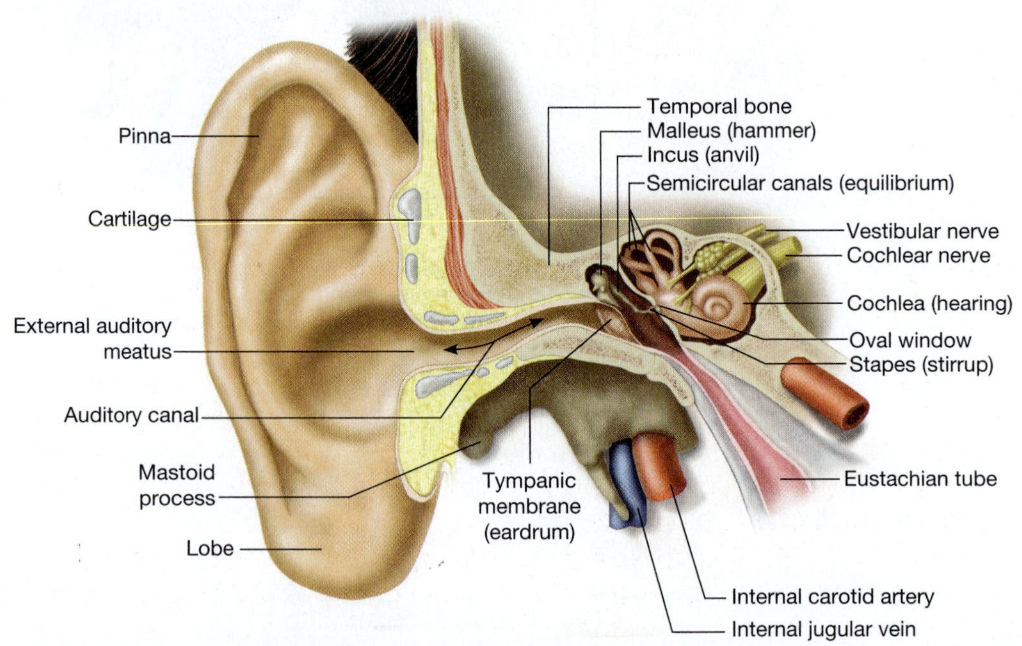

■ **Figure 13-14** The internal structures of the outer, middle, and inner ear.

tympanic membrane (eardrum) to vibrate. The tympanic membrane actually separates the external ear from the middle ear. Earwax or **cerumen** is produced in oil glands in the auditory canal. This wax helps to protect and lubricate the ear. It is also just barely liquid at body temperature. This causes cerumen to slowly flow out of the auditory canal, carrying dirt and dust with it. Therefore, the auditory canal is self-cleaning.

> **Med Term Tip**
> The term *tympanic membrane* comes from the Greek word for *drumhead.* The tympanic membrane or eardrum vibrates to sound waves like a drum head.

Middle Ear

auditory tube (AW-dih-tor-ee)
eustachian tube (yoo-STAY-shee-en)
incus (ING-kus)
malleus (MAL-ee-us)
ossicles (OSS-ih-kls)
oval window
stapes (STAY-peez)

The middle ear is located in a small cavity in the temporal bone of the skull. This air-filled cavity contains three tiny bones called **ossicles** (see Figure 13-15■). These three bones—the **malleus, incus**, and **stapes**—are vital to the hearing process. They amplify the vibrations in the middle ear and transmit them to the inner ear from the malleus to the incus and finally to the stapes. The stapes, the last of the three ossicles, is attached to a very thin membrane that covers the opening to the inner ear called the **oval window**.

The **eustachian tube** or **auditory tube** connects the nasopharynx with the middle ear (see again Figure 13-14). Each time a person swallows, the eustachian tube opens. This connection allows pressure to equalize between the middle ear cavity and the atmospheric pressure.

> **Med Term Tip**
> The three ossicles in the middle ear are the tiniest bones in the body and are sometimes referred to by terms that are similar to their shape. Thus, the malleus is called the hammer, the incus is the anvil, and the stapes is the stirrup (see again Figure 13-15).

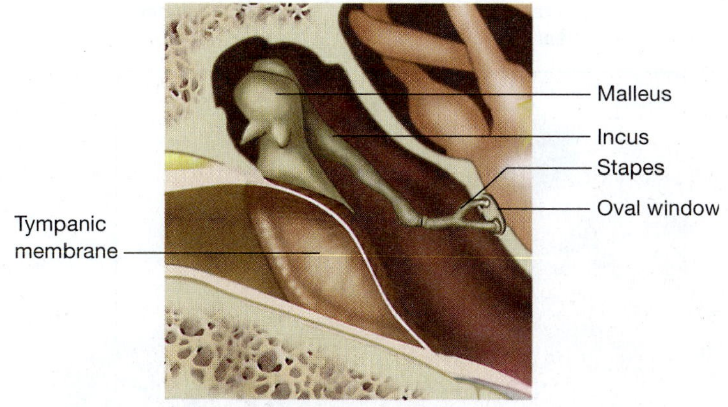

■ **Figure 13-15** Close-up view of the ossicles within the middle ear. These three bones extend from the tympanic membrane to the oval window.

Inner Ear

cochlea (KOH-klee-ah)
labyrinth (LAB-ih-rinth)
organ of Corti (KOR-tee)
saccule (SAK-yool)
semicircular canals
utricle (YOO-trih-kl)
vestibule (VES-tih-byool)

> **What's In A Name?**
> Look for these word parts:
> **-ar** = pertaining to
> **-ule** = small
> **semi-** = partial

The inner ear is also located in a cavity within the temporal bone (see again Figure 13-14). This fluid-filled cavity is referred to as the **labyrinth** because of its shape. The first structure of the inner ear is the **vestibule**. Each of the remaining inner ear structures—the **cochlea** (the sensory organ for hearing) and the **semicircular canals, utricle**, and **saccule** (the sensory organs for equilibrium)—open off the vestibule. Each of these organs contains hair cells, which are the actual sensory receptor cells. In the cochlea, the hair cells are referred to collectively as the **organ of Corti**.

> **Med Term Tip**
> The term *vestibule* comes from the Latin word *vestibulum*, meaning *entrance.* It received this name because it is the entryway into the inner ear.

How Hearing Works

conductive hearing loss (kon-DUK-tiv)

sensorineural hearing loss (sen-soh-ree-NOO-ral)

Figure 13-16 ■ outlines the path of sound through the outer ear and middle ear and into the cochlea of the inner ear. Sound waves traveling down the external auditory canal strike the eardrum, causing it to vibrate. The ossicles conduct these vibrations across the middle ear from the eardrum to the oval window. Oval window movements initiate vibrations in the fluid that fills the cochlea. As the fluid vibrations strike a hair cell, they bend the small hairs and stimulate the nerve ending. The nerve ending then sends an electrical impulse to the brain on the cochlear portion of the vestibulocochlear nerve.

Hearing loss can be divided into two main categories: **conductive hearing loss** and **sensorineural hearing loss**. Conductive refers to disease or malformation of the outer or middle ear. All sound is weaker and muffled in conductive hearing loss since it is not conducted correctly to the inner ear. Sensorineural hearing loss is the result of damage or malformation of the inner ear (cochlea) or the cochlear nerve. In this hearing loss, some sounds are distorted and heard incorrectly. There can also be a combination of both conductive and sensorineural hearing loss.

What's In A Name?

Look for these word parts:
neur/o = nerve
-al = pertaining to

Med Term Tip

Hearing impairment is becoming a greater problem for the general population for several reasons. First, people are living longer. Hearing loss can accompany old age, and there are a greater number of people over age 50 requiring hearing assistance. In addition, sound technology has produced music quality that was never available before. However, listening to loud music either naturally or through earphones can cause gradual damage to the hearing mechanism.

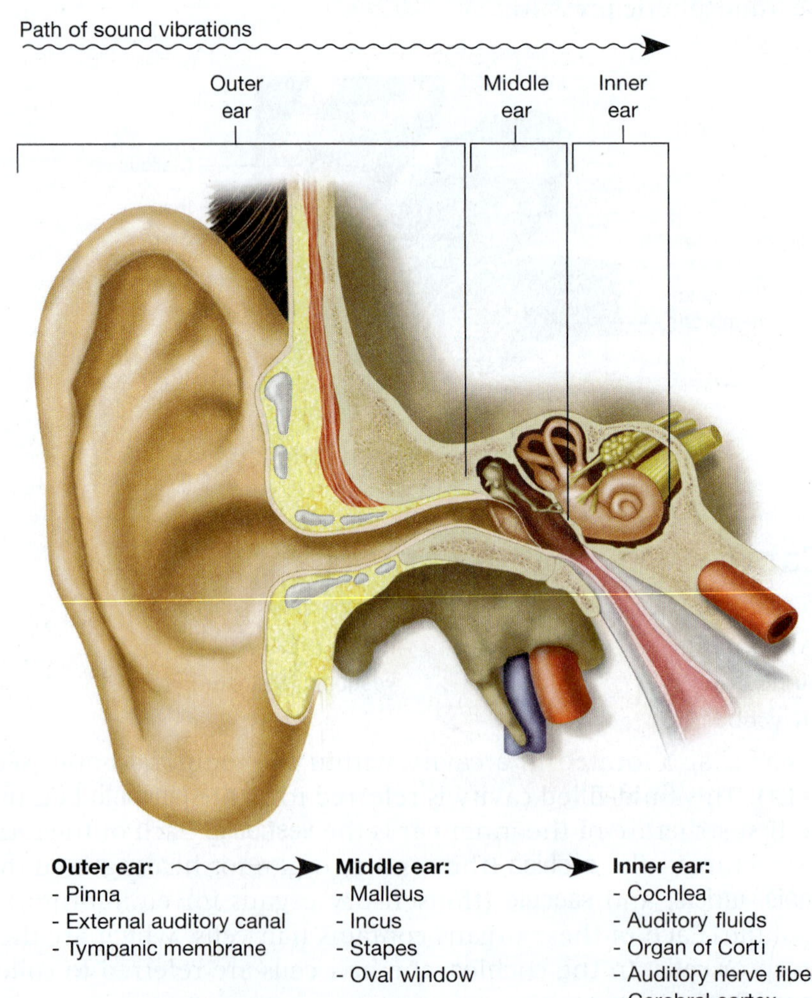

■ **Figure 13-16** The path of sound waves through the outer, middle, and inner ear.

PRACTICE AS YOU GO

F. Complete the Statement

1. The three bones in the middle ear are the ____________________, ____________________, and ____________________.
2. The study of the ear is called ____________________.
3. Another term for the eardrum is ____________________.
4. ____________________ is produced in the oil glands in the auditory canal.
5. The ____________________ tube connects the nasopharynx with the middle ear.
6. The ____________________ is responsible for conducting impulses from the ear to the brain.
7. The ear is responsible for the senses of ____________________ and ____________________.
8. ____________________ hearing loss refers to disease or malformation of the outer or middle ear.

Terminology

Word Parts Used to Build Ear Terms

The following lists contain the combining forms, suffixes, and prefixes used to build terms in the remaining sections of this chapter.

Combining Forms

acous/o	hearing	**cochle/o**	cochlea	**presby/o**	old age
audi/o	hearing	**labyrinth/o**	labyrinth	**py/o**	pus
audit/o	hearing	**laryng/o**	larynx	**rhin/o**	nose
aur/o	ear	**myc/o**	fungus	**salping/o**	auditory tube
auricul/o	ear	**myring/o**	tympanic membrane	**staped/o**	stapes
bi/o	life	**neur/o**	nerve	**tympan/o**	tympanic membrane
cerumin/o	cerumen	**ot/o**	ear	**vestibul/o**	vestibule

Suffixes

-al	pertaining to	**-logy**	study of	**-rrhagia**	abnormal flow
-algia	pain	**-meter**	instrument to measure	**-rrhea**	discharge
-ar	pertaining to	**-metry**	process of measuring	**-rrhexis**	rupture
-cusis	hearing	**-oma**	mass; tumor	**-sclerosis**	hardening
-ectomy	surgical removal	**-ory**	pertaining to	**-scope**	instrument to visually examine
-emetic	pertaining to vomiting	**-osis**	abnormal condition	**-scopy**	process of visually examining
-gram	record	**-otia**	ear condition	**-tic**	pertaining to
-ic	pertaining to	**-otomy**	cutting into		
-itis	inflammation	**-plasty**	surgical repair		

Prefixes					
an-	without	bi-	two	micro-	small
anti-	against	macro-	large	mono-	one

Adjective Forms of Anatomical Terms

Term	Word Parts	Definition
acoustic (ah-KOOS-tik)	acous/o = hearing -tic = pertaining to	Pertaining to hearing
auditory (AW-dih-tor-ee)	audit/o = hearing -ory = pertaining to	Pertaining to hearing
aural (AW-ral)	aur/o = ear -al = pertaining to	Pertaining to the ear

Word Watch

Be careful when using two terms that sound very similar—*aural* meaning *pertaining to the ear* and *oral* meaning *pertaining to the mouth.*

Term	Word Parts	Definition
auricular (aw-RIK-yoo-lar)	auricul/o = ear -ar = pertaining to	Pertaining to the ear
binaural (bye-NOR-al)	bi- = two aur/o = ear -al = pertaining to	Pertaining to both ears
cochlear (KOH-klee-ar)	cochle/o = cochlea -ar = pertaining to	Pertaining to cochlea
monaural (mon-AW-ral)	mono- = one aur/o = ear -al = pertaining to	Pertaining to one ear
otic (OH-tik)	ot/o = ear -ic = pertaining to	Pertaining to the ear
tympanic (tim-PAN-ik)	tympan/o = tympanic membrane -ic = pertaining to	Pertaining to tympanic membrane
vestibular (ves-TIB-yoo-lar)	vestibul/o = vestibule -ar = pertaining to	Pertaining to vestibule

PRACTICE AS YOU GO

G. Give the adjective form for each term.

1. The cochlea ______________________
2. The ear ____________, ____________, or ____________
3. The vestibule ______________________
4. Hearing ______________ or ______________
5. One ear ______________________

Pathology

Term	Word Parts	Definition
Medical Specialties		
audiology (aw-dee-ALL-oh-jee)	audi/o = hearing -logy = study of	Medical specialty involved with measuring hearing function and identifying hearing loss; specialist is an *audiologist*
otorhinolaryngology (ENT) (oh-toh-rye-noh-lair-in-GALL-oh-jee)	ot/o = ear rhin/o = nose laryng/o = larynx -logy = study of	Branch of medicine involving the diagnosis and treatment of conditions and diseases of the ear, nose, and throat; also referred to as *ENT*; physician is an *otorhinolaryngologist*
Signs and Symptoms		
macrotia (mah-KROH-shee-ah)	macro- = large -otia = ear condition	Condition of having abnormally large ears
microtia (my-KROH-shee-ah)	micro- = small -otia = ear condition	Condition of having abnormally small ears
otalgia (oh-TAL-jee-ah)	ot/o = ear -algia = pain	Ear pain
otopyorrhea (oh-toh-pye-oh-REE-ah)	ot/o = ear py/o = pus -rrhea = discharge	Discharge of pus from the ear
otorrhagia (oh-toh-RAY-jee-ah)	ot/o = ear -rrhagia = abnormal flow	Bleeding from the ear
presbycusis (prez-bih-KYOO-sis)	presby/o = old age -cusis = hearing condition	Normal loss of hearing that can accompany aging process
residual hearing (rih-ZID-joo-al)	-al = pertaining to	Amount of hearing still present after damage has occurred to auditory mechanism
tinnitus (tin-EYE-tus)		Ringing in the ears
tympanorrhexis (tim-pan-oh-REK-sis)	tympan/o = tympanic membrane -rrhexis = rupture	Rupture of the tympanic membrane
vertigo (VER-tih-goh)		Dizziness caused by sensation that room is spinning
Hearing Loss		
anacusis (an-ah-KYOO-sis)	an- = without -cusis = hearing	Total absence of hearing; inability to perceive sound; also called *deafness*
deafness		Inability to hear or having some degree of hearing impairment
External Ear		
ceruminosis (seh-roo-mih-NOH-sis)	cerumin/o = cerumen -osis = abnormal condition	Excessive accumulation of earwax resulting in hard wax plug; sound becomes muffled
otitis externa (OE) (oh-TYE-tis / eks-TER-nah)	ot/o = ear -itis = inflammation	External ear infection; may be caused by bacteria or fungus; also called *otomycosis* and commonly referred to as *swimmer's ear*

Pathology (continued)

Term	Word Parts	Definition
otomycosis (oh-toh-my-KOH-sis)	**ot/o** = ear **myc/o** = fungus **-osis** = abnormal condition	Fungal infection of the ear; one type of otitis externa
Middle Ear		
myringitis (mir-in-JYE-tis)	**myring/o** = tympanic membrane **-itis** = inflammation	Inflammation of the tympanic membrane
otitis media (OM) (oh-TYE-tis / MEE-dee-ah)	**ot/o** = ear **-itis** = inflammation	Seen frequently in children; commonly referred to as *middle ear infection*; often preceded by upper respiratory infection during which pathogens move from the pharynx to the middle ear via the eustachian tube; fluid accumulates in the middle ear cavity; fluid may be watery, *serous otitis media*, or full of pus, *purulent otitis media*
otosclerosis (oh-toh-sklair-OH-sis)	**ot/o** = ear **-sclerosis** = hardening	Loss of mobility of the stapes bone, leading to progressive hearing loss
salpingitis (sal-pin-JIGH-tis)	**salping/o** = auditory tube **-itis** = inflammation **Word Watch** Be careful using the combining form **salping/o**, which can mean either *eustachian tube* or *fallopian tube*.	Inflammation of the auditory tube
tympanitis (tim-pan-EYE-tis)	**tympan/o** = tympanic membrane **-itis** = inflammation	Inflammation of the tympanic membrane
Inner Ear		
acoustic neuroma (ah-KOOS-tik / noo-ROH-mah)	**acous/o** = hearing **-tic** = pertaining to **neur/o** = nerve **-oma** = tumor	Benign tumor of eighth cranial nerve sheath; pressure causes symptoms such as tinnitus, headache, dizziness, and progressive hearing loss
labyrinthitis (lab-ih-rin-THIGH-tis)	**labyrinth/o** = labyrinth **-itis** = inflammation	May affect both hearing and equilibrium portions of inner ear; also referred to as *inner ear infection*
Ménière's disease (may-nee-AIRZ)		Abnormal condition within the labyrinth of inner ear that can lead to progressive loss of hearing; symptoms are vertigo, hearing loss, and tinnitus (ringing in the ears); named for French physician Prosper Ménière

PRACTICE AS YOU GO

H. Terminology Matching

Match each term to its definition.

1. ____________ anacusis
2. ____________ otitis externa
3. ____________ microtia

a. small ears
b. dizziness
c. ringing in the ears

4. ____________ otopyorrhea
5. ____________ labyrinthitis
6. ____________ tinnitus
7. ____________ otosclerosis
8. ____________ vertigo
9. ____________ otomycosis
10. ____________ tympanorrhexis

d. a fungal infection
e. absence of hearing
f. ruptured eardrum
g. pus discharge from the ear
h. swimmer's ear
i. loss of mobility of stapes
j. inner ear infection

Diagnostic Procedures

Term	Word Parts	Definition
Audiology Tests		
audiogram (AW-dee-oh-gram)	audi/o = hearing -gram = record	Graphic record that illustrates results of audiometry
audiometer (aw-dee-OM-eh-ter)	audi/o = hearing -meter = instrument to measure	Instrument to measure hearing
audiometry (aw-dee-OM-eh-tree)	audi/o = hearing -metry = process of measuring	Test of hearing ability by determining lowest and highest intensity (decibels) and frequencies (hertz) that person can distinguish; patient may sit in soundproof booth and receive sounds through ear-phones as technician decreases sound or lowers tones
decibel (dB) (DES-ih-bel)		Measures intensity or loudness of a sound; zero decibels is quietest sound measured and 120 dB is loudest sound commonly measured
hertz (Hz)		Measurement of frequency or pitch of sound; lowest pitch on audiogram is 250 Hz; mea-surement can go as high as 8000 Hz, which is highest pitch measured

■ **Figure 13-17** Audiometry exam being administered to a young child who is wearing the earphones through which sounds are given. *(Capifrutta/Shutterstock)*

Diagnostic Procedures (continued)

Term	Word Parts	Definition
Rinne and Weber tuning-fork tests (RIN-eh / VAY-ber)		Tests that assess both nerve and bone conduction of sound; physician holds a tuning fork, an instrument that produces a constant pitch when struck, against or near bones on side of the head
Otology Tests		
otoscope (OH-toh-skohp)	ot/o = ear -scope = instrument to visually examine	Instrument to view inside the ear canal
otoscopy (oh-TOSS-koh-pee)	ot/o = ear -scopy = process of visually examining	Examination of ear canal, eardrum, and outer ear using *otoscope*
tympanogram (TIM-pah-noh-gram)	tympan/o = tympanic membrane -gram = record	Graphic record that illustrates results of tympanometry
tympanometer (tim-pah-NOM-eh-ter)	tympan/o = tympanic membrane -meter = instrument to measure	Instrument used to measure the movement of the tympanic membrane
tympanometry (tim-pah-NOM-eh-tree)	tympan/o = tympanic membrane -metry = process of measuring	Measurement of the movement of the tympanic membrane; can indicate the presence of pressure in the middle ear
Balance Test		
falling test		Test used to observe balance and equilibrium; patient is observed balancing on one foot, then with one foot in front of the other, and then walking forward with eyes open; same test is conducted with patient's eyes closed; swaying and falling with the eyes closed can indicate ear and equilibrium malfunction

■ **Figure 13-18** An otoscope, used to visually examine the external auditory ear canal and tympanic membrane. *(Patrick Watson/Pearson Education, Inc.)*

Med Term Tip

Small children are prone to placing objects in their ears. In some cases, as with peas and beans, these become moist in the ear canal and swell, which makes removal difficult. *Otoscopy*, or the examination of the ear using an *otoscope*, can aid in identifying and removing the cause of hearing loss if it is due to foreign bodies.

Therapeutic Procedures

Term	Word Parts	Definition
Audiology Procedures		
American Sign Language (ASL)		Nonverbal method of communicating in which the hands and fingers are used to indicate words and concepts; used by both persons who are deaf and persons with speech impairments ■ **Figure 13-19** Two women having a conversation using American Sign Language. *(Vladimir Mucibabic/Shutterstock)*
hearing aid		Apparatus or mechanical device used by persons with impaired hearing to amplify sound; also called *amplification device*
Surgical Procedures		
cochlear implant (KOH-klee-ar)	cochle/o = cochlea -ar = pertaining to	Mechanical device surgically placed under the skin behind outer ear (pinna) that converts sound signals into electrical impulses to stimulate the cochlear nerve; can be beneficial for those with profound sensorineural hearing loss ■ **Figure 13-20** Photograph of a child with a cochlear implant. This device sends electrical impulses directly to the brain. *(George Dodson/Pearson Education, Inc.)*
labyrinthectomy (lab-ih-rin-THEK-toh-mee)	labyrinth/o = labyrinth -ectomy = surgical removal	Surgical removal of the labyrinth
labyrinthotomy (lab-ih-rin-THOT-oh-mee)	labyrinth/o = labyrinth -otomy = cutting into	To cut into the labyrinth
myringectomy (mir-in-JEK-toh-mee)	myring/o = tympanic membrane -ectomy = surgical removal	Surgical removal of the tympanic membrane
myringoplasty (mir-IN-goh-plas-tee)	myring/o = tympanic membrane -plasty = surgical repair	Surgical repair of the tympanic membrane

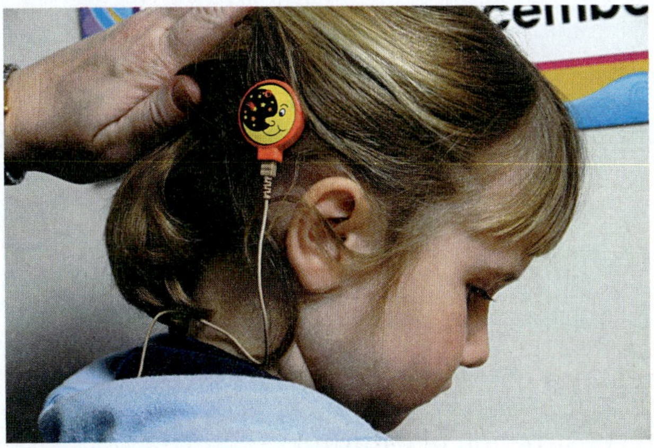

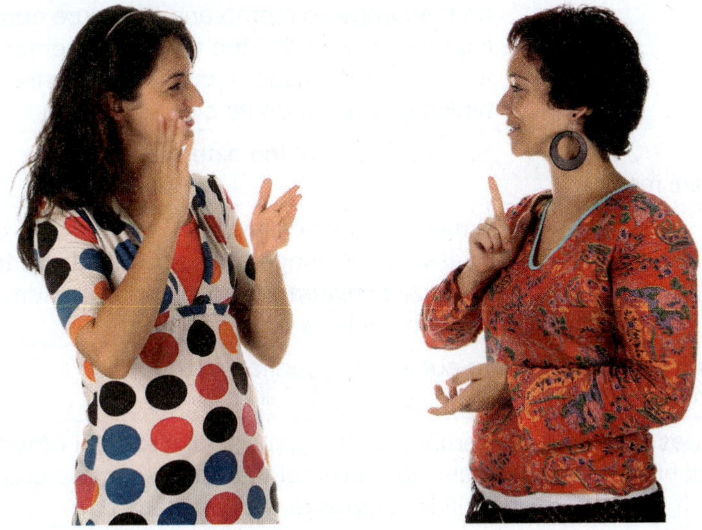

Therapeutic Procedures (continued)

Term	Word Parts	Definition
myringotomy (mir-in-GOT-oh-mee)	**myring/o** = tympanic membrane **-otomy** = cutting into	Surgical puncture of the eardrum with removal of fluid and pus from middle ear to eliminate persistent ear infection and excessive pressure on the tympanic membrane; pressure equalizing tube is placed in the tympanic membrane to allow for drainage of middle ear cavity; tube typically falls out on its own
otoplasty (OH-toh-plas-tee)	**ot/o** = ear **-plasty** = surgical repair	Surgical repair of the external ear
pressure equalizing tube (PE tube)		Small tube surgically placed in child's eardrum to assist in drainage of trapped fluid and to equalize pressure between middle ear cavity and atmosphere
salpingotomy (sal-pin-GOT-oh-mee)	**salping/o** = auditory tube **-otomy** = cutting into	To cut into the auditory tube
stapedectomy (stay-peh-DEK-toh-mee)	**staped/o** = stapes **-ectomy** = pertaining to	Removal of the stapes bone to treat otosclerosis (hardening of the bone); a prosthesis or artificial stapes may be implanted
tympanectomy (tim-pah-NEK-toh-mee)	**tympan/o** = tympanic membrane **-ectomy** = surgical removal	Surgical removal of the tympanic membrane
tympanoplasty (TIM-pah-noh-plas-tee)	**tympan/o** = tympanic membrane **-plasty** = surgical repair	Surgical repair of the tympanic membrane
tympanotomy (tim-pah-NOT-oh-mee)	**tympan/o** = tympanic membrane **-otomy** = cutting into	To cut into the tympanic membrane

PRACTICE AS YOU GO

I. Procedure Matching

Match each procedure term to its definition.

1. ________ myringotomy	**a.** removal of stapes bone
2. ________ tympanoplasty	**b.** reconstruction of eardrum
3. ________ otoplasty	**c.** surgical puncture of eardrum
4. ________ stapedectomy	**d.** repairs external ear
5. ________ Rinne and Weber	**e.** drains off fluid
6. ________ falling test	**f.** treats sensorineural hearing loss
7. ________ PE tube	**g.** tuning-fork tests
8. ________ cochlear implant	**h.** balance test

Pharmacology

Classification	Word Parts	Action	Examples
antibiotic otic solution (OH-tik)	anti- = against bi/o = life -tic = pertaining to ot/o = ear -ic = pertaining to	Eardrops to treat otitis externa	Neomycin, polymyxin B and hydrocortisone solution, Otocort, Cortisporin, Otic Care
antiemetic (an-tye-ee-MEH-tik)	anti- = against -emetic = pertaining to vomiting	Effective in treating nausea associated with vertigo	meclizine, Antivert, Meni-D; prochlorperazine, Compazine
wax emulsifiers		Substances used to soften earwax to prevent buildup within the external ear canal	carbamide peroxide, Debrox Drops, Murine Ear Wax Removal Drops

Abbreviations

ASL	American Sign Language	**OE**	otitis externa
BC	bone conduction	**OM**	otitis media
dB	decibel	**Oto**	otology
EENT	eyes, ears, nose, and throat	**PE tube**	pressure equalizing tube
ENT	ears, nose, and throat	**PORP**	partial ossicular replacement prosthesis
HEENT	head, eyes, ears, nose, and throat	**SOM**	serous otitis media
Hz	hertz	**TORP**	total ossicular replacement prosthesis

PRACTICE AS YOU GO

J. What's the Abbreviation?

1. otitis externa ______________________
2. eyes, ears, nose, and throat ______________________
3. bone conduction ______________________
4. pressure equalizing tube ______________________
5. otitis media ______________________

Chapter Review

Real-World Applications

Medical Record Analysis

This Ophthalmology Consultation Report contains 11 medical terms. Underline each term and write it in the list below the report. Then explain each term as you would to a nonmedical person.

Ophthalmology Consultation Report

Reason for Consultation:	Evaluation of progressive loss of vision in right eye
History of Present Illness:	Patient is a 79-year-old female who has noted gradual deterioration of vision and increasing photophobia during the past year, particularly in the right eye. She states that it feels like there is a film over her right eye. She denies any change in vision in her left eye. Patient has used corrective lenses her entire adult life for hyperopia.
Results of Physical Examination:	Visual acuity test showed no change in this patient's long-standing hyperopia. The pupils react properly to light. Intraocular pressure is normal. Ophthalmoscopy after application of mydriatic drops revealed presence of large opaque cataract in lens of right eye. There is a very small cataract forming in the left eye. There is no evidence of retinopathy, macular degeneration, or keratitis.
Assessment:	Diminished vision in right eye secondary to cataract
Recommendations:	Phacoemulsification of cataract followed by prosthetic lens implant.

	Term	Explanation
1.	__________	__________
2.	__________	__________
3.	__________	__________
4.	__________	__________
5.	__________	__________
6.	__________	__________
7.	__________	__________
8.	__________	__________
9.	__________	__________
10.	__________	__________
11.	__________	__________

Chart Note Transcription

The chart note below contains 10 phrases that can be reworded with a medical term presented in this chapter. Each phrase is identified with an underline. Determine the medical term and write your answers in the space provided.

Pearson General Hospital Consultation Report

Task Edit View Time Scale Options Help Download Archive Date: 17 May 2017

Current Complaint:	An eight-year-old female was referred to the specialist in the treatment of diseases of the ears, nose, and throat **1** by her pediatrician for evaluation of chronic left middle ear infection. **2**
Past History:	Patient's mother reports that her daughter began to experience recurrent ear infections at approximately six months of age. Frequency of the infections has increased during the past two years, and she is missing school. Mother also reports the child's teacher feels she is having difficulty hearing in the classroom.
Signs and Symptoms:	Both ears **3** visual examination of the external ear canal and eardrum **4** revealed that the membrane between the external ear canal and middle ear **5** is normal on the right and bulging on the left. An excessive amount of earwax **6** was noted in both ears. Measurement of the movement of the eardrum **7** indicates that there is a buildup of fluid in the left middle ear. Tests of hearing ability **8** report normal hearing on the right and loss of hearing as a result of the blocking of sound transmission in the middle ear **9** on the left. Patient also noted to have acute pharyngitis with purulent drainage at time of evaluation.
Diagnosis:	Hearing loss secondary to chronic left middle ear infection
Treatment:	Left eardrum incision **10** with placement of pressure equalizing tube for drainage.

1. ______________________________

2. ______________________________

3. ______________________________

4. ______________________________

5. ______________________________

6. ______________________________

7. ______________________________

8. ______________________________

9. ______________________________

10. ______________________________

Case Study

Below is a case study presentation of a patient with a condition discussed in this chapter. Read the case study and answer the questions below. Some questions will ask for information not included within this chapter. Use your text, a medical dictionary, or any other reference material you choose to answer these questions.

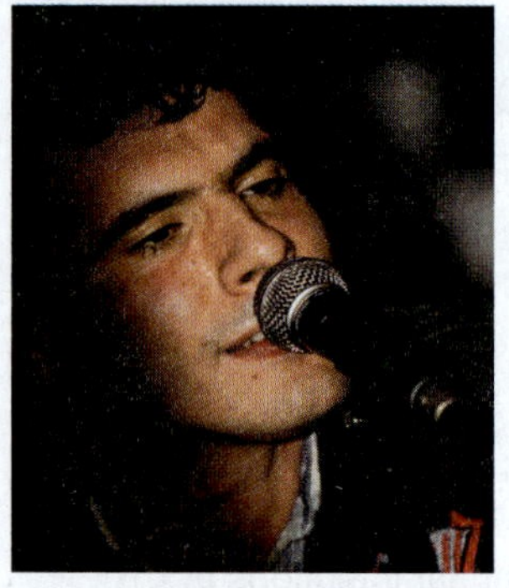

(MY - Music/Alamy Stock Photo)

This 35-year-old male musician was seen in the EENT clinic complaining of a progressive hearing loss over the past 15 years. He is now unable to hear what is being said if there is any environmental noise present. He states that he has played with a group of musicians using amplified instruments and no earplugs for the past 20 years. External ear structures appear normal bilaterally with otoscopy. Tympanometry is normal bilaterally. Audiometry reveals diminished hearing bilaterally. Rinne and Weber tuning-fork tests indicate that the patient has a moderate amount of conductive hearing loss but rule out sensorineural hearing loss. Diagnosis is moderate bilateral conductive hearing loss as a result of prolonged exposure to loud noise. Patient is referred for evaluation for a hearing aid.

Questions

1. Which type of hearing loss does this patient appear to have? Look this condition up in a reference source and include a short description of it.

___

___

2. Explain how the other type of hearing loss (the type ruled out by the Rinne and Weber tuning-fork tests) is different from what this patient has.

___

___

3. What diagnostic tests did the physician perform? Describe them in your own words.

___

___

4. Explain the difference between a hearing aid and a cochlear implant.

___

___

5. How do you think this patient could have avoided this hearing loss?

___

___

Practice Exercises

A. Pharmacology Challenge

Fill in the classification for each drug description, then match the brand name.

	Drug Description	Classification	Brand Name
1.	________ treats dry eyes	____________________	a. Atropine-Care
2.	________ reduces intraocular pressure	____________________	b. Visine
3.	________ eardrops for ear infection	____________________	c. Timoptic
4.	________ dilates pupil	____________________	d. Opticaine
5.	________ treats nausea from vertigo	____________________	e. Debrox Drops
6.	________ eyedrops for bacterial infection	____________________	f. Eserine Sulfate
7.	________ reduces eye redness	____________________	g. Antivert
8.	________ constricts pupil	____________________	h. Refresh Plus
9.	________ softens cerumen	____________________	i. Otocort
10.	________ eyedrops for pain	____________________	j. Del-Mycin

B. Word Building Practice

The combining form **blephar/o** refers to the *eyelid*. Use it to write a term that means:

1. inflammation of the eyelid ____________________
2. surgical repair of the eyelid ____________________
3. drooping of the upper eyelid ____________________

The combining form **retin/o** refers to the *retina*. Use it to write a term that means:

4. a disease of the retina ____________________
5. surgical fixation of the retina ____________________

The combining form **ophthalm/o** refers to the *eye*. Use it to write a term that means:

6. the study of the eye ____________________
7. pertaining to the eye ____________________
8. an eye examination using a scope ____________________

The combining form **irid/o** refers to the *iris*. Use it to write a term that means:

9. iris paralysis ____________________
10. removal of the iris ____________________

The combining form **ot/o** refers to the *ear*. Write a word that means:

11. ear surgical repair ____________________
12. pus flow from the ear ____________________
13. pain in the ear ____________________
14. inflammation of the ear ____________________

The combining form **tympan/o** refers to the *eardrum*. Write a word that means:

15. eardrum rupture ______________________________
16. eardrum incision ______________________________
17. eardrum inflammation ______________________________

The combining form **audi/o** refers to *hearing*. Write a word that means:

18. record of hearing ______________________________
19. instrument to measure hearing ______________________________
20. study of hearing ______________________________

C. Complete the Term

For each definition given below, fill in the blank with the word part that completes the term.

Definition	Term
1. instrument to visually examine the ear	____________scope
2. surgical fixation of the retina	____________pexy
3. without hearing	ana____________
4. drooping eyelid	____________ptosis
5. specialist in measuring vision	____________metrist
6. instrument to measure eardrum	____________meter
7. cutting into the cornea	____________otomy
8. old-age vision condition	presby____________
9. surgical removal of the iris	____________ectomy
10. process of measuring hearing	____________metry
11. eye pain	____________algia
12. hardening of the ear	____________sclerosis
13. inflammation of the conjunctiva	____________itis
14. large ear condition	macr____________
15. state of one color	mono____________ism

D. Using Abbreviations

Fill in each blank with the appropriate abbreviation.

1. __________ is a condition in which light rays focus unevenly on the retina because of an uneven cornea.
2. __________ is a branch of medicine that diagnoses and treats conditions of the ears, nose, and throat.
3. A(An) __________ test measures the sharpness of vision.
4. __________ may be caused by bacteria or fungus in the external ear.
5. __________ is commonly called *cross-eyed* because the eye is turned inward.
6. __________ tubes equalize pressure between the middle ear and the external atmosphere.
7. __________ surgery uses a laser to correct myopia.

8. __________ is commonly called *nearsightedness.*
9. __________, a common infection in children, causes fluid to accumulate in the middle ear cavity.
10. Cataracts are commonly corrected by replacing the lens with a(n) __________ implant.

E. Fill in the Blank

emmetropia	tonometry	Ménière's disease
hyperopia	cataract	hordeolum
acoustic neuroma	strabismus	myopia
otorhinolaryngologist	presbycusis	
conjunctivitis	inner ear	

1. Cheri is having a regular eye checkup. The pressure-reading test that the physician will do to detect glaucoma is ____________________.
2. Carlos's ophthalmologist tells him that he has normal vision. This is called ____________________.
3. Ana has been given an antibiotic eye ointment for pinkeye. The medical term for this condition is ____________________.
4. Adrian is nearsighted and cannot read signs in the distance. This is called ____________________.
5. Ivan is scheduled to have surgery to have the opaque lens of his right eye removed. This condition is a(n) ____________________.
6. Roberto has developed a stye on the corner of his left eye. He has been told to treat it with hot compresses. This condition is called a(n) ____________________.
7. Judith has twin boys with crossed eyes that will require surgical correction. The medical term for this condition is ____________________.
8. Beth is farsighted and has difficulty reading textbooks. Her eyeglass correction will be for ____________________.
9. Grace was told by her physician that her hearing loss was a part of the aging process. The term for this is ____________________.
10. Stacey is having frequent middle ear infections and wishes to be treated by a specialist. She would go to a(n) ____________________.
11. Warren was told that his dizziness may be caused by a problem in the ____________________ area.
12. Shantel is suffering from an abnormal condition of the inner ear, vertigo, and tinnitus. She may have ____________________.
13. Keisha was told that her tumor of the eighth cranial nerve was benign, but she still experienced a hearing loss as a result of the tumor. This tumor is called a(n) ____________________.

F. Define the Term

1. amblyopia ____________________
2. diplopia ____________________
3. mydriatic ____________________
4. miotic ____________________
5. presbyopia ____________________
6. tinnitus ____________________

7. stapes ______________________
8. tympanometry ______________________
9. eustachian tube ______________________
10. labyrinth ______________________
11. audiogram ______________________
12. otitis media ______________________

G. Anatomical Adjectives

Fill in the blank with the missing noun or adjective.

Noun	Adjective
1. conjunctiva	______________
2. ______________	auditory
3. cornea	______________
4. ______________	auricular
5. within the eye	______________
6. ______________	otic
7. tears	______________
8. ______________	iridal
9. one ear	______________
10. sclera	______________
11. ______________	ocular
12. retina	______________
13. eardrum	______________
14. ______________	ophthalmic
15. cochlea	______________

H. Spelling Practice

Some of the following terms are misspelled. Identify the incorrect terms and spell them correctly in the blank provided.

1. opthalmology ______________________
2. otosclerosis ______________________
3. dacryoadenitis ______________________
4. emetropia ______________________
5. labyrinthtitis ______________________
6. presbyopia ______________________
7. stapedectomy ______________________
8. monochromism ______________________
9. otopyorhea ______________________
10. astigmatism ______________________

I. Complete the Statement

1. In order, the structures light rays pass through to strike the retina are: ________________, ________________, ________________, ________________, and ________________.
2. Tears ultimately drain into the ________________.
3. ________________ eye muscles pull the eyeball left, right, up, or down in a straight line. ________________ eye muscles move the eyeball diagonally.
4. The ________________ is a mucous membrane that covers and protects the front of the eyeball.
5. Eyelashes are called ________________.
6. The ciliary body is part of the ________________ layer of the eyeball.
7. The three ossicles are ________________, ________________, and ________________.
8. With ________________ hearing loss, the problem is with the outer or middle ear and sound is muffled. In ________________ hearing loss, the problem is with the inner ear or cochlear nerve and impulses are not successfully sent to the brain.
9. The blind spot in each eyeball is caused by the ________________.
10. The ________________ nerve carries hearing information and the ________________ nerve carries equilibrium information.

MyLab Medical Terminology™

MyLab Medical Terminology is a premium online homework management system that includes a host of features to help you study. Registered users will find:

- A multitude of activities and assignments built within the MyLab platform
- Powerful tools that track and analyze your results—allowing you to create a personalized learning experience
- Videos and audio pronunciations to help enrich your progress
- Streaming lesson presentations (Guided Lectures) and self-paced learning modules
- A space where you and your instructors can check your progress and manage your assignments

Labeling Exercises

Image A

Write the labels for this figure on the numbered lines provided.

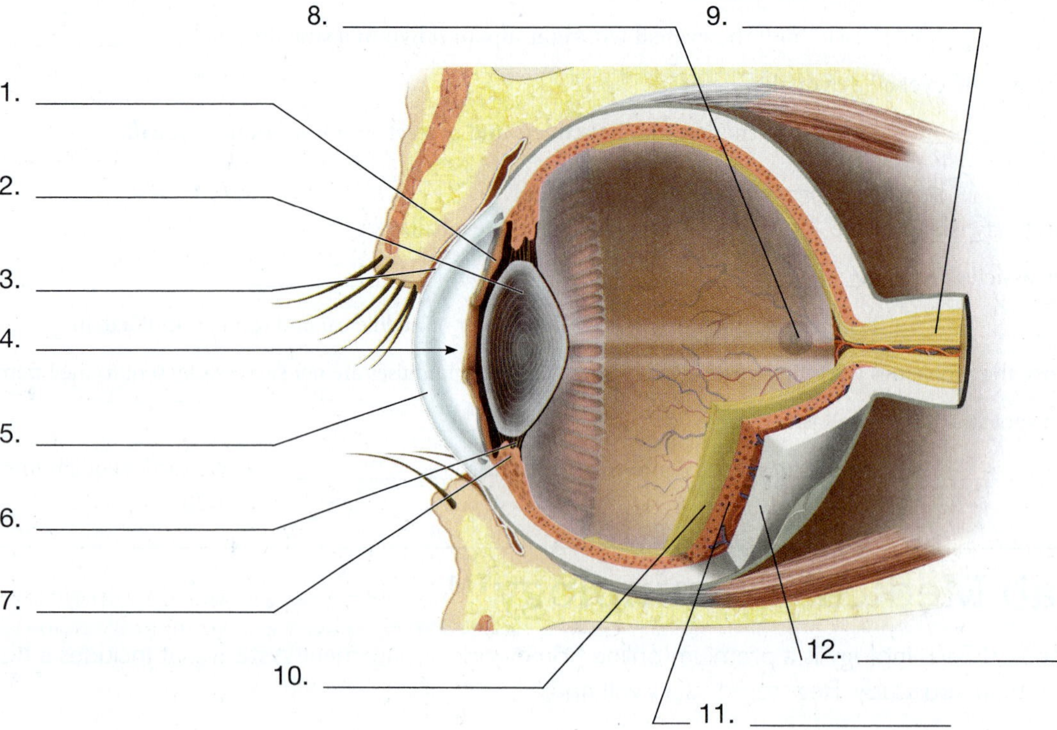

Image B

Write the labels for this figure on the numbered lines provided.

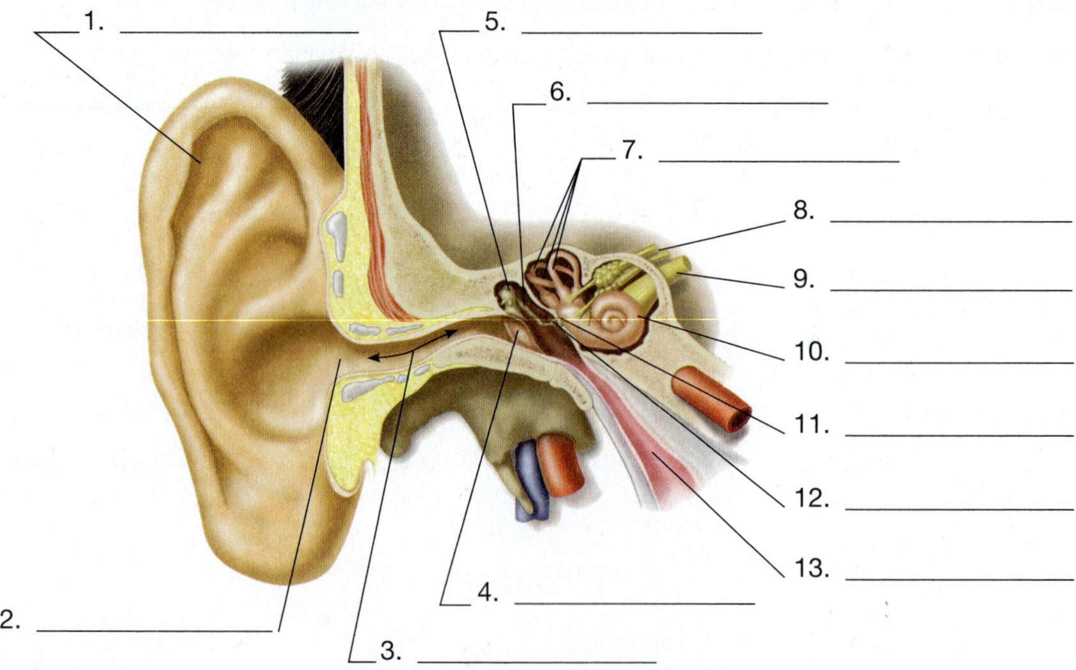

Appendices

Appendix I

Word Parts Arranged Alphabetically and Defined

The word parts that have been presented in this textbook are summarized here with their definitions for quick reference. Prefixes are listed first, followed by combining forms and suffixes.

Prefix	Definition
a-	without
ab-	away from
ad-	toward
allo-	other, different from usual
an-	without
ante-	before, in front of
anti-	against
auto-	self
bi-	two
brady-	slow
circum-	around
contra-	against
de-	without
di-	two
dis-	apart
dys-	painful; difficult; abnormal
e-	outward
endo-	within; inner
epi-	above
eso-	inward
eu-	normal
ex-	outward
exo-	outward
extra-	outside of
hemi-	half
hetero-	different
homo-	same
hyper-	excessive
hypo-	below; insufficient
in-	not; inward
inter-	between
intra-	within

Prefix	Definition
macro-	large
micro-	small
mono-	one
multi-	many
myo-	to shut
neo-	new
non-	not
nulli-	none
pan-	all
para-	beside; abnormal; two like parts of a pair
per-	through
peri-	around
poly-	many
post-	after
pre-	before
primi-	first
pro-	before
pseudo-	false
quadri-	four
re-	again
retro-	backward; behind
semi-	partial
sub-	under
tachy-	fast
tetra-	four
trans-	across
tri-	three
ultra-	beyond
un-	not
xeno-	foreign

Combining Form	Definition
abdomin/o	abdomen
acous/o	hearing
acr/o	extremities
aden/o	gland
adenoid/o	adenoids

Combining Form	Definition
adip/o	fat
adren/o	adrenal glands
adrenal/o	adrenal glands
aer/o	air
agglutin/o	clumping

Combining Form	Definition
albin/o	white
alges/o	sense of pain
alveol/o	alveolus
ambly/o	dull, dim
amnes/o	forgetfulness
amni/o	amnion
an/o	anus
andr/o	male
angi/o	vessel
ankyl/o	stiff joint
anter/o	front
anthrac/o	coal
anxi/o	fear, worry
aort/o	aorta
append/o	appendix
appendic/o	appendix
aque/o	water
arteri/o	artery
arteriol/o	arteriole
arthr/o	joint
articul/o	joint
astr/o	star
atel/o	incomplete
ather/o	fatty substance
atri/o	atrium
audi/o	hearing
audit/o	hearing
aur/o	ear
auricul/o	ear
axill/o	axilla
azot/o	nitrogenous waste
bacteri/o	bacteria
balan/o	glans penis
bar/o	weight
bas/o	base
bi/o	life
blast/o	immature
blephar/o	eyelid
brachi/o	arm
bronch/o	bronchus
bronchi/o	bronchus
bronchiol/o	bronchiole
bucc/o	cheek
burs/o	sac
calc/o	calcium
carcin/o	cancer
cardi/o	heart
carp/o	carpus
caud/o	tail
cauter/o	to burn
cec/o	cecum
centr/o	center
cephal/o	head
cerebell/o	cerebellum

Combining Form	Definition
cerebr/o	cerebrum
cerumin/o	cerumen
cervic/o	neck, cervix
chem/o	chemical, drug
chol/e	bile, gall
cholangi/o	bile duct
cholecyst/o	gallbladder
choledoch/o	common bile duct
chondr/o	cartilage
chori/o	chorion
chrom/o	color
chromat/o	color
cirrh/o	yellow
cis/o	to cut
clavicul/o	clavicle
cleid/o	clavicle
clon/o	rapid contracting and relaxing
coagul/o	clotting
coccyg/o	coccyx
cochle/o	cochlea
col/o	colon
colon/o	colon
colp/o	vagina
compuls/o	drive, compel
concuss/o	to shake violently
coni/o	dust
conjunctiv/o	conjunctiva
corne/o	cornea
coron/o	heart
corpor/o	body
cortic/o	outer layer
cost/o	rib
crani/o	skull
crin/o	to secrete
crur/o	leg
cry/o	cold
crypt/o	hidden
culd/o	cul-de-sac
cutane/o	skin
cyan/o	blue
cycl/o	ciliary body
cyst/o	sac, urinary bladder
cyt/o	cell
dacry/o	tears
delus/o	false belief
dent/o	tooth
depress/o	to press down
derm/o	skin
dermat/o	skin
diaphor/o	profuse sweating
diaphragmat/o	diaphragm
dilat/o	to widen
dipl/o	double
dist/o	away from

Combining Form	Definition
diverticul/o	pouch
dors/o	back
duct/o	to bring
duoden/o	duodenum
dur/o	dura mater
electr/o	electricity
embol/o	plug
embry/o	embryo
emmetr/o	correct, proper
encephal/o	brain
enter/o	small intestine
eosin/o	rosy red
epididym/o	epididymis
epiglott/o	epiglottis
episi/o	vulva
epitheli/o	epithelium
erythr/o	red
esophag/o	esophagus
esthesi/o	sensation, feeling
estr/o	female
extens/o	to stretch out
fasci/o	fibrous band
femor/o	femur
fet/o	fetus
fibr/o	fibers
fibrin/o	fibers
fibul/o	fibula
flex/o	to bend
fus/o	pouring
gastr/o	stomach
genit/o	genital
gingiv/o	gums
glauc/o	gray
gli/o	glue
glomerul/o	glomerulus
gloss/o	tongue
gluc/o	glucose
glute/o	buttock
glyc/o	sugar
glycos/o	sugar, glucose
gonad/o	sex glands
granul/o	granules
gynec/o	female
habilitat/o	ability
hal/o	to breathe
hallucin/o	imagined perception
hem/o	blood
hemat/o	blood
hepat/o	liver
hidr/o	sweat
hist/o	tissue
home/o	sameness
humer/o	humerus
hydr/o	water

Combining Form	Definition
hymen/o	hymen
hyster/o	uterus
iatr/o	physician, medicine, treatment
ichthy/o	scaly, dry
idi/o	distinctive
ile/o	ileum
ili/o	ilium
immun/o	protection
infer/o	below
inguin/o	groin
iod/o	iodine
ir/o	iris
irid/o	iris
isch/o	to hold back
ischi/o	ischium
jejun/o	jejunum
kal/i	potassium
kerat/o	hard, horny, cornea
ket/o	ketones
keton/o	ketones
kinesi/o	movement
klept/o	to steal
kyph/o	hump
labi/o	lip
labyrinth/o	labyrinth (inner ear)
lacrim/o	tears
lact/o	milk
lamin/o	lamina (part of vertebra)
lapar/o	abdomen
laryng/o	larynx
later/o	side
leuk/o	white
lingu/o	tongue
lip/o	fat
lith/o	stone
lob/o	lobe
lord/o	bent backward
lumb/o	loin (low back)
lymph/o	lymph
lymphaden/o	lymph node
lymphangi/o	lymph vessel
macul/o	macula lutea
mamm/o	breast
mandibul/o	mandible
mast/o	breast
maxill/o	maxilla
meat/o	meatus
medi/o	middle
medull/o	inner region, medulla oblongata
melan/o	black
men/o	menses, menstruation
mening/o	meninges

Combining Form	Definition
meningi/o	meninges
ment/o	mind
metacarp/o	metacarpus
metatars/o	metatarsus
metr/o	uterus
mi/o	lessening
mineral/o	minerals, electrolytes
morph/o	shape
muc/o	mucus
muscul/o	muscle
my/o	muscle
myc/o	fungus
mydr/i	widening
myel/o	bone marrow, spinal cord
myocardi/o	heart muscle
myos/o	muscle
myring/o	tympanic membrane
narc/o	stupor, sleep
nas/o	nose
nat/o	birth
natr/o	sodium
necr/o	death
nephr/o	kidney
neur/o	nerve
neutr/o	neutral
noct/i	night
nucle/o	nucleus
nyctal/o	night
o/o	ovum
obsess/o	besieged by thoughts
ocul/o	eye
odont/o	tooth
olig/o	scanty
onych/o	nail
oophor/o	ovary
ophthalm/o	eye
opt/o	eye, vision
optic/o	eye, vision
or/o	mouth
orch/o	testis
orchi/o	testis
orchid/o	testis
orth/o	straight
oste/o	bone
ot/o	ear
ov/i	ovum
ov/o	ovum
ovari/o	ovary
ox/i	oxygen
ox/o	oxygen
palat/o	palate
pancreat/o	pancreas
papill/o	optic disk
parathyroid/o	parathyroid gland

Combining Form	Definition
pareun/o	sexual intercourse
pariet/o	cavity wall
patell/o	patella
path/o	disease
pector/o	chest
ped/o	child; foot
pedicul/o	lice
pelv/o	pelvis
pen/o	penis
perine/o	perineum
peripher/o	away from center
peritone/o	peritoneum
phac/o	lens
phag/o	eat, swallow
phalang/o	phalanges
pharmac/o	drug
pharyng/o	pharynx
phleb/o	vein
phob/o	irrational fear
phon/o	sound
phot/o	light
phren/o	mind
physic/o	body
pineal/o	pineal gland
pituit/o	pituitary gland
pituitar/o	pituitary gland
plant/o	sole of foot
pleur/o	pleura
pneum/o	lung, air
pneumon/o	lung, air
pod/o	foot
poli/o	gray matter
polyp/o	polyp
pont/o	pons
poster/o	back
presby/o	old age
proct/o	rectum and anus
prostat/o	prostate gland
prosthet/o	addition
protein/o	protein
proxim/o	near to
psych/o	mind
pub/o	genital region, pubis
pulmon/o	lung
pupill/o	pupil
py/o	pus
pyel/o	renal pelvis
pylor/o	pylorus
pyr/o	fire
radi/o	radius; ray (X-ray)
radic/o	root
radicul/o	nerve root
rect/o	rectum
ren/o	kidney

Combining Form	Definition
retin/o	retina
rhin/o	nose
rhytid/o	wrinkle
rotat/o	to revolve
sacr/o	sacrum
salping/o	uterine (fallopian) tubes, auditory tube (eustachian tube)
sanguin/o	blood
sarc/o	flesh
scapul/o	scapula
schiz/o	split
scler/o	hard, sclera
scoli/o	crooked
seb/o	oil
sept/o	wall
septic/o	infection
sialaden/o	salivary gland
sigmoid/o	sigmoid colon
sinus/o	sinus
soci/o	society
somat/o	body
somn/o	sleep
son/o	sound
spermat/o	sperm
sphygm/o	pulse
spin/o	spine
spir/o	breathing
splen/o	spleen
spondyl/o	vertebrae
staped/o	stapes
stern/o	sternum
steth/o	chest
stigmat/o	point
super/o	above
synov/o	synovial membrane
synovi/o	synovial membrane
system/o	system
tars/o	tarsus
ten/o	tendon
tend/o	tendon
tendin/o	tendon
testicul/o	testes
thalam/o	thalamus
thec/o	sheath (meninges)

Combining Form	Definition
therm/o	heat
thorac/o	chest
thromb/o	clot
thym/o	thymus gland
thyr/o	thyroid gland
thyroid/o	thyroid gland
tibi/o	tibia
tom/o	to cut
ton/o	tone
tonsill/o	tonsils
topic/o	a specific area
tox/o	poison
toxic/o	poison
trache/o	trachea
trich/o	hair
tuss/o	cough
tympan/o	tympanic membrane
uln/o	ulna
ungu/o	nail
ur/o	urine
ureter/o	ureter
urethr/o	urethra
urin/o	urine
uter/o	uterus
uve/o	choroid
vagin/o	vagina
valv/o	valve
valvul/o	valve
varic/o	dilated vein
vas/o	vessel, vas deferens
vascul/o	blood vessel
ven/o	vein
ventr/o	belly
ventricul/o	ventricle
venul/o	venule
vers/o	to turn
vertebr/o	vertebra
vesic/o	sac, bladder
vesicul/o	seminal vesicle
vestibul/o	vestibule
viscer/o	internal organ
vitre/o	glassy
vulv/o	vulva
xer/o	dry

Suffix	Definition
-ac	pertaining to
-al	pertaining to
-algia	pain
-an	pertaining to
-apheresis	removal, carry away
-ar	pertaining to
-arche	beginning
-ary	pertaining to

Suffix	Definition
-asthenia	weakness
-atic	pertaining to
-blast	immature
-capnia	carbon dioxide
-cardia	heart condition
-cele	protrusion
-centesis	puncture to withdraw fluid
-cide	to kill

Suffix	Definition
-clasia	to surgically break
-crit	separation of
-cusis	hearing
-cyesis	state of pregnancy
-cyte	cell
-cytic	pertaining to cells
-cytosis	more than the normal number of cells
-derma	skin condition
-desis	to fuse
-dipsia	thirst
-dynia	pain
-eal	pertaining to
-ectasis	dilation
-ectomy	surgical removal
-edema	swelling
-emesis	vomiting
-emetic	pertaining to vomiting
-emia	blood condition
-emic	pertaining to a blood condition
-gen	that which produces
-genesis	produces
-genic	producing
-globin	protein
-globulin	protein
-gram	record
-graph	to record
-graphy	process of recording
-gravida	pregnant woman
-ia	condition
-iac	pertaining to
-iasis	abnormal condition
-iatric	pertaining to medical treatment
-iatrist	physician
-iatry	medical treatment
-ic	pertaining to
-ical	pertaining to
-ician	specialist
-ile	pertaining to
-ine	pertaining to
-ion	action
-ior	pertaining to
-ism	state of
-ist	specialist
-istry	specialty of
-itis	inflammation
-kinesia	movement
-lepsy	seizure
-listhesis	slipping
-lith	stone
-lithiasis	condition of stones
-logic	pertaining to study of
-logist	one who studies
-logy	study of

Suffix	Definition
-lysis	to destroy (to break down)
-lytic	destruction
-malacia	abnormal softening
-mania	frenzy
-manometer	instrument to measure pressure
-megaly	enlarged
-meter	instrument for measuring
-metrist	specialist in measuring
-metry	process of measuring
-nic	pertaining to
-oid	resembling
-ole	small
-oma	tumor, mass
-opia	vision condition
-opsia	vision condition
-opsy	view of
-orexia	appetite
-ory	pertaining to
-ose	pertaining to
-osis	abnormal condition
-osmia	smell
-ostomy	surgically create an opening
-otia	ear condition
-otomy	cutting into
-ous	pertaining to
-para	to bear (offspring)
-paresis	weakness
-partum	childbirth
-pathy	disease
-penia	abnormal decrease, too few
-pepsia	digestion
-pexy	surgical fixation
-phage	to eat
-phagia	eat, swallow
-phasia	speech
-phil	attracted to
-philia	condition of being attracted to
-philic	pertaining to being attracted to
-phobia	fear
-phonia	voice
-phoresis	carrying
-phoria	condition to bear
-phylaxis	protection
-plasia	formation of cells
-plasm	formation
-plastic	pertaining to formation
-plastin	formation
-plasty	surgical repair
-plegia	paralysis
-pnea	breathing
-poiesis	formation
-porosis	porous
-prandial	pertaining to a meal

Suffix	Definition
-pressor	to press down
-ptosis	drooping
-ptysis	spitting
-rrhage	abnormal flow
-rrhagia	abnormal flow condition
-rrhagic	pertaining to abnormal flow
-rrhaphy	to suture
-rrhea	discharge
-rrhexis	rupture
-salpinx	uterine tube
-sclerosis	hardening
-scope	instrument for viewing
-scopic	pertaining to visually examining
-scopy	process of visually examining
-spasm	involuntary muscle contraction
-spermia	condition of sperm
-stasis	standing still
-stenosis	narrowing

Suffix	Definition
-taxia	muscle coordination
-tension	pressure
-therapy	treatment
-thorax	chest
-tic	pertaining to
-tocia	labor, childbirth
-tome	instrument to cut
-tonia	tone
-tonic	pertaining to tone
-toxic	pertaining to poison
-tripsy	surgical crushing
-trophic	pertaining to development
-trophy	development
-tropia	turned condition
-tropic	pertaining to stimulating
-tropin	to stimulate
-ule	small
-uria	condition of the urine

Appendix II

Word Parts Arranged Alphabetically by Definition

The definitions of the word parts that have been presented in this textbook are presented here and are arranged alphabetically. Prefixes are listed first, followed by combining forms and suffixes.

Definition	Prefix
abnormal	dys-, para-
above	epi-
across	trans-
after	post-
again	re-
against	anti-, contra-
all	pan-
apart	dis-
around	circum-, peri-
away from	ab-
backward	retro-
before	ante-, pre-, pro-
behind	retro-
below	hypo-
beside	para-
between	inter-
beyond	ultra-
different	hetero-
different from usual	allo-
difficult	dys-
excessive	hyper-
false	pseudo-
fast	tachy-
first	primi-
foreign	xeno-
four	quadri-, tetra-
half	hemi-
in front of	ante-
inner	endo-
insufficient	hypo-
inward	eso-, in-
large	macro-
many	multi-, poly-
new	neo-
none	nulli-
normal	eu-
not	in-, non-, un-
one	mono-
other	allo-
outside of	extra-
outward	e-, ex-, exo-
painful	dys-
partial	semi-
same	homo-
self	auto-
slow	brady-
small	micro-
three	tri-
through	per-
to shut	myo-
toward	ad-
two	bi-, di-
two like parts of a pair	para-
under	sub-
within	endo-, intra-
without	a-, an-, de-

Definition	Combining Form
ability	habilitat/o
above	super/o
addition	prosthet/o
adenoids	adenoid/o
adrenal glands	adren/o, adrenal/o
air	aer/o, pneum/o
alveolus	alveol/o
amnion	amni/o
anus	an/o
aorta	aort/o
appendix	append/o, appendic/o
arm	brachi/o
arteriole	arteriol/o
artery	arteri/o
atrium	atri/o
auditory tube (eustachian tube)	salping/o
away from	dist/o
away from center	peripher/o
axilla	axill/o
back	dors/o, poster/o
bacteria	bacteri/o
base	bas/o
belly	ventr/o
below	infer/o
to bend	flex/o
bent backward	lord/o
besieged by thoughts	obsess/o
bile	chol/e
bile duct	cholangi/o
birth	nat/o
black	melan/o
bladder	vesic/o

Definition	Combining Form
blood	**hem/o, hemat/o, sanguin/o**
blood vessel	**vascul/o**
blue	**cyan/o**
body	**corpor/o, physic/o, somat/o**
bone	**oste/o**
bone marrow	**myel/o**
brain	**encephal/o**
breast	**mamm/o, mast/o**
to breathe	**hal/o**
breathing	**spir/o**
to bring	**duct/o**
bronchiole	**bronchiol/o**
bronchus	**bronch/o, bronchi/o**
to burn	**cauter/o**
buttock	**glute/o**
calcium	**calc/o**
cancer	**carcin/o**
carpus	**carp/o**
cartilage	**chondr/o**
cavity wall	**pariet/o**
cecum	**cec/o**
cell	**cyt/o**
center	**centr/o**
cerebellum	**cerebell/o**
cerebrum	**cerebr/o**
cerumen	**cerumin/o**
cervix	**cervic/o**
cheek	**bucc/o**
chemical	**chem/o**
chest	**pector/o, steth/o, thorac/o**
child	**ped/o**
chorion	**chori/o**
choroid	**uve/o**
ciliary body	**cycl/o**
clavicle	**clavicul/o, cleid/o**
clot	**thromb/o**
clotting	**coagul/o**
clumping	**agglutin/o**
coal	**anthrac/o**
coccyx	**coccyg/o**
cochlea	**cochle/o**
cold	**cry/o**
colon	**col/o, colon/o**
color	**chrom/o, chromat/o**
common bile duct	**choledoch/o**
compel	**compuls/o**
conjunctiva	**conjunctiv/o**
cornea	**corne/o, kerat/o**
correct	**emmetr/o**
cough	**tuss/o**
crooked	**scoli/o**

Definition	Combining Form
cul-de-sac	**culd/o**
to cut	**cis/o, tom/o**
death	**necr/o**
diaphragm	**diaphragmat/o**
dilated vein	**varic/o**
dim	**ambly/o**
disease	**path/o**
distinctive	**idi/o**
double	**dipl/o**
drive	**compuls/o**
drug	**chem/o, pharmac/o**
dry	**ichthy/o, xer/o**
dull	**ambly/o**
duodenum	**duoden/o**
dura mater	**dur/o**
dust	**coni/o**
ear	**aur/o, auricul/o, ot/o**
eat	**phag/o**
electricity	**electr/o**
electrolytes	**mineral/o**
embryo	**embry/o**
epididymis	**epididym/o**
epiglottis	**epiglott/o**
epithelium	**epitheli/o**
esophagus	**esophag/o**
extremities	**acr/o**
eye	**ocul/o, ophthalm/o, opt/o, optic/o**
eyelid	**blephar/o**
false belief	**delus/o**
fat	**adip/o, lip/o**
fatty substance	**ather/o**
fear	**anxi/o**
feeling	**esthesi/o**
female	**estr/o, gynec/o**
femur	**femor/o**
fetus	**fet/o**
fibers	**fibr/o, fibrin/o**
fibrous band	**fasci/o**
fibula	**fibul/o**
fire	**pyr/o**
flesh	**sarc/o**
foot	**ped/o, pod/o**
forgetfulness	**amnes/o**
front	**anter/o**
fungus	**myc/o**
gall	**chol/e**
gallbladder	**cholecyst/o**
genital	**genit/o**
genital region	**pub/o**
gland	**aden/o**
glans penis	**balan/o**
glassy	**vitre/o**

Definition	Combining Form
glomerulus	**glomerul/o**
glucose	**gluc/o, glycos/o**
glue	**gli/o**
granules	**granul/o**
gray	**glauc/o**
gray matter	**poli/o**
groin	**inguin/o**
gums	**gingiv/o**
hair	**trich/o**
hard	**kerat/o, scler/o**
horny	**kerat/o**
head	**cephal/o**
hearing	**acous/o, audi/o, audit/o**
heart	**cardi/o, coron/o**
heart muscle	**myocardi/o**
heat	**therm/o**
hidden	**crypt/o**
to hold back	**isch/o**
humerus	**humer/o**
hump	**kyph/o**
hymen	**hymen/o**
ileum	**ile/o**
ilium	**ili/o**
imagined perception	**hallucin/o**
immature	**blast/o**
incomplete	**atel/o**
infection	**septic/o**
inner region	**medull/o**
internal organ	**viscer/o**
iodine	**iod/o**
iris	**ir/o, irid/o**
irrational fear	**phob/o**
ischium	**ischi/o**
jejunum	**jejun/o**
joint	**arthr/o, articul/o**
ketones	**ket/o, keton/o**
kidney	**nephr/o, ren/o**
labyrinth (inner ear)	**labyrinth/o**
lamina (part of vertebra)	**lamin/o**
larynx	**laryng/o**
leg	**crur/o**
lens	**phac/o**
lessening	**mi/o**
lice	**pedicul/o**
life	**bi/o**
light	**phot/o**
lip	**labi/o**
liver	**hepat/o**
lobe	**lob/o**
loin (low back)	**lumb/o**
lung	**pneum/o, pneumon/o, pulmon/o**
lymph	**lymph/o**
lymph node	**lymphaden/o**

Definition	Combining Form
lymph vessel	**lymphangi/o**
macula lutea	**macul/o**
male	**andr/o**
mandible	**mandibul/o**
maxilla	**maxill/o**
meatus	**meat/o**
medicine	**iatr/o**
medulla oblongata	**medull/o**
meninges	**mening/o, meningi/o**
menses, menstruation	**men/o**
metacarpus	**metacarp/o**
metatarsus	**metatars/o**
middle	**medi/o**
milk	**lact/o**
mind	**ment/o, phren/o, psych/o**
minerals	**mineral/o**
mouth	**or/o**
movement	**kinesi/o**
mucus	**muc/o**
muscle	**muscul/o, my/o, myos/o**
nail	**onych/o, ungu/o**
near to	**proxim/o**
neck	**cervic/o**
nerve	**neur/o**
nerve root	**radicul/o**
neutral	**neutr/o**
night	**noct/i, nyctal/o**
nitrogenous waste	**azot/o**
nose	**nas/o, rhin/o**
nucleus	**nucle/o**
oil	**seb/o**
old age	**presby/o**
optic disk	**papill/o**
outer layer	**cortic/o**
ovary	**oophor/o, ovari/o**
ovum	**o/o, ov/o, ov/i**
oxygen	**ox/o, ox/i**
pain	**alges/o**
palate	**palat/o**
pancreas	**pancreat/o**
parathyroid gland	**parathyroid/o**
patella	**patell/o**
pelvis	**pelv/o**
penis	**pen/o**
perineum	**perine/o**
peritoneum	**peritone/o**
phalanges	**phalang/o**
pharynx	**pharyng/o**
physician	**iatr/o**
pineal gland	**pineal/o**

Definition	Combining Form
pituitary gland	pituitar/o
pleura	pleur/o
plug	embol/o
point	stigmat/o
poison	tox/o, toxic/o
polyp	polyp/o
pons	pont/o
potassium	kal/i
pouch	diverticul/o
pouring	fus/o
to press down	depress/o
profuse sweating	diaphor/o
proper	emmetr/o
prostate gland	prostat/o
protection	immun/o
protein	protein/o
pubis	pub/o
pulse	sphygm/o
pupil	pupill/o
pus	py/o
pylorus	pylor/o
radius	radi/o
radiation	radi/o
rapid contracting and relaxing	clon/o
rectum	rect/o
ray (X-ray)	radi/o
rectum and anus	proct/o
red	erythr/o
renal pelvis	pyel/o
retina	retin/o
to revolve	rotat/o
rib	cost/o
root	radic/o
rosy red	eosin/o
sac	burs/o, cyst/o, vesic/o
sacrum	sacr/o
salivary gland	sialaden/o
sameness	home/o
scaly	ichthy/o
scanty	olig/o
scapula	scapul/o
sclera	scler/o
to secrete	crin/o
seminal vesicle	vesicul/o
sensation	esthesi/o
sense of pain	alges/o
sex glands	gonad/o
sexual intercourse	pareun/o
to shake violently	concuss/o
shape	morph/o
sheath (meninges)	thec/o
side	later/o
sigmoid colon	sigmoid/o
sinus	sinus/o
skin	cutane/o, derm/o, dermat/o
skull	crani/o
sleep	narc/o, somn/o
small intestine	enter/o
society	soci/o
sodium	natr/o
sole of foot	plant/o
sound	phon/o, son/o
specific area	topic/o
sperm	spermat/o
spinal cord	myel/o
spine	spin/o
spleen	splen/o
split	schiz/o
stapes	staped/o
star	astr/o
to steal	klept/o
sternum	stern/o
stiff joint	ankyl/o
stomach	gastr/o
stone	lith/o
straight	orth/o
to stretch out	extens/o
stupor	narc/o
sugar	glyc/o, glycos/o
swallow	phag/o
sweat	hidr/o
synovial membrane	synov/o, synovi/o
system	system/o
tail	caud/o
tarsus	tars/o
tears	dacry/o, lacrim/o
tendon	ten/o, tend/o, tendin/o
testes	testicul/o
testis	orch/o, orchi/o, orchid/o
thalamus	thalam/o
thymus gland	thym/o
thyroid gland	thyr/o, thyroid/o
tibia	tibi/o
tissue	hist/o
tone	ton/o
tongue	gloss/o, lingu/o
tonsils	tonsill/o
tooth	dent/o, odont/o
trachea	trache/o
treatment	iatr/o

Definition	Combining Form	Definition	Combining Form
tympanic membrane	tympan/o, myring/o	venule	venul/o
ulna	uln/o	vision	opt/o, optic/o
ureter	ureter/o	water	hydr/o
urethra	urethr/o	worry	anxi/o
urinary bladder	cyst/o	to widen	dilat/o
urine	ur/o, urin/o	yellow	cirrh/o
uterine (fallopian) tubes	salping/o		

Definition	Suffix	Definition	Suffix
abnormal condition	-iasis, -osis	drooping	-ptosis
abnormal decrease	-penia	ear condition	-otia
abnormal flow	-rrhage	to eat	-phage
abnormal flow (pertaining to)	-rrhagic	eat	-phagia
abnormal flow condition	-rrhagia	enlarged	-megaly
abnormal softening	-malacia	fear	-phobia
action	-ion	fixation (surgical)	-pexy
appetite	-orexia	flow condition (abnormal)	-rrhagia
attracted to	-phil	formation	-plasm, -plastin, -poiesis
to bear (offspring)	-para		
beginning	-arche	formation (pertaining to)	-plastic
being attracted to (condition of)	-philia	formation of cells	-plasia
being attracted to (pertaining to)	-philic	frenzy	-mania
		to fuse	-desis
blood condition	-emia	hardening	-sclerosis
blood condition (pertaining to a)	-emic	hearing	-cusis
breathing	-pnea	heart condition	-cardia
carbon dioxide	-capnia	immature	-blast
carry away	-apheresis	inflammation	-itis
carrying	-phoresis	instrument for measuring	-meter
cell	-cyte	instrument for viewing	-scope
cells (pertaining to)	-cytic	instrument to cut	-tome
chest	-thorax	instrument to measure pressure	-manometer
childbirth	-partum, -tocia		
condition	-ia	involuntary muscle contraction	-spasm
condition (abnormal)	-iasis, -osis	to kill	-cide
condition of being attracted to	-philia	labor	-tocia
condition of sperm	-spermia	laws (pertaining to)	-nomics
condition of stones	-lithiasis	mass	-oma
condition of the urine	-uria	meal (pertaining to a)	-prandial
condition to bear	-phoria	measure pressure (instrument to)	-manometer
crushing (surgical)	-tripsy		
cut (instrument to)	-tome	measuring (instrument for)	-meter
cutting into	-otomy	measuring (process of)	-metry
decrease, too few (abnormal)	-penia	medical treatment	-iatry
to destroy (to break down)	-lysis	medical treatment (pertaining to)	-iatric
destruction	-lytic		
development	-trophy	more than the normal number of cells	-cytosis
development (pertaining to)	-trophic		
digestion	-pepsia	movement	-kinesia
dilation	-ectasis	muscle coordination	-taxia
discharge	-rrhea	narrowing	-stenosis
disease	-pathy	one who studies	-logist

Definition	Suffix
opening (surgically create an)	-ostomy
pain	-algia, -dynia
paralysis	-plegia
pertaining to	-ac, -al, -an, -ar, -ary, -atic, -eal, -ia, -iac, -ic, -ical, -ile, -ine, -ior, -nic, -ory, -ose, -ous, -tic
pertaining to a blood condition	-emic
pertaining to a meal	-prandial
pertaining to abnormal flow	-rrhagic
pertaining to being attracted to	-philic
pertaining to cells	-cytic
pertaining to development	-trophic
pertaining to formation	-plastic
pertaining to medical treatment	-iatric
pertaining to poison	-toxic
pertaining to stimulating	-tropic
pertaining to study of	-logic
pertaining to tone	-tonic
pertaining to visually examining	-scopic
pertaining to vomiting	-emetic
physician	-iatrist
poison (pertaining to)	-toxic
porous	-porosis
pregnant woman	-gravida
pressure	-tension
process of measuring	-metry
process of recording	-graphy
process of visually examining	-scopy
produces	-genesis
producing	-genic
protection	-phylaxis
protein	-globin, -globulin
protrusion	-cele
puncture to withdraw fluid	-centesis
recording (process of)	-graphy
record	-gram
removal	-apheresis
removal (surgical)	-ectomy
repair (surgical)	-plasty
resembling	-oid
rupture	-rrhexis
seizure	-lepsy
separation of	-crit
to shine through	-lucent
skin condition	-derma
slipping	-listhesis
small	-ole, -ule, -osmia
softening (abnormal)	-malacia
specialist	-ician, -ist
specialist in measuring	-metrist
specialty of	-istry

Definition	Suffix
speech	-phasia
sperm (condition of)	-spermia
spitting	-ptysis
standing still	-stasis
state of	-ism
state of pregnancy	-cyesis
to stimulate	-tropin
stimulating (pertaining to)	-tropic
stone	-lith
stones (condition of)	-lithiasis
study of	-logy
study of (pertaining to)	-logic
surgical crushing	-tripsy
surgical fixation	-pexy
surgical removal	-ectomy
surgical repair	-plasty
surgically create an opening	-ostomy
to suture	-rrhaphy
swallow	-phagia
swelling	-edema
that which produces	-gen
thirst	-dipsia
to bear (offspring)	-para
to destroy (to break down)	-lysis
to eat	-phage
to fuse	-desis
to kill	-cide
to press down	-pressin, -pressor
to record	-graph
to shine through	-lucent
to stimulate	-tropin
to suture	-rrhaphy
tone	-tonia
tone (pertaining to)	-tonic
too few	-penia
treatment	-therapy
tumor	-oma
turned condition	-tropia
the urine (condition of)	-uria
uterine tube	-salpinx
view of	-opsy
viewing (instrument for)	-scope
vision condition	-opia, -opsia
visually examining (pertaining to)	-scopic
visually examining (process of)	-scopy
voice	-phonia
vomiting	-emesis
vomiting (pertaining to)	-emetic
weakness	-asthenia, -paresis

Appendix III

Abbreviations

Abbreviation	Meaning
i̇	one
i̇i̇	two
i̇i̇i̇	three
#	number
α	alpha
ā	before
AB	abortion
ABGs	arterial blood gases
ac	before meals
ACR	albumin/creatinine ratio
ACTH	adrenocorticotropic hormone
AD	Alzheimer's disease
ad lib	as desired
ADD	attention-deficit disorder
ADH	antidiuretic hormone
ADHD	attention-deficit/hyperactivity disorder
ADLs	activities of daily living
AE	above elbow
AED	automated external defibrillator
AF	atrial fibrillation
AGN	acute glomerulonephritis
AHT	abusive head trauma
AI	artificial insemination
AIDS	acquired immunodeficiency syndrome
AK	above knee
AKI	acute kidney injury
ALL	acute lymphocytic leukemia
ALS	amyotrophic lateral sclerosis
ALT	alanine transaminase
AMI	acute myocardial infarction
AML	acute myeloid leukemia
ANA	antinuclear antibody
Angio	angiography
ANS	autonomic nervous system
ante	before
AP	anteroposterior
APAP	acetaminophen (Tylenol)
aq	aqueous (water)
ARC	AIDS-related complex
ARDS	adult (or acute) respiratory distress syndrome
ARF	acute renal failure
ARMD	age-related macular degeneration
AROM	active range of motion
AS	arteriosclerosis
ASD	atrial septal defect
ASHD	arteriosclerotic heart disease
ASL	American Sign Language
AST	aspartate transaminase
Astigm	astigmatism
ATN	acute tubular necrosis
AV, A-V	atrioventricular
β	beta
Ba	barium
basos	basophils
BBB	bundle branch block (L for left; R for right)
BC	bone conduction
BCC	basal cell carcinoma
BDT	bone density testing
BE	barium enema, below elbow
bid	twice a day
BK	below knee
BM	bowel movement
BMI	body mass index
BMR	basal metabolic rate
BMT	bone marrow transplant
BNO	bladder neck obstruction
BP	blood pressure
BPD	bipolar disorder
BPH	benign prostatic hyperplasia
BPM, bpm	beats per minute
Bronch	bronchoscopy
BS	bowel sounds
BSE	breast self-examination
BUN	blood urea nitrogen
bx, BX	biopsy
c̄	with
C&S	culture and sensitivity
c.gl.	correction with glasses
C1, C2, etc.	first cervical vertebra, second cervical vertebra, etc.
Ca	calcium
CA	cancer; chronological age
CABG	coronary artery bypass graft
CAD	coronary artery disease
cap(s)	capsule(s)
CAPD	continuous ambulatory peritoneal dialysis
CAT	computerized axial tomography
cath	catheterization
CBC	complete blood count
CBD	common bile duct
CC	chief complaint, clean catch urine specimen
CCU	coronary care unit

Abbreviation	Meaning
C. diff	*Clostridium difficile*
CF	cystic fibrosis
CHF	congestive heart failure
Cl^-	chloride
CK	creatine kinase
CLL	chronic lymphocytic leukemia
CML	chronic myeloid leukemia
CNS	central nervous system
CO_2	carbon dioxide
CoA	coarctation of the aorta
COPD	chronic obstructive pulmonary disease
CPAP	continuous positive airway pressure
CP	cerebral palsy, chest pain
CPK	creatine phosphokinase
CPR	cardiopulmonary resuscitation
CRE	carbapenem-resistant Enterobacteriaceae
CRF	chronic renal failure
crit	hematocrit
CS, C-section	cesarean section
CSD	congenital septal defect
CSF	cerebrospinal fluid
CT	calcitonin, computerized tomography
CTA	clear to auscultation
CTE	chronic traumatic encephalopathy
CTS	carpal tunnel syndrome
CV	cardiovascular
CVA	cerebrovascular accident
CVD	cerebrovascular disease
CVS	chorionic villus sampling
Cx	cervix
CXR	chest X-ray
cysto	cystoscopy
D	diopter (lens strength)
d	day
D&C	dilation and curettage
dB	decibel
d/c, dc, DC	discontinue
DEA	Drug Enforcement Administration
decub	decubitus ulcer, lying down
Derm, derm	dermatology
DEXA	dual-energy X-ray absorptiometry
DI	diabetes insipidus, diagnostic imaging
diff	differential
dil	dilute
DISC, disc	discontinue
disp	dispense
DJD	degenerative joint disease
DM	diabetes mellitus
DOE	dyspnea on exertion
DPT	diphtheria, pertussis, tetanus injection
DRE	digital rectal exam

Abbreviation	Meaning
DSA	digital subtraction angiography
DSM	*Diagnostic and Statistical Manual of Mental Disorders*
DTR	deep tendon reflex
DVA	distance visual acuity
DVT	deep vein thrombosis
DXA	dual-energy X-ray absorptiometry
ECC	extracorporeal circulation
ECCE	extracapsular cataract extraction
ECG	electrocardiogram
ECHO	echocardiography
ECT	electroconvulsive therapy
ED	erectile dysfunction
EDD	estimated date of delivery
EEG	electroencephalogram, electroencephalography
EENT	eyes, ears, nose, and throat
EGD	esophagogastroduodenoscopy
eGFR	estimated glomerular filtration rate
EKG	electrocardiogram
EM	emmetropia
EMB	endometrial biopsy
EMG	electromyogram
ENT	ears, nose, and throat
EOM	extraocular movement
eos	eosinophils
eosins	eosinophils
ERCP	endoscopic retrograde cholangiopancreatography
ERT	estrogen replacement therapy
ERV	expiratory reserve volume
ESR	erythrocyte sedimentation rate
ESRD	end-stage renal disease
ESWL	extracorporeal shockwave lithotripsy
et	and
ET	esotropia
EU	excretory urography
FBS	fasting blood sugar
FDA	Food and Drug Administration
FEKG	fetal electrocardiogram
FHR	fetal heart rate
FHT	fetal heart tone
fib	fibrillation
flu	influenza
FOBT	fecal occult blood test
FRC	functional residual capacity
FS	frozen section
FSH	follicle-stimulating hormone
FTM	female to male
FTND	full-term normal delivery
Fx, FX	fracture
GI	gastrointestinal
GI	first pregnancy
GA	general anesthesia

Abbreviation	Meaning
GB	gallbladder X-ray
GC	gonorrhea
GERD	gastroesophageal reflux disease
GH	growth hormone
gm	gram
gr	grain
grav I	first pregnancy
gt	drop
GTT	glucose tolerance test
gtt	drops
GU	genitourinary
GVHD	graft versus host disease
GYN	gynecology
H_2O	water
HA	headache
HAI	healthcare-associated infection
HAV	hepatitis A virus
Hb	hemoglobin
HBV	hepatitis B virus
HCG, hCG	human chorionic gonadotropin
HCl	hydrochloric acid
HCO_3^-	bicarbonate
HCT, Hct	hematocrit
HCV	hepatitis C virus
HD	Hodgkin's disease, hemodialysis
HDN	hemolytic disease of the newborn
HDV	hepatitis D virus
heart cath	cardiac catheterization
HEENT	head, ears, eyes, nose, and throat
HEV	hepatitis E virus
Hgb	hemoglobin
HIPAA	Health Insurance Portability and Accountability Act
HIV	human immunodeficiency virus
HMD	hyaline membrane disease
HNP	herniated nucleus pulposus
HPV	human papillomavirus
H. pylori	*Helicobacter pylori*
HRT	hormone replacement therapy
HSG	hysterosalpingography
HSV-1	herpes simplex virus type 1
HTN	hypertension
Hz	hertz
I&D	incision and drainage
I&O	intake and output
IBD	inflammatory bowel disease
IBS	irritable bowel syndrome
IC	inspiratory capacity
ICCE	intracapsular cataract extraction
ICD	implantable cardioverter-defibrillator
ICP	intracranial pressure
ICU	intensive care unit
ID	intradermal
IDDM	insulin-dependent diabetes mellitus

Abbreviation	Meaning
Ig	immunoglobulins (IgA, IgD, IgE, IgG, IgM)
IM	intramuscular
inj	injection
IOL	intraocular lens
IOP	intraocular pressure
IPD	intermittent peritoneal dialysis
IPPB	intermittent positive pressure breathing
IRDS	infant respiratory distress syndrome
IRV	inspiratory reserve volume
IUD	intrauterine device
IV	intravenous
IVC	intravenous cholangiography
IVF	*in vitro* fertilization
IVP	intravenous pyelogram
JRA	juvenile rheumatoid arthritis
K^+	potassium
kg	kilogram
KS	Kaposi's sarcoma
KUB	kidneys, ureters, bladder
L	liter
L1, L2, etc.	first lumbar vertebra, second lumbar vertebra, etc.
LASIK	laser-assisted in situ keratomileusis
lat	lateral
LBW	low birth weight
LE	lower extremity
LH	luteinizing hormone
LLE	left lower extremity
LLL	left lower lobe
LLQ	left lower quadrant
LMP	last menstrual period
LP	lumbar puncture
LUE	left upper extremity
LUL	left upper lobe
LUQ	left upper quadrant
LVH	left-ventricular hypertrophy
lymphs	lymphocytes
MA	mental age
mcg	microgram
MD	muscular dystrophy
MDI	metered-dose inhaler
mEq	milliequivalent
MERS	Middle East respiratory syndrome
mg	milligram
MI	myocardial infarction, mitral insufficiency
mL	milliliter
MM	malignant melanoma
mm Hg	millimeters of mercury
MMPI	Minnesota Multiphasic Personality Inventory
mono	mononucleosis

Abbreviation	Meaning
monos	monocytes
MR	mitral regurgitation
MRSA	methicillin-resistant *Staphylococcus aureus*
MS	musculoskeletal, mitral stenosis, multiple sclerosis
MSH	melanocyte-stimulating hormone
MTF	male to female
MTX	methotrexate
MUA	manipulation under anesthesia
MVP	mitral valve prolapse
N&V	nausea and vomiting
Na^+	sodium
NB	newborn
NF	necrotizing fasciitis
NG	nasogastric (tube)
NHL	non-Hodgkin's lymphoma
NIDDM	non-insulin-dependent diabetes mellitus
NK	natural killer cells
noc	night
NPH	neutral protamine Hagedorn (insulin)
NPO	nothing by mouth
NS	nephrotic syndrome, normal saline
NSAID	nonsteroidal anti-inflammatory drug
O&P	ova and parasites
O_2	oxygen
OA	osteoarthritis
OB	obstetrics
OCD	obsessive–compulsive disorder
OCPs	oral contraceptive pills
od, OD	overdose
OE	otitis externa
oint	ointment
OM	otitis media
Ophth	ophthalmology
OR	operating room
ORIF	open reduction–internal fixation
Orth, Ortho	orthopedics
OT	occupational therapy
OTC	over the counter
Oto	otology
oz	ounce
p̄	after
P	phosphorus, pulse
PI	first delivery
PA	posteroanterior, pernicious anemia
PAC	premature atrial contraction
Pap	Papanicolaou test
para I	first delivery
PBI	protein-bound iodine
pc	after meals
PCP	pneumocystis pneumonia
PCV	packed cell volume

Abbreviation	Meaning
PDA	patent ductus arteriosus
PDR	*Physician's Desk Reference*
PE	pulmonary embolism
PE tube	pressure equalizing tube
per	by, through, with
PERRLA	pupils equal, round, reactive to light and accommodation
PET	positron emission tomography
PFT	pulmonary function test
pH	acidity or alkalinity of a solution
PharmD	doctor of pharmacy
PID	pelvic inflammatory disease
PIH	pregnancy-induced hypertension
PMN	polymorphonuclear neutrophil
PMS	premenstrual syndrome
PNS	peripheral nervous system
po	by mouth
PO	phone order
polys	polymorphonuclear neutrophil
PORP	partial ossicular replacement prosthesis
pp	postprandial
PPD	purified protein derivative
PRK	photorefractive keratectomy
PRL	prolactin
prn	as needed
pro-time	prothrombin time
PROM	passive range of motion
prot	protocol
PSA	prostate-specific antigen
pt	patient
PT	physical therapy, prothrombin time
PTC	percutaneous transhepatic cholangiography
PTCA	percutaneous transluminal coronary angioplasty
PTH	parathyroid hormone
PTSD	posttraumatic stress disorder
PUD	peptic ulcer disease
PVC	premature ventricular contraction
PVD	peripheral vascular disease
q	every
qam	every morning
qh	every hour
qid	four times a day
R	respiration, roentgen
RA	rheumatoid arthritis, room air
RAI	radioactive iodine
RBC	red blood cell
RDS	respiratory distress syndrome
REM	rapid eye movement
Rh+	Rh-positive
Rh-	Rh-negative
RIA	radioimmunoassay
RK	radial keratotomy

Abbreviation	Meaning
RLE	right lower extremity
RLL	right lower lobe
RLQ	right lower quadrant
RML	right middle lobe
ROM	range of motion
RP	retrograde pyelogram
RPh	registered pharmacist
RPR	rapid plasma reagin (test for syphilis)
RUE	right upper extremity
RUL	right upper lobe
RUQ	right upper quadrant
RV	reserve volume
Rx	prescription, treatment
$\bar{s}$	without
s.gl.	without correction or glasses
S1	first heart sound
S2	second heart sound
SA, S-A	sinoatrial
SAD	seasonal affective disorder
SARS	severe acute respiratory syndrome
SBS	shaken baby syndrome
SCC	squamous cell carcinoma
SCI	spinal cord injury
SCID	severe combined immunodeficiency
sed rate	erythrocyte sedimentation rate
segs	segmented neutrophils
SG	skin graft, specific gravity
SIDS	sudden infant death syndrome
Sig	label as follows/directions
SK	streptokinase
sl	sublingual
SLE	systemic lupus erythematosus
SMD	senile macular degeneration
SOB	shortness of breath
sol	solution
SOM	serous otitis media
sp. gr.	specific gravity
SPP	suprapubic prostatectomy
SSD	somatic symptom disorder
stat, STAT	at once/immediately
STD	sexually transmitted disease
STI	sexually transmitted infection
STSG	split-thickness skin graft
subcut	subcutaneous
suppos, supp	suppository
susp	suspension
syr	syrup
T & A	tonsillectomy and adenoidectomy
T	tablespoon; temperature
t	teaspoon
T1, T2, etc.	first thoracic vertebra, second thoracic vertebra, etc.
T_3	triiodothyronine
T_4	thyroxine

Abbreviation	Meaning
tab(s)	tablet(s)
TAH-BSO	total abdominal hysterectomy–bilateral salpingo-oophorectomy
TB	tuberculosis
TBI	traumatic brain injury
tbsp	tablespoon
TENS	transcutaneous electrical nerve stimulation
TFT	thyroid function test
THA	total hip arthroplasty
THR	total hip replacement
TIA	transient ischemic attack
tid	three times a day
TKA	total knee arthroplasty
TKR	total knee replacement
TLC	total lung capacity
TO	telephone order
top	apply topically
TORP	total ossicular replacement prosthesis
tPA	tissue plasminogen activator
TPN	total parenteral nutrition
TPR	temperature, pulse, and respiration
TSH	thyroid-stimulating hormone
tsp	teaspoon
TSS	toxic shock syndrome
tTG	tissue transglutaminase
TUR	transurethral resection
TURP	transurethral resection of the prostate
TV	tidal volume
U/A, UA	urinalysis
UC	urine culture, uterine contractions
UE	upper extremity
UGI	upper gastrointestinal series
URI	upper respiratory infection
US	ultrasound
UTI	urinary tract infection
UV	ultraviolet
V fib	ventricular fibrillation
VA	visual acuity
VC	vital capacity
VCUG	voiding cystourethrography
VD	venereal disease
VF	visual field
VO	verbal order
VS	vital signs
VSD	ventricular septal defect
VT, V-tach	ventricular tachycardia
WBC	white blood cell
wt	weight
x	times
XT	exotropia

Abbreviations to Be Avoided

Abbreviations make writing notes faster, but they also create the possibility of being misunderstood. For this reason, the Joint Commission on Accreditation of Healthcare Organizations (JCAHO) and the Institute for Safe Medication Practices (ISMP) publishes lists of error-prone abbreviations that are not to be used. The following table presents these abbreviations and what should be used instead. The Joint Commission (TJC) has determined that the first seven abbreviations (marked with an *) must appear on an accredited institution's "Do Not Use" list of abbreviations.

Abbreviation	Intended Meaning	Potential Problem	Recommendation
IU*	International Unit	Mistaken for "IV" or "10"	Write "international unit"
MS, MSO_4, and $MgSO_4$*	morphine sulfate, magnesium sulfate	Mistaken for each other	Write "morphine sulfate" or "magnesium sulfate"
Not using a zero before a decimal point (0.X)*	.X mg	Decimal point is missed	Always write a zero before a decimal point (0.X mg)
q.d. or QD*	every day	Mistaken for "qid"	Write "daily"
q.o.d. or QOD*	every other day	Mistaken for "qd" or for "qid"	Write "every other day"
U or u*	unit	Mistaken for "0," "4," or "cc"	Write "unit"
Using a zero after a decimal point*	X.0 mg	Decimal point is missed	Never write a zero by itself after a decimal point (X mg is correct)
@	at	Mistaken for "2"	Write "at"
&	and	Mistaken for "2"	Write "and"
< and >	lesser than and greater than	Mistakenly read as the opposite symbol	Write "lesser than" and "greater than"
+	and	Mistaken for "4"	Write "and"
°	hour	Mistaken for "0"	Write "hr," "h," or "hour"
i/d	one daily	Mistaken for "tid"	Write "one daily"
µg	microgram	Mistaken for "mg"	Write "mcg"
ʒ	dram	Mistaken for "3"	Use the metric system
AS, AD, AU and OS, OD, OU	left ear, right ear, both ears and left eye, right eye, both eyes	Mistaken for each other (for example, "AS" and "OS")	Write "left ear," "right ear," "both ears," "left eye," "right eye," and "both eyes"
BT	bedtime	Mistaken for "bid"	Write "bedtime"
cc	cubic centimeter	Mistaken for "U" (units) Meanings can be mistaken for each other.	Since a cubic centimeter is equal to a milliliter, write "mL"
D/C	discharge or discontinue	Mistaken for each other	Write "discharge" or "discontinue"
Dose and unit of measure run together (such as 10mg or 100mL)	10 mg or 100 mL	Mistaken for "100 mg" or "1000 mL"	Use adequate space between dose and unit of measure
Drug name and dose run together (such as Inderal40 mg)	Inderal 40 mg	Mistaken for "Inderal 140 mg"	Use adequate space between drug name and dose
hs or HS	half-strength or at bedtime	Meanings can be mistaken for each other	Write "half-strength" or "at bedtime"
IJ	injection	Mistaken for "IV"	Write "injection"
IN	intranasal	Mistaken for "IM" or "IV"	Write "intranasal" or "NAS"

Abbreviation	Intended Meaning	Potential Problem	Recommendation
Large numbers without proper comma (such as 100000)	100,000	Mistaken for "1,000,000"	Always use commas in large numbers or use words such as "100 thousand"
o.d. or OD	once daily	Mistaken for "right eye (OD)" or "overdose"	write "daily"
OJ	orange juice	Mistaken for "right eye (OD)"	write "orange juice"
Per os	by mouth	"os" can be mistaken to mean "left eye"	write "PO," "orally," or "by mouth"
Period following abbreviation such as mg. or mL.	mg or mL	Period mistaken for "1"	Write "mg" or "mL"
qhs	every bedtime	Mistaken for "qhr"	Write "bedtime"
qn	every night	Mistaken for "qh"	Write "nightly"
q1d	every day	Mistaken for "qid"	Write "daily"
q6PM	every day at 6:00 p.m.	Mistaken to mean "every 6 hours"	Write "daily at 6 p.m."
SC, SQ, sub q	subcutaneous	SC mistaken for "SL," SQ mistaken for "5 every," the separate q mistaken for "every"	Write "subcut" or "subcutaneous"
ss	sliding scale or one-half	Mistaken for each other and for "55"	Write "sliding scale," "one-half," or "1/2"
SSRI and SSI	sliding scale regular insulin and sliding scale insulin	Mistaken for "selective-serotonin reuptake inhibitor" and "strong solution of iodine"	Write "sliding scale (insulin)"
tiw or TIW	three times a week	Mistaken for "three times a day" or "twice weekly"	Write "3 times weekly"
UD	as directed (*ut dictum*)	Mistaken for unit dose	Write "as directed"
x3d	for three days	Mistaken to mean "for 3 doses"	Write "for three days"

Source: Institute for Safe Medicine Practices: ISMP's list of error prone abbreviations, symbols, and dose designations. Available at: www.ismp.org/recommendations/error-prone-abbreviations-list

Answer Keys

Chapter 1 Answers

Practice As You Go

A. **1.** word root, combining vowel, prefix, suffix **2.** combining form **3.** o **4.** suffix **5.** prefix

B. **1.** cardiology **2.** gastrology **3.** dermatology **4.** ophthalmology **5.** immunology **6.** nephrology **7.** hematology **8.** gynecology **9.** neurology **10.** pathology

C. **1.** tachy-, fast **2.** pseudo-, false **3.** hypo-, insufficient **4.** inter-, between **5.** eu-, normal **6.** post-, after **7.** mono-, one **8.** sub-, under

D. **1.** pulmonology **2.** rhinorrhea **3.** nephromalacia **4.** cardiomegaly **5.** gastrotomy **6.** dermatitis **7.** laryngectomy **8.** arthroplasty

E. **1.** metastases **2.** ova **3.** nuclei **4.** phalanges **5.** appendices **6.** vertebrae

F. **1.** c **2.** a **3.** e **4.** d **5.** b

G. **1.** c **2.** a **3.** b

H. **1.** true **2.** false **3.** true **4.** false **5.** true

I. **1.** e **2.** d **3.** f **4.** a **5.** c **6.** b

Practice Exercises

A. **1.** l **2.** e **3.** j **4.** f **5.** d **6.** k **7.** m **8.** o **9.** g **10.** n **11.** b **12.** h **13.** a **14.** c **15.** i

B. **1.** without **2.** slow **3.** without **4.** normal **5.** excessive **6.** between **7.** before **8.** under **9.** not **10.** many **11.** within **12.** outside **13.** two **14.** all **15.** above **16.** against **17.** fast **18.** insufficient **19.** through **20.** around

C. **1.** study of **2.** paralysis **3.** discharge **4.** narrowing **5.** treatment **6.** pertaining to **7.** that which produces **8.** destruction **9.** view of **10.** surgical removal **11.** hardening **12.** pertaining to **13.** pain **14.** surgical fixation **15.** process of measuring **16.** pertaining to **17.** surgical repair **18.** cutting into **19.** instrument for viewing **20.** pertaining to

D. **1.** cardiomalacia **2.** gastrostomy **3.** rhinoplasty **4.** hypertrophy **5.** pathology **6.** neuroma **7.** gastroenterology **8.** otitis **9.** chemotherapy **10.** carcinogen

E. **1.** life **2.** cancer **3.** heart **4.** chemical **5.** to cut **6.** skin **7.** small intestine **8.** stomach **9.** female **10.** blood **11.** protection **12.** voice box **13.** kidney **14.** nerve **15.** eye **16.** ear **17.** disease **18.** lung **19.** nose

F. **1.** diagnoses **2.** diverticula **3.** bursae **4.** bronchi **5.** arteries

G. **1.** *Physician's Desk Reference* (PDR) **2.** pharmacist **3.** generic or nonproprietary **4.** brand or proprietary **5.** the chemical formula **6.** Drug Enforcement Administration

H. **1.** Pravachol, 20 milligrams each, label instructions, take one every night, supply with 30, refill three times with no substitutions **2.** Lanoxin, 0.125 milligrams each, label instructions, take 3 now and then 2 every morning, supply with 100 and may refill as needed **3.** Synthroid, 0.075 milligrams each, label instructions, take 1 every day, supply with 100 and may refill four times **4.** Norvasc, 5 milligrams each, label instructions, take 1 every morning, supply with 60 and no refills

Chapter 2 Answers

Practice As You Go

A. **1.** cells, tissues, organs, systems, body **2.** cytoplasm, nucleus, cell membrane **3.** epithelial **4.** cardiac, skeletal, smooth **5.** connective **6.** neurons

B. **1.** integumentary, d **2.** cardiovascular, i **3.** digestive, g **4.** female reproductive, b **5.** musculoskeletal (skeletal), a **6.** respiratory, j **7.** urinary, c **8.** male reproductive, f **9.** nervous, h **10.** musculoskeletal (muscular), e

C. **1.** c **2.** a **3.** b

D. **1.** cephalic **2.** pubic **3.** crural **4.** gluteal **5.** cervical **6.** brachial **7.** dorsum **8.** thoracic

E. **1.** anatomical **2.** right lower **3.** cranial, spinal **4.** nine **5.** right inguinal **6.** pleural, pericardial

F. **1.** inferior or caudal **2.** supine **3.** lateral **4.** ventral or anterior **5.** deep **6.** apex **7.** distal **8.** posterior or dorsal **9.** cephalic or superior

G. **1.** d **2.** f **3.** a **4.** b **5.** c **6.** e

Practice Exercises

A. **1.** epi-, above **2.** peri-, around **3.** hypo-, insufficient or below **4.** retro-, behind or backward

B. **1.** j **2.** i **3.** f **4.** g **5.** a **6.** c **7.** d **8.** b **9.** h **10.** l **11.** e **12.** m **13.** f **14.** m **15.** k

C. **1.** MS **2.** lat **3.** RUQ **4.** CV **5.** GI **6.** AP **7.** OB **8.** LLQ

D. **1.** thoracic **2.** head **3.** neck **4.** brachial **5.** gluteal **6.** leg **7.** spine **8.** dorsum **9.** abdominal **10.** skull

E. **1.** proxim/o, proximal **2.** super/o, superior **3.** medi/o, medial **4.** ventr/o, ventral **5.** caud/o, caudal **6.** anter/o, anterior **7.** later/o, lateral **8.** dors/o, dorsal **9.** infer/o, inferior **10.** poster/o, posterior

F. **1.** a **2.** c **3.** f **4.** e **5.** a **6.** d **7.** b **8.** e **9.** c **10.** b

G. **1.** sublingual **2.** rectal **3.** topical **4.** intradermal **5.** intramuscular **6.** intravenous **7.** oral

H. **1.** spelled correctly **2.** hypochondriac **3.** integumentary **4.** spelled correctly **5.** spelled correctly **6.** spelled correctly **7.** intravenous **8.** sagittal **9.** spelled correctly **10.** epithelium

I. **1.** otorhinolaryngology **2.** cardiology **3.** gynecology **4.** orthopedics **5.** ophthalmology **6.** urology **7.** dermatology **8.** gastroenterology

Labeling Exercises

A. **1.** cephalic **2.** cervical **3.** thoracic **4.** brachial **5.** abdominal **6.** pelvic **7.** pubic **8.** crural **9.** trunk **10.** vertebral **11.** dorsum **12.** gluteal

B. **1.** frontal or coronal plane **2.** sagittal or median plane **3.** transverse or horizontal plane

Chapter 3 Answers

Practice As You Go

A. **1.** epidermis, dermis **2.** hypodermis or subcutaneous layer **3.** basal cell **4.** fat cells or lipocytes **5.** dermis **6.** keratin **7.** melanin **8.** corium **9.** nail bed **10.** sebaceous, sweat

B. **1.** ungual **2.** dermal, cutaneous, or dermic **3.** epidermal **4.** hypodermic, subcutaneous **5.** intradermal

C. **1.** e **2.** f **3.** i **4.** j **5.** a **6.** c **7.** l **8.** g **9.** k **10.** h **11.** d **12.** b

D. **1.** h **2.** i **3.** j **4.** e **5.** c **6.** a **7.** f **8.** g **9.** b **10.** d

E. **1.** FS **2.** I&D **3.** ID **4.** Subq or Subc **5.** UV **6.** BX or bx **7.** C&S **8.** BCC **9.** decub **10.** Derm or derm

Real-World Applications

Medical Record Analysis

1. basal cell carcinoma—Cancerous tumor of the basal cell layer of the epidermis. A frequent type of skin cancer that rarely metastasizes or spreads. These cancers can arise on sun-exposed skin.
2. lesions—A general term for a wound, injury, or abnormality.
3. biopsies—A piece of tissue is removed by syringe and needle, knife, punch, or brush to examine under a microscope. Used to aid in diagnosis.
4. excised—To surgically cut out.
5. pruritus—Severe itching.
6. anterior—Pertaining to the front side of the body.
7. erythema—Redness or flushing of the skin.
8. depigmentation—Loss of normal skin color or pigment.
9. epidermis—The superficial layer of the skin.
10. dermis—The deeper layer of the skin.
11. dermatoplasty—Skin grafting; transplantation of skin.

Chart Note Transcription

1. ulcer **2.** dermatologist **3.** pruritus **4.** erythema **5.** pustules **6.** dermis **7.** necrosis **8.** culture and sensitivity **9.** cellulitis **10.** debridement

Case Study

1. Systemic lupus erythematosus; another example is rheumatoid arthritis.
2. Erythema—Skin redness; photosensitivity—Intolerance to strong light; alopecia—Baldness; stiffness in joints.
3. Exfoliative cytology and fungal scrapings—in both tests cells are scraped away from the skin and examined under a microscope in order to make a diagnosis; in order to make sure the rash was not caused by something else like a fungal infection.
4. Internist—oral anti-inflammatory medication to reduce pain, swelling, and stiffness in joints; dermatologist—anti-inflammatory corticosteroid cream to reduce the red rash.
5. Completing examinations and various diagnostic tests in order to collect information necessary for a diagnosis.

Practice Exercises

A. **1.** cryosurgery **2.** onychomalacia **3.** allograft **4.** necrosis **5.** diaphoresis **6.** xenograft **7.** anhidrosis **8.** seborrhea **9.** pediculosis **10.** liposuction **11.** dermatology **12.** trichomycosis **13.** ichthyosis **14.** rhytidectomy **15.** xeroderma

B. **1.** redness involving superficial layer of skin **2.** burn damage through epidermis and into dermis causing vesicles **3.** burn damage to full thickness of epidermis and dermis

C. **1.** flat, discolored area **2.** small, solid raised spot less than 0.5 cm **3.** fluid-filled sac **4.** cracklike lesion **5.** raised spot containing pus **6.** small, round swollen area **7.** fluid-filled blister **8.** open sore **9.** firm, solid mass larger than 0.5 cm **10.** torn or jagged wound

D. **1.** dermatitis **2.** dermatosis **3.** dermatome **4.** dermatologist **5.** dermatoplasty **6.** dermatology **7.** melanoma **8.** melanocyte **9.** scleroderma **10.** leukoderma **11.** erythroderma **12.** onychomalacia **13.** paronychia **14.** onychophagia **15.** onychectomy

E. **1.** decub **2.** SLE **3.** C&S **4.** MM **5.** SG **6.** I&D **7.** SCC, BCC **8.** Derm or derm

F. **1.** xeroderma **2.** petechiae **3.** tinea **4.** scabies **5.** paronychia **6.** Kaposi's sarcoma **7.** impetigo **8.** keloid **9.** exfoliative cytology **10.** frozen section

G. **1.** antifungal, e **2.** antipruritic, c **3.** antiparasitic, a **4.** corticosteroid cream, b **5.** anesthetic, f **6.** antibiotic, d

H. **1.** spelled correctly **2.** chemabrasion **3.** rhytidectomy **4.** spelled correctly **5.** hyperhidrosis **6.** paronychia **7.** spelled correctly **8.** spelled correctly **9.** decubitus **10.** spelled correctly

I. **1.** sweat glands, sebaceous glands, hair, nails **2.** basal layer **3.** melanin **4.** collagen **5.** fat **6.** keratin **7.** sebum **8.** sudoriferous

Labeling Exercises

A. **1.** epidermis **2.** dermis **3.** subcutaneous layer **4.** sweat gland **5.** sweat duct **6.** hair shaft **7.** sebaceous gland **8.** arrector pili muscle **9.** sensory receptors

B. **1.** epidermis **2.** dermis **3.** subcutaneous layer **4.** sebaceous gland **5.** arrector pili muscle **6.** hair shaft **7.** hair follicle **8.** hair root **9.** papilla

C. **1.** free edge **2.** lateral nail groove **3.** lunula **4.** nail bed **5.** nail body **6.** cuticle **7.** nail root

Chapter 4 Answers

Practice As You Go

A. **1.** osseous **2.** joint, ligaments **3.** diaphysis, epiphysis **4.** head, condyle, epicondyle, trochanter, tubercle, tuberosity **5.** sinus, foramen, fossa, fissure

B. **1.** patella **2.** tarsus **3.** clavicle **4.** femur **5.** phalanges **6.** carpus **7.** tibia **8.** scapula **9.** phalanges

C. **1.** femoral **2.** sternal **3.** clavicular **4.** coccygeal **5.** maxillary **6.** tibial **7.** patellar **8.** phalangeal **9.** humeral **10.** pubic

D. **1.** e **2.** d **3.** j **4.** b **5.** g **6.** i **7.** a **8.** c **9.** f **10.** h

E. **1.** e **2.** c **3.** f **4.** a **5.** d **6.** b

F. **1.** TKR **2.** HNP **3.** UE **4.** L5 **5.** AK **6.** Fx or FX **7.** NSAID

G. **1.** smooth **2.** myoneural or neuromuscular **3.** skeletal, smooth, cardiac

H. **1.** e **2.** d **3.** b **4.** c **5.** a **6.** h **7.** g **8.** f

I. **1.** d **2.** g **3.** a **4.** h **5.** e **6.** c **7.** f **8.** b

J. **1.** IM **2.** DTR **3.** MD **4.** EMG **5.** CTS

Real-World Applications

Medical Record Analysis

1. osteoarthritis—Joint inflammation resulting in degeneration of the bones and joints, especially those bearing weight. Results in bone rubbing against bone.
2. bilateral—Pertaining to both sides.
3. TKA—Surgical reconstruction of a knee joint by implanting a prosthetic knee joint. Also called *total knee replacement (TKR)*.
4. orthopedic surgeon—Physician that specializes in the diagnosis and treatment of conditions of the musculoskeletal system using surgical means.
5. Radiographs — An X-ray image.
6. physical therapy—Treats disorders using physical means and methods; includes joint motion and muscle strength.
7. therapeutic exercise — Specific exercises planned to improve range of motion and muscle strength
8. gait training—Learning how to walk.
9. occupational therapy—Assists patients to regain, develop, and improve skills that are important for independent functioning.
10. ADLs—Activities of daily living.

Chart Note Transcription

1. Colles' fracture (fx) **2.** cast **3.** fracture **4.** orthopedist **5.** osteoporosis **6.** dual-energy X-ray absorptiometry (DXA, DEXA) **7.** flexion **8.** extension **9.** comminuted fracture (FX, Fx) **10.** femur **11.** total hip arthroplasty (THA)

Case Study

1. Rheumatoid arthritis.
2. Cartilage damage and crippling deformities.
3. Osteoarthritis.
4. Bone scan—Radioactive dye is used to visualize the body; erythrocyte sedimentation rate—A blood test that can determine if a person has an inflammatory disease.
5. Anti-inflammatory medication to reduce inflammation and provide some pain relief; physical therapy—Treatment using warm water and exercises to maintain the flexibility of the joints.
6. Acute—Brief disease, also used to mean sudden and severe disease; chronic—Disease of a long duration.

Practice Exercises

A. **1.** osteocyte **2.** osteoblast **3.** osteoporosis **4.** osteopathy **5.** osteotomy **6.** osteotome **7.** osteomyelitis **8.** osteomalacia **9.** osteochondroma **10.** myopathy **11.** myoplasty **12.** myorrhaphy **13.** electromyogram **14.** myasthenia **15.** tenodynia **16.** tenorrhaphy **17.** arthrodesis **18.** arthroplasty **19.** arthrotomy **20.** arthritis **21.** arthrocentesis **22.** arthralgia **23.** chondrectomy **24.** chondroma **25.** chondromalacia

B. **1.** cervical, 7 **2.** thoracic, 12 **3.** lumbar, 5 **4.** sacrum, 1 (5 fused) **5.** coccyx, 1 (3–5 fused)

C. **1.** osteoporosis **2.** myorrhexis **3.** scoliosis **4.** dystonia **5.** kinesiology **6.** lordosis **7.** spondylolisthesis **8.** arthrocentesis **9.** abduction **10.** osteoarthritis **11.** osteoclasia **12.** chondromalacia **13.** muscular **14.** myasthenia **15.** tendinitis **16.** bursitis **17.** myeloma **18.** arthrodesis

D. **1.** osteoporosis **2.** rickets **3.** lateral epicondylitis **4.** herniated nucleus pulposus **5.** osteogenic sarcoma **6.** scoliosis **7.** pseudohypertrophic muscular dystrophy **8.** systemic lupus erythematosus **9.** spondylolisthesis **10.** carpal tunnel syndrome

E. **1.** axial, 1, upper jaw **2.** appendicular, 16, wrist bones **3.** appendicular, 2, shoulder blade **4.** appendicular, 2, kneecap **5.** axial, 1, breast bone **6.** appendicular, 2, thigh bone **7.** appendicular, 10, forefoot bone **8.** appendicular, 2, shin bone **9.** appendicular, 2, collar bone **10.** axial, 2, cheek bone

F. **1.** CTS **2.** DEXA or DXA **3.** MD **4.** THA or THR **5.** EMG **6.** RA **7.** Fx or FX **8.** NSAID

G. **1.** surgical repair of cartilage **2.** slow movement **3.** porous bone **4.** abnormal increase in lumbar spine curve (swayback) **5.** lack of development **6.** bone marrow tumor **7.** artificial substitute for a body part **8.** cutting into skull **9.** puncture of a joint to withdraw fluid **10.** bursa inflammation

H. **1.** nonsteroidal anti-inflammatory drugs, b **2.** corticosteroids, e **3.** skeletal muscle relaxants, a **4.** bone reabsorption inhibitors, c **5.** calcium supplements, d

I. **1.** massage **2.** mobilization **3.** hydrotherapy **4.** ultrasound **5.** thermotherapy **6.** phonophoresis **7.** cryotherapy **8.** gait training

J. **1.** c **2.** h **3.** f **4.** g **5.** d **6.** e **7.** a **8.** b

K. **1.** spelled correctly **2.** pseudohypertrophic **3.** polymyositis **4.** spelled correctly **5.** spelled correctly **6.** osteochondroma **7.** spondylosis **8.** spelled correctly **9.** spelled correctly **10.** exostosis

Labeling Exercises

A. **1.** skull **2.** cervical vertebrae **3.** sternum **4.** ribs **5.** thoracic vertebrae **6.** lumbar vertebrae **7.** ilium **8.** pubis **9.** ischium **10.** femur **11.** patella **12.** tibia **13.** fibula **14.** tarsus **15.** metatarsus **16.** phalanges **17.** maxilla **18.** mandible **19.** scapula **20.** humerus **21.** ulna **22.** radius **23.** sacrum **24.** coccyx **25.** carpus **26.** metacarpus **27.** phalanges

B. **1.** proximal epiphysis **2.** diaphysis **3.** distal epiphysis **4.** articular cartilage **5.** epiphyseal line **6.** spongy or cancellous bone **7.** compact or cortical bone **8.** medullary cavity

C. **1.** periosteum **2.** synovial membrane **3.** articular cartilage **4.** joint cavity **5.** joint capsule

Chapter 5 Answers

Practice As You Go

A. **1.** cardiology **2.** endocardium, myocardium, epicardium **3.** sinoatrial node **4.** away from **5.** tricuspid, pulmonary, mitral (bicuspid), aortic **6.** atria, ventricles **7.** pulmonary **8.** apex **9.** septum **10.** systole, diastole

B. **1.** arteries, veins, capillaries **2.** veins **3.** arteries **4.** capillaries **5.** systolic, diastolic

C. **1.** cardiac or coronary **2.** interventricular **3.** arterial **4.** venular **5.** myocardial **6.** atrial

D. **1.** f **2.** h **3.** d **4.** g **5.** b **6.** i **7.** a **8.** c **9.** e **10.** j

E. **1.** c **2.** g **3.** j **4.** a **5.** d **6.** b **7.** i **8.** e **9.** f **10.** h

F. **1.** MVP **2.** VSD **3.** PTCA **4.** V fib **5.** DVT **6.** ASHD **7.** CoA **8.** tPA **9.** CV **10.** ECC

Real-World Applications

Medical Record Analysis

1. hypertension—Blood pressure above the normal range.
2. tachycardia—The condition of having a fast heart rate, typically more than 100 beats/minute while at rest.
3. congestive heart failure (CHF)—Pathological condition of the heart in which there is a reduced outflow of blood from the left side of the heart because the left ventricle myocardium has become too weak to efficiently pump blood. Results in weakness, breathlessness, and edema.
4. mitral valve prolapse—Condition in which the cusps or flaps of the heart valve are too loose and fail to shut tightly, allowing blood to flow backward through the valve when the heart chamber contracts. Most commonly occurs in the mitral valve, but may affect any of the heart valves.
5. palpitations—Pounding, racing heartbeats.
6. electrocardiography (EKG)—Process of recording the electrical activity of the heart. Useful in the diagnosis of abnormal cardiac rhythm and heart muscle (myocardium) damage.
7. cardiac biomarkers—Blood test to determine the level of proteins specific to heart muscles in the blood. An increase in these proteins may indicate heart muscle damage such as a myocardial infarction. These proteins include creatine kinase (CK) and troponin.
8. echocardiography—Noninvasive diagnostic method using ultrasound to visualize internal cardiac structures. Cardiac valve activity can be evaluated using this method.

9. stress test—Method for evaluating cardiovascular fitness. The patient is placed on a treadmill or a bicycle and then subjected to steadily increasing levels of work. An EKG and oxygen levels are taken while the patient exercises. The test is stopped if abnormalities occur on the EKG. Also called an *exercise test* or a *treadmill test*.
10. angiocardiography—X-rays taken after the injection of an opaque material into a blood vessel. Can be performed on the aorta as an aortic angiogram, on the heart as an angiocardiogram, and on the brain as a cerebral angiogram.
11. coronary artery disease (CAD)—Insufficient blood supply to the heart muscle due to an obstruction of one or more coronary arteries. May be caused by atherosclerosis and may cause angina pectoris and myocardial infarction.
12. myocardial infarction—Condition caused by the partial or complete occlusion or closing of one or more of the coronary arteries. Symptoms include a squeezing pain or heavy pressure in the middle of the chest (angina pectoris). A delay in treatment could result in death. Also referred to as a *heart attack*.
13. mitral valvoplasty—Removal of a diseased heart valve and replacement with an artificial valve.

Chart Note Transcription

1. angina pectoris **2.** bradycardia **3.** hypertension **4.** myocardial infarction (MI) **5.** electrocardiogram (EKG, ECG) **6.** cardiac biomarkers **7.** coronary artery disease (CAD) **8.** cardiac catheterization **9.** stress test (treadmill test) **10.** percutaneous transluminal coronary angioplasty (PTCA) **11.** coronary artery bypass graft (CABG)

Case Study

1. Heart attack; condition caused by the partial or complete occlusion or closing of one or more of the coronary arteries. Symptoms include a squeezing pain or heavy pressure in the middle of the chest (angina pectoris). A delay in treatment could result in death.
2. The main complaint, the one the patient is most aware of or most anxious about.
3. Angina pectoris—Condition in which there is severe pain with a sensation of constriction around the heart; caused by a deficiency of oxygen to the heart muscle.
4. Nausea—Feeling of need to vomit; dyspnea—Difficulty breathing; diaphoresis—Profuse sweating.
5. Cardiac biomarkers; angiocardiography; cardiac scan; electrocardiography; stress testing; cardiac catheterization; Holter monitor.
6. Smokes; overweight; family history; sedentary lifestyle. He can stop smoking, lose weight, and become more active.

Practice Exercises

A. **1.** cardiac **2.** cardiomyopathy **3.** cardiomegaly **4.** tachycardia **5.** bradycardia **6.** electrocardiogram **7.** angiostenosis **8.** angiitis **9.** angiospasm **10.** arterial **11.** arteriosclerosis **12.** arteriole **13.** endocarditis **14.** epicarditis **15.** myocarditis

B. **1.** aortic **2.** atrial **3.** heart **4.** venous **5.** arteriole **6.** ventricle **7.** valvular **8.** myocardial **9.** venular **10.** heart **11.** blood vessel **12.** artery

C. **1.** angiogram **2.** tachycardia **3.** cardiomyopathy **4.** endocarditis **5.** arteriosclerosis **6.** hypertension **7.** atheroma **8.** phlebitis **9.** thrombolytic **10.** embolectomy **11.** intracoronary **12.** valvoplasty

D. **1.** pulmonary, systemic **2.** myocardium **3.** septum **4.** tricuspid, mitral or bicuspid, pulmonary, aortic **5.** sinoatrial node **6.** coronary **7.** Blood pressure **8.** capillary bed

E. **1.** BBB **2.** MI **3.** PAC **4.** EKG or ECG **5.** ECHO **6.** PTCA **7.** ECC **8.** DVT **9.** CHF **10.** CSD

F. **1.** thin flexible tube **2.** an area of dead tissue **3.** a blood clot **4.** pounding heartbeat **5.** backflow **6.** weakened and ballooning arterial wall **7.** complete stoppage of heart activity **8.** serious cardiac arrhythmia **9.** heart attack **10.** varicose veins in anal region

G. **1.** murmur **2.** defibrillation **3.** hypertension **4.** pacemaker **5.** varicose veins **6.** angina pectoris **7.** CCU **8.** MI **9.** angiography **10.** echocardiogram **11.** Holter monitor **12.** CHF

H. **1.** antiarrhythmic, e **2.** antilipidemic, g **3.** cardiotonic, f **4.** diuretic, h **5.** anticoagulant, b **6.** fibrinolytic, a **7.** vasodilator, d **8.** calcium channel blocker, c

I. **1.** cardiomyopathy **2.** tachycardia **3.** spelled correctly **4.** spelled correctly **5.** spelled correctly **6.** spelled correctly **7.** spelled correctly **8.** infarction **9.** arrhythmia **10.** angiitis

Labeling Exercises

A. **1.** pulmonary arteries **2.** vena cavae **3.** right atrium **4.** right ventricle **5.** systemic veins **6.** capillary bed of lungs **7.** pulmonary veins **8.** aorta **9.** left atrium **10.** left ventricle **11.** systemic arteries **12.** systemic capillary beds

B. **1.** superior vena cava **2.** aorta **3.** pulmonary trunk **4.** pulmonary valve **5.** right atrium **6.** tricuspid valve **7.** right ventricle **8.** inferior vena cava **9.** pulmonary artery **10.** pulmonary vein **11.** left atrium **12.** aortic valve **13.** mitral or bicuspid valve **14.** left ventricle **15.** endocardium **16.** myocardium **17.** pericardium

Chapter 6 Answers

Practice As You Go

A. **1.** phagocytosis **2.** erythrocytes (red blood cells), leukocytes (white blood cells), platelets (thrombocytes) **3.** plasma **4.** hemostasis **5.** ABO system, Rh factor

B. **1.** hematic or sanguineous **2.** leukocytic **3.** thrombocytic **4.** fibrinous **5.** erythrocytic

C. **1.** d **2.** e **3.** c **4.** b **5.** a

D. **1.** c **2.** e **3.** a **4.** b **5.** d

E. **1.** ALL **2.** BMT **3.** eosins or eos **4.** HCT or Hct or crit **5.** PA **6.** CBC **7.** diff **8.** WBC **9.** noc **10.** pc

F. **1.** spleen, tonsils, thymus **2.** thoracic duct, right lymphatic duct **3.** axillary, cervical, mediastinal, inguinal **4.** active acquired **5.** antibody-mediated

G. **1.** splenic **2.** lymphatic **3.** tonsillar **4.** thymic 5. lymphangial

H. **1.** c **2.** a **3.** d **4.** e **5.** b

I. **1.** e **2.** c **3.** d **4.** a **5.** b

J. **1.** AIDS **2.** ARC **3.** HIV **4.** mono **5.** KS **6.** Ig **7.** SCIDS **8.** PCP

Real-World Applications

Medical Record Analysis

1. splenomegaly—An enlarged spleen.
2. non-Hodgkin's lymphoma—Cancer of the lymphatic tissues other than Hodgkin's lymphoma.
3. spleen—An organ located in the upper left quadrant of the abdomen. Consists of lymphatic tissue that is highly infiltrated with blood vessels. It filters out and destroys old red blood cells.
4. splenectomy—The surgical removal of the spleen.
5. Monospot—A blood test for infectious mononucleosis.
6. HIV antigen/antibody immunoassay —A blood test for HIV infection. HIV antigen (foreign viral proteins) can be detected shortly after exposure and antibodies produced by the body in response to an HIV infection can be detected 2–8 weeks after exposure.
7. Magnetic resonance imaging (MRI)—Medical imaging that uses radio-frequency radiation as its source of energy. It does not require the injection of contrast medium or exposure to ionizing radiation. The technique is useful for visualizing large blood vessels, the heart, the brain, and soft tissues.
8. tumor—Abnormal growth of tissue that may be benign or malignant.
9. biopsy—A piece of tissue is removed by syringe and needle, knife, punch, or brush to examine under a microscope. Used to aid in diagnosis.
10. chemotherapy—Treating diseases, especially cancer, with chemicals that are toxic to cells of the body.

Chart Note Transcription

1. hematologist **2.** HIV antigen/antibody immunoassay **3.** prothrombin time **4.** complete blood count (CBC) **5.** erythropenia **6.** thrombopenia **7.** leukocytosis **8.** bone marrow aspiration **9.** leukemia **10.** homologous transfusion

Case Study

1. Acute lymphocytic leukemia.
2. High fever; thrombopenia—Too few platelets; epistaxis—Nosebleed; gingival bleeding—Gums bleeding; petechiae—Pinpoint bruises; ecchymoses—Large black and blue bruises.
3. Bone marrow aspiration—Sample of bone marrow is removed by aspiration with a needle and examined for diseases.
4. A diagnosis based on the results of the physician's direct examination rather than based on other tests like X-rays and labwork.
5. Chemotherapy—Treating disease by using chemicals that have a toxic effect on the body, especially cancerous tissue.
6. Remission—A period during which the symptoms of a disease or disorder leave. Can be temporary.

Practice Exercises

A. **1.** splenomegaly **2.** splenectomy **3.** splenotomy **4.** lymphocytes **5.** lymphoma **6.** lymphadenopathy **7.** lymphadenoma **8.** lymphadenitis **9.** immunologist **10.** immunoglobulin **11.** immunology **12.** hematic **13.** hematoma **14.** hematopoiesis **15.** hemolytic **16.** hemoglobin **17.** leukopenia **18.** erythropenia **19.** pancytopenia **20.** leukocytosis **21.** erythrocytosis **22.** thrombocytosis **23.** erythrocyte **24.** leukocyte **25.** lymphocyte

B. **1.** HCT or Hct or crit **2.** HIV, AIDS **3.** ESR or sed rate **4.** GVHD **5.** C&S **6.** PCP **7.** Pro-time or PT **8.** AML, ALL **9.** RBC, WBC **10.** PA

C. **1.** erythrocytosis **2.** hyperlipidemia **3.** leukopenia **4.** hemoglobin **5.** phlebotomy **6.** fibrinolytic **7.** morphology **8.** hematocrit **9.** pathology **10.** lymphedema **11.** lymphangioma **12.** immunotherapy **13.** tonsillectomy **14.** myeloma **15.** splenomegaly

D. **1.** polycythemia vera **2.** mononucleosis **3.** anaphylactic shock **4.** HIV **5.** Kaposi's sarcoma **6.** autoimmune diseases **7.** Hodgkin's disease **8.** pneumocystis **9.** aplastic **10.** pernicious

E. **1.** reverse transcriptase inhibitor, e **2.** anticoagulant, a **3.** antihemorrhagic, d **4.** antihistamine, h **5.** immunosuppressant, f **6.** fibrinolytic, b **7.** hematinic, g **8.** corticosteroid, c **9.** antiplatelet agent, i

F. **1.** d **2.** f **3.** b **4.** g **5.** a **6.** e **7.** c

G. **1.** treatment with an antibody injection **2.** blood test for mononucleosis **3.** infections seen in immunocompromised patients **4.** intense itching **5.** tissue's response to injury **6.** blood transfusion from another person **7.** caused by vitamin B_{12} deficiency **8.** cancer of blood-forming bone marrow **9.** rapid flow of blood, bleeding **10.** blood poisoning

H. **1.** axillary **2.** sanguineous or hematic **3.** lymph vessel **4.** fibers **5.** spleen **6.** thymus gland **7.** thrombocytic **8.** leukocytic **9.** erythrocytic **10.** tonsils

I. **1.** tonsillitis **2.** spelled correctly **3.** spelled correctly **4.** spelled correctly **5.** inflammation **6.** spelled correctly **7.** autologous **8.** spelled correctly **9.** pancytopenia **10.** dyscrasia

J. **1.** hemoglobin **2.** eosinophils, basophils, neutrophils, monocytes, lymphocytes **3.** Platelet **4.** donor, recipient **5.** lacteals **6.** Lymph nodes **7.** spleen **8.** cellular

Labeling Exercises

A. **1.** plasma **2.** red blood cells or erythrocytes **3.** platelets or thrombocytes **4.** white blood cells or leukocytes

B. **1.** cervical nodes **2.** mediastinal nodes **3.** axillary nodes **4.** inguinal nodes

C. **1.** thymus gland **2.** lymph node **3.** tonsil **4.** spleen **5.** lymphatic vessels

Chapter 7 Answers

Practice As You Go

A. **1.** nasal cavity, pharynx, larynx, trachea, bronchial tubes, lungs **2.** pharynx **3.** epiglottis **4.** 3, 2 **5.** alveoli **6.** pleura **7.** bronchioles, alveoli

B. **1.** c **2.** f **3.** a **4.** h **5.** g **6.** b **7.** e **8.** d

C. **1.** laryngeal **2.** pulmonary **3.** paranasal **4.** alveolar **5.** nasal **6.** diaphragmatic

D. **1.** e **2.** i **3.** h **4.** a **5.** j **6.** d **7.** b **8.** g **9.** f **10.** c

E. **1.** f **2.** c **3.** e **4.** a **5.** d **6.** b

F. **1.** URI **2.** PFT **3.** O_2 **4.** CO_2 **5.** COPD **6.** Bronch **7.** TB **8.** IRDS

Real-World Applications

Medical Record Analysis

1. asthma—Disease caused by various conditions, such as allergens, and resulting in constriction of the bronchial airways, dyspnea, coughing, and wheezing. Can cause violent spasms of the bronchi (bronchospasms) but is generally not a life-threatening condition. Medication can be very effective.
2. dyspnea—Term describing difficult or labored breathing.
3. cyanosis—Refers to the bluish tint of skin that is receiving an insufficient amount of oxygen or circulation.
4. expiration—To breathe out; exhale.
5. phlegm—Thick mucus secreted by the membranes that line the respiratory tract. When phlegm is coughed through the mouth, it is called *sputum*. Phlegm is examined for color, odor, and consistency.
6. auscultation—To listen to body sounds, usually using a stethoscope.
7. rhonchi—Somewhat musical sound during expiration, often found in asthma or infection. Caused by spasms of the bronchial tubes. Also called *wheezing*.
8. arterial blood gases (ABGs)—Testing for the gases present in the blood. Generally used to assist in determining the levels of oxygen (O_2) and carbon dioxide (CO_2) in the blood.
9. hypoxemia—The condition of having an insufficient amount of oxygen in the bloodstream.
10. spirometry—Procedure to measure lung capacity using a *spirometer*.
11. Proventil—Medication that relaxes muscle spasms in bronchial tubes. Used to treat asthma.
12. bronchospasms—An involuntary muscle spasm of the smooth muscle in the wall of the bronchus.

Chart Note Transcription

1. dyspnea **2.** tachypnea **3.** arterial blood gases (ABGs) **4.** hypoxemia **5.** auscultation **6.** crackles **7.** purulent **8.** sputum **9.** CXR **10.** pneumonia **11.** endotracheal intubation

Case Study

1. Pneumonia.
2. Dyspnea—Difficulty breathing; dizziness; orthopnea—Comfortable breathing only while sitting up; elevated temperature, cough.
3. Auscultation (listening to the body sounds) revealed crackles (abnormal sound); chest X-ray revealed fluid in the upper lobe of the right lung.
4. A method of determining a patient's general health and heart and lung function by measuring pulse (100 BPM and rapid), respiratory rate (24 breaths/min and labored), temperature (102°F), and blood pressure (180/110).
5. IV antibiotics—Medicine to kill bacteria given into a vein; intermittent positive pressure breathing—Method of assisting patients in breathing by using a machine that produces an increased pressure.

6. The IV antibiotics were changed to oral antibiotics—she started taking pills.

Practice Exercises

A. **1.** exchange of O_2 and CO_2 **2.** ventilation **3.** exchange of O_2 and CO_2 in the lungs **4.** exchange of O_2 and CO_2 at cellular level **5.** diaphragm **6.** volume of air in the lungs after a maximal inhalation or inspiration **7.** amount of air entering lungs in a single inspiration or leaving lungs in single expiration of quiet breathing **8.** air remaining in the lungs after a forced expiration **9.** nasal cavity, pharynx, larynx, trachea, bronchial tubes, lungs **10.** respiratory rate, temperature, heart rate, blood pressure

B. **1.** rhinitis **2.** rhinorrhea **3.** rhinoplasty **4.** laryngitis **5.** laryngospasm **6.** laryngoscopy **7.** laryngeal **8.** laryngectomy **9.** laryngoplasty **10.** laryngoplegia **11.** bronchial **12.** bronchitis **13.** bronchoscopy **14.** bronchogenic **15.** bronchospasm **16.** thoracotomy **17.** thoracalgia **18.** thoracic **19.** tracheotomy **20.** tracheostenosis **21.** endotracheal **22.** dyspnea **23.** tachypnea **24.** orthopnea **25.** apnea

C. **1.** anosmia **2.** bradypnea **3.** laryngoplegia **4.** hemoptysis **5.** rhinorrhagia **6.** dysphonia **7.** pharyngitis **8.** bronchiectasis **9.** anthracosis **10.** pneumothorax **11.** oximeter **12.** laryngoscopy **13.** pleurocentesis **14.** cardiopulmonary **15.** tracheostenosis

D. **1.** inhalation or inspiration **2.** hemoptysis **3.** pulmonary emboli **4.** sinusitis **5.** pharyngitis **6.** pneumothorax **7.** pertussis **8.** pleurotomy **9.** pleurodynia **10.** nasopharyngitis

E. **1.** ENT **2.** COPD **3.** CF **4.** IRDS **5.** PE **6.** SIDS **7.** ABGs **8.** CXR **9.** PFT **10.** CPAP

F. **1.** cardiopulmonary resuscitation **2.** thoracentesis **3.** respirator **4.** supplemental oxygen **5.** patent **6.** ventilation-perfusion scan **7.** sputum cytology **8.** hyperventilation **9.** rhonchi **10.** anthracosis

G. **1.** decongestant, f **2.** antitussive, a **3.** antibiotic, c **4.** expectorant, g **5.** mucolytic, h **6.** bronchodilator, d **7.** antihistamine, e **8.** corticosteroid, b

H. **1.** alveolar **2.** lung **3.** thoracic **4.** bronchus **5.** tracheal **6.** epiglottis **7.** mucous **8.** pharyngeal **9.** bronchiole **10.** septum

I. **1.** nasopharyngeal **2.** spelled correctly **3.** cannula **4.** hemoptysis **5.** bronchodilator **6.** spelled correctly **7.** spelled correctly **8.** spelled correctly **9.** spelled correctly **10.** pneumoconiosis

Labeling Exercises

A. **1.** pharynx and larynx **2.** trachea **3.** nasal cavity **4.** bronchial tubes **5.** lungs

B. **1.** nares **2.** paranasal sinuses **3.** nasal cavity **4.** hard palate **5.** soft palate **6.** palatine tonsil **7.** epiglottis **8.** vocal cords **9.** esophagus **10.** trachea

C. **1.** trachea **2.** right upper lobe **3.** right middle lobe **4.** right lower lobe **5.** apex of lung **6.** left upper lobe **7.** left lower lobe **8.** diaphragm

Chapter 8 Answers

Practice As You Go

A. **1.** gastrointestinal (GI) **2.** gut, alimentary canal, gastrointestinal tract, mouth, anus **3.** digesting food, absorbing nutrients, eliminating waste **4.** incisors, cuspids or canines **5.** bicuspids or premolars, molars **6.** crown, root **7.** enamel **8.** deciduous, permanent

B. **1.** oropharynx **2.** peristalsis **3.** hydrochloric acid, chyme **4.** duodenum, jejunum, ileum **5.** villi **6.** ileocecal valve, anus, cecum, colon, rectum **7.** sigmoid **8.** defecation

C. **1.** salivary glands, liver, gallbladder, pancreas **2.** amylase, carbohydrates **3.** bile, emulsification, gallbladder **4.** duodenum, buffers, pancreatic enzymes

D. **1.** duodenal **2.** nasogastric **3.** hepatic **4.** pancreatic **5.** cholecystic or cystic **6.** sublingual **7.** esophageal **8.** sigmoidal

E. **1.** i **2.** f **3.** c **4.** a **5.** j **6.** l **7.** e **8.** b **9.** k **10.** d **11.** g **12.** o **13.** h **14.** n **15.** m

F. **1.** f **2.** g **3.** e **4.** h **5.** b **6.** a **7.** d **8.** c

G. **1.** NG **2.** GI **3.** HBV **4.** FOBT **5.** IBD **6.** HSV-1 **7.** AST **8.** pc **9.** PUD **10.** GERD

Real-World Applications

Medical Record Analysis

1. epigastric—Pertaining to the area above the stomach.
2. anemia—A large group of conditions characterized by a reduction in the number of red blood cells or the amount of hemoglobin in the blood; results in less oxygen reaching the tissues.
3. melena—Passage of dark tarry stool. Color is the result of digestive enzymes working on blood in the gastrointestinal tract.
4. dyspepsia—An "upset stomach."
5. antacids—Medication to neutralize stomach acid.
6. complete blood count (CBC)—A combination of blood tests including red blood cell count, white blood cell count, hemoglobin, hematocrit, white blood cell differential, and platelet count.

7. fecal occult blood—Laboratory test on the feces to determine if microscopic amounts of blood are present. Also called *hemoccult* or *stool guaiac*.
8. *Helicobacter pylori*—A bacteria that may damage the lining of the stomach setting up the conditions for peptic ulcer disease to develop.
9. gastroscopy—Procedure in which a flexible *gastroscope* is passed through the mouth and down the esophagus in order to visualize inside the stomach. Used to diagnose peptic ulcers and gastric carcinoma.
10. ulcer—An open sore or lesion in the skin or mucous membrane.
11. peptic ulcer disease—Ulcer occurring in the lower portion of the esophagus, stomach, and/or duodenum; thought to be caused by the acid of gastric juices. Initial damage to the protective lining of the stomach may be caused by a *Helicobacter pylori* (*H. pylori*) bacterial infection. If the ulcer extends all the way through the wall of the stomach, it is called a *perforated ulcer*, which requires immediate surgery to repair.
12. gastrectomy—Surgical removal of the stomach.

Chart Note Transcription

1. gastroenterologist **2.** constipation **3.** cholelithiasis **4.** cholecystectomy **5.** gastroesophageal reflux disease **6.** ascites **7.** lower gastrointestinal series **8.** polyposis **9.** colonoscopy **10.** sigmoid colon **11.** colectomy **12.** colostomy

Case Study

1. Severe RUQ pain—Severe pain is located in the upper right corner of the abdomen; nausea—Feeling the urge to vomit; scleral jaundice—The whites of the eye have a yellowish cast to them.
2. Gallbladder, right kidney, majority of the liver, a small portion of the pancreas, portion of colon and small intestine.
3. Gallstones blocking the common bile duct so bile can't drain into the small intestine.
4. Abdominal ultrasound—The use of high-frequency sound waves to produce an image of an organ, such as the gallbladder; percutaneous transhepatic cholangiography (PTC)—Procedure in which contrast medium is injected directly into the liver to visualize the bile ducts; used to detect obstructions such as gallstones in the common bile duct.
5. Cholelithiasis is the condition of having gallstones present in the gallbladder, they may not be causing any symptoms; cholecystitis is the inflammation of the gallbladder that occurs when gallstones block the flow of bile out of the gallbladder.
6. Laparoscopic cholecystectomy—The gallbladder was removed through a very small abdominal incision with the assistance of a laparoscope.

Practice Exercises

A. **1.** gastritis **2.** gastroenterology **3.** gastrectomy **4.** gastroscopy **5.** gastralgia **6.** gastromegaly **7.** gastrotomy **8.** esophagitis **9.** esophagoscopy **10.** esophagoplasty **11.** esophageal **12.** esophagectomy **13.** proctopexy **14.** proctoptosis **15.** proctitis **16.** proctologist **17.** cholecystectomy **18.** cholecystolithiasis **19.** cholecystolithotripsy **20.** cholecystitis **21.** laparoscope **22.** laparotomy **23.** laparoscopy **24.** hepatoma **25.** hepatomegaly **26.** hepatic **27.** hepatitis **28.** pancreatitis **29.** pancreatic **30.** colostomy **31.** colitis

B. **1.** pharyngoplasty **2.** hepatoma **3.** gastrectomy **4.** polyposis **5.** sigmoidoscope **6.** postprandial **7.** cholecystogram **8.** pancreatitis **9.** sialadenitis **10.** anorexia **11.** hematemesis **12.** bradypepsia **13.** gastroenterology **14.** dysphagia **15.** periodontal

C. **1.** TPN, NG **2.** UGI **3.** O&P **4.** IBS **5.** PUD **6.** GERD **7.** N&V **8.** AST, ALT **9.** FOBT **10.** BM

D. **1.** visual exam of the colon **2.** tooth X-ray **3.** bright red blood in the stool **4.** blood test to determine amount of waste product bilirubin in the bloodstream **5.** weight loss and wasting from a chronic illness **6.** use of NG tube to wash out stomach **7.** surgical repair of hernia **8.** pulling teeth **9.** surgical crushing of common bile duct stone **10.** surgically create a connection between two organs or vessels

E. **1.** liver biopsy **2.** colostomy **3.** barium swallow **4.** lower GI series **5.** colectomy **6.** fecal occult blood test **7.** choledocholithotripsy **8.** total parenteral nutrition **9.** gastric stapling **10.** intravenous cholecystography **11.** colonoscopy **12.** ileostomy

F. **1.** d **2.** g **3.** h **4.** e **5.** f **6.** b **7.** c **8.** a

G. **1.** antidiarrheal, f **2.** proton pump inhibitor, h **3.** antiemetic, d **4.** H_2-receptor antagonist, a **5.** anorexiant, b **6.** laxative, c **7.** antacid, e **8.** antiviral, g

H. **1.** spelled correctly **2.** salivary **3.** ileocecal **4.** submandibular **5.** spelled correctly **6.** spelled correctly **7.** spelled correctly **8.** proctoptosis **9.** spelled correctly **10.** antidiarrheal

I. **1.** buccal **2.** cholecystic **3.** jejunum **4.** colon and rectum **5.** hypoglossal or sublingual **6.** small intestine **7.** pancreas **8.** dental **9.** lip **10.** sigmoid colon **11.** pharyngeal **12.** gastric **13.** duodenum **14.** hepatic **15.** oral

J. **1.** buffers, pancreatic enzymes **2.** bile, liver **3.** amylase **4.** ileocecal valve, anus **5.** small intestine **6.** pyloric sphincter **7.** peristalsis **8.** epiglottis **9.** cuspids or canines, incisors, bicuspids or premolars, molars **10.** gingiva

Labeling Exercises

A. **1.** salivary glands **2.** esophagus **3.** pancreas **4.** small intestine **5.** oral cavity **6.** stomach **7.** liver and gallbladder **8.** colon

B. **1.** esophagus **2.** cardiac or lower esophageal sphincter **3.** pyloric sphincter **4.** duodenum **5.** antrum **6.** fundus of stomach **7.** rugae **8.** body of stomach

C. **1.** cystic duct **2.** common bile duct **3.** gallbladder **4.** duodenum **5.** liver **6.** hepatic duct **7.** pancreas **8.** pancreatic duct

Chapter 9 Answers

Practice As You Go

A. **1.** nephrons **2.** Bowman's capsule, loop of Henle **3.** smooth muscle **4.** retroperitoneal **5.** glomerulus **6.** calyx **7.** two, one **8.** micturition, voiding

B. **1.** homeostasis **2.** filtration, reabsorption, secretion **3.** electrolytes **4.** peritubular **5.** Specific gravity **6.** muscle

C. **1.** ureteral **2.** renal **3.** glomerular **4.** urinary **5.** urethral

D. **1.** c **2.** g **3.** h **4.** i **5.** f **6.** e **7.** d **8.** b **9.** a **10.** j

E. **1.** f **2.** e **3.** h **4.** a **5.** g **6.** c **7.** d **8.** b

F. **1.** kidneys, ureters, bladder **2.** catheterization **3.** cystoscopy **4.** genitourinary **5.** extracorporeal shockwave lithotripsy **6.** urinary tract infection **7.** urine culture **8.** retrograde pyelogram **9.** acute renal failure **10.** blood urea nitrogen **11.** chronic renal failure **12.** water

Real-World Applications

Medical Record Analysis

1. hematuria—The presence of blood in the urine.
2. pyelonephritis—Inflammation of the renal pelvis and the kidney. One of the most common types of kidney disease. It may be the result of a lower urinary tract infection that moved up to the kidney by way of the ureters. There may be large quantities of white blood cells and bacteria in the urine. Blood (hematuria) may even be present in the urine in this condition. Can occur with any untreated or persistent case of cystitis.
3. chronic cystitis—Urinary bladder inflammation.
4. dysuria—Difficult or painful urination.
5. clean catch urinalysis—Laboratory test that consists of the physical, chemical, and microscopic examination of urine.
6. pyuria—The presence of pus in the urine.
7. culture and sensitivity—Laboratory test of urine for bacterial infection. Attempt to grow bacteria on a culture medium in order to identify it and determine which antibiotics it is sensitive to.
8. pathogen—Anything, such as bacteria, viruses, fungi, or toxins, that may cause disease.
9. antibiotic—Medication used to treat bacterial infections of the urinary tract.
10. cystoscopy—Visual examination of the urinary bladder using an instrument called a *cystoscope*.
11. bladder neck obstruction—Blockage of the bladder outlet. Often caused by an enlarged prostate gland in males.
12. congenital—Present from birth.
13. catheterized—Insertion of a tube through the urethra and into the urinary bladder for the purpose of withdrawing urine or inserting dye.

Chart Note Transcription

1. urologist **2.** hematuria **3.** cystitis **4.** clean-catch specimen **5.** urinalysis (U/A, UA) **6.** pyuria **7.** retrograde pyelogram **8.** ureter **9.** ureterolith **10.** extracorporeal shockwave lithotripsy (ESWL) **11.** calculi

Case Study

1. Cystitis—Inflammation of the urinary bladder; pyelonephritis—Inflammation of the renal pelvis and the kidney. One of the most common types of kidney disease. It may be the result of a lower urinary tract infection that moved up to the kidney by way of the ureters. There may be large quantities of white blood cells and bacteria in the urine. Blood (hematuria) may even be present in the urine in this condition. Can occur with any untreated or persistent case of cystitis.
2. Fever; chills; fatigue; urgency—Feeling the need to urinate immediately; frequency—Urge to urinate more often than normal; dysuria—Difficult or painful urination; hematuria—Blood in the urine; cloudy urine with a fishy smell—Urine was not clear and smelled bad.
3. Clean catch specimen—Urine sample obtained after cleaning off the urinary opening and catching or collecting a urine sample in midstream (halfway through the urination process) to minimize contamination from the genitalia; U/A (urinalysis)—A physical, chemical, and microscopic examination of the urine; urine C&S (culture & sensitivity)—Test for the presence and identification of bacteria in

the urine; KUB (kidneys, ureters, and bladder)—An X-ray of the urinary organs.

4. Pyuria—Pus in the urine; bacteriuria—Bacteria in the urine; acidic pH—Indicates a urinary tract infection; culture and sensitivity—Revealed a common type of bacteria; KUB—Pyelonephritis.
5. Antibiotic—To kill the bacteria; push fluids—To flush out the bladder.
6. Clear, pale yellow to deep gold color, aromatic odor, specific gravity between 1.010–1.030, pH between 5.0–8.0, very little protein, no glucose, ketones, or blood.

Practice Exercises

A. **1.** nephropexy **2.** nephrogram **3.** nephrolithiasis **4.** nephrectomy **5.** nephritis **6.** nephropathy **7.** nephrosclerosis **8.** cystitis **9.** cystorrhagia **10.** cystoplasty **11.** cystoscope **12.** cystalgia **13.** pyeloplasty **14.** pyelitis **15.** pyelogram **16.** ureterolith **17.** ureterectasis **18.** ureterostenosis **19.** urethritis **20.** urethroscope **21.** oliguria **22.** hematuria **23.** proteinuria **24.** glycosuria **25.** pyuria

B. **1.** cystopexy **2.** lithotripsy **3.** pyeloplasty **4.** urinalysis **5.** nephroptosis **6.** pyuria **7.** ureterectasis **8.** glomerulonephritis **9.** meatotomy **10.** urethralgia

C. **1.** antispasmodic, b **2.** antibiotic, c **3.** diuretic, a

D. **1.** urination or voiding urine **2.** increases urine production **3.** pain associated with kidney stone **4.** inserting a tube through urethra into the bladder **5.** inflammation of renal pelvis **6.** inflammation of glomeruli in the kidney **7.** cutting into an organ to remove stone **8.** bedwetting **9.** enlargement of urethral opening **10.** damage to glomerulus secondary to diabetes mellitus **11.** lab test of chemical composition of urine **12.** decrease in force of urine stream

E. **1.** anuria **2.** hematuria **3.** calculus or nephrolith **4.** lithotripsy **5.** urethritis **6.** pyuria **7.** bacteriuria **8.** dysuria **9.** ketonuria **10.** proteinuria **11.** polyuria

F. **1.** HD **2.** ESWL **3.** cysto **4.** IVP **5.** KUB **6.** C&S **7.** BNO **8.** UTI

G. **1.** renal transplant **2.** nephropexy **3.** urinary tract infection **4.** pyelolithectomy **5.** renal biopsy **6.** ureterectomy **7.** cystostomy **8.** cystoscopy **9.** IVP

H. **1.** bladder **2.** ureteral **3.** urine **4.** renal **5.** glomerulus **6.** renal pelvis **7.** meatal **8.** urethral

I. **1.** spelled correctly **2.** nephrosclerosis **3.** spelled correctly **4.** spelled correctly **5.** incontinence **6.** spelled correctly **7.** cystocele **8.** catheterization **9.** spelled correctly **10.** lithotripsy

J. **1.** nitrogenous wastes **2.** renal corpuscle **3.** electrolytes **4.** rugae **5.** loop of Henle **6.** urethra, ureters **7.** hilum **8.** cortex, medulla

Labeling Exercises

A. **1.** kidney **2.** urinary bladder **3.** ureter **4.** male urethra **5.** female urethra

B. **1.** cortex **2.** medulla **3.** calyx **4.** renal pelvis **5.** renal papilla **6.** renal pyramid **7.** ureter

C. **1.** efferent arteriole **2.** glomerular (Bowman's) capsule **3.** glomerulus **4.** afferent arteriole **5.** proximal convoluted tubule **6.** descending nephron loop **7.** distal convoluted tubule **8.** collecting tubule **9.** ascending nephron loop **10.** peritubular capillaries

Chapter 10 Answers

Practice As You Go

A. **1.** uterine tubes **2.** vulva **3.** estrogen, progesterone **4.** menopause **5.** ovum **6.** endometrium **7.** hymen **8.** lactation

B. **1.** placenta, umbilical cord **2.** gestation **3.** dilation, expulsion, placental **4.** crowning **5.** breech **6.** amnion, chorion

C. **1.** embryonic **2.** fetal **3.** uterine **4.** ovarian **5.** mammary **6.** vaginal

D. **1.** b **2.** h **3.** g **4.** c **5.** a **6.** i **7.** j **8.** d **9.** e **10.** f

E. **1.** e **2.** g **3.** d **4.** a **5.** h **6.** c **7.** b **8.** f

F. **1.** GI or grav I **2.** AI **3.** UC **4.** FTND **5.** IUD **6.** D&C **7.** HRT **8.** gyn or GYN **9.** AB **10.** OCPs

G. **1.** urinary, reproductive **2.** testes, epididymis, penis **3.** foreskin **4.** testes **5.** bulbourethral glands **6.** testosterone **7.** perineum

H. **1.** testicular **2.** spermatic **3.** vesicular **4.** penile **5.** prostatic

I. **1.** b **2.** e **3.** a **4.** c **5.** f **6.** d

J. **1.** c **2.** a **3.** d **4.** b **5.** e

K. **1.** ED **2.** GC **3.** DRE **4.** TURP **5.** STI

Real-World Applications

Medical Record Analysis

1. gestation—The length of time of pregnancy, normally about 40 weeks.
2. amniocentesis—Puncturing of the amniotic sac using a needle and syringe for the purpose of withdrawing amniotic fluid for testing. Can assist in determining fetal maturity, development, and genetic disorders.
3. fetus—The unborn infant from approximately week 9 until birth.
4. obstetrician—Branch of medicine specializing in the diagnosis and treatment of women during pregnancy and childbirth, and immediately after childbirth. Physician is called an *obstetrician*.
5. multigravida—A woman who has been pregnant two or more times.

6. nullipara—A woman who has not given birth to a live infant.
7. miscarriage—Unplanned loss of a pregnancy due to the death of the embryo or fetus before the time it is viable, also referred to as a *spontaneous abortion*.
8. pelvic ultrasound—Use of high-frequency sound waves to produce an image or photograph of an organ, such as the uterus, ovaries, or fetus.
9. placenta previa—A placenta that is implanted in the lower portion of the uterus and, in turn, blocks the birth canal.
10. abruptio placentae—Emergency condition in which the placenta tears away from the uterine wall prior to delivery of the infant. Requires immediate delivery of the baby.
11. placenta—The organ that connects the fetus to the mother's uterus, supplies fetus with oxygen and nutrients.
12. C-section—Surgical delivery of a baby through an incision into the abdominal and uterine walls.

Chart Note Transcription

1. ejaculation **2.** cryptorchidism **3.** orchidopexy **4.** vasectomy **5.** ejaculation **6.** digital rectal exam (DRE) **7.** prostate cancer **8.** prostate-specific antigen (PSA) **9.** benign prostatic hyperplasia (BPH) **10.** transurethral resection of the prostate (TUR, TURP)

Case Study

1. Genital herpes.
2. Fever—She has a temperature; malaise—A feeling of general discomfort; dysuria—Painful urination; vaginal leukorrhea—A white discharge or flow from the vagina.
3. Vesicles—Small fluid-filled blisters; ulcers—Craterlike erosions of the skin; erythema—Redness; edema—Swelling.
4. An abnormality located on the body in some area outside of the genital region.
5. To feel with your hands.
6. There is a risk of passing the virus to the baby as it passes through the birth canal.

Practice Exercises

A. **1.** GYN, OB **2.** PMS **3.** HDN **4.** CVS **5.** OCPs, IUD **6.** HPV **7.** STI **8.** PSA **9.** TUR or TURP **10.** TSS

B. **1.** the formation of mature sperm **2.** accumulation of fluid within the testes **3.** surgical removal of the prostate gland by inserting a device through the urethra and removing prostate tissue **4.** inability to father children due to a problem with spermatogenesis **5.** surgical removal of the testes **6.** surgical removal of part or all of the vas deferens **7.** removal of the testicles in the male or the ovaries in the female **8.** the normal length of time of pregnancy, about 40 weeks **9.** first bowel movement of newborn **10.** a woman who has never been pregnant **11.** difficult labor and childbirth **12.** discharge from the uterus other than the menstrual flow **13.** a benign fibrous growth **14.** benign cysts forming in the breast **15.** placenta implants in lower uterus and blocks birth canal

C. **1.** colposcopy **2.** colposcope **3.** cervicectomy **4.** cervicitis **5.** hysteropexy **6.** hysterectomy **7.** hysterorrhexis **8.** oophoritis **9.** oophorectomy **10.** mammogram **11.** mammoplasty **12.** amniotomy **13.** amniorrhea **14.** prostatectomy **15.** prostatitis **16.** orchiectomy **17.** orchioplasty **18.** orchiotomy **19.** aspermia **20.** oligospermia **21.** spermatogenesis **22.** spermatolysis

D. **1.** balanoplasty **2.** hyperplasia **3.** cryptorchidism **4.** varicocele **5.** oligospermia **6.** oophorectomy **7.** colposcope **8.** salpingocyesis **9.** lactorrhea **10.** endometriosis **11.** pyosalpinx **12.** neonatology **13.** menorrhagia **14.** primigravida **15.** hysterorrhexis

E. **1.** conization **2.** stillbirth **3.** puberty **4.** premenstrual syndrome **5.** laparoscopy **6.** fibroid tumor **7.** D&C **8.** eclampsia **9.** endometriosis **10.** cesarean section

F. **1.** e **2.** i **3.** h **4.** c **5.** a **6.** d **7.** g **8.** b **9.** f

G. **1.** androgen therapy, f **2.** oxytocin, a **3.** antiprostatic agent, b **4.** birth control pills, g **5.** spermatocide, d **6.** erectile dysfunction agent, h **7.** hormone replacement therapy, i **8.** abortifacient, e **9.** fertility drug, c

H. **1.** amniotic **2.** cervical **3.** embryonic **4.** endometrium **5.** mammary **6.** ovary **7.** uterus **8.** fetus **9.** vesicular **10.** sperm **11.** testicular **12.** glans penis **13.** epididymal **14.** prostate gland **15.** penile

I. **1.** spelled correctly **2.** epispadias **3.** spelled correctly **4.** circumcision **5.** spelled correctly **6.** spelled correctly **7.** mammogram **8.** preeclampsia **9.** spelled correctly **10.** premenstrual

J. **1.** follicle-stimulating hormone, luteinizing hormone, estrogen, progesterone **2.** ovulation **3.** uterine tube or fallopian tube **4.** lactation **5.** embryo **6.** expulsion **7.** spermatogenesis **8.** prostate gland

Labeling Exercises

A. **1.** uterine tube or fallopian tube **2.** ovary **3.** fundus of uterus **4.** corpus (body) of uterus **5.** cervix **6.** vagina **7.** clitoris **8.** labium majora **9.** labium minora

B. **1.** seminal vesicle **2.** vas deferens **3.** prostate gland **4.** bulbourethral gland **5.** urethra **6.** epididymis **7.** glans penis **8.** testis

C. **1.** areola **2.** nipple **3.** lactiferous gland **4.** lactiferous duct **5.** fat

Chapter 11 Answers

Practice As You Go

A. **1.** d **2.** g **3.** i **4.** a **5.** j **6.** b **7.** e **8.** f **9.** h **10.** c

B. **1.** endocrinology **2.** pituitary **3.** gonads **4.** corticosteroids **5.** circadian rhythm **6.** iodine **7.** insulin, glucagon **8.** thymus gland

C. **1.** thymic **2.** pancreatic **3.** thyroidal **4.** ovarian **5.** testicular

D. **1.** b **2.** a **3.** e **4.** h **5.** j **6.** i **7.** f **8.** g **9.** c **10.** d

E. **1.** e **2.** d **3.** a **4.** f **5.** c **6.** b **7.** h **8.** g

F. **1.** NIDDM **2.** IDDM **3.** ACTH **4.** PTH **5.** T_3 **6.** TSH **7.** FBS **8.** PRL

Real-World Applications

Medical Record Analysis

1. hyperglycemia—The condition of having a high level of sugar in the blood; associated with diabetes mellitus.
2. ketoacidosis—Acidosis due to an excess of acidic ketone bodies (waste products). A serious condition requiring immediate treatment that can result in death for the diabetic patient if not reversed. Also called *diabetic acidosis.*
3. glycosuria—Having a high level of sugar excreted in the urine.
4. type 1 diabetes mellitus—Also called *insulin-dependent diabetes mellitus.* It develops early in life when the pancreas stops insulin production. Patient must take daily insulin injections.
5. polyuria—The condition of producing an excessive amount of urine.
6. polydipsia—Excessive feeling of thirst.
7. fasting blood sugar—Blood test to measure the amount of sugar circulating throughout the body after a 12-hour fast.
8. insulin—Medication administered to replace insulin for type 1 diabetics or to treat severe type 2 diabetics.
9. glucose tolerance test—Test to determine the blood sugar level. A measured dose of glucose is given to a patient either orally or intravenously. Blood samples are then drawn at certain intervals to determine the ability of the patient to use glucose. Used for diabetic patients to determine their insulin response to glucose.
10. glucometer—A device designed for a diabetic to use at home to measure the level of glucose in the bloodstream.

Chart Note Transcription

1. endocrinologist **2.** obesity **3.** hirsutism **4.** radioimmunoassay (RIA) **5.** cortisol **6.** adenoma **7.** adrenal cortex **8.** Cushing's syndrome **9.** adenoma **10.** adrenal cortex **11.** adrenalectomy

Case Study

1. Diabetes mellitus.
2. Diaphoresis—Profuse sweating; rapid respirations—Breathing fast; rapid pulse—Fast heart rate; disorientation—Confused about his surroundings.
3. Blood serum test—Lab test to measure the levels of different substances in the blood, used to determine the function of endocrine glands.
4. Hyperglycemia—Blood level of glucose is too high; ketoacidosis—An excessive amount of acidic ketone bodies in the body.
5. Type 1, insulin-dependent, or juvenile diabetes mellitus because he has had it since childhood and he is taking insulin shots.
6. Type 2, non-insulin-dependent diabetes mellitus typically develops later in life. The pancreas produces normal to high levels of insulin, but the cells fail to respond to it. Patients may take oral hypoglycemic agents to improve insulin function, or may eventually have to take insulin.

Practice Exercises

A. **1.** thyroidectomy **2.** thyroidal **3.** hyperthyroidism **4.** pancreatic **5.** pancreatitis **6.** pancreatectomy **7.** pancreatotomy **8.** adrenal **9.** adrenomegaly **10.** adrenopathy **11.** thymoma **12.** thymectomy **13.** thymic **14.** thymitis

B. **1.** thyroidectomy **2.** glucometer **3.** postprandial **4.** hypothyroidism **5.** hyperpituitarism **6.** acromegaly **7.** hyponatremia **8.** polydipsia **9.** adrenalitis **10.** hypercalcemia **11.** glycosuria **12.** thymoma

C. **1.** HRT **2.** RIA **3.** FBS **4.** DM **5.** FSH, LH **6.** PTH **7.** ACTH **8.** TSH **9.** ADH **10.** T_3, T_4

D. **1.** hormone obtained from cortex of adrenal gland **2.** having excessive hair **3.** a nerve condition characterized with spasms of extremities; can occur from imbalance of pH and calcium or disorder of parathyroid gland **4.** disorder of the retina occurring with diabetes mellitus **5.** increase in blood sugar level **6.** decrease in blood sugar level **7.** another term for epinephrine; produced by inner portion of adrenal gland **8.** hormone produced by pancreas; essential for metabolism of blood sugar **9.** toxic condition due to hyperactivity of thyroid gland **10.** a condition resulting when the endocrine gland secretes more hormone than is needed by the body

E. **1.** insulinoma **2.** ketoacidosis **3.** panhypopituitarism **4.** pheochromocytoma **5.** Hashimoto's thyroiditis **6.** gynecomastia

F. **1.** corticosteroids, e **2.** human growth hormone therapy, a **3.** oral hypoglycemic agent, d **4.** antithyroid agent, c **5.** insulin, f **6.** thyroid replacement hormone, b

G. **1.** f **2.** i **3.** a **4.** c **5.** j **6.** e **7.** b **8.** g **9.** d **10.** h

H. **1.** spelled correctly **2.** glycosuria **3.** spelled correctly **4.** adrenalitis **5.** spelled correctly **6.** spelled correctly **7.** Recklinghausen **8.** hyperpituitarism **9.** spelled correctly **10.** radioimmunoassay

I. **1.** ovarian **2.** pancreatic **3.** testicular **4.** thymic **5.** thyroidal **6.** parathyroidal

J. **1.** homeostasis **2.** exocrine, endocrine **3.** adrenal **4.** islet, glucagon, insulin **5.** calcium **6.** pituitary **7.** thymosin **8.** basal metabolic rate (BMR)

Labeling Exercises

A. **1.** pineal gland **2.** thyroid and parathyroid glands **3.** adrenal glands **4.** pancreas **5.** pituitary gland **6.** thymus gland **7.** ovary **8.** testis

B. **1.** pituitary gland **2.** bone and soft tissue **3.** GH **4.** testes **5.** FSH, LH **6.** ovary **7.** FSH, LH **8.** thyroid gland **9.** TSH **10.** adrenal cortex **11.** ACTH **12.** breast **13.** PRL

C. **1.** liver **2.** stomach **3.** pancreas **4.** beta cell **5.** alpha cell **6.** islets of Langerhans

Chapter 12 Answers

Practice As You Go

A. **1.** brain, spinal cord **2.** cranial, spinal **3.** dendrites, nerve cell body, axon **4.** myelin **5.** cerebrum **6.** cerebellum **7.** eyesight **8.** hearing, smell

B. **1.** ascending, descending **2.** efferent or motor, afferent or sensory **3.** dura mater, arachnoid layer, pia mater **4.** parasympathetic, sympathetic **5.** somatic

C. **1.** cerebrospinal **2.** meningeal **3.** subdural **4.** encephalic **5.** neural **6.** intracranial

D. **1.** b **2.** f **3.** g **4.** h **5.** i **6.** j **7.** e **8.** c **9.** d **10.** a

E. **1.** e **2.** c **3.** g **4.** b **5.** a **6.** d **7.** h **8.** f

F. **1.** CSF **2.** CVD **3.** EEG **4.** ICP **5.** PET **6.** CVA **7.** ANS

G. **1.** d **2.** g **3.** j **4.** a **5.** c **6.** i **7.** f **8.** e **9.** h **10.** b

Real-World Applications

Medical Record Analysis

1. paraplegia—Paralysis of the lower portion of the body and both legs.
2. comminuted fracture—Fracture in which the bone is shattered, splintered, or crushed into many small pieces or fragments.
3. epidural hematoma—Mass of blood in the space outside the dura mater of the brain and spinal cord.
4. spinal cord injury—Damage to the spinal cord as a result of trauma. Spinal cord may be bruised or completely severed.
5. unconscious—State of being unaware of surroundings, with the inability to respond to stimuli.
6. anesthesia—The lack of feeling or sensation.
7. paralysis—Temporary or permanent loss of function or voluntary movement.
8. computed tomography scan (CT scan)—An imaging technique that is able to produce a cross-sectional view of the body.
9. laminectomy—Removal of a portion of a vertebra, called the *lamina*, in order to relieve pressure on the spinal nerve.
10. spinal fusion—Surgical immobilization of adjacent vertebrae. This may be done for several reasons, including correction for a herniated disk.
11. physical therapy (PT)—Treats disorders using physical means and methods; includes joint motion and muscle strength.
12. occupational therapy (OT)—Assists patients to regain, develop, and improve skills that are important for independent functioning.

Chart Note Transcription

1. neurologist **2.** dysphasia **3.** hemiplegia **4.** convulsions **5.** electroencephalography (EEG) **6.** lumbar puncture (LP) **7.** brain scan **8.** cerebral cortex **9.** astrocytoma **10.** craniotomy **11.** cryosurgery

Case Study

1. Cerebrovascular accident (CVA or stroke).
2. aphasia—Inability to speak; hemiparesis—Weakness on one side of the body; syncope—Fainting; delirium—Abnormal mental state with confusion, disorientation, and agitation.
3. hypertension—High blood pressure; atherosclerosis—Hardening of arteries due to buildup of yellow fatty substances; diabetes mellitus—Inability to make or use insulin properly to control blood sugar levels.
4. brain scan—An image of the brain after injection of radioactive isotopes into the circulation; revealed an infarct in the right cerebral hemisphere.
5. infarct—An area of tissue within an organ that undergoes necrosis (death) following the loss of its blood supply.
6. hemorrhage—Ruptured blood vessel; thrombus—Stationary clot; embolus—Floating clot; compression—Pinching off a blood vessel.

Practice Exercises

A. **1.** h **2.** k **3.** d **4.** g **5.** a **6.** b **7.** f **8.** j **9.** e **10.** l **11.** i **12.** c

B. **1.** neuritis **2.** neurologist **3.** neuralgia **4.** polyneuritis **5.** neurectomy **6.** neuroplasty **7.** neuroma **8.** neurorrhaphy **9.** meningitis **10.** meningocele **11.** myelomeningocele **12.** encephalogram **13.** encephalopathy **14.** encephalitis **15.** encephalocele **16.** cerebrospinal **17.** cerebral

C. **1.** ADHD **2.** OCD **3.** LP **4.** PET **5.** MS **6.** SCI **7.** ALS **8.** TIA **9.** CP **10.** CVA

D. **1.** injecting radiopaque dye into spinal canal to examine under X-ray the outlines made by the dye **2.** X-ray of the blood vessels of the brain after the injection of radiopaque dye **3.** reflex test on bottom of foot to detect lesion and abnormalities of nervous system **4.** test that measures how fast an impulse travels along a nerve to pinpoint an area of nerve damage **5.** laboratory examination of fluid taken from the brain and spinal cord **6.** positron emission tomography to measure cerebral blood flow, blood volume, oxygen, and glucose uptake **7.** recording the ultrasonic echoes of the brain **8.** needle puncture into the spinal cavity to withdraw fluid

E. **1.** psychotherapy **2.** dementia **3.** analgesic **4.** myelogram **5.** electroencephalography **6.** subdural **7.** meningitis **8.** polyneuritis **9.** sclerosis **10.** concussion **11.** radiculopathy **12.** anesthetic **13.** pyromania **14.** insomnia

F. **1.** tumor of astrocyte cells **2.** seizure **3.** without sensation **4.** weakness of one-half of body **5.** physician that treats nervous system with surgery **6.** without sense of pain **7.** localized seizure of one limb **8.** paralysis of all four limbs **9.** accumulation of blood in the subdural space **10.** within the meninges

G. **1.** d **2.** e **3.** f **4.** g **5.** b **6.** a **7.** c **8.** j **9.** h **10.** i

H. **1.** delirium **2.** amyotrophic lateral sclerosis **3.** Bell's palsy **4.** cerebral aneurysm **5.** Parkinson's disease **6.** cerebrospinal fluid shunt **7.** transient ischemic attack **8.** subdural hematoma **9.** cerebral palsy **10.** nerve conduction velocity

I. **1.** anesthetic, e **2.** dopaminergic drugs, a **3.** hypnotic, d **4.** analgesic, g **5.** sedative, b **6.** narcotic analgesic, c **7.** anticonvulsant, f

J. **1.** i **2.** k **3.** h **4.** j **5.** e **6.** f **7.** b **8.** a **9.** d **10.** c **11.** g

K. **1.** minor tranquilizers **2.** humanistic psychotherapy **3.** lithium **4.** antipsychotic drugs **5.** psychoanalysis **6.** antidepressant drugs

L. **1.** general anesthesia **2.** local anesthesia **3.** topical anesthesia **4.** regional anesthesia

M. **1.** cerebellar **2.** thalamus **3.** cerebrum **4.** vertebra **5.** intracranial **6.** spine **7.** encephalic **8.** pontine **9.** medullary **10.** nerve **11.** meningeal **12.** ventricle

N. **1.** spelled correctly **2.** cephalalgia **3.** spelled correctly **4.** posttraumatic **5.** spelled correctly **6.** spelled correctly **7.** quadriplegia **8.** hydrocephalus **9.** amyotrophic **10.** spelled correctly

O. **1.** psychology, psychiatry **2.** somatic **3.** autonomic **4.** sensory, motor **5.** subarachnoid **6.** brainstem **7.** vision **8.** myelin

Labeling Exercises

A. **1.** brain **2.** spinal nerves **3.** spinal cord

B. **1.** dendrites **2.** nerve cell body **3.** unmyelinated region **4.** myelinated axon **5.** nucleus **6.** axon **7.** terminal end fibers

C. **1.** cerebrum **2.** diencephalon **3.** thalamus **4.** hypothalamus **5.** brainstem **6.** midbrain **7.** cerebellum **8.** pons **9.** medulla oblongata

Chapter 13 Answers

Practice As You Go

A. **1.** ophthalmology **2.** cilia **3.** lacrimal **4.** cornea **5.** retina **6.** iris **7.** choroid **8.** cones, rods **9.** rectus, oblique **10.** conjunctiva

B. **1.** pupillary **2.** optic or optical **3.** retinal **4.** lacrimal **5.** intraocular **6.** extraocular

C. **1.** h **2.** g **3.** a **4.** d **5.** b **6.** i **7.** c **8.** f **9.** e **10.** j

D. **1.** d **2.** a **3.** f **4.** e **5.** b **6.** c

E. **1.** IOL **2.** EM **3.** XT **4.** MY **5.** EOM **6.** VA

F. **1.** malleus, incus, stapes **2.** otology **3.** tympanic membrane **4.** cerumen **5.** eustachian or auditory **6.** vestibulocochlear nerve **7.** hearing, equilibrium **8.** conductive

G. **1.** cochlear **2.** otic or aural or auricular **3.** vestibular **4.** acoustic or auditory **5.** monaural

H. **1.** e **2.** h **3.** a **4.** g **5.** j **6.** c **7.** i **8.** b **9.** d **10.** f

I. **1.** c **2.** b **3.** d **4.** a **5.** g **6.** h **7.** e **8.** f

J. **1.** OE **2.** EENT **3.** BC **4.** PE tube **5.** OM

Real-World Applications

Medical Record Analysis

1. photophobia—Although the term translates into *fear of light*, it actually means a strong sensitivity to bright light.
2. hyperopia—With this condition a person can see things in the distance but has trouble reading material at close range. Also known as *farsightedness.* This condition is corrected with converging or biconvex lenses.
3. visual acuity test—Measurement of the sharpness of a patient's vision. Usually, a Snellen chart is used for this test in which the patient identifies letters from a distance of 20 feet.
4. intraocular—Pertaining to inside the eye.
5. ophthalmoscopy—Examination of the interior of the eyes using an instrument called an

ophthalmoscope. The physician dilates the pupil in order to see the cornea, lens, and retina. Used to identify abnormalities in the blood vessels of the eye and some systemic diseases.

6. mydriatic drops—Any substance that causes the pupil to dilate by paralyzing the iris and/or ciliary body muscles. Particularly useful during eye examinations and eye surgery.
7. cataract—Damage to the lens causing it to become opaque or cloudy, resulting in diminished vision. Treatment is usually surgical removal of the lens with the cataract and replacement with a prosthetic lens.
8. retinopathy—A general term for disease affecting the retina.
9. macular degeneration—Deterioration of the macular area of the retina of the eye. May be treated with laser surgery to destroy the blood vessels beneath the macula.
10. phacoemulsification—Use of high-frequency sound waves to emulsify (liquefy) a lens with a cataract, which is then aspirated (removed by suction) with a needle.
11. prosthetic lens implant—The use of an artificial lens to replace the lens removed during cataract surgery.

Chart Note Transcription

1. otorhinolaryngologist (ENT) **2.** otitis media (OM) **3.** binaural **4.** otoscopy **5.** tympanic membrane **6.** cerumen **7.** tympanometry **8.** audiometry test **9.** conductive hearing loss **10.** myringotomy or tympanotomy

Case Study

1. Conductive hearing loss results from disease or malformation of the outer or middle ear; all sound is weaker because it is not conducted correctly to the inner ear.
2. Sensorineural hearing loss as a result of damage or malformation of the inner ear or the cochlear nerve.
3. Otoscopy examination of the auditory canal and middle ear; tympanometry measurement of the movement of the tympanic membrane; audiometry test for hearing ability; Rinne and Weber tuning-fork tests assess both the nerve and bone conduction of sound.
4. Hearing aids or amplification devices amplify sound and will work best for conductive hearing loss; cochlear implant is a device that converts sound signals into magnetic impulses to stimulate the auditory nerve and is used to treat profound sensorineural hearing loss.
6. Protect his ears better during playing music by wearing earplugs.

Practice Exercises

A. **1.** artificial tears, h **2.** antiglaucoma medication, c **3.** antibiotic otic solution, i **4.** mydriatic, a **5.** antiemetic, g **6.** antibiotic ophthalmic solution, j **7.** ophthalmic decongestant, b **8.** miotic, f **9.** wax emulsifier, e **10.** anesthetic ophthalmic solution, d

B. **1.** blepharitis **2.** blepharoplasty **3.** blepharoptosis **4.** retinopathy **5.** retinopexy **6.** ophthalmology **7.** ophthalmic **8.** ophthalmoscopy **9.** iridoplegia **10.** iridectomy **11.** otoplasty **12.** otopyorrhea **13.** otalgia **14.** otitis **15.** tympanorrhexis **16.** tympanotomy **17.** tympanitis **18.** audiogram **19.** audiometer **20.** audiology

C. **1.** otoscope **2.** retinopexy **3.** anacusis **4.** blepharoptosis **5.** optometrist **6.** tympanometer **7.** keratotomy **8.** presbyopia **9.** iridectomy **10.** audiometry **11.** ophthalmalgia **12.** otosclerosis **13.** conjunctivitis **14.** macrotia **15.** monochromatism

D. **1.** Astigm **2.** ENT **3.** VA **4.** OE **5.** ET **6.** PE **7.** LASIK **8.** MY **9.** OM **10.** IOL

E. **1.** tonometry **2.** emmetropia **3.** conjunctivitis **4.** myopia **5.** cataract **6.** hordeolum **7.** strabismus **8.** hyperopia **9.** presbycusis **10.** otorhinolaryngologist **11.** inner ear **12.** Ménière's disease **13.** acoustic neuroma

F. **1.** dull/dim vision **2.** double vision **3.** enlarge or widen pupil **4.** constrict pupil **5.** vision changes due to normal aging **6.** ringing in the ears **7.** middle-ear bone **8.** measures movement in eardrum **9.** auditory tube **10.** inner ear **11.** results of hearing test **12.** middle ear infection

G. **1.** conjunctival **2.** hearing **3.** corneal **4.** ear **5.** intraocular **6.** ear **7.** lacrimal **8.** iris **9.** monaural **10.** scleral **11.** eye **12.** retinal **13.** tympanic **14.** eye **15.** cochlear

H. **1.** ophthalmology **2.** spelled correctly **3.** spelled correctly **4.** emmetropia **5.** labyrinthitis **6.** spelled correctly **7.** spelled correctly **8.** monochromatism **9.** otopyorrhea **10.** spelled correctly

I. **1.** cornea, pupil; aqueous humor, lens, vitreous humor **2.** nasal cavity **3.** rectus, oblique **4.** conjunctiva **5.** cilia **6.** choroid **7.** incus, malleus, stapes **8.** conductive, sensorineural **9.** optic disk **10.** auditory, vestibular

Labeling Exercises

A. **1.** iris **2.** lens **3.** conjunctiva **4.** pupil **5.** cornea **6.** suspensory ligaments **7.** ciliary body **8.** fovea centralis **9.** optic nerve **10.** retina **11.** choroid **12.** sclera

B. **1.** pinna **2.** external auditory meatus **3.** auditory canal **4.** tympanic membrane **5.** malleus **6.** incus **7.** semicircular canals **8.** vestibular nerve **9.** cochlear nerve **10.** cochlea **11.** oval window **12.** stapes **13.** Eustachian tube

Glossary/Index

Note: Headings in **bold** indicate definitions. Page numbers with *t* indicate tables; those with *f* indicate figures.

A

Adhesion, scar tissue forming in fascia surrounding a muscle making it difficult to stretch muscle, 129
Adipose, type of connective tissue; also called *fat*; stores energy and provides protective padding for underlying structures, 30*f*, 31
Adjective suffixes, 9
Adrenal, pertaining to adrenal glands, 406
Adrenal cortex, outer layer of adrenal glands; secretes several families of hormones: mineralocorticoids, glucocorticoids, and steroid sex hormones, 396*t*, 398, 398*f*
Adrenalectomy, surgical removal of one or both adrenal glands, 413
Adrenal feminization, development of female secondary sexual characteristics (such as breasts) in a male; often as a result of increased estrogen secretion by adrenal cortex, 408
Adrenal glands, pair of glands in endocrine system located just above each kidney; composed of two sections, cortex and medulla, that function independently of each other; cortex secretes steroids, such as aldosterone, cortisol, androgens, estrogens, and progestins; medulla secretes epinephrine and norepinephrine; regulated by adrenocorticotropic hormone, which is secreted by pituitary gland, 396, 398–399, 408–409
Adrenaline, hormone produced by adrenal medulla; also known as epinephrine; some of its actions include increasing heart rate and force of contraction, bronchodilation, and relaxation of intestinal muscles, 396*t*, 398–399
Adrenalitis, inflammation of adrenal gland, 409
Adrenal medulla, inner portion of adrenal gland; secretes epinephrine and norepinephrine, 396*t*, 398, 398*f*
Adrenal virilism, development of male secondary sexual characteristics (such as deeper voice and facial hair) in a female; often as a result of increased androgen secretion by adrenal cortex, 408
Adrenocorticotropic hormone (ACTH), hormone secreted by anterior pituitary; regulates function of adrenal gland cortex, 397*t*, 401–402, 402*f*
Adrenomegaly, enlarged adrenal gland, 407
Adrenopathy, adrenal gland disease, 407
Adult respiratory distress syndrome (ARDS), acute respiratory failure in adults characterized by tachypnea, dyspnea, cyanosis, tachycardia, and hypoxemia; also called *acute respiratory distress syndrome*, 245
Adverse reaction. *See* Side effect
Aerosol, drugs inhaled directly into nose and mouth, 45
Aerosol therapy, medication suspended in mist intended to be inhaled; delivered by a nebulizer, which delivers mist for period of time while patient breathes, or a metered-dose inhaler (MDI), which delivers a single puff of mist, 46*f*, 251
Afferent, moving toward, 315
Afferent arteriole, arteriole that carries blood into glomerulus, 315, 316*f*
Afferent neurons, nerve that carries impulses to brain and spinal cord from skin and sense organs; also called *sensory neurons,* 433–434, 435*f*
Agglutinate, clumping together to form small clusters; platelets agglutinate to start clotting process, 189–190
Agranulocytes, nongranular white blood cells; one of two types found in plasma that are classified as either monocytes or lymphocytes, 189, 189*t*
AIDS-related complex (ARC), early stage of AIDS; there is a positive test for virus but only mild symptoms of weight loss, fatigue, skin rash, and anorexia, 212
Alanine transaminase (ALT), enzyme normally present in blood; levels are increased in persons with liver disease, 292
Albinism, genetic condition in which person is not able to produce melanin; an albino has white hair and skin and pupils of eyes are red, 70
Albumin, protein normally found circulating in bloodstream; it is abnormal for albumin to be in urine, 188, 319
Albumin/creatinine ratio (ACR), screening test for persons at risk (for example, diabetics) for developing kidney disease, 328
Aldosterone, hormone produced by adrenal cortex; regulates levels of sodium and potassium in body and as a side effect volume of water lost in urine, 396*t*, 398
Alimentary canal, also known as gastrointestinal system or digestive system; covers area between mouth and anus and includes 30 feet of intestinal tubing; has a wide range of functions; serves to store and digest food, absorb nutrients, and eliminate waste; major organs include mouth, pharynx, esophagus, stomach, small intestine, and large intestine, 270
Allergen, antigen capable of causing a hypersensitivity or allergy in body, 210
Allergic asthma, inflammation and narrowing of airways triggered by inhaling an allergen, 210
Allergic conjunctivitis, inflammation of conjunctiva caused by allergens in the air, 210
Allergic rhinitis, sneezing, runny nose, congestion, cough, itchy eyes due to allergic reaction to an allergen, 210
Allergist, physician who specializes in testing for and treating allergies, 209
Allergy, hypersensitivity to a substance in environment or medication, 210
Allergy shots, type of immunotherapy in which person receives very tiny doses of allergen to which he or she is allergic; over time, person's sensitivity to allergen reduces, 215
Allograft, skin graft from one person to another; donor is usually a cadaver, 77
Alopecia, absence or loss of hair, especially of head, 75
Alveolar, pertaining to alveoli, 239
Alveoli, tiny air sacs at end of each bronchiole; surrounded by capillary network; gas exchange takes place as oxygen and carbon dioxide diffuse across alveolar and capillary walls, 233, 233*f*
Alzheimer's disease (AD), chronic, organic mental disorder consisting of dementia, which is more prevalent in adults after 65 years of age; involves progressive disorientation, apathy, speech and gait disturbances, and loss of memory, 440, 455

Amblyopia, loss of vision not as a result of eye pathology; usually occurs in patients who see two images; in order to see only one image, brain will no longer recognize image being sent to it by one of eyes; may occur if strabismus is not corrected; commonly referred to as *lazy eye*, 482

Ambulatory care center, facility that provides services that do not require overnight hospitalization; services range from simple surgeries, to diagnostic testing, to therapy; also called a *surgical center* or *outpatient clinic*, 15*t*

Amenorrhea, absence of menstruation, which can be result of many factors, including pregnancy, menopause, and dieting, 359

American Sign Language (ASL), nonverbal method of communicating in which hands and fingers are used to indicate words and concepts; used by people who are deaf or speech impaired, 503, 503*f*

Amino acids, organic substances found in plasma, used by cells to build proteins, 188

Amniocentesis, puncturing of amniotic sac using a needle and syringe for purpose of withdrawing amniotic fluid for testing; can assist in determining fetal maturity, development, and genetic disorders, 366

Amnion, innermost of two membranous sacs surrounding fetus; amniotic sac contains amniotic fluid in which baby floats, 353–354

Amniorrhea, discharge of amniotic fluid, 359

Amniotic, pertaining to amnion, 357

Amniotic fluid, fluid inside amniotic sac, 353–354, 353*f*

Amniotomy, incision into amniotic sac; commonly referred to as *breaking the water,* 367

Amplification device. *See* Hearing aid

Amputation, partial or complete removal of a limb for a variety of reasons, including tumors, gangrene, intractable pain, crushing injury, or uncontrollable infection, 116

Amylase, digestive enzyme found in saliva that begins digestion of carbohydrates, 278

Amyotrophic lateral sclerosis (ALS), condition with muscular weakness and atrophy due to degeneration of motor neurons of spinal cord; also called *Lou Gehrig's disease,* after New York Yankees' baseball player who died from this disease, 443

Anacusis, total absence of hearing; unable to perceive sound; also called *deafness,* 499

Anal, pertaining to anus, 282

Anal canal, passageway between rectum and anus for feces to exit the body, 277

Anal fistula, abnormal tube-like passage from surface around anal opening directly into rectum, 288

Analgesia, reduction in perception of pain or sensation due to neurological condition or medication, 438

Analgesic, substance that relieves pain without loss of consciousness; may be either narcotic or nonnarcotic; narcotic drugs are derived from opium poppy and act on brain to cause pain relief and drowsiness, 450

Anal sphincter, rings of muscles that control defecation, 277

Anaphylactic shock, life-threatening condition resulting from ingestion of food or medications that produce severe allergic response; circulatory and respiratory problems occur, including respiratory distress, hypotension, edema, tachycardia, and convulsions, 210

Anaphylaxis. *See* Anaphylactic shock

Anastomosis, to surgically create a connection between two organs or vessels, 296

Anatomical divisions of the abdomen, method of dividing the abdominopelvic cavity into nine regions: right and left hypochondriac, epigastric, right and left lumbar, umbilical, right and left inguinal, and hypogastric, 41t

Anatomical position, used to describe positions and relationships of a structure in human body; for descriptive purposes, assumption is always that person is in anatomical position; body standing erect with arms at sides of body, palms of hands facing forward, and eyes looking straight ahead; legs are parallel with feet and toes pointing forward, 36–37, 37*f*

Ancillary reports, report in patient's medical record from various treatments and therapies patient has received, such as rehabilitation, social services, or respiratory therapy, 14*t*

Androgen, class of steroid hormones secreted by adrenal cortex and testes; these hormones, such as testosterone, produce a masculinizing effect, 373–374, 396*t*, 398–399

Androgen therapy, replacement male hormones to treat patients who produce insufficient hormone naturally, 382

Anemia, reduction in number of red blood cells (RBCs) or amount of hemoglobin in blood; results in less oxygen reaching tissues, 194

Anencephaly, congenital defect in which portions of the brain do not develop; child born missing portions of brain, cranium, and scalp; usually fatal within a few hours of birth, 440

Anesthesia, partial or complete loss of sensation with or without loss of consciousness as a result of drug, disease, or injury, 448–449

Anesthesiologist, physician who has specialization in practice of administering anesthetics, 14*t*, 438

Anesthesiologist's report, medical record document that relates details regarding substances given to patient and patient's response to anesthesia, and vital signs during surgery, 14*t*

Anesthesiology, branch of medicine specializing in all aspects of anesthesia, including for surgical procedures, resuscitation measures, and management of acute and chronic pain; physician is *anesthesiologist*, 438

Anesthetic, substance that produces a lack of feeling that may be of local or general effect, depending on type of administration, 79, 450

Anesthetic ophthalmic solution, eyedrops for pain relief associated with eye infections, corneal abrasions, or surgery, 490

Aneurysm, weakness in wall of artery that results in localized widening of artery, 166, 166*f*
Aneurysmectomy, surgical removal of aneurysm, 171
Angiitis, inflammation of vessels, 162
Angina pectoris, severe chest pain with sensation of constriction around heart; caused by a deficiency of oxygen to heart muscle, 163
Angiogram, X-ray record of a vessel, 169
Angiography, process of taking X-ray of blood or lymphatic vessels after injection of a radiopaque substance, 169
Angiospasm, involuntary muscle contraction of a vessel, 162
Angiostenosis, narrowing of a vessel, 162
Anhidrosis, abnormal condition of no sweat, 65
Ankylosing spondylitis, inflammatory spinal condition that resembles rheumatoid arthritis; results in gradual stiffening and fusion of vertebrae; more common in men than in women, 111
Anorchism, absence of one or both testes; may be congenital or result of accident or surgery, 377
Anorexia, loss of appetite that can accompany other conditions such as gastrointestinal (GI) upset, 284
Anorexia nervosa, type of eating disorder characterized by distorted body image, a pathological fear of becoming fat, and severe weight loss due to excessive dieting, 455, 455*f*
Anorexiant, substance that treats obesity by suppressing appetite, 298
Anosmia, loss of sense of smell, 240
Anoxia, lack of oxygen, 241
Antacid, substance that neutralizes acid in stomach, 298
Antagonistic pairs, pair of muscles arranged around a joint that produce opposite actions, 124, 125*f*, 126*f*, 126*t*–127*t*, 127*f*
Anteflexion, while uterus is normally in this position, exaggeration of forward bend of uterus is abnormal; forward bend is near neck of uterus; position of cervix, or opening of uterus, remains normal, 350
Antepartum, before birth, 358
Anterior, directional term meaning more toward the front or belly side of body; akin to *ventral*, 43*f*, 43*t*
Anterior lobe, anterior portion of pituitary gland; secretes adrenocorticotropic hormone, follicle-stimulating hormone, growth hormone, luteinizing hormone, melanocyte-stimulating hormone, prolactin, and thyroid-stimulating hormone, 401, 401*f*
Anterior pituitary gland, 348, 401*f*, 402, 402*f*
Anterior tibial artery, 157*f*
Anterior tibial vein, 158*f*
Anthracosis, type of pneumoconiosis that develops from collection of coal dust in lung; also called *black lung* or *miner's lung*, 245
Antiarrhythmic, controls cardiac arrhythmias by altering nerve impulses within heart, 173
Antibiotic, substance that destroys or prohibits growth of microorganisms; used to treat bacterial infections; not found effective in treating viral infections; to be effective, it must be taken regularly for specified period, 79, 254, 333
Antibiotic ophthalmic solution, eyedrops for treatment of bacterial eye infections, 490
Antibiotic otic solution, eardrops to treat otitis externa, 505
Antibody, protein material produced in body as a response to invasion of foreign substance, 206
Antibody-mediated immunity, production of antibodies by B cells in response to an antigen; also called *humoral immunity*, 206
Anticoagulant, substance that prevents or delays clotting or coagulation of blood; commonly called *blood thinner*, 173, 197
Anticonvulsant, prevents or relieves convulsions; drugs such as phenobarbital reduce excessive stimulation in brain to control seizures and other symptoms of epilepsy, 450
Antidepressant drugs, medications classified as stimulants that alter patient's mood by affecting levels of neurotransmitters in brain, 458
Antidiarrheal, prevents or relieves diarrhea, 298
Antidiuretic hormone (ADH), hormone secreted by posterior pituitary; promotes water reabsorption by kidney tubules, 397*t*, 401–402, 402*f*
Antidote, substance that will neutralize poisons or their side effects, 333
Antiemetic, substance that treats nausea, vomiting, and motion sickness, 298, 505
Antifungal, substance that kills fungi infecting skin, 79
Antigen, substance capable of inducing formation of antibody; antibody then interacts with antigen in antigen-antibody reaction, 206
Antigen-antibody complex, combination of antigen with its specific antibody; increases susceptibility to phagocytosis and immunity, 206–207
Antiglaucoma medications, group of drugs that reduce intraocular pressure by lowering amount of aqueous humor in eyeball; may achieve this by either reducing production of aqueous humor or increasing its outflow, 490
Antihemorrhagic, substance that prevents or stops hemorrhaging, 198
Antihistamine, substance that acts to control allergic symptoms by counteracting histamine, which exists naturally in body and is released in allergic reactions, 215, 254
Antilipidemic, substance that reduces amount of cholesterol and lipids in bloodstream; treats hyperlipidemia, 173
Antinuclear antibody (ANA) **test,** blood test to assist in diagnosis of autoimmune diseases, 214
Antiparasitic, substance that kills mites or lice, 79
Antiplatelet agent, substance that interferes with action of platelets; prolongs bleeding time; used to prevent heart attacks and strokes, 173, 198
Antiprostatic agent, medication to treat early cases of benign prostatic hypertrophy; may prevent surgery for mild cases, 382
Antipruritic, substance that reduces severe itching, 79
Antipsychotic drugs, major tranquilizer drugs that have transformed treatment of patients with psychoses and schizophrenia by reducing patient agitation and panic and shortening schizophrenic episodes, 458

Antiseptic, substance used to kill bacteria in skin cuts and wounds or at a surgical site, 79
Antisocial personality disorder, patient engages in behaviors that are illegal or outside of social norms, 456
Antispasmodic, medication to prevent or reduce bladder muscle spasms, 333
Antithyroid agents, medication given to block production of thyroid hormones in patients with hypersecretion disorders, 414
Antitussive, substance that controls or relieves coughing; codeine is an ingredient in many prescription cough medicines that acts upon the brain to control coughing, 254
Antrum, tapered distal end of the stomach, 275, 275*f*
Anuria, complete suppression of urine formed by kidneys and complete lack of urine excretion, 323
Anus, terminal opening of digestive tube, 270
Anvil. *See* Incus
Anxiety disorders, a classification of psychiatric disorders in the DSM-5 characterized by persistent worry and apprehension; includes panic disorder, general anxiety disorder, and phobias, 453
Aorta, largest artery in body; located in mediastinum and carries oxygenated blood away from left side of heart, 152, 153*f*, 157*f*
Aortic, pertaining to aorta, 160
Aortic arch, 157*f*
Aortic valve, semilunar valve between left ventricle of heart and aorta in heart; prevents blood from flowing backward into ventricle, 151–152, 151*f*, 153*f*
Apex, directional term meaning tip or summit; an area of lungs and heart, 44*f*, 149, 149*f*, 153*f*, 234, 234*f*
Apgar score, evaluation of neonate's adjustment to outside world; observes color, heart rate, muscle tone, respiratory rate, and response to stimulus, 366
Aphagia, being unable to swallow or eat, 284
Aphasia, inability to communicate due to brain damage, 438
Aphonia, no voice, 241
Aphthous ulcers, painful ulcers in mouth of unknown cause; commonly called *canker sores*, 286
Aplastic anemia, severe form of anemia that develops as consequence of loss of functioning red bone marrow; results in decrease in number of all formed elements; treatment may eventually require bone marrow transplant, 194
Apnea, condition of not breathing, 241
Apocrine gland, type of sweat gland that opens into hair follicles located in pubic and underarm areas; glands secrete substance that can produce odor when it comes into contact with bacteria on skin causing what is commonly referred to as *body odor*, 62
Appendectomy, surgical removal of appendix, 296
Appendicitis, inflammation of appendix, 288
Appendicular skeleton, consists of bones of upper and lower extremities, shoulder, and pelvis, 95, 98–100, 99*f*, 100*f*, 101*f*
Appendix. *See* Vermiform appendix
Aquaretics, medication that inserts water channels in the nephron to treat hyponatremia, 414
Aqueous humor, watery fluid filling spaces between cornea and lens, 474*f*, 475
Arachnoid layer, delicate middle layer of meninges, 433, 433*f*
Areola, pigmented area around nipple of breast, 352, 352*f*
Arrector pili, small slip of smooth muscle attached to hairs; when this muscle contracts hair shaft stands up and results in "goose bumps," 59*f*, 60, 61*f*
Arrhythmia, irregularity in heartbeat or action, 165
Arterial, pertaining to artery, 160
Arterial anastomosis, surgical joining together of two arteries; performed if artery is severed or if damaged section of artery is removed, 171
Arterial blood gases (ABGs), lab test that measures amount of oxygen and carbon dioxide in blood, 249
Arteriolar, pertaining to arteriole, 161
Arteriole, smallest branch of an artery; carries blood to capillaries, 155–156
Arteriorrhexis, ruptured artery, 166
Arteriosclerosis (AS), condition with thickening, hardening, and loss of elasticity of walls of arteries, 166
Artery, blood vessel that carries blood away from heart, 148, 148*f*, 155–156, 155*f*, 156*f*, 157*f*
Arthralgia, pain in a joint, 107
Arthrocentesis, removal of synovial fluid with needle from joint space, such as in knee, for examination, 116
Arthroclasia, surgically breaking loose a fused joint, 116
Arthrodesis, procedure to stabilize a joint by fusing bones together, 116
Arthrogram, record of a joint, 114
Arthrography, visualization of joint by radiographic study after injection of contrast medium into joint space, 114
Arthroscope, instrument to view inside joint, 115
Arthroscopic surgery, use of arthroscope to facilitate performing surgery on joint, 116
Arthroscopy, examination of interior of joint by entering joint with arthroscope; arthroscope contains small television camera allowing physician to view interior of joint on monitor during procedure, 116
Arthrotomy, surgically cutting into a joint, 116
Articular cartilage, layer of cartilage covering ends of bones; acts as cushion and prevents bones in joint from rubbing directly on each other, 92, 93*f*, 102*f*
Articulation, another term for a joint, point where two bones meet, 101
Artificial tears, medications, many of them over-the-counter, to treat dry eyes, 490
Asbestosis, type of pneumoconiosis developing from collection of asbestos fibers in lungs; may lead to development of lung cancer, 245
Ascending colon, section of colon following cecum; ascends right side of abdomen, 276*f*, 277, 277*f*
Ascending nephron loop, 316*f*
Ascending tracts, nerve tracts carrying sensory information up spinal cord to brain, 432–433

Azotemia, accumulation of nitrogenous waste in bloodstream; occurs when kidney fails to filter these wastes from blood, 323

B

B cells, common name for B lymphocytes, respond to foreign antigens by producing protective antibodies, 206
B lymphocytes, humoral immunity cells, which respond to foreign antigens by producing protective antibodies; simply referred to as *B cells, 206*
Babinski's reflex, reflex test to determine lesions and abnormalities in nervous system; Babinski's reflex is present if great toe extends instead of flexes when lateral sole of foot is stroked; normal response to this stimulation would be flexion, or upward movement, of toe, 447
Baby teeth. *See* Deciduous teeth
Bacteria, primitive, single-celled microorganisms that are present everywhere; some are capable of causing disease in humans, 205
Bacteriuria, bacteria in urine, 323
Balanic, pertaining to glans penis, 376
Balanitis, inflammation of skin covering glans penis, 378
Balanoplasty, surgical repair of glans penis, 380
Balanorrhea, discharge from glans penis, 377
Balloon angioplasty. *See* Percutaneous transluminal coronary angioplasty
Bariatric surgery, group of surgical procedures designed to treat morbid (extreme) obesity by reducing size of stomach or diverting food from portion of alimentary canal, 296
Barium enema (BE). *See* Lower gastrointestinal series
Barium swallow. *See Upper gastrointestinal series*
Barrier contraception, prevention of pregnancy using a device to prevent sperm from meeting ovum; includes condoms, diaphragms, and cervical caps, 367
Bartholin's glands, glands located on either side of vaginal opening that secrete mucus for vaginal lubrication, 351, 351*f*
Basal cell carcinoma (BCC), tumor of basal cell layer of epidermis; frequent type of skin cancer that rarely metastasizes or spreads; these cancers can arise on sun-exposed skin, 70, 70*f*
Basal layer, deepest layer of epidermis; this living layer constantly multiplies and divides to supply cells to replace cells that are sloughed off skin surface,58, 60
Basal metabolic rate (BMR), minimum rate of metabolism necessary to support functions of body at rest, 403–404
Base, directional term meaning bottom or lower part, 44*t*, 234
Basilic vein, 158*f*
Basophil (basos), granulocyte white blood cell that releases histamine and heparin in damaged tissues, 189*f*, 189*t*
Basophilic, pertaining to a leukocyte that attracts a basic pH stain, 192
Bell jar apparatus, 236*f*
Bell's palsy, one-sided facial paralysis due to inflammation of facial nerve, 444
Benign prostatic hyperplasia (BPH), enlargement of prostate gland commonly seen in males over age, 50, 378
Beta-blocker drugs, medications that treat hypertension and angina pectoris by lowering heart rate, 173
Biceps, arm muscle named for number of attachment points; *bi-* means *two* and biceps have two heads attached to bone, 119*f*, 124, 125*f*
Bicuspid valve, valve between left atrium and ventricle; prevents blood from flowing backward into atrium; has two cusps or flaps; also called *mitral valve*, 151–152, 153*f*
Bicuspids, premolar permanent teeth having two cusps or projections that assist in grinding food; humans have eight bicuspids, 271*f*, 272, 273*f*
Bilateral, pertaining to two sides, 5, 7
Bile, substance produced by liver and stored in gallbladder; added to chyme in duodenum and functions to emulsify fats so they can be digested and absorbed, 279
Bile duct, 279, 279*f*, 280
Bilirubin, waste product produced from destruction of worn-out red blood cells; disposed of by liver, 188
Binaural, referring to both ears, 498
Biopsy (BX, bx), piece of tissue is removed by syringe and needle, knife, punch, or brush to examine under a microscope; used to aid in diagnosis, 77
Bipolar disorder (BPD), mental disorder in which patient has alternating periods of depression and mania, 454
Bipolar and related disorders, a classification of psychiatric disorders in the DSM-5 characterized by alternation between periods of deep depression and mania; includes bipolar disorder (BPD),
Bitewing X-ray, X-ray taken with part of film holder held between teeth, and film held parallel to teeth, 293
Black lung. *See* Anthracosis
Bladder, 316*f*
Bladder cancer, cancerous tumor that arises from cells lining bladder; major symptom is hematuria, 327
Bladder neck obstruction (BNO), blockage of bladder outlet into urethra, 327
Blepharectomy, surgical removal of eyelid, 488
Blepharitis, inflammatory condition of eyelash follicles and glands of eyelids that results in swelling, redness, and crusts of dried mucus on lids; can be result of allergy or infection, 485
Blepharoplasty, surgical repair of eyelid, 488
Blepharoptosis, drooping eyelid, 481
Blind spot. *See* Optic disk
Blood, major component of hematic system; consists of watery plasma, red blood cells, and white blood cells, 33*t*, 186–199
  abbreviations, 198–199
  ABO system, 190
  adjective forms of anatomical terms, 192
  anatomy and physiology, 187*f*, 188–190, 189*f*, 189*t*, 190*f*
  diagnostic procedures, 196, 196*f*

Bradypnea, slow breathing, 241
Brain, one of the largest organs in body and coordinates most body activities; center for all thought, memory, judgment, and emotion; each part of brain is responsible for controlling different body functions, such as temperature regulation and breathing; four sections include cerebrum, cerebellum, diencephalon, and brainstem, 30*f*, 31, 428, 429–431, 430*f*, 431*f*, 440–443, 440*f*, 441*f*, 442*f*
Brain scan, injection of radioactive isotopes into circulation to determine function and abnormality of brain, 447
Brainstem, area of brain with three components: medulla oblongata, pons, and midbrain; pathway for impulses to be conducted between brain and spinal cord; also contains centers that control respiration, heart rate, and blood pressure; in addition, 12 pairs of cranial nerves begin in brainstem, 429, 431
Brain tumor, intracranial mass, either benign or malignant; benign tumor of brain can be fatal since it will grow and cause pressure on normal brain tissue, 440, 440*f*
Brand name, name a pharmaceutical company chooses as trademark or market name for its drug; also called *proprietary* or *trade name*, 16
Breaking the water. *See* Amniotomy
Breast cancer, malignant tumor of breast; usually forms in milk-producing gland tissue or lining of milk ducts, 362, 362*f*
Breasts, milk-producing glands to provide nutrition for newborn; also called *mammary glands*, 348, 352, 352*f*, 362
Breech birth, placement of fetus in which buttocks or feet are presented first for delivery rather than head, 354, 355*f*
Bridge, dental appliance attached to adjacent teeth for support to replace missing teeth, 295
Broad spectrum, ability of drug to be effective against a wide range of microorganisms, 79
Bronchial, pertaining to the bronchi, 239
Bronchial tree, 233*f*
Bronchial tube, organ of respiratory system that carries air into each lung, 230, 233–234, 233*f*
Bronchiectasis, results from dilation of bronchus or bronchi that can result from infection; this abnormal stretching can be irreversible and result in destruction of bronchial walls; major symptom is large amount of purulent (pus-filled) sputum; rales (bubbling chest sound) and hemoptysis may be present, 241, 245
Bronchiolar, pertaining to a bronchiole, 239
Bronchioles, narrowest air tubes in lungs; each bronchiole terminates in tiny air sacs called *alveoli*, 233, 233*f*
Bronchitis, acute or chronic inflammation of lower respiratory tract that often occurs after other childhood infections such as measles, 245
Bronchodilator, medication that dilates or opens bronchi (airways in lungs) to improve breathing, 254
Bronchogenic carcinoma, malignant lung tumor that originates in bronchi; usually associated with history of cigarette smoking, 245, 245*f*
Bronchogram, X-ray record of lungs and bronchial tubes, 249
Bronchography, process of taking X-ray of lung after radiopaque substance has been placed into trachea or bronchial tube, 249
Bronchoplasty, surgical repair of a bronchial defect, 251
Bronchoscope, instrument to view inside a bronchus, 249
Bronchoscopy (Bronch), using bronchoscope to visualize bronchi; instrument can also be used to obtain tissue for biopsy and to remove foreign objects, 249, 250*f*
Bronchospasm, involuntary muscle spasm in bronchi, 241
Bronchus, distal end of trachea splits into left and right main bronchi as it enters each lung; each main bronchus is subdivided into smaller branches; smallest bronchi are bronchioles; each bronchiole ends in tiny air sacs called *alveoli*, 233
Bruise. *See* Hematoma
Buccal, (1) pertaining to cheeks; (2) drugs that are placed under lip or between cheek and gum, 45, 47*f*, 282
Buccolabial, pertaining to cheeks and lips, 282
Buffers, chemicals that neutralize acid, particularly stomach acid, 280
Bulbourethral gland, also called *Cowper's gland*; these two small male reproductive system glands are located on either side of urethra just distal to prostate; secretion from these glands neutralizes acidity in urethra and vagina, 373, 373*f*, 375
Bulimia, eating disorder characterized by recurrent binge eating and then purging of food with laxatives and vomiting, 455
Bulla, large blister; larger than a vesicle, 65
Bundle branch block (BBB), occurs when electrical impulse is blocked from travelling down atrioventricular bundle or bundle branches; results in ventricles beating at a different rate than atria; also called a *heart block*, 165
Bundle branches, part of conduction system of heart; electrical signal travels down interventricular septum, 153, 154*f*
Bundle of His. *See* Atrioventricular bundle
Bunion, inflammation of bursa of the great toe, 113
Bunionectomy, removal of bursa at joint of great toe, 116
Burn, damage to skin caused by heat, electricity, ultraviolet light, or caustic chemicals; full-thickness burn exists when all layers are burned, called *third-degree burn*; partial-thickness burn exists when first layer of skin, epidermis, is burned, and second layer of skin, dermis, is damaged, called *second-degree burn*; first-degree burn damages only epidermis, 70–72, 71*f*, 72*f*
Bursa, saclike connective tissue structure found in some joints; protects moving parts from friction; some common bursa locations are elbow, knee, and shoulder joints, 101, 102
Bursectomy, surgical removal of a bursa, 116
Bursitis, inflammation of bursa between bony prominences and muscles or tendons; common in shoulder and knee, 107

C

Cachexia, loss of weight and generalized wasting that occurs during a chronic disease, 284

Calcitonin (CT), hormone secreted by thyroid gland; stimulates deposition of calcium into bone, 397*t*, 403–404

Calcium inorganic substance found in plasma; important for bones, muscles, and nerves, 188, 400

Calcium channel blocker drugs, medications that treat hypertension, angina pectoris, and congestive heart failure by causing heart to beat less forcefully and less often, 173

Calcium supplements, maintaining high blood levels of calcium in association with vitamin D helps maintain bone density and treats osteomalacia, osteoporosis, and rickets, 118

Calculus, stone formed within organ by accumulation of mineral salts; found in kidney, renal pelvis, ureters, bladder, or urethra; plural is *calculi*, 323, 323*f*

Callus, mass of bone tissue that forms at fracture site during its healing, 107

Calyx, duct that connects renal papilla to renal pelvis; urine flows from collecting tubule through calyx and into renal pelvis, 314, 315*f*

Cancellous bone, bony tissue found inside a bone; contains cavities that hold red bone marrow; also called *spongy bone*, 92–93, 93*f*

Cancerous tumors, malignant growths in the body, 205

Candidiasis, yeastlike infection of skin and mucous membranes that can result in white plaques on tongue and vagina, 361

Canines, also called *cuspid teeth* or *eyeteeth*; permanent teeth located between incisors and bicuspids that assist in biting and cutting food; humans have four canine teeth, 272

Canker sores. *See* Aphthous ulcers

Capillaries, smallest blood or lymphatic vessels; blood capillaries are very thin to allow gas, nutrient, and waste exchange between blood and tissues; lymph capillaries collect lymph fluid from tissues and carry it to larger lymph vessels, 148, 148*f*, 155*f*, 156

Capillary bed, network of capillaries found in a given tissue or organ, 156

Carbapenem-resistant Enterobacteriaceae (CRE) **infection,** infection by group of bacteria resistant to powerful antibiotics, frequently occurs in healthcare settings, 213

Carbon dioxide waste product of cellular energy production; removed from cells by blood and eliminated from body by lungs, 148–149, 148*f*, 230

Carbuncle, inflammation and infection of skin and hair follicle that may result from several untreated boils; most commonly found on neck, upper back, or head, 75

Cardiac, pertaining to the heart, 161

Cardiac arrest, when heart stops beating and circulation ceases, 163

Cardiac biomarkers, blood test to determine level of proteins specific to heart muscles in blood; increase in these proteins may indicate heart muscle damage such as myocardial infarction; proteins include creatine kinase (CK) and troponin, 169

Cardiac catheterization (heart cath), passage of thin tube (catheter) through arm vein and blood vessel leading into heart; used to detect abnormalities, to collect cardiac blood samples, and to determine pressure within cardiac area, 169

Cardiac muscle, involuntary muscle found in heart, 122–123, 122*f*, 123*f*, 149

Cardiac scan, patient is given radioactive thallium intravenously and then scanning equipment is used to visualize heart; especially useful in determining myocardial damage, 169

Cardiac sphincter, also called *lower esophageal sphincter* or *gastroesophageal sphincter*; prevents food and gastric juices from backing up into esophagus, 275, 275*f*

Cardiac tamponade, pressure on heart resulting from fluid buildup inside pericardial sac, 163

Cardiologist, physician specializing in treating diseases and conditions of cardiovascular system, 162

Cardiology, branch of medicine specializing in conditions of cardiovascular system, 32*t*, 162

Cardiomegaly, abnormally enlarged heart, 163

Cardiomyopathy, general term for disease of myocardium that may be caused by alcohol abuse, parasites, viral infection, and congestive heart failure, 163

Cardiopulmonary resuscitation (CPR), emergency treatment provided by trained persons and given to patients when their respirations and heart stop; provides oxygen to brain, heart, and other vital organs until medical treatment can restore normal heart and pulmonary function, 170, 253

Cardiotonic, substance that strengthens the heart muscle, 173

Cardiovascular, pertaining to the heart and blood vessels, 32

Cardiovascular system (CV), system that transports blood to all areas of body; organs include heart and blood vessels (arteries, veins, and capillaries); also called *circulatory system*, 145–175
- abbreviations, 174–175
- adjective forms of anatomical terms, 160–161
- anatomy and physiology, 147*f*, 148–159
- diagnostic procedures, 168–170
- functions, 32*t*, 146
- medical specialties, 32*t*
- pathology, 162–167
- pharmacology, 173
- terminology, 146, 159–160
- therapeutic procedures, 170–172

Cardiovascular technologist/technician, healthcare professional trained to perform a variety of diagnostic and therapeutic procedures including electrocardiography, echocardiography, and exercise stress tests, 162

Cardioversion. *See* Defibrillation

Carotid artery, 157*f*

Carotid endarterectomy, surgical procedure for removing obstruction within carotid artery, major artery in neck that carries oxygenated blood to brain; developed to prevent strokes but found to be useful only in severe stenosis with TIA, 449

Carpal, pertaining to the carpus or wrist, 104

Carpal tunnel release, surgical cutting of ligament in wrist to relieve nerve pressure caused by carpal tunnel syndrome, which can be caused by repetitive motion such as typing, 133

Carpal tunnel syndrome (CTS), painful disorder of wrist and hand, induced by compression of median nerve as it passes under ligaments on palm side of wrist; symptoms include weakness, pain, burning, tingling, and aching in forearm, wrist, and hand, 130

Carpals, wrist bones in upper extremity, 92, 104

Carpus, collective name for the eight wrist bones in each upper extremity, 91*f*, 98, 99*f*, 100, 100*f*, 100*t*

Cartilage, strong, flexible connective tissue found in several locations in body, such as covering ends of bones in synovial joint, nasal septum, external ear, eustachian tube, larynx, trachea, bronchi, and intervertebral disks, 30*f*, 31, 92

Cartilaginous joints, allow slight movement but hold bones firmly in place by solid piece of cartilage; example is pubic symphysis; fetal skeleton is composed of cartilaginous tissue, 101, 102*f*

Cast, application of solid material to immobilize extremity or portion of body as a result of fracture, dislocation, or severe injury; most often made of plaster of Paris or fiberglass, 117

Castration, surgical removal of testicles in male or ovaries in female, 380

Cataract, diminished vision resulting from lens of eye becoming opaque or cloudy; treatment is usually surgical removal of lens with cataract and replacement with prosthetic lens, 482, 482*f*

Catheter (cath), flexible tube inserted into body for purpose of moving fluids into or out of body; used in cardiovascular system to place dye into blood vessels so they may be visualized on X-rays; used in urinary system to drain urine from bladder, 169, 330

Catheterization, insertion of a tube through urethra and into urinary bladder for purpose of withdrawing urine or inserting dye, 330

Caudal, directional term meaning toward feet or tail, or below; akin to *inferior*, 43*f*, 43*t*

Cauterization, destruction of tissue by using caustic chemicals, electric currents, or by heating or freezing, 78

Cecal, pertaining to the cecum, 282

Cecum, first portion of colon; a blind pouch off beginning of large intestine; appendix originates at end, 276*f*, 277, 277*f*

Celiac disease, autoimmune condition affecting small intestine; caused by reaction to gluten; symptoms may include abdominal bloating and pain, diarrhea, and nutritional deficiencies, 288

Cell, basic unit of all living things; composes all tissues and organs in body; performs survival functions such as reproduction, respiration, metabolism, and excretion; some also able to carry on specialized functions, such as contraction by muscle cells and electrical impulse transmission by nerve cells, 27*f*, 28, 30*f*

Cell-mediated immunity, immunity resulting from activation of sensitized T lymphocytes; immune response causes antigens to be destroyed by direct action of cells; also called *cellular immunity*, 206

Cell membrane, outermost boundary of the cell, 28, 29*f*

Cellular immunity, also called *cell-mediated immunity*; process results in production of T cells and natural killer (NK) cells that directly attach to foreign cells; immune response fights invasion by viruses, bacteria, fungi, and cancer, 206–207

Cellulitis, inflammation of cellular or connective tissues, 72

Cementum, anchors root of a tooth into socket of jaw, 272, 273*f*

Central canal, canal that extends down length of spinal cord; contains cerebrospinal fluid, 432

Central nervous system (CNS), portion of nervous system consisting of brain and spinal cord; receives impulses from all over body, processes information, and then responds with action; consists of both gray and white matter, 428–429

- brain, 30*f*, 31, 428, 429–431, 430*f*, 431*f*, 440–443, 440*f*, 441*f*, 442*f*
- meninges, 428–429, 433, 433*f*, 445–446, 446*f*
- spinal cord, 30*f*, 31, 428, 431*f*, 432–433, 432*f*, 435*f*, 443–444, 444*f*

Cephalalgia, a headache, 439

Cephalic, 1) pertaining to the head; 2) directional term meaning toward the head, or above, 39*f*, 43*f*, 43*t*, 437

Cephalic region, head region of the body, 38*t*, 39*f*

Cephalic vein, 158*f*

Cerebellar, pertaining to cerebellum, 437

Cerebellitis, inflammation of cerebellum, 440

Cerebellum, second largest portion of brain, located beneath posterior portion of cerebrum; part of brain that aids in coordinating voluntary body movements and maintaining balance and equilibrium; attached to brainstem by pons; refined muscular movement is initiated in cerebrum, 429, 431*f*

Cerebral, pertaining to the cerebrum, 437

Cerebral aneurysm, localized abnormal dilatation of blood vessel, usually artery; result of congenital defect or weakness in wall of vessel; ruptured aneurysm is a common cause for hemorrhagic CVA, 440, 441*f*

Cerebral angiography, X-ray of blood vessels of brain after injection of radiopaque dye, 447

Cerebral contusion, bruising of brain from blow or impact; symptoms last longer than 24 hours and include unconsciousness, dizziness, vomiting, unequal pupil size, and shock, 441

Cerebral cortex, outer layer of cerebrum; composed of folds of gray matter called *gyri*, which are separated by sulci, 429

Cerebral hemispheres, divisions of cerebrum into right and left halves, 429–430

Cerebral palsy (CP), brain damage resulting from a defect, trauma, infection, or lack of oxygen before, during, or shortly after birth, 441

Cerebrospinal, pertaining to cerebrum and spine, 437

Cerebrospinal fluid (CSF), watery, clear fluid found in ventricles of brain; provides protection from shock or sudden motion to brain, 429, 431

Cerebrospinal fluid analysis, laboratory examination of clear, watery, colorless fluid from within brain and spinal cord; can detect infections and abnormal presence of blood, 447

Cerebrospinal fluid shunt, surgical procedure in which bypass is created to drain cerebrospinal fluid; used to treat hydrocephalus by draining excess cerebrospinal fluid from brain and diverting it to abdominal cavity, 449

Cerebrovascular accident (CVA), also called a *stroke*; development of infarct due to loss in blood supply to area of brain; blood flow can be interrupted by ruptured blood vessel (hemorrhage), floating clot (embolus), stationary clot (thrombosis), or compression; extent of damage depends on size and location of infarct and often includes speech problems and muscle paralysis, 441, 441*f*

Cerebrum, largest section of brain; located in upper portion, and possesses thoughts, judgment, memory, association skills, and ability to discriminate between items; outer layer is cerebral cortex, which is composed of folds of gray matter; elevated portions, or convolutions, are called *gyri* and are separated by fissures or sulci; has both a left and right division or hemisphere, each with its own four lobes: frontal, parietal, occipital, and temporal, 429–430, 430*f*

Cerumen, also called *earwax*; thick, waxy substance produced by oil glands in auditory canal; helps to protect and lubricate ear, 494–495, 494*f*

Ceruminosis, excessive accumulation of earwax in ear canal, 499

Cervical, (1) pertaining to neck; (2) pertaining to cervix, 39*f*, 104, 357

Cervical biopsy, taking a sample of tissue from cervix to test for presence of cancer cells, 366

Cervical cancer, malignant growth in cervix; main cause is infection by *human papillomavirus* (HPV), a sexually transmitted virus for which there is now a vaccine; Pap smear tests have helped with early detection, 36

Cervical nerve, 435*f*

Cervical nodes, 203*t*, 204*f*

Cervical region, neck region of body, 38*t*, 39*f*

Cervical vertebrae (C1, C2, etc.), seven vertebrae in neck region, 91*f*, 95, 97, 98*f*, 98*t*

Cervicectomy, surgical removal of cervix, 367

Cervix (Cx), narrow, distal portion of uterus that joins to vagina, 348*f*, 350, 350*f*, 351*f*, 353*f*

Cesarean section (CS, C-section), surgical delivery of baby through incision into abdominal and uterine walls; legend has it that Roman emperor Julius Caesar was first person born by this method, 367

Chancroid, highly infectious nonsyphilitic venereal ulcer, 378, 378*f*

Cheeks, form lateral walls of oral cavity, 270–271

Chemabrasion, abrasion using chemicals; also called a *chemical peel*, 78

Chemical name, name for a drug based on its chemical formula or molecular structure, 16

Chemical thyroidectomy, large dose of radioactive iodine is given in order to kill thyroid gland cells without having to actually do surgery, 413

Chest tube. *See* Thoracostomy

Chest X-ray (CXR), taking radiographic picture of lungs and heart from back and sides, 249

Cheyne-Stokes respiration, abnormal breathing pattern in which there are long periods (10-60 seconds) of apnea followed by deeper, more rapid breathing, 241

Chickenpox. *See* Varicella

Chiropractic, healthcare profession concerned with diagnosis and treatment of spine and musculoskeletal system with intention of affecting nervous system and improving health; healthcare practitioner is a *chiropractor*, 106

Chiropractor, 106

Chlamydia, parasitic microorganism causing genital infections in males and females; can lead to pelvic inflammatory disease in females and eventual infertility, 379

Choked disk. *See* Papilledema

Cholecystalgia, gallbladder pain, 284

Cholecystectomy, surgical removal of gallbladder; removal of gallbladder through laparoscope is newer procedure with fewer complications than more invasive abdominal surgery; laparoscope requires a small incision into abdominal cavity, 296

Cholecystic, pertaining to gallbladder, 282

Cholecystitis, inflammation of gallbladder, 291

Cholecystogram, dye given orally to patient is absorbed and enters gallbladder, and then X-ray is taken, 293

Choledocholithotripsy, crushing of a gallstone in common bile duct, 296

Cholelithiasis, formation or presence of stones or calculi in gallbladder or common bile duct, 291, 291*f*

Chondrectomy, surgical removal of cartilage, 116

Chondroma, cartilage tumor, 110

Chondromalacia, softening of cartilage, 107

Chondroplasty, surgical repair of cartilage, 116

Chorion, outer of two membranous sacs surrounding fetus; helps to form placenta, 353–354

Chorionic, pertaining to chorion, 357

Chorionic villus sampling (CVS), removal of small piece of chorion for genetic analysis; may be done at earlier stage of pregnancy than amniocentesis, 366

Choroid, middle layer of eyeball; provides blood supply for eye, 474–475, 474*f*

Choroid layer, 473*f*, 475, 480, 485

Chronic obstructive pulmonary disease (COPD), progressive, chronic, and usually irreversible group of conditions in which lungs have diminished capacity for inhalation and exhalation; person may have difficulty breathing on exertion (dyspnea) and a cough, 246

Chronic traumatic encephalopathy (CTE), progressive brain degeneration caused by severe blow or repeated less severe blows to the head, 441

Chyme, semisoft mixture of food and digestive fluids that pass from stomach into small intestines, 275, 280

Cicatrix, a scar, 72
Cilia, term for eyelashes that protect eye from foreign particles or for nasal hairs that help filter dust and bacteria out of inhaled air, 230–231, 476
Ciliary body, intraocular eye muscles that change shape of the lens, 474*f*, 475
Circadian rhythm, 24-hour clock that governs periods of wakefulness and sleepiness, 400
Circle of Willis, 441*f*
Circulatory system, system that transports blood to all areas of body; organs include heart and blood vessels (arteries, veins, and capillaries); also called *cardiovascular system*, 148, 148*f*
Circumcision, surgical removal of prepuce, or foreskin of penis; generally performed on newborn male at request of parents; primary reason is for ease of hygiene; also a ritual practice in some religions, 374, 380
Circumduction, movement in a circular direction from a central point, 126*t*
Cirrhosis, chronic disease of the liver, 291
Clavicle, also called *collar bone*; bone of pectoral girdle, 98, 99*f*, 100, 100*f*, 100*t*
Clavicular, pertaining to clavicle or collar bone, 104
Clean catch specimen (CC), urine sample obtained after cleaning off urinary opening and catching or collecting a sample in midstream (halfway through urination process) to minimize contamination from genitalia, 328
Cleft lip, congenital anomaly in which upper lip fails to come together; often seen along with cleft palate; corrected with surgery, 286
Cleft palate, congenital anomaly in which roof of mouth has split or fissure; corrected with surgery, 286
Clinical divisions of the abdomen, method of dividing the abdominopelvic cavity into 4 regions: right upper quadrant, left upper quadrant, right lower quadrant, and left lower quadrant, 42
Clinical psychologist, diagnoses and treats mental disorders; specializes in using individual and group counseling to treat patients with mental and emotional disorders, 453
Clitoris, small organ containing erectile tissue covered by labia minora; contains sensitive tissue aroused during sexual stimulation and is similar to penis in male, 348*f*, 351, 351*f*
Closed fracture, simple fracture with no open skin wound; also called a *simple fracture*, 108, 108*f*
Closed reduction. *See* Reduction
Clostridium difficile (C. diff) **infection,** bacterial infection causing colon inflammation; spread through contact with contaminated feces, 213
Clubbing, abnormal widening and thickening of ends of fingers and toes associated with chronic oxygen deficiency; seen in patients with chronic respiratory conditions or circulatory problems, 241
Clubfoot. *See* Talipes
Coagulate, convert liquid to gel or solid, as in blood coagulation, 193
Coarctation of the aorta (CoA), severe congenital narrowing of aorta, 167
Coccygeal, pertaining to coccyx or tailbone, 104
Coccyx, tailbone, three to five very small vertebrae attached to sacrum; often become fused, 91*f*, 95, 96*f*, 97, 98*f*, 98*t*
Cochlea, portion of labyrinth associated with hearing; rolled in shape of snail shell; lined by organ of Corti, 494*f*, 495
Cochlear, pertaining to cochlea, 498
Cochlear implant, mechanical device surgically placed under skin behind outer ear (pinna); converts sound signals into magnetic impulses to stimulate auditory nerve; can be beneficial for those with profound sensorineural hearing loss, 503, 503*f*
Cochlear nerve, branch of vestibulocochlear nerve that carries hearing information to brain, 494, 494*f*
Coitus, sexual intercourse, 374
Cold sores. *See* Herpes labialis
Colectomy, surgical removal of colon, 296
Collagen fibers, fibers made up of insoluble fibrous protein present in connective tissue that forms flexible mat to protect skin and other parts of body, 60
Collecting tubule, portion of renal tubule, 315, 316*f*
Colles' fracture, specific type of wrist fracture,108, 108*f*
Colon, section of large intestine; functions to reabsorb most of fluid in digested food; material that remains after water reabsorption is feces; sections include cecum, ascending colon, transverse colon, descending colon, and sigmoid colon, 275–277, 276*f*, 277*f*
Colonic, pertaining to colon, 282
Colonoscope, instrument to view inside colon, 294
Colonoscopy, flexible fiberscope passed through anus, rectum, and colon used to examine upper portion of colon; polyps and small growths can be removed during procedure, 294
Color vision tests, use of polychromic (multicolored) charts to determine ability of patient to recognize color, 486, 486*f*
Colorectal, pertaining to colon and rectum, 282
Colorectal carcinoma, cancerous tumor originating in the colon or rectum, 288
Colostomy, surgical creation of opening in some portion of colon through abdominal wall to outside surface; fecal material (stool) drains into bag worn on abdomen, 296, 296*f*
Colostrum, thin fluid first secreted by breast after delivery; does not contain much protein, but is rich in antibodies, 358
Colposcope, instrument to view inside vagina, 365
Colposcopy, visual examination of cervix and vagina using colposcope, 365
Coma, profound unconsciousness resulting from illness or injury, 439
Combining form, word root plus combining vowel; always written with a "/" between word root and combining vowel; for example, in *cardi/o*, *cardi* is word root and *o* is combining vowel, 4
Combining vowel, vowel inserted between word parts to make it possible to pronounce long medical terms; usually the vowel *o*, 2–4

Coronary artery disease (CAD), insufficient blood supply to heart muscle due to obstruction of one or more coronary arteries; may be caused by atherosclerosis and may cause angina pectoris and myocardial infarction, 164, 164*f*
Corporeal, pertaining to body, 161
Corpus, body or central portion of uterus, 348*f*, 350
Corpus albicans, 349*f*
Corpus luteum, 349*f*
Cortex, outer layer of organ; within endocrine system, refers to outer layer of adrenal glands; within urinary system, refers to outer layer of kidney, 314, 315*f*
Cortical, pertaining to cortex or outer layer, 104
Cortical bone, hard exterior surface bone; also called *compact bone*, 92–93
Corticosteroid cream, powerful anti-inflammatory cream, 79
Corticosteroids, natural or synthetic adrenal cortex hormones; include mineralocorticoid hormones, glucocorticoid hormones, and steroid sex hormones; used as medication for its strong anti-inflammatory properties, 118, 215, 254, 398, 414
Cortisol, glucocorticoid hormone secreted by adrenal cortex; regulates carbohydrate metabolism, 396*t*, 398–399
Costal, pertaining to rib, 98*f*, 104
Cowper's glands, also called *bulbourethral glands*; these two small male reproductive system glands are located on either side of urethra just distal to prostate; secretion from these glands neutralizes acidity in urethra and vagina, 375
Crackles, abnormal sound made during inspiration; usually indicates presence of fluid or mucus in small airways; also called *rales*, 241
Cranial, pertaining to skull, 104, 437
Cranial bones, 95*t*
Cranial cavity, dorsal body cavity; within skull and contains brain, 40, 40*f*, 41*t*
Cranial nerves, nerves that arise from brain, 428, 433–434, 434*t*
Craniotomy, incision into skull, 116
Cranium, skull; bones that form protective covering over brain, 95, 96*f*
Creatinine, waste product of muscle metabolism, 188, 328
Creatinine clearance, test of kidney function; creatinine is waste product cleared from bloodstream by kidneys; for test, urine is collected for 24 hours and amount of creatinine in urine is compared to amount of creatinine that remains in bloodstream, 328
Creatine kinase (CK), muscle enzyme found in skeletal muscle and cardiac muscle; blood levels become elevated in disorders such as heart attack, muscular dystrophy, and other skeletal muscle pathologies; also called *creatine phosphokinase*, 129
Creatine phosphokinase. *See* Creatine kinase
Crepitation, noise produced by bones or cartilage rubbing together, 107
Cretinism. *See* Congenital hypothyroidism
Crick in the neck, 130
Crohn's disease, form of chronic inflammatory bowel disease affecting ileum and/or colon; also called *regional ileitis*, 288
Cross-eyed. *See* Esotropia
Cross infection, occurs when person, either patient or healthcare worker, acquires pathogen from another patient or healthcare worker, 207
Cross-section, internal view of body produced by slice perpendicular to long axis of structure, 37–38, 37*f*
Croup, acute viral respiratory infection common in infants and young children and characterized by hoarse cough, 244
Crown, portion of tooth covered by enamel; also artificial covering for tooth created to replace original enamel, 272, 273*f*, 295
Crowning, when head of baby is visible through vaginal opening; a sign that birth is imminent, 354, 355*f*
Crural, pertaining to leg, 39*f*
Crural region, lower extremity region of body, 38*t*, 39*f*
Cryopexy, surgical fixation of retina by using extreme cold, 488
Cryosurgery, exposing tissues to extreme cold in order to destroy them; used in treating malignant tumors and to control pain and bleeding, 78
Cryotherapy, using cold for therapeutic purposes, 132
Cryptorchidism, failure of testes to descend into scrotal sac before birth; usually the testes will descend before birth; surgical procedure called *orchidopexy* may be required to bring testes down into scrotum permanently; failure of testes to descend could result in sterility in male, 377
Culdoscopy, examination of a blind pouch-like area of the female pelvic cavity by introducing endoscope through wall of vagina, 365
Culture and sensitivity (C&S), laboratory test in which colony of pathogens that have been removed from infected area are grown to identify pathogen and then determine its sensitivity to a variety of antibiotics, 77
Cumulative action, action that occurs in body when drug is allowed to accumulate or stay in body, 254
Curettage, removal of superficial skin lesions with curette (surgical instrument shaped like spoon) or scraper, 78
Cushing's syndrome, set of symptoms that result from hypersecretion of adrenal cortex; may be result of tumor of adrenal glands; symptoms include weakness, edema, excess hair growth, skin discoloration, and osteoporosis, 408
Cuspids, permanent teeth located between incisors and bicuspids that assist in biting and cutting food; humans have four cuspids; also called *canine teeth* or *eyeteeth*, 271*f*, 272, 273*f*
Cusps, leaflets or flaps of heart valve, 151
Cutaneous, pertaining to skin, 58, 64
Cutaneous membrane, another term for skin, 58
Cuticle, thin skinlike layer overlapping base of nail, 61, 61*f*
Cyanosis, slightly bluish color of skin due to deficiency of oxygen and excess of carbon dioxide in blood; caused by a variety of disorders, ranging from

D

Dermatome, instrument for cutting skin or thin transplants of skin, 78
Dermatoplasty, surgical repair of skin, 78
Dermatosis, abnormal condition of skin, 72
Dermic, pertaining to the skin, 64
Dermis, living layer of skin located between epidermis and subcutaneous layer; also referred to as *corium*; contains hair follicles, sweat glands, sebaceous glands, blood vessels, lymph vessels, sensory receptors, nerve fibers, and muscle fibers, 58, 59*f*, 60, 61*f*
Descending aorta, 153*f*
Descending colon, section of colon that descends left side of abdomen, 276*f*, 277, 277*f*
Descending nephron loop, 316*f*
Descending tracts, nerve tracts carrying motor signals down spinal cord to muscles, 432
Diabetes insipidus (DI), disorder caused by inadequate secretion of hormone by posterior lobe of pituitary gland; there may be polyuria and polydipsia, 410*f*
Diabetes mellitus (DM), serious disease in which pancreas fails to produce insulin or insulin does not work properly; consequently, patient has very high blood sugar; kidney will attempt to lower high blood sugar level by excreting excess sugar in urine, 409
Diabetic acidosis. *See* Ketoacidosis
Diabetic nephropathy, accumulation of damage to glomerulus capillaries due to chronic high blood sugars of diabetes mellitus, 325
Diabetic retinopathy, secondary complication of diabetes affecting blood vessels of retina, resulting in visual changes and even blindness, 409
Diagnostic and Statistical Manual of Mental Disorders, Fifth Edition (DSM-5), 453
Diagnostic reports, found in patient's medical record; consist of results of all diagnostic tests performed on patient, principally from clinical lab and medical imaging (e.g., X-ray and ultrasound), 14*t*
Diaphoresis, excessive or profuse sweating, 65
Diaphragm, major muscle of inspiration; separates thoracic from abdominal cavity, 40, 40*f*, 235–236, 236*f*
Diaphragmatic, pertaining to diaphragm, 239
Diaphragmatocele. *See* Hiatal hernia
Diaphysis, shaft portion of long bone, 92, 93*f*
Diarrhea, passing of frequent, watery bowel movements; usually accompanies gastrointestinal (GI) disorders, 284
Diastole, period of time during which heart chamber is relaxed, 152
Diastolic pressure, lower pressure within blood vessels during relaxation phase of heartbeat, 159
Diencephalon, portion of brain that contains two most critical areas of brain, thalamus and hypothalamus, 429, 430*f*
Digestive system, system that digests food and absorbs nutrients; organs include mouth, pharynx, esophagus, stomach, small and large intestines, liver, gallbladder, pancreas, and salivary glands; also called *gastrointestinal system*, 34*t*, 263–299, 268–299
- abbreviations, 299
- accessory organs of, 278–280, 279*f*
- adjective forms of anatomical terms, 282–283
- anatomy and physiology, 269*f*, 270–280
- colon, 275–277, 276*f*, 277*f*
- diagnostic procedures, 292–295
- esophagus, 270, 271*f*, 272*f*, 274, 275*f*, 286
- function, 268
- gallbladder, 270, 279–279, 279*f*
- liver, 270, 279, 279*f*
- medical specialties, 34*t*
- oral cavity, 270–271, 271*f*, 272*f*, 286
- pancreas, 270, 279*f*, 280, 396, 397*t*, 399–400, 400*f*, 409
- pathology, 284–291
- pharmacology, 298–299
- pharynx, 121, 205, 231–232, 231*f*, 272*f*, 274, 286
- salivary glands, 270, 278, 279*f*
- small intestine, 270, 275–277, 276*f*, 288–290
- stomach, 270, 275, 275*f*, 286
- teeth, 270–271, 271*f*, 272*f*, 273*f*
- terminology, 268, 270, 280–281
- therapeutic procedures, 295–298

Digital rectal exam (DRE), manual examination for enlarged prostate gland performed by palpating (feeling) prostate gland through wall of rectum, 380
Digital veins, 158*f*
Dilation and curettage (D&C), surgical procedure in which opening of cervix is dilated and uterus is scraped or suctioned of its lining or tissue; often performed after spontaneous abortion and to stop excessive bleeding from other causes, 367
Dilation stage, first stage of labor; begins with uterine contractions that press fetus against cervix causing it to dilate to 10 cm and become thin; thinning of cervix is called *effacement*, 354, 355*f*
Diphtheria, bacterial infection characterized by severe inflammation that can form membrane coating in upper respiratory tract that can cause marked difficulty breathing, 244
Diplopia, double vision, 481
Directional terms, 42–43, 43*t*–44*t*
Discharge summary, part of patient's medical record; comprehensive outline of patient's entire hospital stay; includes condition at time of admission, admitting diagnosis, test results, treatments and patient's response, final diagnosis, and follow-up plans, 14*t*
Dislocation, occurs when bones in joint are displaced from their normal alignment, 113
Disruptive, impulse control, and conduct disorders, a classification of psychiatric disorders in the DSM-5 characterized by the inability to resist impulses to perform some act harmful to individual or others; includes kleptomania, pyromania, and explosive disorder, 454
Dissociative amnesia, loss of memory, 454
Dissociative disorders, a classification of psychiatric disorders in the DSM-5 in which severe emotional conflict is so repressed that split in personality or memory loss occurs; includes dissociative amnesia and dissociative identity disorder, 454

Dissociative identity disorder, having two or more distinct personalities, 454
Distal, directional term meaning located farthest from point of attachment to body, 43*f*, 44*t*
Distal convoluted tubule, portion of renal tubule, 315, 316*f*
Diuresis, abnormal secretion of large amounts of urine, 323
Diuretic, substance that increases excretion of urine, which promotes loss of water and salt from body; can assist in lowering blood pressure, 173, 333
Diverticulectomy, surgical removal of diverticulum, 297
Diverticulitis, inflammation of diverticulum or sac in intestinal tract, especially in colon, 288, 288*f*
Diverticulosis, abnormal condition of having diverticula (outpouches off gut), 288
Diverticulum, an outpouching off the gut, 288, 288*f*, 297
Dopaminergic drugs, group of medications to treat Parkinson's disease by either replacing dopamine that is lacking or increasing strength of dopamine that is present, 450
Doppler ultrasonography, measurement of sound-wave echoes as they bounce off tissues and organs to produce image; within cardiovascular system, used to measure velocity of blood moving through blood vessels to look for blood clots, 169
Dorsal, directional term meaning more toward the back or spinal cord side of the body; akin to *posterior*, 43*f*, 43*t*
Dorsal cavities, 41*t*
Dorsiflexion, backward bending, as of hand or foot, 126*f*, 126*t*
Dorsum, refers to posterior region of back of body, 38*t*, 39*f*
Drug Enforcement Administration (DEA), government agency that enforces regulation of controlled substances, 17
Drug interaction, occurs when effect of one drug is altered because it was taken at same time as another drug, 197
Drugs. *See* Pharmacology
Dry gangrene, late stages of gangrene characterized by affected area becoming black and leathery, 72
Dual-energy X-ray absorptiometry (DXA, DEXA), measurement of bone density using low-dose X-ray for purpose of detecting osteoporosis, 115
Duchenne's muscular dystrophy. *See* Pseudohypertrophic muscular dystrophy
Duodenal, pertaining to duodenum, 282
Duodenum, first section of small intestine; location where digestion is completed after chyme mixes with digestive juices from pancreas and gallbladder, 275–276, 276*f*, 280
Dura mater, term means *tough mother*; fibrous outermost meninges layer that forms a tough protective layer, 433, 433*f*
Dwarfism, condition of being abnormally small; may be hereditary condition or endocrine dysfunction, 410
Dyscrasia, general term indicating presence of disease affecting blood, 193
Dysentery, disease characterized by diarrhea, often with mucus and blood, severe abdominal pain, fever, and dehydration, 288
Dyskinesia, difficult or painful movement, 129
Dysmenorrhea, painful cramping associated with menstruation, 359
Dysorexia, abnormal appetite, 284
Dyspareunia, condition of having painful sexual intercourse, 359
Dyspepsia, indigestion, 285
Dysphagia, having difficulty eating, 285, 438
Dysphasia, impairment of speech as a result of brain lesion, 439
Dysphonia, abnormal voice, 242
Dyspnea, difficult, labored breathing, 242
Dystocia, abnormal or difficult labor and childbirth, 359
Dystonia, abnormal tone, 129
Dysuria, painful or difficult urination; symptom in many disorders, such as cystitis, urethritis, enlarged prostate in male, and prolapsed uterus in female, 323

E

Eardrops, substance placed directly into ear canal for purpose of relieving pain or treating infection, 45
Eardrum. *See* Tympanic membrane
Earwax. *See* Cerumen
Ecchymosis, skin discoloration or bruise caused by blood collecting under skin, 65, 65*f*
Echocardiography (ECHO), noninvasive diagnostic method using ultrasound to visualize internal cardiac structures; cardiac valve activity can be evaluated using this method, 169
Echoencephalography, recording of ultrasonic echoes of brain; useful in determining abnormal patterns of shifting in brain, 447
Eclampsia, convulsive seizures and coma that can occur in woman between 20th week of pregnancy and up to six weeks postpartum; often associated with hypertension, 362
Ectopic pregnancy. *See* Salpingocyesis
Eczema, superficial dermatitis accompanied by papules, vesicles, and crusting, 72
Edema, condition in which body tissues contain excessive amounts of fluid, 407
Effacement, thinning of cervix during labor, 354, 355*f*

terminology, 394, 405–406
testes, 373–374, 373*f*, 377–378, 396, 397*t*, 403, 403*f*
therapeutic procedures, 413
thymus gland, 202, 205, 205*f*, 396, 397*t*, 403, 404*f*, 410–411
thyroid gland, 231*f*, 396, 397*t*, 401*f*, 403–404, 404*f*, 411
Endocrinologist, physician who specializes in treatment of endocrine glands, 407
Endocrinology, branch of medicine specializing in conditions of endocrine system, 35*t*, 407
Endocrinopathy, disease of endocrine system, 407
Endometrial, pertaining to the endometrium, 357
Endometrial biopsy (EMB), taking sample of tissue from lining of uterus to test for abnormalities, 366
Endometrial cancer, cancer of endometrial lining of uterus, 360
Endometriosis, abnormal condition of endometrium tissue appearing throughout pelvis or on abdominal wall; this tissue is usually found within uterus, 362
Endometritis, inflammation of endometrial lining of uterus, 360
Endometrium, inner lining of uterus; contains rich blood supply and reacts to hormonal changes every month, which results in menstruation; during pregnancy, lining of uterus does not leave body but remains to nourish unborn child, 350, 350*f*
Endoscopic retrograde cholangiopancreatography (ERCP), using endoscope to X-ray bile and pancreatic ducts, 294
Endothelium, 153*f*
Endotracheal intubation, placing tube through mouth to create airway, 251, 251*f*
Enema, injection of fluid through rectum and into large intestine for purpose of cleansing bowel for testing, treating constipation, or administering drugs, 295
Enteric, pertaining to small intestine, 282
Enteritis, inflammation of only small intestine, 288
Enucleated, loss of cell's nucleus, 188
Enucleation, surgical removal of an eyeball, 488
Enuresis, elimination disorder characterized by the involuntary discharge of urine after age by which bladder control should have been established; usually occurs by age 5; *nocturnal enuresis* refers to bed-wetting at night, 324, 454
Eosinophil (eosins, eos), granulocyte white blood cells that destroy parasites and increase during allergic reactions, 189*f*, 189*t*
Eosinophilic, pertaining to [a leukocyte] that attracts a rosy red stain, 192
Epicardium, outer layer of heart; forms part of pericardium, 150, 150*f*
Epicondyle, projection located above or on condyle, 94, 95*f*
Epidermal, pertaining to above [upon] the skin, 64
Epidermis, superficial layer of skin; is composed of squamous epithelium cells; these are flat scalelike cells that are arranged in layers, called *stratified squamous epithelium*; many layers of epidermis create a barrier to infection; epidermis does not have a blood supply, so is dependent on deeper layers of skin for nourishment; however, deepest epidermis layer is called *basal layer*; these cells are alive and constantly dividing; older cells are pushed out toward surface by new cells forming beneath; during this process, they shrink and die, becoming filled with a protein called *keratin*; keratin-filled cells are sloughed off as dead cells, 58–60, 59*f*, 61*f*
Epididymal, pertaining to epididymis, 376
Epididymectomy, surgical removal of epididymis, 380
Epididymis, coiled tubule that lies on top of testes within scrotum; stores sperm as they are produced and turns into vas deferens, 373, 373*f*, 374, 378, 403*f*
Epididymitis, inflammation of epididymis causing pain and swelling in inguinal area, 378
Epidural hematoma, mass of blood in space outside dura mater of brain and spinal cord, 445
Epidural space, 433*f*
Epigastric, anatomical division of abdomen, middle section of upper row, 41*f*, 41*t*
Epiglottic, pertaining to epiglottis, 239
Epiglottis, flap of cartilage that covers larynx when swallowing; prevents food and drink from entering larynx and trachea, 231*f*, 232, 272*f*, 274
Epilepsy, recurrent disorder of brain in which convulsive seizures and loss of consciousness occur, 442
Epinephrine, hormone produced by adrenal medulla; also known as *adrenaline*; actions include increased heart rate and force of contraction, bronchodilation, and relaxation of intestinal muscles, 396*t*, 398–399
Epiphyseal line, 93*f*
Epiphysis, wide ends of a long bone, 92, 93*f*
Episiorrhaphy, to suture perineum after birth, 367
Episiotomy, surgical incision of perineum to facilitate delivery process; can prevent irregular tearing of tissue during birth, 367
Epispadias, congenital opening of urethra on dorsal surface of penis, 378
Epistaxis, nosebleed, 242
Epithelial tissue, tissue found throughout body as skin, outer covering of organs, and inner lining for tubular or hollow structures, 28, 30*f*
Epithelium, epithelial tissue composed of close-packed cells that form covering for and lining of body structures, 29, 30*f*
Equilibrium, sense of balance, 494
Erectile dysfunction (ED), inability to copulate due to inability to maintain erection; also called *impotence*, 378, 456
Erectile dysfunction agents, medications that temporarily produce erection in patients with erectile dysfunction, 382
Erectile tissue, tissue with numerous blood vessels and nerve endings; becomes filled with blood and enlarges in size in response to sexual stimulation, 351, 374
Eructation, burping of gas or stomach acid into mouth; belching, 285
Erythema, redness or flushing of skin, 66
Erythroblastosis fetalis. *See* Hemolytic disease of the newborn
Erythrocyte, also called *red blood cells* (RBCs); cells that contain hemoglobin, an iron-containing pigment that

F

Fimbriae, fingerlike extensions on end of uterine (fallopian) tubes; drape over each ovary in order to direct ovum into uterine tube after being expelled by ovary, 349–350, 349*f*, 350*f*, 399*f*
First-degree burn. *See* Burn
Fissure, 1) crack-like skin lesion; 2) slit-shaped opening in a bone, 66, 66*f*, 94
Fistulectomy, surgical removal of a fistula, 297
Fixation, procedure to stabilize fractured bone while it heals; external fixation includes casts, splints, and pins inserted through skin; internal fixation includes pins, plates, rods, screws, and wires that are applied during an open reduction, 117
Flat bone, type of bone with thin flattened shape; examples include scapula, ribs, and pelvic bones, 92, 93*f*
Flat-plate abdomen. *See* Kidneys, ureters, bladder (KUB)
Flatulence, excess gas in stomach or intestines; may be passed through anus 285
Flesh-eating disease. *See* Necrotizing fasciitis
Flexion, act of bending or being bent, 125*f*, 125*t*
Flexor carpi, muscle named for its action, flexion, 124
Floating kidney. *See* Nephroptosis
Flu. *See* Influenza
Fluorescein angiography, process of injecting dye (fluorescein) to observe movement of blood for detecting lesions in macular area of retina; used to determine if there is detachment of retina, 486
Fluorescein staining, applying dye eyedrops of bright green fluorescent color; used to look for corneal abrasions or ulcers, 486
Flutter, arrhythmia in which atria beat too rapidly, but in regular pattern, 166
Focal seizure, localized epileptic seizure often affecting one limb, 439
Follicle-stimulating hormone (FSH), hormone secreted by anterior pituitary gland; stimulates growth of eggs in females and sperm in males, 348–349, 397*t*, 401–402, 402*f*
Foramen, passage or opening through bone for nerves and blood vessels, 94
Formed elements, solid, cellular portion of blood; consists of erythrocytes, leukocytes, and platelets, 188
Fossa, shallow cavity or depression within or on surface of a bone, 94
Fovea capitis, 95*f*
Fovea centralis, area of retina that has sharpest vision, 474*f*, 475
Fracture (FX, Fx), injury to bone that causes it to break; named to describe type of damage to bone, 108–109, 108*f*, 109*f*, 117–118
Fraternal twins, twins that develop from two different ova fertilized by two different sperm; although twins, these siblings do not have identical DNA, 358
Free edge, exposed edge of a nail that is trimmed when nails become too long, 61, 61*f*
Frequency, greater than normal occurrence in urge to urinate, without increase in total daily volume of urine; frequency is indication of inflammation of bladder or urethra, 324
Frontal bone, forehead bone of skull, 95, 97, 97*f*, 97*t*
Frontal lobe, one of four cerebral hemisphere lobes; controls motor functions, 429–430, 431*f*
Frontal plane, vertical plane that divides body into front (anterior or ventral) and back (posterior or dorsal) sections; also called *coronal plane*, 37–38, 37*f*
Frontal section, sectional view of body produced by cut along frontal plane; also called *coronal section*, 37–38, 37*f*
Frozen section (FS), thin piece of tissue is cut from frozen specimen for rapid examination under a microscope, 77
Full-term pregnancy, 353*f*
Functional bowel disorder. *See* Irritable bowel syndrome
Functional residual capacity (FRC), air that remains in lungs after normal exhalation has taken place, 235*t*
Fundus, domed upper portion of organ such as stomach or uterus, 275, 275*f*, 348*f*, 350, 350*f*, 353*f*
Fungal scrapings, scrapings, taken with curette or scraper, of tissue from lesions are placed on a growth medium and examined under a microscope to identify fungal growth, 77
Fungi, organisms found in Kingdom Fungi; some are capable of causing disease in humans, such as yeast infections or histoplasmosis, 205
Furuncle, staphylococcal skin abscess with redness, pain, and swelling; also called a *boil*, 75

G

Gait training, assisting patient to learn to walk again or how to use assistive device (such as crutches or walker) to walk, 132
Gallbladder (GB), small organ located just under liver; functions to store bile produced by liver; releases bile into duodenum through common bile duct, 270, 279–280, 279*f*
Gambling disorder, addictive disorder in which patient is unable to control urge to gamble, 457
Gametes, reproductive sex cells—ova and sperm, 399
Gamma globulin, protein component of blood containing antibodies that help to resist infection, 188
Ganglion, knotlike mass of nerve tissue located outside brain and spinal cord, 433–434
Ganglion cyst, cyst that forms on tendon sheath, usually on hand, wrist, or ankle, 131
Gangrene, necrosis of skin usually due to deficient blood supply, 72
Gastralgia, stomach pain, 285
Gastrectomy, surgical removal of stomach, 297
Gastric, pertaining to stomach, 282
Gastric banding, laparoscopic bariatric surgical procedure; places restrictive band around top portion of stomach; results in being able to eat only small meals and losing weight, 297
Gastric bypass, bariatric surgical procedure; divides stomach into small upper portion and larger lower portion; small intestine is connected to small upper portion, bypassing large stomach; limits amount of food eaten, 297
Gastric carcinoma, cancerous tumor of stomach, 286

Gastric stapling, procedure that closes off large section of stomach with rows of staples; results in much smaller stomach to assist very obese patients to lose weight, 297
Gastritis, inflammation of stomach that can result in pain, tenderness, nausea, and vomiting, 286
Gastroenteritis, inflammation of stomach and small intestine, 286
Gastroenterologist, physician specialized in treating diseases and conditions of gastrointestinal tract, 284
Gastroenterology, branch of medicine specializing in conditions of gastrointestinal system, 34*t*, 284
Gastroesophageal reflux disease (GERD), acid from stomach backs up into esophagus, causing inflammation and pain, 286
Gastroesophageal sphincter. *See* Cardiac sphincter
Gastrointestinal, pertaining to the stomach and intestines, 282
Gastrointestinal system (GI), digests food and absorbs nutrients; organs include oral cavity, pharynx, esophagus, stomach, small and large intestines, liver, gallbladder, pancreas, and salivary glands; also called *digestive system*, 34*t*, 270
Gastroscope, instrument for viewing inside stomach, 294
Gastroscopy, flexible gastroscope is passed through mouth and down esophagus in order to visualize inside stomach; used to diagnose peptic ulcers and gastric carcinoma, 294
Gastrostomy, surgical creation of gastric fistula or opening through abdominal wall; opening is used to place food into stomach when esophagus is not entirely open (esophageal stricture), 297
Gavage, using nasogastric tube to place liquid nourishment directly into stomach, 295
Gender dysphoria, person identifies as gender contrary to the gender of his or her birth, 455
General anesthesia (GA), produces a loss of consciousness including absence of pain sensation; administered to patient by either intravenous or inhalation method; patient's vital signs must be carefully monitored when in use, 448
General anxiety disorder, feeling dread in absence of clearly identifiable stress trigger, 453
General hospital, hospital that typically provides services to diagnose (laboratory, diagnostic imaging) and treat (surgery, medications, therapy) diseases for a short period of time; in addition, usually provides emergency and obstetrical care; also called *acute care hospital*, 15*t*
Generic name, recognized and accepted official name for a drug; each drug has only one generic name; this name is not subject to trademark, so may be used by any pharmaceutical manufacturer; also called *nonproprietary name*, 16
Genital herpes, spreading skin disease that can appear like a blister or vesicle, caused by sexually transmitted virus, 379
Genital warts, growths and elevations of warts on genitalia of both males and females that can lead to cancer of cervix in females, 379
Genitalia, male and female reproductive organs, 348
Genitourinary (GU) **system,** organs of the urinary system and female or male sexual organs, 314, 373
German measles (rubella), 74
Gestation, length of time from conception to birth, generally nine months; calculated from first day of last menstrual period, with a range of from 259 days to 280 days, 353
Gigantism, excessive development of body due to overproduction of growth hormone by pituitary gland; opposite of dwarfism, 410
Gingiva, tissue around teeth; also called *gums*, 270–271, 271*f*, 272*f*, 273*f*
Gingival, pertaining to gums, 282
Gingivectomy, surgical removal of gum tissue that has pulled away from the teeth, 295
Gingivitis, inflammation of gums characterized by swelling, redness, and tendency to bleed, 286
Glands, organs of body that release secretions; exocrine glands, like sweat glands, release their secretions into ducts; endocrine glands, such as thyroid gland, release their hormones directly into bloodstream, 396, 428
  adrenal, 396, 398–399, 408–409
  apocrine, 62
  bulbourethral, 373, 373*f*, 375
  lymph, 202, 203, 203*t*, 204*f*
  parathyroid, 396, 397*t*, 400, 401*f*, 409–410
  pineal, 396, 397*t*, 400, 401*f*
  pituitary, 396, 401–402, 401*f*, 402*f*, 410
  prostate, 316*f*, 317*f*, *373*, 373*f*, 375, 378
  salivary, 270, 278, 279*f*
  sebaceous, 58, 59*f*, 61*f*, 62, 476
  sudoriferous, 62
  sweat, 58, 59*f*, 62
  thymus, 202, 205, 205*f*, 396, 397*t*, 403, 404*f*, 410–411
  thyroid, 231*f*, 396, 397*t*, 401*f*, 403–404, 404*f*, 411
Glans penis, larger and softer tip of penis; protected by covering called *prepuce* or *foreskin*, 374
Glaucoma, increase in intraocular pressure that, if untreated, may result in atrophy (wasting away) of optic nerve and blindness; treated with medication and surgery; increased risk of developing in persons over 60 years of age, people of African ancestry, persons who have sustained serious eye injury, and anyone with family history of diabetes or glaucoma, 482
Globulins, one type of protein found dissolved in plasma, 188
Glomerular, pertaining to a glomerulus, 322
Glomerular capsule, also called *Bowman's capsule*; part of renal corpuscle; double-walled cuplike structure that encircles glomerulus; within filtration stage of urine production, waste products filtered from blood enter Bowman's capsule as glomerular filtrate, 315, 316*f*
Glomerular filtrate, product of filtration stage of urine production; water, electrolytes, nutrients, wastes, and toxins that are filtered from blood passing through glomerulus; filtrate enters Bowman's capsule, 318–319, 318*f*
Glomerulonephritis, inflammation of kidney (primarily of glomerulus); since glomerular membrane is inflamed,

it becomes more permeable and will allow protein and blood cells to enter filtrate; results in protein in urine (proteinuria) and hematuria, 325

Glomerulus, ball of capillaries encased by Bowman's capsule; within filtration stage of urine production, wastes filtered from blood leave glomerulus capillaries and enter Bowman's capsule, 315, 316*f*

Glossal, pertaining to tongue, 282

Glossopharyngeal nerve, 434*t*

Glottis, opening between vocal cords; air passes through glottis as it moves through larynx; changing tension of vocal cords changes size of opening, 232

Glucagon, hormone secreted by pancreas; stimulates liver to release glucose into blood, 280, 397*t* 399–400, 400*f*

Glucocorticoids, group of hormones secreted by adrenal cortex; regulate carbohydrate levels in body; cortisol is an example, 396*t*, 398

Glucometer, device for measuring level of glucose in bloodstream, 413

Glucose, form of sugar used by cells of body to make energy; transported to cells in blood, 188

Glucose tolerance test (GTT), determines blood sugar level; a measured dose of glucose is given to patient either orally or intravenously; blood samples are then drawn at certain intervals to determine ability of patient to utilize glucose; used for diabetic patients to determine their insulin response to glucose, 412

Gluteal, pertaining to buttocks, 39*f*

Gluteal region, refers to buttock region of body, 38*t*, 39*f*

Gluteus maximus, muscle named for its size and location; gluteus means "rump area" and maximus means "large," 124

Glycosuria, presence of sugar in the urine, 324, 407

Goiter, enlargement of thyroid gland, 411, 411*f*

Gonadotropins, general name for two anterior pituitary hormones, follicle-stimulating hormone and luteinizing hormone, 397*t*, 401–402, 402*f*

Gonads, organs responsible for producing sex cells; female gonads are ovaries, and they produce ova; male gonads are testes, and they produce sperm, 399

Gonorrhea, sexually transmitted inflammation of mucous membranes of either sex; can be passed on to infant during birth process, 379

Gout, type of arthritis; usually in first metatarsophalangeal joint; caused by high uric acid blood level, 113

Graft versus host disease (GVHD), serious complication of bone marrow transplant; immune cells from donor bone marrow (graft) attack recipient's (host's) tissues, 212

Grand mal seizure. *See* Tonic-clonic seizure

Granulocytes, granular polymorphonuclear leukocytes; three types: neutrophil, eosinophil, and basophil, 189, 189*t*

Graves' disease, condition resulting in overactivity of thyroid gland and can result in crisis situation; a type of *hyperthyroidism*, 411

Gray matter, tissue within central nervous system; consists of unsheathed or uncovered nerve cell bodies and dendrites, 428–429

Great saphenous vein, 158*f*

Greenstick fracture, fracture in which there is incomplete break; one side of bone is broken and other side is bent; commonly found in children due to their softer and more pliable bone structure, 109

Growth hormone (GH), hormone secreted by anterior pituitary that stimulates growth of body, 397*t*, 401–402, 402*f*

Guillain-Barré syndrome, disease of nervous system in which nerves lose their myelin covering; may be caused by autoimmune reaction; characterized by loss of sensation and/or muscle control in arms and legs; symptoms then move toward trunk and may even result in paralysis of diaphragm, 444

Gums, tissue around teeth; also called *gingiva*, 270–271, 271*f*

Gut, name for continuous muscular tube that stretches between mouth and anus; also called *alimentary canal*, 270

Gynecologist, physician specialized in treating conditions and diseases of female reproductive system, 359

Gynecology (GYN, gyn), branch of medicine specializing in conditions of female reproductive system, 34*t*, 359

Gynecomastia, development of breast tissue in males; may be symptom of adrenal feminization, 407

Gyri, convoluted, elevated portions of cerebral cortex; separated by fissures or sulci; singular is *gyrus*, 429–430, 431*f*

H

***H. pylori* antibody test,** used to diagnose *H. pylori* infection causing peptic ulcer disease; may be performed on stool, breath, or tissue sample, 292

H_2-receptor antagonist, blocks production of stomach acids, 299

Hair, structure in integumentary system, 58, 59*f*, 60, 61*f*, 75

Hair follicle, cavities in dermis that contain hair root; hair grows longer from root, 60, 61*f*

Hair root, deeper cells that divide to grow hair longer, 60, 61*f*

Hair shaft, older keratinized cells that form most of length of a hair, 60, 61*f*

Hallucination, perception of something that is not there; may be visual, auditory, gustatory, or tactile, 456

Hammer. *See* Malleus

Hard palate, 95*t*, 231*f*, 267*f*, 272*f*

Hashimoto's thyroiditis, chronic form of thyroiditis, 411

Head, large ball-shaped end of a bone; may be separated from shaft of bone by area called *neck*, 94

Healthcare-associated infection (HAI), infection acquired from patients or healthcare workers; also called *nosocomial infection*, 207

Healthcare settings, 15, 15*t*

Health Insurance Portability and Accountability Act (HIPAA), 16

Health Maintenance Organization (HMO), organization that contracts with group of physicians and other healthcare workers to provide care exclusively for its members, 15*t*

Herpes zoster virus, virus responsible for causing shingles, 445, 445*f*

Hertz (Hz), measurement of frequency or pitch of sound; lowest pitch on audiogram is 250 Hz; measurement can go as high as 8000 Hz, which is highest pitch measured, 501

Hesitancy, decrease in force of urine stream, often with difficulty initiating flow; often a symptom of blockage along urethra, such as enlarged prostate gland, 324

Heterograft, skin graft from animal of another species (usually a pig) to a human; also called a *xenograft*, 6, 78

Hiatal hernia, protrusion of stomach through diaphragm and extending into thoracic cavity; gastroesophageal reflux disease is a common symptom, 287, 287*f*

Hilum, controlled entry/exit point of an organ such as kidney or lung, 234, 314, 315*f*

Hipbone, 99*f*

Hirsutism, excessive hair growth over body, 66, 407

Histology, study of tissues, 28

Histoplasma capsulatum, fungus responsible for causing histoplasmosis, 246

Histoplasmosis, pulmonary infection caused by fungus *Histoplasma capsulatum* found in dust and in droppings of pigeons and chickens, 246

History and physical, medical record document written or dictated by admitting physician; details patient's history, results of physician's examination, initial diagnoses, and physician's plan of treatment, 14*t*

HIV antigen/antibody immunoassay, blood test for HIV infection; antigens are present shortly after exposure; antibodies appear 2–8 weeks after exposure, 214

Hives, appearance of wheals as part of allergic reaction, 210

Hodgkin's disease (HD), also called *Hodgkin's lymphoma*; cancer of lymphatic cells found in concentration in lymph nodes, 211

Hodgkin's lymphoma. *See* Hodgkin's disease

Holter monitor, portable ECG monitor worn by patient for a period of a few hours to a few days to assess heart and pulse activity as person goes through activities of daily living, 170

Home health care, agencies that provide nursing, therapy, personal care, or housekeeping services in patient's own home, 15*t*

Homeostasis, steady state or state of balance within body; kidneys assist in maintaining homeostasis, 318, 396

Homologous transfusion, replacement of blood by transfusion of blood received from another person, 197

Hordeolum, a stye (or sty), a small purulent inflammatory infection of a sebaceous gland of eye, treated with hot compresses and surgical incision, 485

Horizontal plane, divides body into upper (superior) and lower (inferior) sections; also called *transverse plane*, 37–38, 37*f*

Hormonal contraception, use of hormones to block ovulation and prevent contraception; may be in pill form, patch or implant under skin, or injection, 367

Hormone, chemical substance secreted by endocrine gland; enters bloodstream and is carried to target tissue; hormones work to control functioning of target tissue; given to replace loss of natural hormones or to treat disease by stimulating hormonal effects, 396, 396*t*–397*t*

Hormone replacement therapy (HRT), artificial replacement of hormones in patient unable to produce sufficient hormones; example is estrogen replacement in menopausal women, 369, 413

Hospice, organized group of healthcare workers who provide supportive treatment to dying patients and their families, 15*t*

Housemaid's knee. *See* Prepatellar bursitis

Human growth hormone therapy, therapy with human growth hormone in order to stimulate skeletal growth; used to treat children with abnormally short stature, 414

Human immunodeficiency virus (HIV), virus that causes AIDS; also known as a *retrovirus*, 212, 212*f*, 379

Human papillomavirus (HPV), responsible for causing some cases of cervical cancer, 360

Human papillomavirus (HPV) **DNA test,** examination of sample of cervical tissue, obtained by swabbing or scraping cervix, to determine infection by virus responsible for cervical cancer, 364

Humanistic psychotherapy, form of psychological counseling in which therapist does not delve into patients' past; it is believed that patients can learn how to use their own internal resources to deal with their problems, 458

Humeral, pertaining to humerus or upper arm bone, 105

Humerus, upper arm bone in upper extremity, 91*f*, 93*f*, 98, 99*f*, 100, 100*f*, 100*t*

Humoral immunity, responds to antigens, such as bacteria and foreign agents, by producing antibodies; also called *antibody-mediated immunity*, 206

Humpback. *See* Kyphosis

Hunchback. *See* Kyphosis

Hyaline membrane disease (HMD). *See* Infant respiratory distress syndrome

Hydrocele, accumulation of fluid within testes, 377

Hydrocephalus, accumulation of cerebrospinal fluid within ventricles of brain, causing head to be enlarged; treated by creating artificial shunt for fluid to leave brain, 442, 442*f*

Hydrochloric acid (HCl), acid secreted by stomach lining; aids in digestion, 275

Hydronephrosis, distention of pelvis due to urine collecting in kidney resulting from obstruction, 326

Hydrotherapy, using water for treatment purposes, 132

Hymen, thin membranous tissue that covers external vaginal opening or orifice; broken during first sexual encounter of female; can also be broken prematurely by use of tampons or during some sports activities, 351, 351*f*

Hymenectomy, surgical removal of hymen, 368

Hyoid bone, single, U-shaped bone suspended in neck between mandible and larynx; a point of attachment for swallowing and speech muscles, 95, 97

I

Iliac, pertaining to ilium; one of pelvic bones, 105
Ilium, one of three bones that form the os coxae or innominate bone of the pelvis, 91*f*, 98, 100, 101*f*, 101*t*
Immune response, ability of lymphocytes to respond to specific antigens, 205–207, 206*f*
Immunity, body's ability to defend itself against pathogens, 205–207
immune response, 205–207, 206*f*
standard precautions, 207
Immunization, providing protection against communicable diseases by stimulating immune system to produce antibodies against that disease; also called *vaccination*, 205–206
Immunocompromised, having immune system unable to respond properly to pathogens, 212
Immunodeficiency disorder. *See* Immunocompromised
Immunoglobulin (Ig), antibodies secreted by B cells; all antibodies are immunoglobulins; assist in protecting body and its surfaces from invasion of bacteria; for example, immunoglobulin IgA in colostrum, first milk from mother, helps to protect newborn from infection, 206
Immunologist, physician who specializes in treating infectious diseases and other disorders of immune system, 209
Immunology, branch of medicine specializing in conditions of lymphatic and immune systems, 33*t*, 209
Immunosuppressants, substances that block certain actions of immune system; required to prevent rejection of transplanted organ, 215
Immunotherapy, boosting or strengthening of patient's immune system in order to treat disease, 215
Impacted fracture, fracture in which bone fragments are pushed into each other, 109
Impetigo, highly contagious staphylococcal skin infection, most commonly occurring on faces of children; begins as blisters that then rupture and dry into thick, yellow crust, 73, 73*f*
Implant, prosthetic device placed in jaw to which a tooth or denture may be anchored, 295
Implantable cardioverter-defibrillator (ICD), device implanted in heart that delivers electrical shock to restore normal heart rhythm; particularly useful for persons who experience ventricular fibrillation, 171
Incision and drainage (I&D), making incision to create opening for drainage of material such as pus, 78
Incisors, biting teeth in very front of mouth that function to cut food into smaller pieces; humans have eight incisors, 271*f*, 272, 273*f*
Incus, one of three ossicles of middle ear; also called *anvil*, 495, 495*f*
Infant respiratory distress syndrome (IRDS), lung condition most commonly found in premature infants characterized by tachypnea and respiratory grunting; also called *hyaline membrane disease* (HMD) and *respiratory distress syndrome of the newborn*, 246
Infarct, area of tissue within organ that undergoes necrosis (death) following loss of blood supply, 162
Inferior, directional term meaning toward feet or tail, or below; akin to *caudal*, 43*f*, 43*t*
Inferior vena cava, branch of vena cava that drains blood from abdomen and lower body, 152, 153*f*, 158*f*, 398*f*
Infertility, inability to produce children; generally defined as no pregnancy after properly timed intercourse for one year, 363
Inflammation, tissue response to injury from pathogens or physical agents; characterized by redness, pain, swelling, and feeling hot to touch, 210, 210*f*
Inflammatory bowel disease (IBD). *See* Ulcerative colitis
Influenza (flu), viral infection of respiratory system characterized by chills, fever, body aches, and fatigue; commonly called the *flu*, 246
Informed consent, medical record document, voluntarily signed by patient, or responsible party, that clearly describes purpose, methods, procedures, benefits, and risks of diagnostic or treatment procedure, 14*t*
Inguinal, pertaining to groin area; there is a collection of lymph nodes in this region that drain each leg, 209
Inguinal hernia, hernia or protrusion of intestine into inguinal region of body, 289, 289*f*
Inguinal nodes, 203*t*, 204*f*
Inhalation, (1) to breathe air into lungs; also called *inspiration*; (2) to introduce drugs into body by breathing them in, 45, 46*t*, 230
Inhalation anesthesia, general anesthesia administered by breathing it in, 448
Innate immunity. *See* Natural immunity
Inner ear, innermost section of ear; contains cochlea, semicircular canals, saccule, and utricle, 494, 494*f*, 495, 496*f*, 500
Inner ear infection. *See* Labyrinthitis
Innominate bone, also called *os coxae* or *hipbone*; pelvis portion of lower extremity; consists of ilium, ischium, and pubis and unites with sacrum and coccyx to form pelvis, 98, 100
Insertion, attachment of skeletal muscle to more movable bone in joint, 124, 125*f*
Insomnia disorder, sleeping disorder characterized by marked inability to fall asleep, 456
Inspiration. *See* Inhalation
Inspiratory capacity (IC), volume of air inhaled after normal exhale, 235*t*
Inspiratory reserve volume (IRV), air that can be forcibly inhaled after normal respiration has taken place; also called *complemental air*, 235*t*
Insulin, hormone secreted by pancreas; regulates level of sugar in bloodstream; the more insulin present in blood, the lower blood sugar will be, 280, 397*t*, 399–400, 400*f*, 414
Insulin-dependent diabetes mellitus (IDDM), also called *type 1 diabetes mellitus*; develops early in life when pancreas stops insulin production; people with IDDM must take daily insulin injections, 409
Insulinoma, tumor of islets of Langerhans cells of pancreas that secretes excessive amount of insulin, 409
Integument, another term for skin, 58
Integumentary system, skin and its appendages including sweat glands, oil glands, hair, and nails;

Ischemia, localized and temporary deficiency of blood supply due to obstruction of circulation, 162
Ischial, pertaining to ischium, one of pelvic bones, 105
Ischium, one of three bones forming os coxae or innominate bone of pelvis, 91*f*, 98, 100, 101*f*, 101*t*
Islets of Langerhans, regions within pancreas that secrete insulin and glucagon; also called *pancreatic islets*, 399–400, 400*f*
Isthmus, 404*f*

J

Jaundice, yellow cast to skin, mucous membranes, and whites of eyes caused by deposit of bile pigment from too much bilirubin in blood; bilirubin is a waste product produced when worn-out red blood cells are broken down; may be symptom of disorders such as gallstones blocking common bile duct or carcinoma of liver, 285
Jejunal, pertaining to jejunum, 282
Jejunostomy, 277
Jejunum, middle portion of small intestine; site of nutrient absorption, 275–276, 276*f*
Joint, point at which two bones meet; provides flexibility, 92, 101–102, 102*f*, 113–114, 114*f*
Joint capsule, elastic capsule that encloses synovial joints, 101, 102, 102*f*
Jugular vein, 158*f*

K

Kaposi's sarcoma (KS), form of skin cancer frequently seen in acquired immunodeficiency syndrome (AIDS) patients; consists of brownish-purple papules that spread from skin and metastasize to internal organs, 73, 212
Keloid, formation of scar after injury or surgery resulting in raised, thickened red area, 73, 73*f*
Keratin, hard protein substance produced by body; found in hair and nails, and filling inside of epidermal cells, 58, 60
Keratitis, inflammation of cornea, 483
Keratometer, instrument to measure cornea, 486
Keratometry, measurement of curvature of cornea using instrument called a *keratometer*, 487
Keratoplasty, surgical repair of cornea (corneal transplant), 488
Keratosis, overgrowth and thickening of epithelium, 73
Ketoacidosis, acidosis due to excess of ketone bodies (waste products); serious condition requiring immediate treatment as it may result in death for diabetic patient if not reversed, 409
Ketones, waste products in the bloodstream, 315, 320*t*
Ketonuria, ketones in urine, 324
Kidneys, two organs located in lumbar region of back behind parietal peritoneum; under muscles of back, just a little above waist; have concave or depressed area that gives them bean-shaped appearance; center of this concavity is called *hilum*, 313*f*, 314–315, 315*f*, 318
Kidneys, ureters, bladder (KUB), X-ray taken of abdomen demonstrating kidneys, ureters, and bladder without using any contrast dye; also called *flat-plate abdomen*, 329
Kinesiology, study of movement, 129
Kissing disease. *See* Mononucleosis
Kleptomania, impulse control disorder in which patient is unable to refrain from stealing, 454
Kyphosis, abnormal increase in outward curvature of thoracic spine; also known as *hunchback* or *humpback*, 111, 112*f*

L

Labial, pertaining to the lips, 283
Labia majora, outer folds of skin that serves as protection for female external genitalia and urethral meatus, 348*f*, 351, 351*f*
Labia minora, inner folds of skin that serve as protection for female external genitalia and urethral meatus, 348*f*, 351, 351*f*
Labor, period of time beginning with uterine contractions and ending with birth of baby; there are three stages: dilation, expulsion, and placental stage, 354, 355*f*
Labyrinth, refers to inner ear; several fluid-filled cavities within temporal bone; labyrinth consists of cochlea, vestibule, and three semicircular canals; hair cells called *organ of Corti* line inner ear; hair cells change sound vibrations to electrical impulses and send impulses to brain via vestibulocochlear nerve, 494*f*, 495
Labyrinthectomy, surgical removal of labyrinth, 503
Labyrinthitis, labyrinth inflammation, 500
Labyrinthotomy, incision in labyrinth, 503
Laceration, torn or jagged wound; incorrectly used to describe a cut, 73
Lacrimal, pertaining to tears, 480
Lacrimal apparatus, consists of lacrimal gland, lacrimal canals, and nasolacrimal duct, 474, 474*f*, 477, 477*f*, 485
Lacrimal bone, facial bone, 95, 97, 97*f*, 97*t*
Lacrimal canals, located in inner corner of eye socket; collect tears and drain them into lacrimal sac, 477, 477*f*
Lacrimal gland, located in outer corner of each eyelid; washes anterior surface of eye with fluid called *tears*, 477, 477*f*
Lactation, function of secreting milk after childbirth from breasts or mammary glands, 352
Lacteals, lymphatic vessels in intestines that serve to absorb fats from diet, 202
Lactic, pertaining to milk, 358
Lactiferous ducts, carry milk from milk-producing glands to nipple, 352, 352*f*
Lactiferous glands, milk-producing glands in breast, 352, 352*f*
Lactorrhea, discharge of milk, 362
Laminectomy, removal of portion of a vertebra in order to relieve pressure on spinal nerve, 117, 449

Laparoscope, instrument to view inside abdomen, 294, 365
Laparoscopic adrenalectomy, surgical removal of adrenal gland through small incision in abdomen and using endoscopic instruments, 413
Laparoscopic cholecystectomy, surgical removal of gallbladder using laparoscope, 297
Laparoscopy, instrument or scope is passed into abdominal wall through small incision; abdominal cavity is then examined for tumors and other conditions with this lighted instrument; also called *peritoneoscopy*, 294, 365, 365*f*
Laparotomy, incision into abdomen, 297, 368
Large intestine, part of alimentary canal of digestive system extending from ileocecal valve to anus; consists of cecum, colon, rectum, and anal canal; responsible primarily for reabsorption of water; material remaining in large intestine is *feces* ready for defecation, 270, 277, 277*f*, 288–290
Laryngeal, pertaining to larynx, 239
Laryngectomy, surgical removal of larynx; procedure is most frequently performed for surgical removal of cancer, 251
Laryngitis, inflammation of larynx causing difficulty in speaking, 244
Laryngopharynx, inferior section of pharynx; lies at same level in neck as larynx, 231–232, 231*f*, 272*f*, 274
Laryngoplasty, surgical repair of larynx, 252
Laryngoplegia, paralysis of voice box, 243
Laryngoscope, instrument to view larynx, 249
Laryngoscopy, examination of interior of larynx with lighted instrument called *laryngoscope*, 250
Larynx, also called *voice box*; respiratory system organ responsible for producing speech; located just below pharynx, 230, 231*f*, 232
Laser photocoagulation, use of laser beam to destroy very small precise areas of the retina; may be used to treat retinal detachment or macular degeneration, 488
Laser therapy, removal of skin lesions and birthmarks using laser beam that emits intense heat and power at a close range; laser converts frequencies of light into one small, powerful beam, 78
Laser-assisted in situ keratomileusis (LASIK), correction of myopia using laser surgery to remove corneal tissue, 488, 488*f*
Lateral (lat), directional term meaning to the side, 43*f*, 44*t*
Lateral epicondylitis, inflammation of muscle attachment to lateral epicondyle of elbow; often caused by strongly gripping; commonly called *tennis elbow*, 130
Lateral view, positioning patient so that side of body faces X-ray machine, 40*f*, 43*f*, 410*f*
Lavage, using NG tube to wash out stomach, 296
Laxative, mild cathartic, 299
Lazy eye. *See* Amblyopia
Left atrium, 12, 148*f*, 150*f*, 152, 153*f*
Left coronary artery, 156*f*
Left hypochondriac, anatomical division of abdomen, left side of upper row, 41*t*
Left inguinal, anatomical division of abdomen, left side of lower row, 41*t*
Left lower quadrant (LLQ), clinical division of abdomen; contains portions of small and large intestines, left ovary and uterine (fallopian) tube, and left ureter, 42*t*
Left lumbar, anatomical division of abdomen, left side of middle row, 41*t*
Left upper quadrant (LUQ), clinical division of abdomen; contains left lobe of liver, spleen, left kidney, stomach, portion of pancreas, and portions of small and large intestines, 42*t*
Left ventricle, 148*f*, 150*f*, 152, 153*f*, 156
Legally blind, describes person who has severely impaired vision; usually defined as having visual acuity of 20/200, 483
Legionnaires' disease, severe, often fatal bacterial infection characterized by pneumonia and liver and kidney damage; named after people who came down with it at American Legion convention in 1976, 246
Lens, transparent structure behind pupil and iris; functions to bend light rays so they land on retina, 474*f*, 475, 478*f*
Lesion, general term for wound, injury, or abnormality, 66
Leukemia, cancer located in red bone marrow tissue responsible for producing white blood cells; results in large number of abnormal and immature leukocytes circulating in bloodstream, 195
Leukocytes, also called *white blood cells* (WBCs); group of several different types of cells that provide protection against invasion of bacteria and other foreign material; able to leave bloodstream and search out foreign invaders (bacteria, viruses, and toxins), where they perform phagocytosis, 188–189, 189*f*, 189*t*, 195
Leukocytic, pertaining to white blood cells, 192
Leukocytosis, too many white blood cells, 195
Leukoderma, disappearance of pigment from skin in patches, causing milk-white appearance; also called *vitiligo*, 66
Leukopenia, too few white (cells), 195
Leukorrhea, whitish or yellowish vaginal discharge, 360
Ligaments, very strong bands of connective tissue that bind bones together at a joint, 92
Ligation and stripping, surgical treatment for varicose veins; damaged vein is tied off (ligation) and removed (stripping), 172
Lingual, pertaining to the tongue, 283
Lingual tonsils, tonsils located on very posterior section of tongue as it joins with pharynx, 205, 231–232, 272*f*
Lipocytes, medical term for cells that contain fat molecules, 60
Lipoma, fatty tumor that generally does not metastasize, 66
Liposuction, removal of fat beneath skin by means of suction, 78
Lips, anterior opening of oral cavity, 270–271, 271*f*, 272*f*
Lithium, special category of drug used successfully to calm patients who suffer from bipolar disorder, 458
Lithotomy, surgical incision to remove kidney stones, 331

Lithotripsy, physical destruction of stone in urinary system by crushing or sound waves, 331
Liver, large organ located in right upper quadrant of abdomen; serves many functions in body; digestive system role includes producing bile, processing absorbed nutrients, and detoxifying harmful substances, 270, 279, 279*f*
Liver transplant, transplant of a liver from a donor, 297
Lobar, pertaining to a lobe (of the lung), 239
Lobe, ear, 494, 494*f*
Lobectomy, surgical removal of a lobe from an organ, such as a lung; often treatment of choice for lung cancer; may also be removal of one lobe of thyroid gland, 252, 413
Lobes, subdivisions of organ such as lungs or brain, 234, 234*f*
Local anesthesia, substance that produces a loss of sensation in one localized part of body; patient remains conscious when using this type of anesthetic; administered either topically or via subcutaneous route, 448
Long bone, type of bone longer than it is wide; examples include femur, humerus, and phalanges, 92, 93*f*
Longitudinal section, internal view of body produced by lengthwise slice along long axis of structure, 37–38, 37*f*
Long-term care facility, facility that provides long-term care for patients who need extra time to recover from illness or accident before they return home or for persons who can no longer care for themselves; also called a *nursing home*, 15*t*
Loop of Henle, portion of renal tubule; also called *nephron loop*, 315, 316*f*
Lordosis, abnormal increase in forward curvature of lumbar spine; also known as *swayback*, 112, 112*f*
Lower esophageal sphincter, also called *cardiac sphincter* or *gastroesophageal sphincter*; prevents food and gastric juices from backing up into esophagus, 275, 275*f*
Lower extremity (LE), the leg, 98, 99*f*
Lower gastrointestinal series (lower GI series), X-ray image of colon and rectum is taken after administration of barium by enema; also called *barium enema*, 293, 293*f*
Lumbar, pertaining to five low back vertebrae, 105
Lumbar puncture (LP), puncture with needle into lumbar area (usually fourth intervertebral space) to withdraw fluid for examination and for injection of anesthesia; also called *spinal puncture* or *spinal tap*, 448, 448*f*
Lumbar vertebrae, five vertebrae in low back region, 91*f*, 95, 97, 98*f*, 98*t*
Lumbosacral plexus, 435*f*
Lumen, space, cavity, or channel within tube or tubular organ or structure in body, 155
Lumpectomy, surgical removal of only a breast tumor and tissue immediately surrounding it, 368
Lung volumes/capacities, 235, 235*t*
Lungs, major organs of respiration; consist of air passageways, bronchi and bronchioles, and air sacs, or alveoli; gas exchange takes place within alveoli, 230, 234, 234*f*, 235
Lunula, lighter-colored, half-moon region at base of a nail, 61, 61*f*
Luteinizing hormone (LH), secreted by anterior pituitary; regulates function of male and female gonads and plays a role in releasing ova in females, 348–349, 397*t*, 401–402, 402*f*
Lymph, clear, transparent, colorless fluid found in lymphatic vessels, 202
Lymph glands. *See* Lymph nodes
Lymph nodes, small organs in lymphatic system that filter bacteria and other foreign organisms from body fluids; commonly referred to as *lymph glands*, 202, 203, 203*t*, 204*f*
Lymphadenectomy, surgical removal of a lymph node; usually done to test for malignancy, 215
Lymphadenitis, inflammation of lymph glands; referred to as *swollen glands*, 211
Lymphadenopathy, disease of lymph nodes, 211
Lymphangial, pertaining to lymph vessels, 209
Lymphangiogram, X-ray taken of lymph vessels after injection of dye; lymph flow through chest is traced, 214
Lymphangiography, process of taking X-ray of lymph vessels after injection of dye, 214
Lymphangioma, lymph vessel tumor, 211
Lymphatic, pertaining to lymph, 209
Lymphatic and immune system, 200–216
- abbreviations, 216
- adjective forms of anatomical terms, 209
- anatomy and physiology, 201*f*, 202–207, 202*f*, 203*f*, 203*t*, 204*f*, 206*f*
- diagnostic procedures, 214, 214*f*
- functions, 200
- immunity, 205–207
- lymph nodes, 202, 203, 203*t*, 204*f*
- pathology, 209–212, 210*f*, 211*f*, 212*f*
- pharmacology, 215
- spleen, 202, 203, 203*t*, 204*f*
- terminology, 200, 208
- therapeutic procedures, 214–215
- thymus gland, 202, 203, 203*t*, 204*f*
- tonsils, 202, 203, 203*t*, 204*f*

Lymphatic capillaries, smallest lymph vessels; collect excessive tissue fluid, 202
Lymphatic ducts, two largest vessels in lymphatic system, right lymphatic duct and thoracic duct, 202–203
Lymphatic system, helps body fight infection; organs include spleen, lymph vessels, and lymph nodes, 33*t*
Lymphatic vessels, extensive network of vessels throughout entire body; conduct lymph from tissue toward thoracic cavity, 202–203, 202*f*, 203*f*, 204*f*
Lymphedema, edema appearing in extremities due to obstruction of lymph flow through lymphatic vessels, 210
Lymphocyte (lymphs), agranulocyte white blood cell that provides protection through immune response, 189*f*, 189*t*
Lymphocytic, pertaining to a [white] cell formed in lymphatic tissue, 192

M

N

Nucleus, structure within a cell that contains DNA, 28, 29*f*
Nulligravida, woman who has never been pregnant, 359
Nullipara, woman who has never produced a viable baby, 359
Number prefixes, 7
Nurse, to breastfeed a baby, 352
Nurse's notes, medical record document that records patient's care throughout day; includes vital signs, treatment specifics, patient's response to treatment, and patient's condition, 14*t*
Nursing home, facility that provides long-term care for patients who need extra time to recover from illness or accident before they return home or for persons who can no longer care for themselves; also called *long-term care facility*, 15*t*
Nyctalopia, difficulty seeing in dim light; usually due to damaged rods; also called *night blindness*, 481
Nystagmus, jerky-appearing involuntary eye movement, 485

O

Obesity, having too much body fat leading to body weight that is above a healthy level; person whose weight interferes with normal activity and body function has *morbid obesity*, 285, 408
Oblique fracture, fracture at angle to bone, 109, 109*f*
Oblique muscles, oblique means "slanted"; two eye muscles are oblique muscles, 476, 476*f*
Obsessive-compulsive and related disorders, classification of psychiatric disorders in DSM-5 characterized by obsessive preoccupations and repetitive behaviors; caused by persistent thoughts, ideas, or impulses, 455
Obsessive-compulsive disorder (OCD), mental disorder in which person performs repetitive rituals in order to reduce anxiety, 455
Obstetrician, physician specializing in pregnancy and childbirth, 359
Obstetrics (OB), branch of medicine that treats women during pregnancy and childbirth, and immediately after childbirth, 34*t*, 359
Occipital bone, cranial bone, 95, 97, 97*f*, 97*t*
Occipital lobe, one of four cerebral hemisphere lobes; controls eyesight, 429–430, 431*f*
Occupational Safety and Health Administration (OSHA), federal agency that issued mandatory guidelines to ensure that all employees at risk of exposure to body fluids are provided with personal protective equipment, 207
Occupational therapist, healthcare professional that specializes in assisting persons to regain, develop, and improve skills important for independent functioning (activities of daily living), 129, 132*f*
Occupational therapy (OT), assists persons to regain, develop, and improve skills important for independent functioning (activities of daily living), specialist is *occupational therapist*, 129
Ocular, pertaining to eye, 480
Oculomotor nerve, 434*t*
Oculomycosis, condition of eye fungus, 484
Olfactory nerve, 434*t*
Oligomenorrhea, scanty menstrual flow, 360
Oligospermia, condition of having few sperm, 377
Oliguria, condition of scanty amount of urine, 324
Onychectomy, surgical removal of a nail, 78
Onychia, infected nailbed, 76
Onychomalacia, softening of nails, 67
Onychomycosis, abnormal condition of nail fungus, 76
Onychophagia, nail biting, 76
Oocyte, female sex cells or gametes produced in ovary; oocyte fuses with sperm to produce embryo; also called *ovum*, 348–349
Oogenesis, process of producing ova by the ovaries, 348
Oophorectomy, removal of an ovary, 368
Oophoritis, inflammation of an ovary, 360
Open fracture. *See* Compound fracture
Open reduction. *See* Reduction
Operative report, medical record report from surgeon detailing operation; includes pre- and postoperative diagnosis, specific details of surgical procedure itself, and how patient tolerated procedure, 14*t*
Ophthalmalgia, eye pain, 481
Ophthalmic, pertaining to eyes, 480
Ophthalmic decongestants, over-the-counter medications that constrict arterioles of eye, reduce redness and itching of conjunctiva, 490
Ophthalmologist, physician specialized in treating conditions and diseases of eye, 481
Ophthalmology (Ophth), branch of medicine specializing in condition of eye; physician is *ophthalmologist*, 36*t*, 474, 481
Ophthalmoplegia, paralysis of eye, 481
Ophthalmorrhagia, bleeding from the eye, 481
Ophthalmoscope, instrument to view inside eye, 487
Ophthalmoscopy, examination of interior of eyes using instrument called *ophthalmoscope*; pupil is dilated in order to see cornea, lens, and retina; identifies abnormalities in blood vessels of eye and some systemic diseases, 487, 487*f*
Opiates. *See* Narcotic analgesic
Opportunistic infections, infectious diseases associated with patients who have compromised immune systems and lowered resistance to infections and parasites, 212
Opposition, moves thumb away from palm; ability to move thumb into contact with other fingers, 126*t*
Optic, pertaining to eye, 480
Optical, pertaining to eye or vision, 480
Optic disk, area of retina associated with optic nerve; also called *blind spot*, 474*f*, 475, 475*f*
Optic nerve, second cranial nerve that carries impulses from retina to brain, 434*t*, 474, 474*f*, 477, 478*f*
Optician, grinds and fits corrective lenses and contacts as prescribed by physician or optometrist, 481
Optometer, instrument to measure vision, 487
Optometrist, doctor of optometry; provides care for eyes including examining eyes for diseases, assessing visual acuity, prescribing corrective lenses and eye treatments, and educating patients, 481
Optometry, process of measuring vision, 481

Oral, (1) pertaining to mouth; (2) administration of medication through mouth, 45, 45*t*, 283
Oral cavity, the mouth, 270–271, 271*f*, 272*f*, 286
Oral contraceptive pills (OCPs), birth control medication that uses low doses of female hormones to prevent conception by blocking ovulation, 369
Oral hypoglycemic agents, medication taken by mouth that causes decrease in blood sugar; not used for insulin-dependent patients; no proof that medication will prevent long-term complications of diabetes mellitus, 414
Oral surgeon, practitioner of oral surgery, 284
Oral surgery, branch of dentistry that uses surgical means to treat dental conditions; specialist is *oral surgeon*, 284
Orbit, opening in skull formed by portions of frontal, zygomatic, maxillary, ethmoid, sphenoid, lacrimal, and palatine bones; houses and protects eyeball, 474
Orchidectomy, surgical removal of one or both testes, 380
Orchidopexy, surgical fixation to move undescended testes into scrotum and attaching to prevent retraction, 380
Orchiectomy, surgical removal of one or both testes, 380
Orchioplasty, surgical repair of testes, 380
Orchiotomy, to cut into testes, 380
Orchitis, inflammation of a testis, 377
Organs, group of different types of tissue coming together to perform special functions; for example, heart contains muscular fibers, nerve tissue, and blood vessels, 27*f*, 28, 31, 32*t*–36*t*
Organ of Corti, sensory receptor hair cells lining cochlea; these cells change sound vibrations to electrical impulses and send impulses to brain via vestibulocochlear nerve, 495, 496*f*
Origin, attachment of skeletal muscle to less movable bone in joint, 124, 125*f*
Oropharynx, middle section of pharynx that receives food and drink from mouth, 231–232, 231*f*, 272*f*, 274
Orthodontic, pertaining to straight teeth, 272
Orthodontics, dental specialty concerned with straightening teeth, 284
Orthodontist, dental specialist in straightening teeth, 284
Orthopedic surgeon, physician specializing in surgical care of musculoskeletal system, 107
Orthopedic surgery, branch of medicine specializing in surgical treatments of musculoskeletal system, 32*t*
Orthopedics (Orth, ortho), branch of medicine specializing in diagnosis and treatment of conditions of musculoskeletal system, 32*t*, 107
Orthopedist, 107
Orthopnea, term to describe patient who needs to sit up straight in order to breathe comfortably, 243
Orthostatic hypotension, sudden drop in blood pressure person experiences when standing up suddenly, 162
Orthotics, healthcare profession specializing in making orthopedic appliances such as braces and splints; person skilled in making and adjusting these appliances is an *orthotist*, orthotic is the appliance, 107, 116
Orthotist, healthcare professional specializing in making orthopedic appliances such as braces and splints, 107
Os coxae, also called *innominate bone* or *hipbone*; pelvis portion of lower extremity; consists of ilium, ischium, and pubis and unites with sacrum and coccyx to form pelvis, 98, 100
Osseous tissue, bony tissue; one of hardest materials in body, 92
Ossicles, three small bones in middle ear; bones are incus, malleus, and stapes; ossicles amplify and conduct sound waves to inner ear, 495, 495*f*
Ossification, process of bone formation, 92
Ostealgia, bone pain, 107
Osteoarthritis (OA), type of arthritis resulting in degeneration of bones and joints, especially those bearing weight; also called *degenerative joint disease* (DJD), 113
Osteoblast, immature bone cell, 92
Osteochondroma, tumor composed of both cartilage and bony substance, 110
Osteoclasia, intentional breaking of bone in order to correct deformity, 117
Osteocyte, mature bone cell, 92
Osteogenic sarcoma, most common type of bone cancer; usually begins in osteocytes found at ends of long bones; also called *osteosarcoma*, 110
Osteoma, tumor found in bone tissue, 110
Osteomalacia, softening of bones caused by deficiency of calcium; thought to be caused by insufficient sunlight and vitamin D in children, 110
Osteomyelitis, inflammation of bone and bone marrow due to infection; can be difficult to treat, 111
Osteopathy, form of medicine that places great emphasis on musculoskeletal system and body system as a whole; manipulation is also used as part of treatment, 111
Osteoporosis, decrease in bone mass that results in thinning and weakening of bone with resulting fractures; bone becomes more porous, especially in spine and pelvis, 111
Osteotome, instrument to cut bone, 117
Osteotomy, surgical procedure that cuts into a bone, 117
Otalgia, ear pain, 499
Otic, pertaining to ear, 498
Otitis externa (OE), external ear infection; most commonly caused by fungus; also called *otomycosis* and commonly referred to as *swimmer's ear*, 499
Otitis media (OM), commonly referred to as *middle ear infection;* seen frequently in children; often preceded by upper respiratory infection, 500
Otolaryngology. *See* Otorhinolaryngology
Otology (Oto), study of ear, 494
Otomycosis, fungal infection of ear, usually in auditory canal, 500
Otoplasty, surgical repair of external ear, 504
Otopyorrhea, pus discharge from ear, 499
Otorhinolaryngologist, 240
Otorhinolaryngology (ENT), branch of medicine that treats conditions and diseases of ear, nose, and throat; also referred to as *ENT*, 33*t*, 36*t*, 240, 499

P

Pharyngoplasty, surgical repair of pharynx, 298
Pharyngoplegia, paralysis of pharynx, 270, 286
Pharynx, medical term for throat; passageway that conducts air from nasal cavity to trachea and also carries food and drink from mouth to esophagus; divided into three sections: nasopharynx, oropharynx, and laryngopharynx, 205, 231–232, 231*f*, 272*f*, 274, 286
Pheochromocytoma, usually benign tumor of adrenal medulla that secretes epinephrine; symptoms include anxiety, heart palpitations, dyspnea, profuse sweating, headache, and nausea, 409
Phimosis, narrowing of foreskin over glans penis that results in difficulty with hygiene; condition can lead to infection or difficulty with urination; treated with circumcision, surgical removal of foreskin, 378
Phlebitis, inflammation of a vein, 167
Phlebotomist, 196*f*
Phlebotomy, creating opening into vein to withdraw blood, 196, 196*f*
Phlegm, thick mucus secreted by membranes that line respiratory tract; called *sputum* when coughed through mouth; examined for color, odor, and consistency, 243
Phobias, type of anxiety disorder in which person has irrational fears; example is arachnophobia, fear of spiders, 453
Phonophoresis, use of ultrasound waves to introduce medication across skin into subcutaneous tissues, 132
Photophobia, strong sensitivity to bright light, 482
Photorefractive keratectomy (PRK), surgical use of laser to reshape cornea to correct errors of refraction, 489
Photosensitivity, condition in which skin reacts abnormally when exposed to light such as ultraviolet rays of sun, 68
Physiatrist, physician specializing in restoring function; primarily cares for patients with musculoskeletal and nervous system disorders, 129
Physical medicine, branch of medicine focused on restoring function; primarily cares for patients with musculoskeletal and nervous system disorders; physician is *physiatrist*, 129
Physical therapist, healthcare specialist in evaluating and treating disorders and rehabilitating people using physical methods such as heat, cold, massage, and exercise, 129
Physical therapy (PT), evaluation and treatment of disorders and rehabilitation of people using physical methods such as heat, cold, massage, and exercise; specialist is *physical therapist*, 129
Physician's Desk Reference (PDR), 17
Physician's offices, individual or groups of physicians providing diagnostic and treatment services in a private office setting rather than in a hospital, 15*t*
Physician's orders, medical record document that contains complete list of care, medications, tests, and treatments physician orders for patient, 14*t*
Physician's progress notes, part of patient's medical record; physician's daily record of patient's condition, results of physician's examinations, summary of test results, updated assessment and diagnoses, and further plans for patient's care, 14*t*
Pia mater, term means "soft mother"; this thin innermost meninges layer is applied directly to surface of brain, 433, 433*f*
Pineal, pertaining to pineal gland, 406
Pineal gland, gland in endocrine system that produces hormone called *melatonin*, 396, 397*t*, 400, 401*f*
Pinealectomy, surgical removal of pineal gland, 413
Pinna, also called *auricle*; external ear; functions to capture sound waves as they go past outer ear, 494, 494*f*
Pisse prophets, 314
Pituitary, pertaining to pituitary gland, 406
Pituitary anterior lobe, 397*t*
Pituitary gland, endocrine gland located behind optic nerve in brain; also called *master gland* since it controls functions of many other endocrine glands; is divided into two lobes: anterior and posterior; anterior pituitary gland secretes hormones that aid in controlling growth and stimulating thyroid gland, sexual glands, and adrenal cortex; posterior pituitary is responsible for antidiuretic hormone and oxytocin, 396, 401–402, 401*f*, 402*f*, 410
Pituitary posterior lobe, 397*t*
Placebo, inactive, harmless substance used to satisfy patient's desire for medication; also used in research when given to control group of persons in a study in which another group receives a drug; effect of placebo versus drug is then observed, 79
Placenta, also called *afterbirth*; organ attached to uterine wall composed of maternal and fetal tissues; oxygen, nutrients, carbon dioxide, and wastes are exchanged between mother and baby through placenta; baby is attached to placenta by way of umbilical cord, 353–354, 353*f*, 355*f*
Placenta previa, occurs when placenta is in lower portion of uterus and thus blocks birth canal, 363, 363*f*
Placental stage, third stage of labor, which takes place after delivery of infant; uterus resumes strong contractions and placenta detaches from uterine wall and is delivered through vagina, 354, 355*f*
Plantar flexion, bending sole of foot; pointing toes downward, 126*f*, 126*t*
Plaque, yellow, fatty deposit of lipids in artery, 162
Plasma, liquid portion of blood containing 90% water; remaining 10% consists of plasma proteins (serum albumin, serum globulin, fibrinogen, and prothrombin), inorganic substances (calcium, potassium, and sodium), organic components (glucose, amino acids, cholesterol), and waste products (urea, uric acid, ammonia, and creatinine), 188
Plasmapheresis, method of removing plasma from body without depleting formed elements; whole blood is removed and cells and plasma are separated; cells are returned to patient along with donor plasma transfusion, 197
Plasma proteins, found in plasma; includes serum albumin, serum globulin, fibrinogen, and prothrombin, 188

Plastic surgery, surgical specialty involved in repair, reconstruction, or improvement of body structures such as skin that are damaged, missing, or misshapen; physician is plastic surgeon, 32*t*, 65, 78
Platelet count, blood test to determine number of platelets in given volume of blood, 196
Platelets, cells responsible for coagulation of blood; also called *thrombocytes* and contain no hemoglobin, 189–190, 195
Pleura, protective double layer of serous membrane around lungs; parietal membrane is outer layer and visceral layer is inner membrane; secretes thin, watery fluid to reduce friction associated with lung movement, 40, 234
Pleural, pertaining to pleura, 239
Pleural cavity, cavity formed by serous membrane sac surrounding lungs, 40–41, 40*f*, 234
Pleural effusion, abnormal presence of fluid or gas in pleural cavity; physicians can detect presence of fluid by tapping chest (percussion) or listening with stethoscope (auscultation), 248
Pleural rub, grating sound made when two surfaces, such as pleural surfaces, rub together during respiration; caused when one of surfaces becomes thicker as a result of inflammation or other disease conditions; rub can be felt through fingertips when placed on chest wall or heard through stethoscope, 243
Pleurectomy, surgical removal of pleura, 252
Pleurisy, inflammation of pleura; also called *pleuritis*, 248
Pleuritis. *See* Pleurisy
Pleurocentesis, puncture of pleura to withdraw fluid from thoracic cavity in order to diagnose disease, 252
Pleurodynia, pleural pain, 243
Plural endings, 12
Pneumatic retinopexy, surgical injection of gas bubble into eye and positioning head so that bubble presses against area of detached retina, 489
Pneumoconiosis, condition resulting from inhaling environmental particles that become toxic, such as coal dust (anthracosis) or asbestos (asbestosis), 247
Pneumocystis pneumonia (PCP), pneumonia caused by fungus *Pneumocystis jiroveci*; opportunistic infection often seen in those with weakened immune systems, such as AIDS patients, 213
Pneumonectomy, surgical removal of an entire lung, 252
Pneumonia, inflammatory condition of lung, which can be caused by bacterial and viral infections, diseases, and chemicals, 247
Pneumothorax, collection of air or gas in pleural cavity, possibly resulting in collapse of lung, 248, 248*f*
Podiatrist, 107
Podiatry, healthcare profession specializing in diagnosis and treatment of disorders of feet and lower legs; healthcare professional is podiatrist, 107
Poliomyelitis, acute viral disease that causes inflammation of gray matter of spinal cord, resulting in paralysis in some cases; has been brought under almost total control through vaccinations, 443
Polyarteritis, inflammation of many arteries, 167
Polycystic kidneys, formation of multiple cysts (pouches) within kidney tissue; results in destruction of normal kidney tissue and uremia, 326, 326*f*
Polycythemia vera, production of too many red blood cells in bone marrow, 194
Polydipsia, condition of having excessive amount of thirst, such as in diabetes, 408
Polymyositis, disease involving muscle inflammation and weakness from unknown cause, 130
Polyneuritis, inflammation of many nerves, 445
Polyp, small tumor with pedicle or stem attachment; commonly found in vascular organs such as nose, uterus, and rectum, 290, 290*f*
Polyphagia, to eat excessively, 285
Polyposis, small tumors that contain pedicle or footlike attachment in mucous membranes of large intestine (colon), 290, 290*f*
Polysomnography, monitoring a patient while sleeping to identify sleep apnea; also called *sleep apnea study*, 250
Polyuria, condition of having excessive urine production; can be a symptom of disease conditions such as diabetes, 324, 408
Pons, portion of brainstem that forms bridge between cerebellum and cerebrum, 429, 430*f*, 431
Pontine, pertaining to pons, 437
Popliteal artery, 157*f*
Popliteal vein, 158*f*
Positron emission tomography (PET), use of positive radionuclides to reconstruct brain sections; measurements can be taken of oxygen and glucose uptake, cerebral blood flow, and blood volume, 447
Posterior, directional term meaning near or on back or spinal cord side of body; akin to *dorsal*, 43*f*, 43*t*
Posterior lobe, posterior portion of pituitary gland; secretes antidiuretic hormone and oxytocin, 401, 401*f*
Posterior pituitary gland, 401*f*, 402, 402*f*
Posterior tibial artery, 157*f*
Posterior tibial vein, 158*f*
Postpartum, period immediately after delivery or childbirth, 359
Postprandial (pp), pertaining to after a meal, 285
Posttraumatic stress disorder (PTSD), results from exposure to actual or implied death, serious injury, or sexual violence, 457
Postural drainage, draining secretions from bronchi by placing patient in position that uses gravity to promote drainage; used for treatment of cystic fibrosis and bronchiectasis, and before lobectomy surgery, 251
Potassium (K^+), inorganic substance found in plasma; important for bones and muscles, 188, 318, 398, 408
Potentiation, giving patient second drug to boost (potentiate) effect of another drug; total strength of drugs is greater than sum of strength of individual drugs, 197
Preeclampsia, toxemia of pregnancy that, if untreated, can result in true eclampsia; symptoms include hypertension, headaches, albumin in urine, and edema, 363

Protozoans, single-celled organisms that can infect body, 205
Proximal, directional term meaning located closest to point of attachment to body, 43*f*, 44*t*
Proximal convoluted tubule, portion of renal tubule, 315, 316*f*
Pruritus, severe itching, 68
Pseudocyesis, false pregnancy, 363
Pseudohypertrophic muscular dystrophy, one type of inherited muscular dystrophy in which muscle tissue is gradually replaced by fatty tissue, giving the appearance of a strong and healthy muscle; also called *Duchenne's muscular dystrophy*, 130
Psoriasis, chronic inflammatory condition consisting of crusty papules forming patches with circular borders, 74, 74*f*
Psychiatric nurse, nurse with additional training in care of patients with mental, emotional, and behavioral disorders, 453
Psychiatric social worker, social worker with additional training in care of patients with mental, emotional, or behavioral disorders, 453
Psychiatrist, physician with specialized training in diagnosing and treating mental disorders; prescribes medication and conducts counseling, 453
Psychiatry, branch of medicine that deals with the diagnosis, treatment, and prevention of mental disorders, 453
Psychoanalysis, method of obtaining a detailed account of past and present emotional and mental experiences from patient to determine source of problem and eliminate effects, 458
Psychology, study of human behavior and thought process; behavioral science is primarily concerned with understanding how human beings interact with their physical environment and with each other, 453
Psychopharmacology, study of effects of drugs on mind and particularly use of drugs in treating mental disorders; main classes of drugs for treatment of mental disorders are antipsychotic drugs, antidepressant drugs, minor tranquilizers, and lithium, 458
Psychotherapy, method of treating mental disorders by mental rather than chemical or physical means; includes psychoanalysis, humanistic therapies, and family and group therapy, 458
Pterygium, hypertrophied conjunctival tissue in inner corner of eye, 485
Puberty, series of events leading up to a child becoming capable of reproduction, 350–351
Pubic, pertaining to pubis; one of pelvic bones, 39*f*, 105
Pubic region, genital region of body, 38*t*, 39*f*
Pubis, one of three bones that form os coxae or innominate bone, 91*f*, 98, 100, 101*f*, 101*t*
Pulmonary, pertaining to lung, 239
Pulmonary angiography, injecting dye into blood vessel for purpose of taking X-ray of arteries and veins of lungs, 249
Pulmonary artery, large artery that carries deoxygenated blood from right ventricle to lung, 152, 153*f*
Pulmonary capillaries, network of capillaries in lungs that tightly encase each alveolus; site of gas exchange, 233
Pulmonary circulation, transports deoxygenated blood from right side of heart to lungs where oxygen and carbon dioxide are exchanged; then carries oxygenated blood back to left side of heart, 148, 148*f*
Pulmonary edema, condition in which lung tissue retains excessive amount of fluid; results in labored breathing, 247
Pulmonary embolism (PE), blood clot or air bubble in pulmonary artery or one of its branches, 247
Pulmonary fibrosis, formation of fibrous scar tissue in lungs, which leads to decreased ability to expand lungs; may be caused by infections, pneumoconiosis, autoimmune diseases, and toxin exposure, 247
Pulmonary function test (PFT), group of diagnostic tests that give information regarding airflow in and out of the lungs, lung volumes, and gas exchange between the lungs and bloodstream, 235, 250
Pulmonary trunk, 149*f*, 150*f*
Pulmonary valve, semilunar valve between right ventricle and pulmonary artery in heart; prevents blood from flowing backward into ventricle, 151–152, 151*f*
Pulmonary veins, large veins that return oxygenated blood from lungs to left atrium, 152, 153*f*
Pulmonologist, physician specialized in treating diseases and disorders of respiratory system, 240
Pulmonology, branch of medicine specializing in conditions of respiratory system, 33*t*, 240
Pulp cavity, hollow interior of tooth; contains soft tissue made up of blood vessels, nerves, and lymph vessels, 272, 273*f*
Pulse (P), expansion and contraction produced by blood as it moves through artery; can be taken at several pulse points throughout body where artery is close to surface, 159
Punch biopsy, small cylinder of tissue is removed by an instrument that pierces through tissue like a hole punch, 77
Pupil, hole in center of iris; size is changed by iris dilating or constricting, 474*f*, 475, 477, 478*f*
Pupillary, pertaining to pupil, 480
Purified protein derivative (PPD). *See* Tuberculin skin tests
Purkinje fibers, part of conduction system of heart; found in ventricular myocardium, 153, 154*f*
Purpura, hemorrhages into skin and mucous membranes, 68, 68*f*
Purulent, pus-filled sputum, which can be result of infection, 68
Pustule, raised spot on skin containing pus, 68, 68*f*
Pyelitic, pertaining to renal pelvis, 322
Pyelitis, inflammation of renal pelvis, 326
Pyelogram, X-ray record of the renal pelvis, 329
Pyelonephritis, inflammation of renal pelvis and kidney; one of most common types of kidney disease; may be result of lower urinary tract infection that

moved up to kidney by way of ureters; may be large quantities of white blood cells and bacteria in urine, and blood (hematuria) may even be present in urine in this condition; can occur with any untreated or persistent case of cystitis, 326

Pyeloplasty, surgical repair of renal pelvis, 332

Pyloric, pertaining to pylorus, 283

Pyloric sphincter, located at distal end of stomach; controls passage of food into duodenum, 275, 275*f*, 279*f*

Pyoderma, pus-producing skin infection, 68

Pyosalpinx, condition of having pus in uterine (fallopian) tubes, 360

Pyothorax, condition of having pus in chest cavity, 243

Pyromania, impulse control disorder in which patient is unable to control impulse to start fires, 454

Pyrosis, pain and burning sensation usually caused by stomach acid splashing up into the esophagus; commonly called *heartburn*, 286

Pyuria, presence of pus in urine, 324

Q

Quadriplegia, paralysis of all four extremities; same as tetraplegia, 439

R

Radial, pertaining to radius; lower arm bone, 105

Radial artery, 157*f*

Radial keratotomy, spokelike incisions around cornea that result in it becoming flatter; surgical treatment for myopia, 489

Radial nerve, 435*f*

Radial vein, 158*f*

Radical mastectomy, surgical removal of breast tissue plus chest muscles and axillary lymph nodes; term radical is used to describe extensive surgical procedures designed to remove root cause of disease, 368

Radiculitis, nerve root inflammation, 445

Radiculopathy, disease of nerve root, 445

Radiograph, image produced by radiography (i.e., an X-ray), 115

Radiography, making of X-ray pictures, 115

Radioimmunoassay (RIA), test used to measure levels of hormones in plasma of blood, 412

Radius, one of forearm bones in upper extremity, 91*f*, 98, 99*f*, 100, 100*f*, 100*t*

Rales. *See* Crackles

Range of motion (ROM), maximum amount of movement allowed at a joint, from maximum flexion through maximum extension; measured as degrees of a circle, 101–102

Raynaud's phenomenon, periodic ischemic attacks affecting extremities of body, especially fingers, toes, ears, and nose; affected extremities become cyanotic and very painful; attacks are brought on by arterial constriction due to extreme cold or emotional stress, 167

Reabsorption, second phase of urine production; substances needed by body are reabsorbed as filtrate passes through kidney tubules, 318–319, 318*f*

Recklinghausen disease, excessive production of parathyroid hormone, which results in degeneration of bones, 410

Rectal, (1) pertaining to rectum; (2) substances introduced directly into rectal cavity in form of suppositories or solution; drugs may have to be administered by this route if patient is unable to take them by mouth due to nausea, vomiting, and surgery, 45, 47*t*, 283

Rectocele, protrusion or herniation of rectum into vagina, 361

Rectum, area at end of large intestine for storage of feces that leads to anal canal, 277, 277*f*, 348*f*

Rectus abdominis, muscle named for its location and direction of its fibers: rectus means *straight* and abdominis means *abdominal*, 119*f*, 124

Rectus muscles, rectus means *straight*; four of the eye muscles are rectus muscles, 476, 476*f*

Red blood cell count (RBC), blood test to determine number of erythrocytes in volume of blood; decrease in red blood cells may indicate anemia; increase may indicate polycythemia, 196

Red blood cell morphology, determines diseases such as sickle cell anemia through examination of blood for abnormalities in shape (morphology) of erythrocytes, 196

Red blood cells (RBCs), also called *erythrocytes*; contain hemoglobin and iron-containing pigment that binds oxygen in order to transport it to cells of body, 188, 189*f*

Red bone marrow, tissue that manufactures most of blood cells; found in cancellous bone cavities, 92–93

Reduction, correcting a fracture by realigning bone fragments; closed reduction is doing manipulation without entering body; open reduction is process of making surgical incision at site of fracture to do reduction, necessary when bony fragments need to be removed, or *internal fixation*, such as plates or pins, is required, 118

Refract, bending of light rays as they enter eye, 474

Refractive error test, eye examination performed by physician to determine and correct refractive errors in eye, 487

Regional anesthesia, anesthetic interrupts patient's pain sensation in a particular region of body; injected near nerve that will be blocked from sensation; patient usually remains conscious; also referred to as *nerve block*, 448

Regional ileitis. *See* Crohn's disease

Regurgitation, to flow backward; within cardiovascular system refers to blood flowing backward through valve; within digestive system refers to food flowing backward from stomach to mouth, 163, 286

Rehabilitation, process of treatment and exercise that can help person with disability attain maximum function and well-being, 133

Rehabilitation centers, facilities that provide intensive physical and occupational therapy; include inpatient and outpatient treatment, 15*t*

Reinfection, infection that occurs when person becomes infected again with same pathogen, 207
Renal, pertaining to kidney, 322
Renal artery, artery that originates from abdominal aorta and carries blood to nephrons of kidney, 157*f*, 314, 315*f*
Renal cell carcinoma, cancerous tumor that arises from kidney tubule cells, 326
Renal colic, pain caused by kidney stone, which can be excruciating and generally requires medical treatment, 324
Renal corpuscle, part of a nephron; double-walled cuplike structure called *glomerular capsule* or *Bowman's capsule* and contains capillary network called glomerulus; afferent arteriole carries blood to glomerulus and efferent arteriole carries blood away from glomerulus; filtration stage of urine production occurs in renal corpuscle as wastes are filtered from blood in glomerulus and enter Bowman's capsule, 315, 316*f*
Renal failure, inability of kidneys to filter wastes from blood resulting in uremia; may be acute or chronic; major reason for patient being placed on dialysis, 327
Renal papilla, tip of renal pyramid, 314, 315*f*
Renal pelvis, large collecting site for urine within kidney; collects urine from each calyx; urine leaves renal pelvis via ureter, 314, 315*f*
Renal pyramid, triangular-shaped region of renal medulla, 314, 315*f*
Renal transplant, surgical replacement with a donor kidney, 332, 332*f*
Renal tubule, network of tubes found in a nephron; consists of proximal convoluted tubule, nephron loop (loop of Henle), distal tubule, and collecting tubule; where reabsorption and secretion stages of urine production occur; as glomerular filtrate passes through, most of water and some of dissolved substances, such as amino acids and electrolytes, are reabsorbed; at same time, substances that are too large to filter into Bowman's capsule, such as urea, are secreted directly from bloodstream into renal tubule; filtrate that reaches collecting tubule becomes urine, 315, 316*f*
Renal vein, carries blood away from kidneys, 158*f*, 314, 315*f*
Repetitive motion disorder, group of chronic disorders involving tendon, muscle, joint, and nerve damage, resulting from tissue being subjected to pressure, vibration, or repetitive movements for prolonged periods, 131
Reproductive system, 345–382. *See also* Female reproductive system; Male reproductive system
Residual hearing, amount of hearing still present after damage has occurred to auditory mechanism, 499
Residual volume (RV), air remaining in lungs after forced exhalation, 235*t*
Respirator. *See* Ventilator
Respiratory distress syndrome of the newborn. *See* Infant respiratory distress syndrome
Respiratory membrane, formed by tight association of walls of alveoli and capillaries; gas exchange between lungs and blood occurs across this membrane, 233–234
Respiratory muscles, 235–236
Respiratory rate, 236–237, 237*t*
Respiratory system, brings oxygen into lungs and expels carbon dioxide; organs include nose, pharynx, larynx, trachea, bronchial tubes, and lungs, 33*t*, 227–255
- abbreviations, 255
- adjective forms of anatomical terms, 239
- anatomy and physiology, 229*f*, 230–237
- bronchial tubes, 230, 233–234, 233*f*
- diagnostic procedures, 249–250, 250*f*
- function, 228
- larynx, 230, 231*f*, 232
- lungs, 230, 234, 234*f*, 235
- lung volumes/capacities, 235, 235*t*
- medical specialties, 33*t*, 240
- nasal cavity, 33*t*, 230–231, 231*f*
- pathology, 240–248
- pharmacology, 254
- pharynx, 121, 205, 231–232, 231*f*
- respiratory muscles, 235–236, 236*f*
- respiratory rate, 236–237, 237*t*
- terminology, 228, 237–238
- therapeutic procedures, 251–253
- trachea, 230, 232, 232*f*, 233*f*, 236*f*

Respiratory therapist (RT), allied health professional whose duties include conducting pulmonary function tests, monitoring oxygen and carbon dioxide levels in blood, and administering breathing treatments, 235
Respiratory therapy, allied health specialty that assists patients with respiratory and cardiopulmonary disorders, 240
Retina, innermost layer of eye; contains visual receptors called *rods* and *cones* that receive light impulses and transmit them to brain via optic nerve, 474–475, 474*f*, 475*f*, 477, 478*f*
Retinal, pertaining to retina, 480
Retinal arteries, 475*f*, 478*f*
Retinal blood vessels, blood vessels that supply oxygen to rods and cones of retina, 474*f*, 475, 478*f*
Retinal detachment, occurs when retina becomes separated from choroid layer; separation seriously damages blood vessels and nerves, resulting in blindness, 484
Retinitis pigmentosa, progressive disease of eye resulting in retina becoming sclerosed (hard), pigmented (colored), and atrophied (wasting away); no known cure, 484
Retinoblastoma, malignant eye tumor occurring in children, usually under the age of 3; requires enucleation, 484
Retinopathy, retinal disease, 484
Retinopexy, surgical fixation of retina, 489
Retrograde pyelography (RP), diagnostic X-ray in which dye is inserted through urethra to outline bladder, ureters, and renal pelvis, 329, 329*f*
Retroperitoneal, pertaining to behind peritoneum; describes position of kidneys, which is outside of peritoneal sac alongside spine, 314

S

Sarcoidosis, autoimmune disease of unknown cause in which lesions may appear in liver, skin, lungs, lymph nodes, spleen, eyes, and small bones of hands and feet, 213
Scabies, contagious skin disease caused by egg-laying mite that causes intense itching; often seen in children, 74
Scapula, also called *shoulder blade*; upper extremity bone, 91*f*, 93*f*, 98, 99*f*, 100, 100*f*, 100*t*
Scapular, pertaining to scapula or shoulder blade, 105
Schedule I, drugs with highest potential for addiction and abuse; not accepted for medical use; examples are heroin and LSD, 17, 18*t*
Schedule II, drugs with high potential for addiction and abuse; accepted for medical use in United States; examples are codeine, cocaine, morphine, opium, and secobarbital, 17, 18*t*
Schedule III, drugs with moderate-to-low potential for addiction and abuse; examples are butabarbital, anabolic steroids, and acetaminophen with codeine, 17, 18*t*
Schedule IV, drugs with lower potential for addiction and abuse than Schedule III drugs; examples are chloral hydrate, phenobarbital, and diazepam, 17, 18*t*
Schedule V, drugs with low potential for addiction and abuse; example is low-strength codeine combined with other drugs to suppress coughing, 17, 18*t*
Schizophrenia spectrum and other psychotic disorders, classification of psychiatric disorders in DSM-5 characterized by distortions of reality such as delusions and hallucinations, 456
Schwann cell, 429*f*
Sciatic nerve, 435*f*
Sclera, tough protective outer layer of eyeball; commonly referred to as "white of eye," 474, 474*f*
Scleral, pertaining to sclera, 480
Scleral buckling, placing a band of silicone around outside of sclera to stabilize detaching retina, 489
Scleritis, inflammation of sclera, 484
Scleroderma, condition in which skin has lost its elasticity and become hardened, 68
Scleromalacia, softening of sclera, 482
Sclerotherapy, medical treatment for varicose veins; results in veins collapsing and sticking together, 171
Sclerotomy, to cut into the sclera, 489
Scoliosis, abnormal lateral curvature of spine, 112, 112*f*
Scrotum, sac that serves as container for testes; divided by septum, supports testicles and lies between legs and behind penis, 373–374, 373*f*
Sebaceous cyst, sac under skin filled with sebum or oil from sebaceous gland; can grow to large size and may need to be excised, 74
Sebaceous glands, also called *oil glands*; produce substance called *sebum* that lubricates skin surfaces and eyeball, 58, 59*f*, 61*f*, 62, 476
Seborrhea, oily discharge, 68
Sebum, thick, oily substance secreted by sebaceous glands that lubricates skin to prevent drying out, 62
Second-degree burn. *See* Burn
Secretion, third phase of urine production; additional waste products are added to filtrate as it passes through kidney tubules, 318–319, 318*f*
Sedative, produces relaxation without causing sleep, 450
Seizure, sudden, uncontrollable onset of symptoms, such as in an epileptic seizure, 439
Self-inoculation, infection that occurs when person becomes infected in different part of body by pathogen from another part of his or her own body, such as intestinal bacteria spreading to urethra, 207
Semen, contains sperm and fluids secreted by male reproductive system glands; leaves body through urethra, 373
Semen analysis, procedure used when performing fertility workup to determine if male is able to produce sperm; semen is collected by patient after abstaining from sexual intercourse for a period of three to five days; sperm in semen are analyzed for number, swimming strength, and shape; also used to determine if vasectomy has been successful; after a period of six weeks, no sperm should be present in sample from patient, 380
Semicircular canals, portion of labyrinth associated with balance and equilibrium, 494*f*, 495
Semiconscious, state of being aware of surroundings and responding to stimuli only part of time, 440
Semilunar valve, heart valves located between ventricles and great arteries leaving heart; pulmonary valve is located between right ventricle, and pulmonary artery; aortic valve is located between left ventricle and aorta, 151–152, 151*f*
Seminal vesicles, two male reproductive system glands located at base of bladder; secrete fluid that nourishes sperm into vas deferens; fluid plus sperm constitutes much of semen, 373, 373*f*, 374
Seminiferous tubules, network of coiled tubes that make up bulk of testes; sperm development takes place in walls of tubules and mature sperm are released into tubule in order to leave testes, 373–374, 403*f*
Sensorineural hearing loss, type of hearing loss in which sound is conducted normally through external and middle ear but there is a defect in inner ear or with cochlear nerve, resulting in inability to hear; hearing aid may help, 496
Sensory neurons, carry sensory information from sensory receptors to brain; also called *afferent neurons*, 433–434, 435*f*
Sensory receptors, nerve fibers located directly under skin surface; detect temperature, pain, touch, and pressure; messages for these sensations are conveyed to brain and spinal cord from nerve endings in skin, 58, 59*f*, 428
Sepsis. *See* Septicemia
Septal, pertaining to nasal septum, 239
Septicemia, having bacteria in bloodstream; commonly referred to as *sepsis* or *blood poisoning*, 193
Serous fluid, watery secretion of serous membranes, 234
Serum, clear, sticky fluid that remains after blood has clotted, 188

Superior mesenteric vein, 158*f*
Superior vena cava, branch of vena cava that drains blood from chest and upper body, 152, 153*f*, 154*f*, 158*f*
Supination, turning palm or foot upward, 126*t*, 127*f*
Supine, directional term meaning *lying horizontally and facing upward*, 44*t*
Supplemental air. *See* Expiratory reserve volume
Supplemental oxygen therapy, providing patient with additional concentration of oxygen to improve oxygen levels in bloodstream; oxygen may be provided by mask or nasal cannula, 251
Suppositories (suppos), method for administering medication by placing it in substance that will melt after being placed in body cavity, usually rectally, and release medication, 45
Suppurative, containing or producing pus, 68
Surgical center, facility that provides services that range from simple surgeries to diagnostic testing to therapy and do not require overnight hospitalization; also called *ambulatory care center* or *outpatient clinic*, 15*t*
Surgical suffixes, 9–10
Suspensory ligament, 350*f*
Swayback. *See* Kyphosis
Sweat duct, leads from sweat gland to surface of skin; carries sweat, 59*f*, 62
Sweat glands, produce sweat, which assists body in maintaining its internal temperature by creating cooling effect when it evaporates, 58, 59*f*, 62
Sweat pore, surface opening of sweat duct, 59*f*, 62
Sweat test, performed on sweat to determine level of chloride; there is an increase in skin chloride in disease cystic fibrosis, 250
Swimmer's ear. *See* Otitis externa
Sympathetic branch, part of autonomic nervous system; stimulates body in times of stress and crisis by increasing heart rate, dilating airways to allow for more oxygen, increasing blood pressure, inhibiting digestion, and stimulating production of adrenaline during crisis, 434
Symphysis pubis, 348*f*
Synapse, point at which axon of one neuron meets dendrite of next neuron, 428
Synaptic cleft, gap between two neurons, 428
Syncope, fainting, 440
Syndrome, group of symptoms and signs that when combined present clinical picture of disease or condition, 408
Synovectomy, surgical removal of synovial membrane, 117
Synovial fluid, secreted by synovial membrane in synovial joint; lubricates joint and reduces friction, 101–102
Synovial joint, freely moving joint that is lubricated by synovial fluid, 101, 102*f*
Synovial membrane, lines synovial joint; secretes lubricating fluid called *synovial fluid*, 101, 102, 102*f*
Synovitis, inflammation of synovial membrane, 107
Syphilis, infectious, chronic sexually transmitted infection that can involve any organ; may exist for years without symptoms; treated with antibiotic penicillin, 379
System, several organs working in compatible manner to perform complex function or functions; examples include digestive system, cardiovascular system, and respiratory system, 27*f*, 28
Systemic circulation, transports oxygenated blood from left side of heart to cells of body and then back to right side of heart, 148, 148*f*
Systemic lupus erythematosus (SLE), chronic disease of connective tissue that injures skin, joints, kidneys, nervous system, and mucous membranes; may produce characteristic butterfly rash across cheeks and nose, 75, 114
Systemic veins, 148*f*, 156, 158*f*
Systole, period of time during which heart chamber is contracting, 152
Systolic pressure, maximum pressure within blood vessels during heart contraction, 159

T

Tachycardia, condition of having a fast heart rate, typically over 100 bpm while at rest, 166
Tachypnea, rapid breathing rate, 244
Talipes, congenital deformity of foot; also referred to as *clubfoot*, 114
Target organs, hormones act on them to either increase or decrease organ's activity level, 396
Tarsal, pertaining to tarsus or ankle, 93*f*, 105
Tarsus, collective name for the seven ankle and heel bones in each lower extremity, 91*f*, 98, 99*f*, 100, 101*f*, 101*t*
Taste buds, found on surface of tongue; designed to detect bitter, sweet, sour, salty, and umami flavors in foods, 270–271
T cells, lymphocytes active in cellular immunity, 205, 403
Tears, fluid that washes and lubricates anterior surface of eyeball, 477
Teeth, structures in mouth that mechanically break up food into smaller pieces during chewing, 270–271, 271*f*, 272*f*, 273*f*
Temporal bone, cranial bone, 95, 97, 97*f*, 97*t*
Temporal lobe, one of four cerebral hemisphere lobes; controls hearing and smell, 429–430, 431*f*
Tendinitis, inflammation of tendon, 131
Tendinous, pertaining to tendon, 128
Tendons, strong connective tissue cords that attach skeletal muscles to bones, 30*f*, 31, 123
Tendoplasty, surgical repair of a tendon, 133
Tendotomy, incision into a tendon, 133
Tennis elbow. *See* Lateral epicondylitis
Tenodesis, surgical procedure to stabilize a joint by anchoring down tendons of muscles that move joint, 133
Tenodynia, pain in tendon, 130
Tenoplasty, surgical repair of tendon, 133
Tenorrhaphy, suturing a tendon, 133

Thyromegaly, enlarged thyroid, 408
Thyrotoxicosis, condition that results from overproduction of thyroid glands; symptoms include rapid heart action, tremors, enlarged thyroid gland, exophthalmos, and weight loss, 411
Thyroxine (T4), hormone produced by thyroid gland; also known as T4 and requires iodine for production; regulates level of cell metabolism; the greater the level of hormone in the bloodstream, the higher the cell metabolism, 397*t*, 403–404
Tibia, also called *shin bone*; lower extremity bone, 91*f*, 98, 99*f*, 100, 101*f*, 101*t*
Tibial, pertaining to tibia or shin bone, 106
Tic douloureux. *See* Trigeminal neuralgia
Tidal volume (TV), amount of air that enters lungs in single inhalation or leaves lungs in single exhalation of quiet breathing, 235*t*
Tinea, fungal skin disease resulting in itching, scaling lesions, 75
Tinea capitis, fungal infection of scalp; commonly called *ringworm*, 75
Tinea pedis, fungal infection of foot; commonly called *athlete's foot*, 75
Tinnitus, ringing in ears, 499
Tissues, formed when cells of same type are grouped to perform one activity; for example, nerve cells combine to form nerve fibers; there are four types: nervous, muscle, epithelial, and connective
connective, 27*f*, 28–31, 30*f*
epithelial, 28, 30*f*
muscle, 28, 29, 30*f*, 122
nervous, 28, 30*f*, 31, 428
Tissue transglutaminase (tTG) **antibody test,** blood test for celiac disease, 293
T lymphocytes, type of lymphocyte involved with producing cells that physically attack and destroy pathogens, 205
Tongue, muscular organ in floor of mouth; works to move food around inside mouth and is also necessary for speech, 270–271, 271*f*, 272*f*
Tonic-clonic seizure, type of severe epileptic seizure characterized by loss of consciousness and convulsions; seizure alternates between strong continuous muscle spasms (tonic) and rhythmic muscle contraction and relaxation (clonic); also called *grand mal seizure*, 440
Tonometry, measurement of intraocular pressure of eye using tonometer to check for condition of glaucoma; generally part of normal eye exam for adults, 487
Tonsillar, pertaining to tonsils, 209
Tonsillectomy, surgical removal of tonsils, 215
Tonsillitis, inflammation of tonsils, 212
Tonsils, collections of lymphatic tissue located in pharynx to combat microorganisms entering body through nose or mouth; include pharyngeal tonsils, palatine tonsils, and lingual tonsils, 202, 205, 205*f*, 271*f*, 272*f*
Tooth cavity. *See* Dental caries
Topical, applied directly to skin or mucous membranes; distributed in ointment, cream, or lotion form; used to treat skin infections and eruptions, 45, 47*f*
Topical anesthesia, applied using either liquid or gel placed directly onto specific area; patient remains conscious; used on skin, cornea, and mucous membranes in dental work, 449
Torticollis, severe neck spasms pulling head to one side; commonly called *wryneck* or *crick in the neck*, 130
Total abdominal hysterectomy-bilateral salpingo-oophorectomy (TAH-BSO), removal of entire uterus, cervix, both ovaries, and both uterine (fallopian) tubes, 368
Total calcium, blood test to measure total amount of calcium to assist in detecting parathyroid and bone disorders, 413
Total hip arthroplasty (THA), surgical reconstruction of hip by implanting prosthetic or artificial hip joint; also called *total hip replacement*, 117, 117*f*
Total hip replacement (THR). *See* Total hip arthroplasty
Total knee arthroplasty (TKA), surgical reconstruction of knee joint by implanting prosthetic knee joint; also called *total knee replacement*, 117
Total knee replacement (TKR). *See* Total knee arthroplasty
Total lung capacity (TLC), volume of air in lungs after maximal inhalation, 235*t*
Total parenteral nutrition (TPN), providing 100% of patient's nutrition intravenously; used when patient is unable to eat, 296
Toxemia. *See* Preeclampsia
Toxicity, extent or degree to which a substance is poisonous, 333
Toxic shock syndrome (TSS), rare and sometimes fatal staphylococcus infection that generally occurs in menstruating women; initial infection occurs in vagina and is associated with prolonged wearing of super-absorbent tampon; toxins secreted by bacteria then enter bloodstream, 361
Toxins, substances poisonous to body; many are filtered out of blood by kidney, 205
Trachea, also called *windpipe*; conducts air from larynx down to main bronchi in chest, 230, 232, 232*f*, 233*f*, 236*f*, 272*f*
Tracheal, pertaining to trachea, 106, 239
Tracheostenosis, narrowing and stenosis of lumen or opening into trachea, 244
Tracheostomy. *See* Tracheotomy
Tracheotomy, surgical procedure used to make opening in trachea to create airway; tracheostomy tube can be inserted to keep opening patent; also called *tracheostomy*, 253, 253*f*
Tracts, bundles of nerve fibers located within central nervous system, 428–429
Traction, process of pulling or drawing, usually with mechanical device; used in treating orthopedic (bone and joint) problems and injuries, 118
Tractotomy, precision cutting of a nerve tract in spinal cord to treat intractable pain or muscle spasms, 449
Trademark, pharmaceutical company's brand name for drug, 16
Transcutaneous electrical nerve stimulation (TENS), application of mild electrical current by device with electrodes placed on skin over painful area; relieves pain by interfering with nerve signal to brain on pain nerve, 449

Transdermal, route of drug administration; medication coats underside of patch applied to skin; medication is then absorbed across skin, 45, 47*t*

Transfusion reaction. *See* Hemolytic reaction

Transient ischemic attack (TIA), temporary interference with blood supply to brain, causing neurological symptoms such as dizziness, numbness, and hemiparesis; may lead eventually to full-blown stroke (CVA), 443

Transurethral resection of the prostate (TUR, TURP), surgical removal of prostate gland by inserting device through urethra and removing prostate tissue, 380

Transverse colon, section of colon that crosses upper abdomen from right side of body to left, 276*f*, 277, 277*f*

Transverse fracture, complete fracture straight across bone at right angles to long axis of bone, 110, 110*f*

Transverse plane, horizontal plane that divides body into upper (superior) and lower (inferior) sections; also called *horizontal plane*, 37–38, 37*f*

Transverse section, sectional view of body produced by cut along transverse plane, 37–38, 37*f*

Trauma- and Stressor-related disorders, classification of psychiatric disorders in DSM-5 involving exposure to actual or implied death, injury, or violence; includes posttraumatic stress disorder, 457

Traumatic brain injury (TBI), brain damage resulting from impact (such as a car accident), blast waves (such as from an explosion), or a penetrating projectile (such as caused by a bullet); symptoms may be mild, moderate, or severe and may include loss of consciousness, headache, vomiting, loss of motor coordination, and dizziness, 443

Treadmill test. *See* Stress testing

Tremor, involuntary quivering movement of part of body, 440

Trichomoniasis, genitourinary infection usually without symptoms (asymptomatic) in both males and females; disease in women can produce itching and/or burning and foul-smelling discharge, and can result in vaginitis, 379

Trichomycosis, abnormal condition of hair fungus, 75

Tricuspid valve, between right atrium and ventricle of heart; prevents blood from flowing backward into atrium; has three cusps or flaps, 151–152, 151*f*, 153*f*

Trigeminal nerve, 434*t*

Trigeminal neuralgia, chronic disorder characterized by sudden, sharp pain on one side of face in area served by trigeminal cranial nerve; usually caused by pressure on and irritation of nerve or may be sign of multiple sclerosis; also called *tic douloureux*, 445

Triiodothyronine (T3), hormone produced by thyroid gland known as T3 that requires iodine for its production; regulates level of cell metabolism; the greater the level of hormone in bloodstream, the higher the cell metabolism, 397*t*, 403–404

Trochanter, large blunt process that provides attachment for tendons and muscles, 94, 95*f*

Trochlear nerve, 434*t*

Trunk, torso region of body, 39*f*, 39*t*

Tubal ligation, surgical tying-off of uterine (fallopian) tubes to prevent conception from taking place; results in sterilization of female, 368

Tubal pregnancy. *See* Salpingocyesis

Tubercle, small, rounded process that provides attachment for tendons and muscles, 94

Tuberculin skin test (TB test), applying chemical agent under surface of skin to determine if patient has been exposed to tuberculosis; also called *Mantoux test*, 250

Tuberculosis (TB), infectious disease caused by tubercle bacillus, *Mycobacterium tuberculosis*; most commonly affects respiratory system and causes inflammation and calcification of system; incidence is on the increase and is seen in many patients with weakened immune systems, 247

Tuberosity, large, rounded process that provides attachment to tendons and muscles, 94

Two-hour postprandial glucose tolerance test, assists in evaluating glucose metabolism; patient eats high-carbohydrate diet and fasts overnight before test; blood sample is then taken two hours after meal, 413

Tympanectomy, surgical removal of eardrum, 504

Tympanic, pertaining to eardrum, 498

Tympanic membrane, also called *eardrum*; as sound moves along auditory canal, it strikes tympanic membrane causing it to vibrate; this conducts sound wave into middle ear, 494–495, 494*f*

Tympanitis, eardrum inflammation, 500

Tympanogram, graphic record that illustrates results of tympanometry, 502

Tympanometer, instrument to measure eardrum's movement, 502

Tympanometry, measurement of movement of tympanic membrane; can indicate presence of pressure in middle ear, 502

Tympanoplasty, another term for surgical reconstruction of eardrum; also called *myringoplasty*, 504

Tympanorrhexis, ruptured eardrum, 499

Tympanotomy, incision into eardrum, 504

Type 1 diabetes mellitus. *See* insulin-dependent diabetes mellitus

Type 2 diabetes mellitus. *See* non-insulin-dependent diabetes mellitus

Type A blood, one of ABO blood types; person with type A markers on his or her RBCs; type A blood will make anti-B antibodies, 190

Type AB blood, one of ABO blood types; person with both type A and type B markers on his or her RBCs; since it has both markers, it will not make antibodies against either A or B blood, 190

Type and cross-match, lab test performed before person receives blood transfusion; double-checks blood type of both donor's and recipient's blood, 197

Type B blood, one of ABO blood types; person with type B markers on his or her RBCs; type B blood will make anti-A antibodies, 190

Type O blood, one of ABO blood types; person with no markers on his or her RBCs; type O blood will not react with anti-A or anti-B antibodies; therefore, is considered universal donor, 190

U

W

X

Y

Z